Medicine in an Age of Revolution

Medicine in an Age of Revolution

PETER ELMER

OXFORD
UNIVERSITY PRESS

OXFORD
UNIVERSITY PRESS

Great Clarendon Street, Oxford, OX2 6DP,
United Kingdom

Oxford University Press is a department of the University of Oxford.
It furthers the University's objective of excellence in research, scholarship,
and education by publishing worldwide. Oxford is a registered trade mark of
Oxford University Press in the UK and in certain other countries

Published in the United States of America by Oxford University Press
198 Madison Avenue, New York, NY 10016, United States of America

British Library Cataloguing in Publication Data
Data available

Library of Congress Control Number: 2023935833

ISBN 978–0–19–885398–5

DOI: 10.1093/oso/9780198853985.001.0001

Printed and bound in the UK by
TJ Books Limited

Acknowledgements

This book marks the culmination of a project with its roots in another century. It was originally intended as the first in a trilogy of works concerned with the interaction between medicine, religion and politics in early modern Britain. Like the best laid plans, it has appeared in reverse order. This is partly the result of my engagement in a five-year Wellcome Trust funded project, based at Exeter University, which enabled me to look again at the subject matter under consideration and benefit from further research in archives across Britain and America. I am indebted to the various libraries and archives that have facilitated the research of the project team, with special mention to all our wonderful county record offices who currently languish under the effect of cuts to the public sector. I would also like to thank the Director and staff of the Folger Shakespeare Library in Washington DC, who provided a congenial home in which to work on several themes of this book during the summer of 2019.

As ever, I am indebted to the patience of my family, who have had to endure long periods of my absence, both from home and locked away in my 'cupboard', especially as I am meant to be retired. I promise to try harder in future. I would particularly like to thank the members of the project team, especially Dr Alun Withey, Dr Ismini Pells and Dr John Cunningham for their help and assistance with specific aspects of the research. Likewise to Professor Patrick Wallis of the LSE for allowing access to his database on London apothecaries. My special thanks are reserved, however, for Jonathan Barry, who has been the perfect colleague in so many ways. May our collaboration long continue!

Christmas 2022

Contents

The appendices can also be accessed via the Early Modern Medical Practitioners website at practitioners.exeter.ac.uk, where regularly updates will appear.

List of Abbreviations

APC	*Acts of the Privy Council of England, 1542–1631*, 45 vols, ed. J. R. Dasent *et al* (London, 1890–1964).
Besse, *Sufferings*	J. Besse, *A Collection of the Sufferings of the People Called Quakers… from 1650, to… 1689*, 2 vols (London, 1753).
BL	British Library, London.
BLARS	Bedfordshire and Luton Archives and Records Service, Bedford.
Bloom and James	J. H. Bloom and R. R. James, *Medical Practitioners in the Diocese of London… 1529–1725* (Cambridge, 1935).
Bodl.	Bodleian Library, Oxford.
Boyle, *Correspondence*	*The Correspondence of Robert Boyle*, eds M. Hunter, A. Clericuzio and L. M. Principe, 6 vols (London, 2001).
Cal. Rev.	*Calamy Revised. Being a Revision of Edmund Calamy's Account of the Ministers and Others Ejected and Silenced, 1660–2*, ed. A. G. Matthews (Oxford, 1934; reissued 1988).
CCAL	Canterbury Cathedral Archives and Library, Canterbury.
CLRO	Corporation of London Record Office, London.
CSPD	*Calendar of State Papers, Domestic.*
CUL	Cambridge University Library, Cambridge.
DCNQ	*Devon and Cornwall Notes and Queries.*
DHC	Dorset History Centre, Dorchester.
DRO	Devon Record Office, Exeter.
DWL	Doctor Williams' Library, London.
ERO	Essex Record Office, Chelmsford.
ESkRO	East Suffolk Record Office, Ipswich.
ESxRO	East Sussex Record Office, Lewes.
Ewen, *Witch Hunting*	C. L'Estrange Ewen, *Witch Hunting and Witch Trials. The Indictments for Witchcraft from the Records of 1373 Assizes Held for the Home Circuit A. D. 1559–1736* (London, 1929).
FHL	Friends House Library, London.
Firth and Rait	C. H. Firth and R. S. Rait (eds), *Acts and Ordinances of the Interregnum, 1642–1660*, 3 vols (London, 1911).
Foster	J. Foster (ed.), *Alumni Oxonienses: The Members of the University of Oxford, 1500–1714*, 3 vols (Oxford and London, 1891–2).
FSL	Folger Shakespeare Library, Washington DC
Green, *CPCC*	M. A. E. Green (ed.), *Calendar of the Proceedings of The Committee for Compounding, &c, 1643–1660*, 5 vols (London, 1889–92).
GRO	Gloucestershire Record Office, Gloucester.
HALS	Hertfordshire Archives and Local Studies, Hertford.

Henning	B. Henning (ed.), *The History of Parliament: The House of Commons, 1660–1690*, 3 vols (London, 1983).
HLRO	House of Lords Record Office, London.
HMC	*Historical Manuscripts Commission*
Innes Smith	R. W. Innes Smith, *English-Speaking Students of Medicine at the University of Leyden* (Edinburgh & London, 1932).
Innes Smith MSS	Innes Smith MSS, Edinburgh University.
KHLC	Kent History and Library Centre, Maidstone.
LAO	Lincolnshire Archives Office, Lincoln.
LMA	London Metropolitan Archives, London.
Locke, *Correspondence*	De Beer, E.S. (ed), *The Correspondence of John Locke*, 7 vols (Oxford, OUP, 1976–82).
LPL	Lambeth Palace Library, London.
LRRO	Leicestershire and Rutland Record Office, Leicester.
Munk	W. Munk, *The Roll of the Royal College of Physicians of London, 1518–1800*, 3 vols (London, 1878).
NNkRO	Norwich & Norfolk Record Office, Norwich.
NRO	Northamptonshire Record Office, Northampton.
ODNB	*Oxford Dictionary of National Biography*, 60 vols (Oxford, 2004).
Oldenburg, *Correspondence*	*The Correspondence of Henry Oldenburg*, eds A. R. and M. B. Hall, 13 vols (Madison, Milwaukee, London & Philadelphia, 1965–86).
Raach	J. H. Raach, *A Directory of English Country Physicians, 1603–1643* (London, 1962).
RCPL, Annals	Annals, Royal College of Physicians, London, 3 vols.
SAL	Society of Apothecaries, London.
SHC	Surrey History Centre, Woking.
SUL, HP	Sheffield University Library, Hartlib Papers.
TCD	Trinity College, Dublin.
Thurloe, *State Papers*	*A Collection of the State Papers of John Thurloe, Esq.*, ed. T. Birch, 7 vols (London, 1742).
TNA	The National Archives, Kew, London.
VCH	*Victoria County History.*
Venn	J. Venn and J. A. Venn (eds), *Alumni Cantabrigienses... from the Earliest Times to 1751*, 4 vols (Cambridge, 1922).
Wal. Rev.	*Walker Revised Being a Revision of John Walker's* Sufferings of the Clergy During the Grand Rebellion 1642–60, ed. A. G. Matthews (Oxford, 1948).
Wood, *Ath. Ox.*	Anthony Wood, *Athenae Oxonienses*, 4 vols, ed. P. Bliss (London, 1813–20).
Wood, *Fasti*	see Wood, *Athenae Oxonienses.*
WRO	Worcestershire Record Office, Worcester.
WSA	Wiltshire and Swindon Archives, Chippenham.
WSkRO	West Suffolk Record Office, Bury St Edmunds.
WSxRO	West Sussex Record Office, Chichester.

1
Introduction

The idea that medicine today is inextricably linked with developments in the wider world of politics requires little explanation. Ever since the mid-nineteenth century, the two worlds of medicine and politics have grown ever closer as the governments of nation states have striven to foster improvements in the health of their subjects and citizens. In Britain, of course, the creation of a state-funded National Health Service at the end of World War Two marked the culmination of this process and continues to generate much heated debate in political circles. The ever-spiralling cost of medical treatments, exacerbated by the pace of technological change and medical innovation, has inevitably sparked much discussion as to how governments can continue to afford such a system of health care, but regardless of the debate, few question the overall role of the state in such matters. Issues surrounding the health of the nation dominate political discussion, and medical practitioners, either as individuals or through organizations such as the BMA or nursing unions, make a large contribution to that debate. And with the onset of a major, global pandemic in the shape of Covid, the connection between government and medicine has simply intensified. It is impossible here in the West at least to see how medicine could ever be discussed or understood without resort to a wider, political context.

It was not always so. In Britain, prior to the mid-nineteenth century, traditional historiography accords a very limited role to the relationship between medicine and politics. The dominant paradigm describes a health system that was shaped by what has been described as a 'medical marketplace' in which consumers (patients) purchased cures and remedies from a range of providers (healers), whom they chose with few constraints.[1] Politicians, whether at local or national level, had little interest or say in such day-to-day matters and were largely silent on issues such as the regulation of health care or education and training of medical personnel. At the same time, those active in providing a range of medical services rarely argued for a wider role for the state in such matters with the notable exception of state-funded support for medical assistance to the ever-expanding armies and navies of pre-modern Britain. The apolitical nature of the medical world of early modern Britain is perhaps best captured in the recent work of Margaret Pelling, who has argued that physicians in this period largely exempted themselves from political office-holding at all levels of governance—a reflection of the ambiguously gendered nature of the medical 'profession' at this time.[2]

Medicine in an Age of Revolution. Peter Elmer, Oxford University Press. © Peter Elmer 2023.
DOI: 10.1093/oso/9780198853985.003.0001

While the two worlds of medicine and politics may have collided infrequently in this period, historians have nonetheless detected broader ideological patterns at work in early modern British medicine. The ground-breaking work in this respect was undoubtedly undertaken by Charles Webster, who in 1975, put forward a compelling case for puritanism as the prime motor of scientific and medical change in mid-seventeenth-century England.[3] Building on the work of an earlier generation of historians of science who had argued that Protestantism in general, and puritanism in particular, were most congenial to innovation in the natural sciences, Webster's work, despite its critics, continues to inform much general debate as to the place of medicine and science in this period. It has also proved highly influential in shaping the approach of later generations of historians to specific aspects of the medical history of early modern Britain. In what follows, I wish to re-examine some of the suppositions that lie behind the Webster thesis and to address a range of subsidiary questions related to the place of medicine and medical practitioners in the wider political culture of early modern England. Webster himself concluded that the apocalyptic middle decades of the seventeenth century, the period once described as the 'puritan revolution', witnessed a dramatic shift in attitudes towards medicine and natural philosophy that amounted to nothing less than a 'great instauration' of learning on the lines foreseen by the English polymath Francis Bacon (1561–1626). This great awakening had come about as a direct result of the English civil wars in which a resurgent and forward-looking puritanism had provided the ideological underpinning for a movement that saw the collapse of the *ancien régime* in the shape of the Stuarts and the creation of a godly republic.

It is not my intention here to dispute the significance of the events that helped to bring about the intellectual revolution that Webster so elegantly charted in his masterpiece, *The Great Instauration*. The English civil wars undoubtedly marked a great turning point in the history of the British Isles, unleashing powerful forces that would, by the end of the seventeenth century, fully transform the British state. However, the idea that puritanism provided the vital ideological spark to fuel scientific and medical change in the second half of the seventeenth century, as adumbrated by Webster and others, is questionable and open to debate. The key point at issue is largely a definitional one, a point acknowledged by Webster in 1986 when he sought to answer critics of the puritanism-medicine hypothesis who were critical of what they perceived as the all-encompassing and excessively broad definition of puritanism adopted in *The Great Instauration*. Webster now conceded that the puritans of mid-seventeenth-century England were 'never a completely unified group', that they represented 'a whole spectrum of attitudes', and that puritanism itself was 'in a constant state of flux'. He nonetheless remained committed to the idea that puritanism, especially its more radical manifestations, constituted the essential catalyst for medical progress in the seventeenth century.[4]

Webster's focus on the iconoclastic and anti-authoritarian nature of the puritan movement reflects an approach to the subject that has been largely discredited by most recent work in the field. Building on the work of scholars such as Nicholas Tyacke and Patrick Collinson, historians of religion now tend to emphasize the innate conservatism of puritanism, with its characteristic emphasis on order and hierarchy.[5] At the same time, like-minded scholars posited the view that puritanism represented a constantly evolving and fracturing entity, forged in the white heat of debate over the nature of the English Church from the 1560s onwards. Some, like Peter Lake, have stressed the inclusive nature of that Church, which allowed for a spectrum of opinions while at the same time imputing innovation to the Laudian Arminians.[6] Others have focused on puritanism's innate, fissiparous tendencies, especially after 1640. This in turn has encouraged the idea that puritanism is best seen as a movement split between two irreconcilable parts, radical and conservative, that were poles apart on most social, religious and political issues, particularly matters of church governance. The radical wing of the movement thus categorically rejected the idea of a state church while a much larger, conservative, 'mainstream' group sought to remodel, but not destroy, the Anglican Church. This new scholarly consensus, however, has also proven fragile. The work of David Como on antinomianism, for example, and its relationship to 'mainstream' puritanism, has once again called into question any simple dichotomy that might reduce puritanism to one of two mutually exclusive categories of religious belief or identity.[7]

Oddly, these developments have impacted little on recent accounts of the ideological roots of the scientific revolution and medical reform in early modern England.[8] Webster's warning that scholars might best avoid a recourse to head counting to ascertain the relative contribution of well-defined religious groups to scientific and medical advance has, by and large, been heeded. General histories of the seventeenth century continue to allocate a prominent role to puritanism as a dynamic force in science and medicine. And while few now refer to the middle years of the seventeenth century as the age of puritan revolution, most still identify the period from 1640 to 1660 as a critical moment in the emergence of new ideas and practices in the related fields of science and medicine. In what follows, I seek to re-examine these developments in the light of recent research in the burgeoning field of the social history of medicine, as well as a mass of new evidence gleaned from a vast range of sources. In particular, this study is indebted to research undertaken as part of a Wellcome Trust–funded project aimed at creating a database of all medical practitioners in England, Wales and Ireland between the early sixteenth and eighteenth centuries. The advantages of prosopography are manifold. In piecing together, from a variety of sources, the detailed biographies of thousands of early modern healers, it is possible, *pace* Webster, to make a more accurate and detailed assessment of the ways in which religious and political identities impinged upon attitudes to medical practice and beliefs. Critically, such an approach also facilitates greater understanding of the complex web of networks that medical practitioners inhabited, and thus allows one to make firmer judgements as to the ideological roots of medical innovation. Technology, as never before, now allows the historian to gather vast amounts of historical data, with relative ease. In utilizing these developments, it is possible to provide a much fuller picture of the state of the medical 'profession' in early modern England, and to detect underlying themes in the lives and careers of those engaged in the healing arts. It also allows for a major re-assessment of the relationship between medicine, religion and politics in England, which forms the core of this study.[9]

One of the overarching assumptions of this study is that the middle decades of the seventeenth century in England did indeed witness a sea change in attitudes to medicine and healing. While many continue to question the ideological origins of the English Revolution, particularly its debt to the iconoclastic zeal of a puritan minority, few would dispute the extent of the impact of the civil wars upon all aspects of British society after 1640. Medicine and its practitioners were not immune from the winds of change unleashed by military conflict and political and religious upheaval which contemporaries believed had 'turned the world upside down'. The desire for wholesale reform of the organization and practice of medicine as well as support for new approaches to medical thinking permeate much public and private discourse in this period. Evidence for a growing engagement with medicine and medical issues is evident from a variety of sources. Publication of medical books and pamphlets, often in the vernacular, took off after 1649, encouraged in part by the collapse of censorship in the wake of military conflict.[10] As we shall see in chapter 2, the language of medicine and healing permeated religious and political discussion of the crisis engendered by civil war, both at the local and national level, a reflection in part of the general populace's mindset grounded in the Renaissance commonplace of the body politic. Medicine for many held the key as to how best to explain and react to the political crisis unfolding in the 1640s, the word 'crisis' itself replete with medical connotations. The desire for 'healing' was widespread and may have provided a motive for some to engage more closely with medicine, including active participation in the provision of medical care. The collapse of the system of ecclesiastical licensing across England and the inability of the College of Physicians to exert its customary powers over medical interlopers in London almost certainly facilitated this process. Moreover, there is little doubt that the civil wars of the 1640s, followed by the growing military demands of the English state in the 1650s, were critical in encouraging new entrants into the medical 'profession'. As we shall see, many of these new recruits were keen to explore novel avenues of medical research and practice. At the same time, the emergence of the fiscal-military state, which grew exponentially hereafter, provided, as we shall see, a range of opportunities for medical practitioners to acquire enhanced social status and professional credit, more often than not through the assumption of lucrative government posts and office-holding.[11] Apothecaries and surgeons, frequently depicted before 1640 as subservient to the university-educated physician, were particularly well placed to capitalize on this sudden upsurge in demand for medical services. But others too were equally attracted by the lure of a career in medicine. This is especially true for those sons of the gentry and 'middling sort' who opted for a university education. As Robert Frank has shown, the number of students graduating with medical degrees at Oxford spiraled after 1640 and continued to grow thereafter.[12] Medicine proved equally popular in Interregnum Cambridge. To what extent this growth in the numbers of university-educated doctors can be understood as a response to the growth in demand for their services is difficult to determine. But there can be little doubt that the years after 1640 witnessed a marked upsurge in interest in medical study, both within and outside academia, which ultimately transformed early modern attitudes to medicine, natural philosophy and society.

The growth in numbers of medical practitioners of all types after 1640 was matched by a concurrent growth of interest in exploring new channels of research in various fields of medical enquiry including physiology and chemistry. Developments in both fields were to some extent a continuation of earlier interests and discoveries—most notably Harvey's discovery of the circulation of the blood. After 1640, however, the pace of change and innovation accelerated as it became increasingly entrenched in the medical faculties of Oxford and Cambridge. Medical students were now less wedded to the study of the traditional curriculum which emphasized the centrality of Galenic humoralism and were more open to new ideas about the functioning of the body and its potential impact upon the treatment of illness.[13] One by-product of this medical renaissance was a growing focus upon the study of individual diseases, sparked in part by a concomitant revival of interest in Hippocratic medicine recast as empiricism and epitomized by the work of Thomas Sydenham (1624–1689). Another, which can be found both within and outside the universities, was the vast upsurge of interest in the ideas and practices of the iatrochemists or chymical physicians, particularly Paracelsus and van Helmont, which promised at various times to topple Galen and Galenic medicine from its accustomed pedestal.[14] These developments thus helped to spawn what some have seen as a coordinated medical reform movement in the 1650s composed of a group of like-minded scholars and enthusiasts focused on the remarkable figure of the Polish émigré Samuel Hartlib (d.1662).

There can be no doubt as to the significance of the work of Hartlib and his supporters and associates in raising awareness of both the need and potential for wholesale medical reform in mid-seventeenth-century Britain. Hartlib's European connections facilitated a critical exchange of ideas which allowed English advocates of medical change to learn from, and adapt to, developments on the continent. At the same time, home-grown radicals were increasingly calling for the implementation of a range of social reforms many of which focused on the shortcomings of contemporary medicine and its impact upon those least able to pay for the services of medical specialists. The desire for root-and-branch change is epitomized by the career of Nicholas Culpeper (1616–1654) who became the standard bearer for a new form of medical provision which deliberately undercut the closed shop operated by the physicians of the College in London. A religious radical and a republican who had fought in the civil wars, Culpeper utilized the power of print to castigate the privileged physician while at the same time empowering the patient to take greater control over the wellbeing of his or her body.[15] The seeds of medical reform were thus well and truly planted in Interregnum England, but the failure of the various schemes of the Hartlibians and others to come to fruition suggests that the godly authorities who now ruled England did not share the medical reformers' zeal for change. While some puritans, broadly defined, were clearly eager for innovation, others, particularly those in positions of authority, were not. At the same time, as I hope to demonstrate in what follows, various elements of the medical reform programme were to prove especially appealing to medics and others drawn from the ranks of the puritans' staunchest religious and political opponents. It is for this reason that I argue here for the critical role of the period, rather than specific religious groupings, in creating a conducive atmosphere for the promotion of medical change. The English Revolution, medically speaking, transformed the whole population, regardless of religious and political affiliation, and in the process created an opportunity for all to speculate freely as to the merits of a wide range of medical initiatives.

It nonetheless remains true, I believe, that individual members of the medical reform movement were subject, like the generality of the population, to intense politicization because of the events of the civil war and its aftermath. I use this phrase frequently in this study, firstly in the general sense of a people made more aware of the impact of political life and events on their lives and careers. But secondly, to denote the way in which, especially after 1660, political differences and divisions became polarized and facilitated the emergence of two distinct medical communities. None of this is to argue that medicine was entirely free of politics before 1640. The recent study of the furore surrounding the death or 'murder' of James I in 1625 is a powerful reminder of the tightrope that royal physicians were forced to walk when confessional politics intruded on their daily work.[16] Nor am I seeking to devalue or denigrate other studies in the social history of medicine which have adopted a broader definition of the term 'political' to incorporate issues such as gender and their incorporation in the wider literature of the period.[17] My usage here harkens back to earlier studies which sought to demonstrate how 'high' politics may have shaped the medical landscape of the seventeenth century. This study is, above all, an attempt to put politics back into medicine and to show how the latter was both shaped by the political debates and divisions of the period while at the same time suggesting ways in which medicine may have contributed to contemporary understanding of political belief and practices.

In chapter 2, I begin this study by noting the extent to which contemporaries in the 1640s, faced with the calamitous prospect of civil war, articulated their approach to these events through the prism of an early modern commonplace, the body politic. British historians have, by and large, tended to assume that it died on the scaffold along with Charles I in 1649 when the act of regicide fatally exposed the fallacy of a political system built on the idea of divine right.[18] Here, however, I argue not only for its continuing vitality after 1649 but also for its remarkable ability to survive and adapt in a world where political, medical, philosophical and scientific developments, including the onset of Hobbesian materialism and Cartesianism, posed a growing challenge to the old order. At the same time, I argue, *pace* Walzer and others, that puritanism itself was not inherently ill disposed to organicist concepts of the state. On the contrary, I argue that it was the continuing fascination with the idea of a single, unified and organic body politic that encouraged puritan commentators, including those with a medical background, to engage with a host of political issues as contemporaries struggled to come to terms with the consequences of civil war and religious and political upheaval. Medicine and politics were thus natural bedfellows in a providential world in which God frequently spoke to men and women through the analogy of the human body.[19]

The revival of interest in the idea of the body politic, spawned by the debates of the civil war years, provides one explanation for the politicization of healers and healing after 1640. In chapter 3, I discuss the manifold forms that this process took. Medical practitioners were, of course, active in providing support to the two sides in the political conflict on the battlefield. Such support was not restricted, however, to volunteering to fight and serve in the respective armies of Parliament and King. On the parliamentary side, medical men were also active in a range of spheres, supporting the various regimes of Parliament and commonwealth in a range of capacities, including as pamphleteers, propagandists and servants of the state. Many, significantly, opted for the first time to stand for political and judicial office, both at national and local level, a process in marked contrast to the apparent political apathy of medical practitioners before 1640. In doing so, they frequently benefited, acquiring medical posts, status, wealth and property, including church and crown lands, in return for their unstinting support for the cause the parliamentary cause. Likewise, those medical men who fought for and supported the King, and remained loyal to the Stuart cause, were equally politicized by the events of the 1640s and 1650s. In the case of loyal medics or prospective medics, defeat engendered a range of responses including, at its most extreme, a willingness among some to exploit the unique patient–practitioner relationship as an opportunity to engage in espionage and plotting on behalf of the royalist cause. Others turned to medicine through either necessity, as in the case of those clergy who lost their livings, or choice as is evident from the large numbers of loyalist students who opted to study for a medical rather than a clerical career in the 1650s. There is little doubt that as a result of such developments medicine itself underwent acute politicization.

Nonetheless, in this chapter and elsewhere, I argue against the orthodox view espoused by Charles Webster and others who have depicted the medical revolution of the 1640s and 1650s as a by-product of puritanism. In line with Patrick Collinson's view of puritanism as inherently conservative, I suggest, with some caveats, that the cause of medical reform, both in terms of practice and theory, was largely the preserve of radical groups to the 'left' of the puritan mainstream, who instinctively favoured de-regulation of the medical 'profession' combined with a deep-seated antipathy toward Galenic humoralism. The growing interest in new medical theories of the body and its cure, especially those based on the tenets of Paracelsus and van Helmont, were not, however, limited to a radical fringe. During the course of the 1650s, as many royalists and loyal Anglicans embarked upon medical study, often as an alternative to a clerical career, the allure of 'chymistry' was to prove especially attractive to the enemies of the 'good old cause'.

In chapter 4, I discuss these developments further with a major re-evaluation of a landmark moment in seventeenth-century English medicine, namely the attempt in 1665 to overthrow the regulatory authority of the College of Physicians in London and to replace it with a new body that favoured the use of chemical medicines and de-regulation. If successful, the Society of Chemical Physicians would, in all probability, have revolutionized medical practice in the capital and encouraged change throughout the rest of the country. Its principal aim was to create a free market in medicine in London, untrammelled by the regulatory powers of the College of Physicians, and to undermine the historic dependence of the medical elite upon Galenic humoralism. The members of the Society, who claimed the backing of an impressive network of powerful noblemen, courtiers and senior clerics at the court of the recently restored Charles II, agitated to introduce a new approach to medicine and healing based upon the radical tenets of Paracelsus, van Helmont and their iatrochemical followers. Critically, such aspirations, which envisaged the true physician as both the creator and supplier of chemically prepared medicines, threatened to erode the traditional relationship between doctors and apothecaries. Not surprisingly, their opponents responded by depicting the 'chymists' as radically subversive, the heirs of those religious enthusiasts who just a few years earlier had threatened to turn the world upside down. In the event, the iatrochemists failed in their objective, despite the fact that for the most part the majority of their members were men with impeccable loyalist credentials and that the bulk of their influential supporters were drawn from the highest echelons of Restoration society. Here, I discuss the reasons for failure, but also provide an important postscript to this critical moment in English medical history in tracing the continuing encouragement proffered by the King and senior courtiers, including Gilbert Sheldon, archbishop of Canterbury, for the aims of the chymists in the period after 1665.

One important aspect of the affair of the Society of Chemical Physicians was the degree of support offered to the chymists by archbishop Sheldon and other senior clergymen, which, I argue, was partly inspired by Sheldon's antipathy for the puritan dominated College of Physicians, and its covert support for nonconformist physicians in and outside the capital. As such, it provides a good example of the way in which medicine and the medical 'profession' after 1660 had become polarized and politicized as a result of the events of the previous two decades. In chapters 5 and 6, I discuss these developments in more detail so as to demonstrate how all facets of medical practice and thinking had fallen prey to political imperatives. Above all, I wish to show how such a process was increasingly creating a medical world divided into two camps that were defined by religious and political allegiance. In chapter 5, I examine this process by focusing on the impact of the Restoration settlement upon nonconformist medical practitioners, many of whom were drawn from the ranks of ejected puritan ministers or their families. Many, moreover, discouraged or prevented from acquiring a medical education in England, were increasingly attracted to the medical schools of the United Provinces (modern-day Netherlands), where they not only encountered the latest medical thinking but, in many cases, were also inveigled into supporting various plots to overthrow the Stuarts. Indeed, many of the alliances forged by English medical students of a dissenting background in Holland at this time were later to prove long-lasting and significant for many years to come. Following the Glorious Revolution of 1688, most returned home and many were drawn into political disputes with their Tory and high Anglican colleagues, thus further encouraging the process of politicization in the era of the 'rage of party'.

In chapter 6, in contrast to the creation of what some have termed a 'dissenting medical tradition', I focus on the emergence of a pro-Anglican and Tory medical establishment in the four decades after 1660.[20] Here, in particular, I chart the rapid rise to power of the politically active Tory physician, who can be found in growing numbers inhabiting the corridors of power in late seventeenth-century England. This is especially evident at the level of local, corporate government, where university-educated physicians were increasingly active as common councilmen, aldermen and mayors and shared in the judicial as well as political functions of provincial office. As doctors, they were ideally suited to provide advice and expertise in relation to what constituted good governance, frequently comparing the operations of the body politic to that of the human body as well as providing suitable cures for what many perceived as the desperate diseases then flourishing in England's corporations. Some of the more eminent members of the profession went one stage further by producing lengthy and detailed publications defending the political status quo, often with the support and encouragement of the crown which facilitated access to the state's archives. By the end of the seventeenth century, then, physicians of a Tory bent were fully embedded within the political and religious establishment in a way that was inconceivable before 1640. In the remainder of the chapter, I explore further the nature of these networks and their impact on both medicine and politics in the four decades after the Restoration.

Finally, in chapter 7, I briefly touch on how the politicization of medicine after 1660, and the emergence of two contending camps defined by differing religious and political outlooks, impacted on medicine itself. One aspect of this process, which I have discussed more fully elsewhere, relates to divergent attitudes among medics to the age-old problem of the relationship between mind and body, or matter and spirit. The exact nature of this relationship was both complex and controversial, particularly given the materialistic assumptions of much Galenic medicine including Galen's rejection of the idea of an immortal soul. However, since the Middle Ages, philosophers, physicians and others had reached a compromise, whereby the role of spiritual entities, including the soul, within the human body was preserved. A delicate balance of material and spiritual forces was generally understood to pertain, one which came under increasing strain following the outbreak of civil war in England in the 1640s. There ensued what one might term a 'crisis of spirit' which engulfed not only the intellectual world but also that impinged upon all aspects of religious and political life. Anglican loyalists and supporters of divine right rule increasingly depicted puritanical religion as a form of 'enthusiasm' in which excessive weight was allocated to the role of spirit or spiritual enlightenment in the attainment of godliness. Nonconformists were subsequently said to be suffering a form of madness, which, invoking the recent neurological discoveries of Thomas Willis, was widely construed as a form of physical illness. For their part, puritans and their successors after 1660 were equally keen to preserve the role of spirit in everyday life, including physical affliction, preferring a variety of alternative explanations, including bewitchment, to account for their sufferings. As Michael MacDonald pointed out as long ago as 1981, mental breakdown and madness tended to flourish in communities and societies where conflict rather than concord prevailed. It is my contention here that those suffering religious persecution after 1660, nonconformists, were also most prone to a range of what one might loosely term 'spiritual afflictions', which in turn were best treated by 'spiritual physicians' drawn from among the ranks of the ejected clergy. In contrast, Anglican physicians, suspicious of any claim on the role of spirit in disease, were increasingly drawn to 'safer' materialistic explanations for the same ailments. The Restoration, it might be said, had made men and women sick, but physicians now differed as how best to treat such ailments depending upon which side of the political divide they now occupied.

Notes

1. The idea of a medical marketplace was first popularized by early modern scholars in the 1980s. However, the idea is not without its critics; see for example the introductory essay and other essays in M. S. R. Jenner and P. Wallis (eds), *Medicine and the Market in England and Its Colonies, c.1450–c.1850* (Houndmills, Basingstoke, 2007).

2. M. Pelling, 'Politics, Medicine, and Masculinity: Physicians and Office-bearing in Early Modern England', in M. Pelling and S. Mandelbrote (eds), *The Practice of Reform in Health, Medicine and Science, 1500–2000* (Aldershot, 2005), 81–105.
3. C. Webster, *The Great Instauration: Science, Medicine and Reform 1626–1660* (London, 1975).
4. C. Webster, 'Puritanism, Separatism and Science', in R. L. Numbers and D. C. Lindberg (eds), *God and Nature: Historical Essays on the Encounter between Christianity and Science* (Berkeley, CA, 1986), 192–217. For a rejoinder, see W. J. Birken, 'Merton Revisited: English Independency and Medical Conservatism in the Seventeenth Century', in E. L. Furdell (eds), *Textual Healing: Essays on Medieval and Early Modern Medicine* (Leiden & Boston, MA, 2005), 259–83.
5. There is, of course, an enormous literature on this subject. For the current debate surrounding the meaning of the term 'puritan' and its various manifestations, see especially the various essays in J. Coffey and P. C. H. Lim (eds), *The Cambridge Companion to Puritanism* (Cambridge, 2008). I first outlined my reservations with regard to the puritanism-medicine hypothesis in 'Medicine, Religion and the Puritan Revolution', in R. French and A. Wear (eds), *The Medical Revolution of the Seventeenth Century* (Cambridge, 1989), 10–45.
6. See, for example, P. Lake, 'The Laudian Style: Order, Uniformity and the Pursuit of the Beauty of Holiness in the 1630s', in K. Fincham (ed.), *The Early Stuart Church, 1603–1642* (Basingstoke, 1993), 161–85.
7. D. R. Como, *Blown by the Spirit: Puritanism and the Emergence of an Antinomian Underground in Pre-Civil-War England* (Stanford, 2004), especially chapter 1, which contains a very useful and succinct summary of the long-running debate over the role and nature of puritanism in early modern England.
8. It seems telling, for example, that the collection of essays in footnote 5 above contains no essay on, or reappraisal of, the relationship between puritanism, medicine and natural philosophy.
9. Exeter University, 'The Medical World of Early Modern England, Wales and Ireland, *c.*1500–1715'. The first fruits of this research can now be found on the project website at practitioners.exeter.ac.uk. More complete biographies of all the medical practitioners discussed in this work will appear on the site in due course alongside the three appendices cited throughout.
10. Webster, *Great Instauration*, 264–73. For the broader context in which medical publishing took place, see E. L. Furdell, *Publishing and Medicine in Early Modern England* (Rochester, NY, 2002).
11. For innovation in medical provision for combatants in England during and after the civil wars, see E. Gruber von Arni, *Justice to the Maimed Soldier: Nursing, Medical Care and Welfare for Sick and Wounded Soldiers and Their Families during the English Civil Wars and Interregnum, 1642–1660* (Aldershot, 2001). For recent evaluation of medical provision and personnel in that conflict, see especially I. Pells, 'Reassessing Frontline Medical Practitioners of the British Civil Wars in the Context of the Seventeenth-Century Medical World', *Historical Journal*, 62 (2019), 399–425.
12. R. G. Frank Jnr, 'Medicine', in N. Tyacke (ed.), *The History of the University of Oxford. Volume IV. Seventeenth Century Oxford* (Oxford, 1997), 505–58, esp. 511–13. Frank

estimated that by the 1650s Oxford was attracting eight to fifteen times as many recruits to medicine as it did fifty years earlier; ibid., 513.

13. Ibid., 527–34.
14. The old-fashion spelling of 'chymist' and 'chymistry' is preferred throughout this study in line with current scholarly thinking which seeks to acknowledge the somewhat anachronistic sense of the more modern term; see especially L. Principe and W. Newman, 'Alchemy vs Chemistry: The Etymological Origins of a Historiographic Mistake', *Early Science and Medicine*, 3 (1998), 32–65.
15. For a brief biography of the life and achievements of Culpeper, see the article by Patrick Curry in *ODNB*.
16. A. Bellany and T. Cogswell, *The Murder of King James I* (New Haven & London, 2015).
17. See, for example, E. Decamp, *Civic and Medical Worlds in Early Modern England: Performing Barbery and Surgery* (London, 2016).
18. See, for example, R. Zaller, 'Breaking the Vessels: The Desacralization of Monarchy in Early Modern England', *Sixteenth Century Journal*, 29 (1998), 757–78; M. Schoenfeldt, 'Reading Bodies', in K. Sharpe and S. N. Zwicker (eds), *Reading, Society and Politics in Early Modern England* (Cambridge, 2003), 232–3.
19. For the politicization of royal physicians, utilizing the notion of the body politic, in the wake of the French Wars of Religion at the court of Henri IV, see J. Soll, 'Healing the Body Politic: French Royal Doctors, History, and the Birth of a Nation 1560–1634', *Renaissance Quarterly*, 55 (2002), 1259–86. Soll relates this process to the humanist endeavours of Renaissance physicians to write *historiae* or narratives of specific illnesses which encouraged a medical preoccupation with history and writing about the past. I discuss this development more fully in chapter 6 in relation to loyalist and Tory physicians after the Restoration.
20. For the concept of a 'dissenting medical tradition', see W. J. Birken, 'The Dissenting Tradition in English Medicine of the Seventeenth and Eighteenth Centuries', *Medical History*, 39 (1995), 197–218.

2

The Premature Death of a Renaissance Commonplace

The Body Politic in Puritan England, 1640–1660

Introduction

The idea of the body politic has a long history. Indeed, the language of classical medicine, which informed discussion of the body politic for much of our period, continues to shape the way we talk about politics today, even if the meaning of everyday terms such as 'constitution', 'crisis' and 'purging' have lost their original associations with the physical body. In the sixteenth and seventeenth centuries, it is generally acknowledged that recourse to the analogy of the body politic represented an essentially conservative political stance. The orderly and hierarchical organization of the human body was said to act as both a model for, and to imitate, the harmonious operations of the wider cosmos, including the world of politics.[1] Not surprisingly, it became widely associated with monarchical forms of government, in which the role of the King was paralleled in the human body by that of the head or heart. Lesser organs carried out the functions of minor offices of state and government, while the part played by the rest of the population was reserved for the hands, feet and stomach. The organic concept of the state, which was mirrored at all levels of government in early modern Britain, thus provided a blueprint for politicians and political commentators and an overarching metaphysical and analogical justification for maintaining the status quo. In an age in which educated men and women, as well as many of their illiterate inferiors, were well versed in the language of humoral medicine, recourse to the language of the body politic was ubiquitous and can be found in parliamentary debates and private diaries, as well as the burgeoning culture of print and daily newsletters.

Most historians who have focused on the legitimating authority of ideas drawn from the body politic in early modern British political discourse have, however, tended to concentrate almost exclusively on its relevance for the period before 1640. The fate of the concept of the body politic after the onset of civil war and the execution of its head, Charles I, in 1649, has evoked little comment. Moreover, when historians have commented on such matters they have generally assumed as a matter of course that the revolutionary forces unleashed in Britain in the 1640s

Medicine in an Age of Revolution. Peter Elmer, Oxford University Press. © Peter Elmer 2023.
DOI: 10.1093/oso/9780198853985.003.0002

precipitated the demise of organicist forms of discourse and their replacement by new ways of speaking about government and the governed. Typical of this way of thinking is the approach taken by Michael Walzer in his highly influential, though now somewhat outdated, study of civil war politics, *The Revolution of the Saints*, first published in 1966.[2] Walzer portrayed the puritan politicians and preachers of the civil war era as harbingers of a new political order. The old verities and commonplaces, based on an organic image of the state, held no place in their metaphysical or political worldview. Instead, puritanism was depicted by Walzer as a radical and progressive ideology and the post–civil war period as an era of reconstruction in which a new kingdom modelled on the biblical archetype of the New Jerusalem replaced more traditional forms of government based on divine right monarchy. The outcome, despite the setback of the Restoration, was a brave new world in which the radical ideas of Milton, Hobbes and Locke flourished to the detriment of older notions of political order based on natural correspondences and bodily metaphors.

Despite a revolution in historical thinking in the last thirty years in relation to the origins of the English civil war, most historians continue to subscribe to the view that the events of the 1640s marked the demise of the image of the organic state. Even revisionists such as Kevin Sharpe, who has done more than most to resuscitate the image of Charles I as an able and reform-minded, if misunderstood, head of state, continue to promote the view that the period from 1642 to 1660 marked a decisive break in the cultural, political and intellectual life of the nation. Sharpe thus contends that this period witnessed an end to the old verities, analogues and metaphors that construed pre–civil war political thinking, destroyed as they were by the innate radicalism of the puritan agenda.[3] Likewise, cultural historians of the body have been quick to date the death of the body politic to the middle decades of the seventeenth century, even if, as in the case of Jonathan Sawday, this process has been attributed to scientific and philosophical developments rather than the hurly burly of contemporary political events.[4] Here, I would like to suggest that the death of the body politic and related forms of political discourse, like the demise of Mark Twain, has been somewhat exaggerated. Belief in an organic and hierarchical state, shaped by popular understanding of the working of the human body, continued to inform a wide spectrum of opinion, both 'elite' and 'popular', in the period from 1640 to 1660. Most crucially, such ideas were invoked not just by Stuart apologists and sequestrated Anglican ministers, but they were also actively promoted by many people associated with the puritan mainstream or those 'church puritans' who eagerly sought to preserve the idea of a single, unified state church.

On what basis then have historians consigned the concept of the body politic to the dustbin of history by 1660? Two main arguments have been put forward to explain its demise. Firstly, following Walzer, there is the suggestion that organicist notions of the state held no place in a puritan political worldview that was essentially radical and iconoclastic. Such views gained wide currency in the 1960s and 1970s, especially in the work of Marxist historians of the 'English Revolution' such as Christopher Hill and have continued to inform the work of later writers concerned with the political legacy of the 'puritan revolution'. Integral to this explanation is the exceptional emphasis that puritan preachers and propagandists are thought to have placed upon the notion of a social contract between governor and governed, itself a product of the Calvinist preoccupation with covenant theology. According to this view, puritans saw both church and state as 'artificial institutions, created by an act of will of their individual members and subject to change by them'. Here, the emphasis is placed upon the origin of political relations for which 'organic analogies seemed deficient'.[5] A second explanation for the demise of the body politic has focused on the role of the new science, especially Cartesian mechanism, in dismantling the scientific props of a worldview based on structural correspondences and analogous patterns of behaviour in the cosmos. This view has been put forward, for example, by Jonathan Sawday, who has accordingly dated the demise of the body politic to the second half of the seventeenth century.[6]

In many respects, it is hard to deny the validity of these claims in the face of the growing impact of the Scientific Revolution in the second half of the seventeenth century. Some important caveats, however, are worthy of consideration. In the first place, there is little evidence on the ground to suggest that resort to the language of the body politic and similar analogical thinking was limited in the immediate aftermath of the Restoration to the conservative political discourse of triumphant royalists and Anglican ministers. On the contrary, organicist political thinking continued to appeal to a broad cross section of the public after 1660, including many who had formerly served or supported Parliament and the Cromwellian state in the previous two decades. The desire for religious peace and political harmony was both genuine and widespread in the years immediately following the return of Charles II, and the image of the body provided commentators of various backgrounds with a common language to express such aspirations.[7] It would be a mistake, however, to assume that the continued recourse to organicist political ideas represented a conservative reaction on the part of such men and a rejection of their former commitment to the radical overhaul of society. As much recent work on the origins of the English civil wars has suggested, puritanism was not, *pace* Walzer and others, an inherently revolutionary ideology. Nor were most pre- and post-civil war 'puritans' intent on destroying political consensus and the idea of an integrated and unitary state. Indeed, their commitment to the values of a hierarchical and organicist state were evident before the outbreak of civil war in 1642, continued throughout the 1640s and 1650s, and resurfaced again in the 1660s and 1670s when their spokesmen consistently appealed for the re-establishment of traditional political forms based on the ancient constitution of king, aristocracy and commons.

It would be wrong, however, to infer from this that puritan subscription to the consensual language of the body politic meant that there were no differences of opinion or emphasis with their religious and political rivals in church and state. As Kevin Sharpe has noted, 'a common shared language could articulate different, even contrary positions'.[8] Above all, it is necessary to acknowledge that the citation of harmonist thinking and parallels drawn between human and political bodies might as easily articulate criticism of the status quo as much as represent slavish acceptance of the traditional political order. As early as 1614, the court preacher and Calvinist John Rawlinson reminded James I of his duty to his subjects by recourse to the analogy of the body politic. Worried by the effect of excessive taxation on the poor, Rawlinson warned the King that '[s]hould the head in the naturall body draw all the bloud, and marrow, and substance of the other members to it selfe, it must needs turne to the destruction of the heade it selfe. For how should the head continue without a body?'[9] Prior to 1640, however, it was rare for preachers, puritan or otherwise, to criticize the head of the body politic in this fashion. More often than not, the anger of dissidents or critics was directed towards other agents of the state, such as lawyers, who in the words of the Lancashire puritan Christopher Hudson should be 'the Physitians not the horse-leeches or blood-suckers of ye Comonwealth'.[10] Hudson's views echoed those of another puritan minister and radical critic of the government, Thomas Scot, who in 1623 lauded the legal profession as 'the Physitians of the body politique' while at the same time condemning many of their practices.[11]

Significantly, both Hudson and Scot used the public platform of the county assizes as an opportunity to express criticism of the government of the body politic under the early Stuarts. Similar tactics were employed by the puritan lecturer, Thomas Sutton, who in 1622 admonished the judges of the home circuit by reminding them that '[o]f all the parts in the body Naturall the braine is most subject unto diseases, and of all parts in the body Politique the Magistrate most obnoxious to slips and falls'. Preached in a period of relative political calm, Sutton's sermon was not published until 1631 when the changed circumstances brought about by Charles I's rejection of Parliament and onset of the Personal Rule gave his words added bite and menace.[12] The pulpit on occasions such as these enabled puritan critics of the regime to propagate their own distinctive version of the body politic, which differed in emphasis rather than kind from that espoused by their opponents in church and state. In all the examples cited and countless others, the puritan emphasis consistently reiterated the need to preserve order, hierarchy and unity in the godly commonwealth. This entailed, above all, a profound respect for the doctrine of callings, whereby all were expected to perform their allotted role in society in much the same way as the various members or parts of the body were allocated their particular functions.[13] Puritan respect for social order was never more apparent than in the sanctity bestowed upon the three professions: the church, law and medicine. Typically,

Thomas Sutton identified the three principal members of the body politic as the magistrate, lawyer and physician, which he correlated with the role played in the human body by the brain, liver and heart.[14] Others widened this trinity to include the clergy. The Northamptonshire puritan, Joseph Bentham, for example, invoked the analogy of the human body to explain why it was essential that laymen and the unlearned should not intrude themselves into the clerical sphere:

> In a body all members have not the same vigour, neither are the guifts granted to all in the mysticall body. Bodily members intrude not into each others office: neither in the mysticall body should they thrust themselves into another's calling.[15]

Such concern for order and obedience to the doctrine of callings permeated puritan discourse prior to 1640. It was noticeably present in the attitude of puritan physicians to interlopers in the profession of physick. Both John Cotta and James Hart, puritans who practised in Northampton in the first half of the seventeenth century, declaimed in print against those who regularly invaded the medical sphere and called for greater policing in this area. In so doing, they also echoed another common refrain of puritan preachers who repeatedly warned against the dangers of excessive curiosity and transgressing the bounds of one's divinely allotted competence.[16] Such respect for traditional values was typical of puritan social thinking in this period, and contrasts with the very different picture painted by Walzer and others. Though puritan ministers and laymen may have criticized aspects of the various policies of the government of Charles I in the years immediately prior to the outbreak of the civil war, they did so in large part with a deferential attitude to authority in general and in a spirit of conservatism aimed at preserving rather than overturning the existing social order. The inequalities of the Commonwealth, so frequently likened to differences in other aspects of the divine creation, were seen by puritan commentators as a natural by-product of a hierarchically ordered cosmos in which the human body acted as a prime exemplar.

Puritan Conceptions of the Body Politic, 1640–1660

Recourse to such modes of thinking continued to permeate puritan discourse throughout the troubled years of the 1640s and 1650s. Indeed, as Walzer himself noted, '[m]edical terminology provided one of the key themes of the revolutionary period', a point underlined by David Cressy in his in-depth study of the critical years between 1640 and 1642.[17] Now, however, the stress was on diagnosis and cure and there was no shortage of volunteers, on both sides of the growing political divide, to offer medically informed advice to those 'state physicians' who resided at court and sat in Parliament. In the case of the puritanical opposition to the Caroline church and state, recourse to such ideas was most evident in that series of fast sermons preached before Parliament, and imitated elsewhere in England, throughout the 1640s. As early as November 1640, the popular puritan preacher Stephen Marshall had compared Parliament to 'a Colledg of Physicians' to whom 'it may seem unfit to prescribe... a way of cure'.[18] It did not take long, however, for his clerical colleagues to gather up the courage to offer their observations and remedies for the ailing body politic. In February 1643, John Marston, preaching before a large auditory at St Margaret's, Westminster, including numerous members of the House of Commons, expanded on Marshall's analogical train of thought when he declared that 'the State hath long laine sick of a feavour, and we have had more then a Colledge of Physitians in this blest Parliament'. Alluding to the execution of Strafford, he went on to claim that 'to assuage the heat of this distemper, they have let it blood, but discreetly in one vaine onely, lest it bleed to death'.[19] As a moderate and somewhat reluctant supporter of the war, Marston and others like him warned against excessive recourse to phlebotomy or bloodshed in resolving the problems of the body politic.[20] Others were less fastidious when it came to supporting the call for greater bloodletting, and many resorted to medical analogies in order to vindicate the stance of Parliament. The militant Presbyterian John Brinsley, for example, in a fast sermon preached before the godly corporation of Great Yarmouth in December 1642, warmly supported the war by likening God's role in orchestrating the outcome of the conflict to that of a physician superintending a surgeon. In prescribing a detailed account of the necessary procedures to be followed, Brinsley was at pains to absolve Parliament, in the guise of the surgeon, from some degree of responsibility for the escalating conflict by suggesting that it was ultimately God, in the role of the physician, who was responsible for wielding the lancet. He alone decided 'what persons it shall strike, what incision it shall make, how deep it shall go, how many, not only ounces, but dropps of blood it shall draw'.[21]

The analogy of the body politic was a remarkably flexible tool of political analysis in the 1640s and was readily adapted to provide varying degrees of comfort and understanding for those seeking to make sense of, and to respond to, the growing conflict between King and Parliament. Those who wished to see a militant response to the political crisis, such as the Exeter puritan, John Bond, thus resorted to condemning temporizers and moderates by comparing their words and actions to those patients who shun 'violent remedies' and argue that 'such physick is too corrosive, and may endanger the whole politicke body'. In preference to their 'Lenitives, cooling juleps and palliations', Bond prescribed a saw as the 'best salve' for a gangrene, a course of action which disallowed further and dangerous prevarication. Four years later, reflecting on the recent siege of parliamentarian Exeter by the royalist armies of the west, Bond once again resorted to the language of the consulting room when he compared the city to a body that was assaulted with a 'double disease', from without by 'a strong, crafty, pestilential enemie' and within 'with a Malignant putrid fever in her owne blood'.[22] Other puritan ministers, such as Anthony Tuckney, invoked the image of the ruler as physician to gently chide those in authority, including the King, to use their power to heal the infirmities of the body politic. In a sermon delivered before Parliament in August 1643 he thus observed, on the authority of Galen, that in former times kings and emperors prescribed medicines to their subjects with their own hands. The contemporary resonance of this allusion was not lost on his audience, for he went on to say that 'although all Monarches now cure not the Kings evil; yet all both Kings and Magistrates should, as occasion and need shal be, have both skill and will to cure greater and more dangerous diseases in the body Politick'. Alluding to the time of the prophet Isaiah, he concluded, somewhat caustically, 'that in those times although Rulers and Healers were two words, yet they made account that they should bee and doe one and the same thing: and soe indeed if God be with them, they both are and doe accordingly'.[23]

On occasions, godly ministers ostensibly on the same side invoked the analogy of the body politic to articulate and support conflicting courses of action. This was apparent, for example, at the critical moment in early 1645 when the 'peace party' in Parliament, supported by their Scottish allies, made one last ditch attempt to come to terms with the King at Uxbridge. The peace negotiations held there, however, proved highly contentious and were opposed by many within Parliament who wished to see the war fought to a military conclusion. The two opposing views were adumbrated in two contrasting sermons preached at Uxbridge on consecutive days. The first, a fast sermon delivered by John Whincop, set out the aims and wishes of the 'peace party', who hoped to see a truce and a negotiated settlement with the King. Accordingly, Whincop cautioned MPs, whom he addressed as 'our Physitians', to proceed slowly and carefully in the cure of the nation, 'as sick a patient... as ever any had, a poore kingdome, all in a desperate malignant burning fever'. An immediate cure was out of the question, but if the life of the patient was to be saved, Whincop assured his listeners, then it must proceed without further bloodletting. The Treaty of Uxbridge thus resembled a potential death-bed scene:

> In all humane possibility, this is one of the last gentle healing medicines that ever this Land is like to have: purg'd... and bloudied it hath been oft before. How many ounces shall I say, or pounds? How many flouds, how many rivers nay, seas of bloud hath poore England lost within these five years? (it is now grown faint, very faint (God knows) a good cordiall, an happie Accommodation, were the likeliest Physick in the World, to set it right again'.[24]

In contrast, the following day the Presbyterian Christopher Love preached at Uxbridge a sermon radically different in tone, but one that nonetheless resorted throughout to medical and healing metaphors. Asking his auditors what it was that caused distempers in a land, and how these might be detected, Love repeatedly contrasted the natural causes and symptoms of bodily ill health with the irreligious and superstitious doctrines and ceremonies of the Church of England, which he blamed for the nation's ills. That the land was indeed labouring under sickness was evident from a variety of symptoms. Citing among others Hippocrates, Love claimed that not only was the head of the kingdom divided from the body of the people, but the latter were undernourished and could no longer 'digest and relish the Gospell'. The faint beat of the nation's pulse was thus a sure sign that 'the Vitalls are wasting'.[25] If further proof were wanted, one need look no further than the fact that God had sent the people of England physicians, 'our Worthies of Parliament, the healers of our breaches', as well as surgeons in the guise of 'our Military Men', who 'let us blood' and thereby demonstrate that 'there is much corrupt blood running in our veins, and many peccant humors gathering together in the body of our Nation'. None, moreover, were spared the surgeon's lancet for 'God sees that there are prophane Nobles, a corrupt Gentry, and many Malignant humors among the Commonalty, else so much blood had not been spilt, so many veines had not been opened'. Accordingly, the cure of the nation's ills consisted in a continuation of the war effort and the need to stiffen the resolve of the 'war party' in Parliament, which Love repeatedly appealed to as a 'Colledge of Physitians' that had 'discerned the causes of our distempers, propounded Remedies, and…made some good progresse in our cure'. Various medicines had been administered and the early signs were promising. The dismantling of episcopacy, church courts, idolatry and superstition (including the parliamentary orders abolishing crosses, crucifixes 'with abundance of such like trumpery') was taken 'as an undoubted argument that God is beginning to heal us', as was the imposition of 'physic' in the form of the Solemn League and Covenant, prescribed by the 'state physicians' in Parliament. The cure, however, was not yet perfected, and so, for Love, the bloodletting must continue.[26]

The disagreements that erupted among the supporters of the parliamentarian cause, exposed as they were at crucial moments such as this, ultimately proved insoluble. The growing divisions in Parliament, which grew worse after the defeat of the King in 1646, were compounded by the growth of radical sectarianism and what was widely perceived as a descent into religious and political anarchy.[27] The execution of the King, lamented by many former puritans as well as their erstwhile opponents in church and state, and the creation of a republic did little to assuage these anxieties. Consequently, given the unsettled nature of the times, it is perhaps unsurprising that throughout the 1650s opponents as well as supporters of the new regime, continued to invoke organicist imagery to console flagging spirits and to buttress the new order. Before tracing these developments, however, it is worth noting how, in the case of puritan spokesmen for the parliamentary cause in the 1640s, the expression of such ideas was often made on special fast days that were observed throughout those parts of England under parliamentarian control. The fact that these were preached on the occasion of a general *fast*, an act with obvious medical connotations, underlines the sense in which these showpiece events were construed as literal testimonies to the reality of a providential deity and a harmonious and ordered cosmos. The act of fasting was intended to procure good health and was commonly invoked in time of plague as a divine remedy for what was widely regarded as a disease beyond the natural capacity of physicians to cure.[28] Moreover, in extraordinary circumstances fasting was also promoted by puritan ministers as a cure for demonic possession. These, of course, were extreme and exceptional diseases, but the general principle—that all sickness was ultimately a form of divine punishment inflicted on mankind for the sins of Adam—was widely accepted by preachers of all persuasions. Individual sinners were often punished by God for their transgressions with suitably apposite diseases. In much the same way, the corporate sins of a nation, or general disorder in the body politic, were frequently held responsible for engendering ill health in the whole community, as in the case of the plague. The 1640s, of course, witnessed a decade of unprecedented conflict that threatened to tear apart the unity of the three kingdoms. Given the prevalence of belief in the organicist state, many contemporaries became convinced that the catastrophic descent into civil war heralded the appearance of several new diseases that threatened the lives of individual members of the corrupt body politic. And in most cases, it was the supporters of the puritan and parliamentarian cause who were principally responsible for spreading the idea that the breakdown of civil and religious order had initiated an epidemic of new diseases. Thus in 1643, the royalist physician, Edward Greaves, dismissed reports, propagated by parliamentarian sources, that the epidemic then raging in the garrison at Oxford was a new disease. Similar reports circulated in 1645 of a new epidemic ravaging the parliamentary army in the west country.[29]

The most significant new disease to emerge in the 1640s, however, was rickets. It was first referred to as such by the puritan minister at Exeter, John Bond, who in a sermon preached in 1641 condemned the 'arbitrary men' in government (that is the supporters of Charles I) for endangering the health of the nation by threatening to make 'the whole body Politiq; like the child sick of the Rickets'. Bond, who as we have already seen was prone to viewing the events of the early 1640s through the lens of medical metaphors, went on to explain to his audience that:

> The Rickets is a disease in Children, which causeth an extraordinary growth, or rather swelling, in the upper parts of the body toward the head, but the lower members all the while doe pine, languish, and waste away: and therefore 'tis not so much a natural nutrition, as an unnaturall corruption of the whole body.[30]

Other references to the rickets can be found in the sermons of the Presbyterian preacher Jeremiah Whitaker. In April 1645, for example, in a sermon preached before the Lord Mayor of London, he specifically alluded to it, alongside other diseases such as the sweating sickness and the pox, as one of the many 'new diseases' to afflict the contemporary world. Pessimistic as to the physician's ability to find an effective cure, Whitaker again referred to the disease in early 1646, when, in a sermon before Parliament, he compared those children suffering from rickets, 'who in the face look well, and swell in upper parts, but shrinke downwards', to those who promote religious controversy but were otherwise lax in their practice of religious faith.[31] Rickets was the subject of intensive study in England in the 1640s, culminating in the publication of the first large-scale study of the disease, *De Rachidite* (1650), which William Birken has hailed as 'a monument to Puritan medicine in the seventeenth century'.[32] Clerical and other social commentators continued to allude to the disease throughout the 1650s, often using it as a metaphor for spiritual pride or hypocrisy. In 1653, for example, William Sclater, invoked rickets in an assize sermon at Taunton, and compared its trademark symptoms (swollen head and 'a debility downwards') with those religious enthusiasts who professed spiritual wisdom but failed to engage with the emotional aspects of true religion.[33] In a similar vein, the Essex minister, John Beadle, compared religious hypocrites to 'some children that are sick of a disease they call the Rickets, who have great heads, and big bellies, but shrimpled hands, and weak knees'. Beadle's views found an echo in the work of an anonymous chronicler of 'vulgar errors' in 1659. Criticizing those who 'abound in New Notions, but abstain not from their old Vices', he claimed that such people laboured with the 'Spirituall Ricketts'.[34] The idea that new diseases such as rickets may have arisen as a punishment for the peculiar sins of the English in the middle decades of the seventeenth century was given added currency by the Presbyterian John Bird in 1661. Eager to promote the restoration of Charles II, Bird equated the appearance of rickets with the slide towards political and religious anarchy in the 1640s and 1650s. Turmoil in the body politic was mirrored by the outbreak of new complaints in the bodies of Englishmen and women. The cure for the latter lay partly in the hands of physicians, but, as Bird and countless others made clear, it was primarily dependant on a resolution of the kingdom's religious and political problems.[35] This was as true in the early 1660s as it had been throughout the previous two decades, and there is little doubt that most puritan commentators subscribed to such normative beliefs.

Michael Walzer has argued that the kind of analogical reasoning associated with harmonist modes of thinking died with the defeat of the King in the first civil war. Others, not unreasonably, have inclined to the view that it received its death knell with the execution of Charles I in 1649. Neither view is borne out by the evidence, however, for not only did such ways of thinking continue to appeal to a wide cross section of the British public, including many leading parliamentarian and puritan propagandists, but they also proved remarkably versatile in accommodating new political and medical developments. Following the establishment of the Commonwealth in 1649, supporters of the new regime continued to invoke the body as a template for governing the country. In Charles I's place, new figures arose to take up the mantle of state physician. In 1651, for example, the medical writer, Daniel Border, dedicated a self-help manual to John Bradshaw, Lord President of the Council and the man who had presided over the trial of the King. In it, he implored Bradshaw to defend the people from 'the Common Enemy' and to take on the role of 'the great Physitian' in order to 'cleanse and purge the evill and maligne humors, which are apt to arise in the body politick'.[36] New political arrangements, moreover, did not necessarily lead to the disappearance of more traditional modes of political discourse. Bradshaw's legal colleague and fellow regicide, John Cook, for example, combined a commitment to a radical social and political agenda with a continuing respect for the naturalness of a political order based on the organization and operation of the human body.[37] The malleability of the notion of the body politic was particularly evident in the various assize sermons preached by loyal ministers in the 1650s. George Swinnock, for example, consistently invoked the analogy in a sermon originally preached at Hertford assizes in 1653. He thus compared the laws of the nation to the 'nerves and sinews of the Body Politick, or as Physick to the natural body, to prevent diseases and purge out ill humours'. And just as the natural body exhibited order, distinction and a hierarchy of the parts, so too did the government of the nation. In classical fashion, the magistrate was thus compared to the head, which above all other parts of the body natural/politic must be preserved and protected. Swinnock, however, was careful to avoid any suggestion that invocation of the analogy implied support for any specific form of government: 'The Genus of Magistracy is from God, yet the Species, whether Monarchy, Democracy, or Aristocracy may be at the choice of men'.[38] In a passage echoing Swinnock's concerns, the preacher William Thomas opined that false witnesses in court were the bane of the body politic, 'the administration of justice, which depends on the truth of witnesses, being the sinews, nay the vital spirits of a Commonwealth'.[39] Others, such as fellow puritan, John Warren, substituted the belly for the head or heart as the chief organ of government in the reformed commonwealth and allotted pride of place in the body politic to the godly magistrate. In similar fashion, Richard Saunders, in an assize sermon preached in 1651, extolled the administration of the law as the 'very soul and breath of a body politick [which]...can no more be without it, then a naturall body can live without breath, and without a soul'.[40] The dispensation of godly justice thus formed the bedrock of the puritan programme for the reform of society and provided a consistent focus of ministerial concern in the pulpit.

The ability of political commentators concerned with the reform and reorganization of society to cite the example or model of the human body in support of their radical claims in the 1650s may also reflect the availability of new models of the body at this time. This period, as is well documented, witnessed various breakthroughs in the fields of anatomy and physiology (much of it informed by the mechanical philosophy of Descartes), as well as radical developments in the practice of medicine. Some puritan ministers, for example, demonstrated an early familiarity with, and acceptance of, Harvey's discovery of the blood. In a fast sermon preached before the Commons in 1642, Charles Herle referred to the recent dispute among physicians 'whether the motion of the blood be circular or no'.[41] Others alluded to the contemporary dispute between the Galenists and Paracelsians,[42] or invoked the latest anatomical research, which they sought to recruit in the cause of religious and political order. Thus William Sclater, in a sermon preached before the assizes at Winchester in 1652, recommended clemency as a key attribute in a judge, comparing moderation to 'that water observed by Anatomists in the Pericardium, which cools the Ebullitions about the heart'.[43] New medical theories and beliefs also appealed to political commentators. The ideas of the Flemish iatrochemist, Jan Baptist van Helmont (1579–1644), proved particularly fertile territory in this respect. This much is evident in one of the first major treatises in English devoted to Helmontianism penned by the otherwise anonymous proselyte, Noah Biggs.[44] In *The Vanity of the Craft of Physick* (1651), Biggs appealed to the Rump Parliament to initiate a major reform of medicine and medical education along Helmontian lines. Utterly disparaging of the ability of conventional Galenic physicians to heal most diseases, Biggs advocated in their stead a new form of medicine and a new type of practitioner that reflected more accurately the divine nature of the physician's calling.[45] And he did so by constant resort to medico-political analogies that championed the new regime. Adulterated medicines, for example, are referred for judgement to 'the Parliament of our Intellects', which would soon discover such drugs 'to be desperate malignants and Traitors to the present government and Republique of our Body'. In typical Helmontian fashion, Biggs also rejected the mythical nature of 'Prestor-John humours' as well as the related panoply of methods devised by Galenic physicians to remove these fluids from the body, reserving his particular ire for the practice of phlebotomy. In a long and extended metaphor condemning the use of such interventions, Biggs made clear his political allegiance to the Cromwellian regime when he castigated the Galenists' use of cathartic medicines, which:

> profligate, banish, and cast out from the Independency of our vitall Œconomy... not one of the three humours which they say offends, is become malignant, and endeavours to settle a commission of array, to plunder not the petty suburbs but the Westminster-Hall of our sanity and strength, and hath been found, not only pleading for the monarchy and tyranny of diseases and distempers, but in actuall armes against the Re-publique; for which he is adjudged a Delinquent and Traitor, and to be sequestred and thrust out of the lines of Communication, by the back door or port esquiline of our healthfull City; but is onely the honest - round-head, a true and peaceable Commonwealths-man, the bloud who is chosen and ordain'd to be one of the keepers of the liberties, life and health of our bodies.[46]

Biggs' fervent support for van Helmont, moreover, meant that his criticisms of contemporary medicine were not restricted to Galenism. Paracelsus and his followers were equally suspect in Biggs' eyes, as, for example, in their promotion of metallic or mineral-based medicines, which at best were deemed useless and at worse acutely detrimental to some of the central functions of the body. Such receipts were typically indigestible:

> [s]eeing they have refus'd to answer and subscribe to the engagement of the Common-Hall of our œconomy, the stomack (who is made Lord paramount and Surveyor-Generall over all things that's to be receiv'd in) and have not submitted to the present power of digestion... that's conferred on it by the Parliament of our Interiours, in their totality and full season: it is therefore adjudged and voted that they shall not be preferred any further, nor admitted to compound... and therefore are looked upon as Delinquents, and never are converted into true Common-Wealths-men, bloud.[47]

As the example of Biggs suggests, the political rhetoric of the body, and invocation of the body politic, was not intrinsically conservative, but was quite capable of offering, in the words of Andrew Mendelsohn, 'a legitimate way to propose change and revolution, or simply intervention in what was thought to be a natural order'.[48] Another example of this process in action can be seen in the response of the apologist for the 'good old cause', the fifth monarchist, John Rogers, to the publication of Richard Baxter's *Holy Commonwealth*, in 1659. Rogers, who mistakenly assumed that Baxter was arguing in favour of the restoration of government by a single sovereign authority, argued for democracy on the grounds that 'a due and equal temperament of the whole Body, by an even balance and proportion of the four Elements... and Aliments of the Politic Body', was more likely to conduce to good government than the 'Mastery of the One above the other'.[49] Other radical critics of the political status quo such as Henry Stubbe were less deferential to such ideas, though intriguingly, in Stubbe's case, he was more than happy to point out the inconsistencies and flaws in Baxter's position through *ad hominem* attacks on his bodily as well as intellectual integrity. Thus, Stubbe poked fun at Baxter's pretensions to heal the sick, not, as in the days of the apostles by laying on of hands or holy oils, but rather by recourse to the kind of nostrums favoured by empirics such as 'a liquorish stick, or Gascoines powder'. He consistently denigrated his medical knowledge, claiming he was little read in Hippocrates. But above all, he reserved his most caustic remarks for Baxter's renowned hypochondria, which he cited as a token of divine displeasure and a rebuke to Baxter's political principles, 'in fine', concluding 'that the Atrophy of his body is a manifestation of the Sterility of his principles'.[50]

Stubbe's intention in ridiculing Baxter in this way was to point out the absurdity of providentialist accounts of the body, which he believed were invoked by religious conservatives like Baxter to stigmatize their radical opponents. Stubbe was particularly incensed by Baxter's citation of the infamous case of the birth of a monstrous child to the New England antinomian, Mrs Dyer, which he cited as an example of divine judgement on the Vanists or followers of Stubbe's patron, Henry Vane.[51] If anything, however, the outspoken dismissal of such evidences of divine providence by men like Stubbe simply increased the likelihood that others of a more conservative stamp, like Baxter, would grow more, not less, convinced of the need to draw parallels between the natural and the political world. The growing urgency with which preachers invoked the legitimacy of the body politic as a metaphor for government in the 1650s can thus be seen as a reflection of the fear of social, religious and political anarchy unleashed by the civil war and the establishment of a republic. The essential conservatism of mainstream puritan political thinking, evident in the repeated paeans to order that characterized puritan preaching before, during and after the breakdown of monarchical government in the early 1640s, was clearly a factor here. By the late 1650s, the majority of moderate puritans were eager to promote monarchy as a panacea for the nation's ills, often invoking traditional images derived from harmonist modes of thought, including the virtues of the body politic, to vindicate their stance. As pressure grew in the 1650s to persuade Cromwell to accept the offer of the crown, the Lord Protector found himself heralded as 'the universal medicine' and 'the body politic's doctor'.[52] Following his death in 1658, and the rapid collapse of the protectorate, puritan preachers once again retreated to the safety of medical metaphors to explain the current crisis in the Commonwealth. In October 1658, for example, the Presbyterian Samuel Slater used the occasion of a special fast day following the inauguration of Richard Cromwell as his father's successor to call for greater order in church and state and an end to the anarchy of unfettered religious freedom. Typically, he did so by repeatedly reminding his audience of the merits of a well ordered and inclusive body politic, in which it was as much incumbent upon the prince to seek the welfare of his subjects as it was part of the duty of the latter to pray for, and attend to, the demands of their superiors:

> And so it is in the natural body; there is not the meanest member, but it shares in the care of the other members, if one member suffers saith the Apostle, all the members suffer with it; but they will all much more joyn together and unite their forces, and act for the good and welfare of the Head. So it is in a Nation, the Body Politick; the meanest and lowest persons in it should be prayed for, and their good should be studied and promoted... how much more then ought this to be done for him who is the Head of this Body, from whom the whole hath guidance & direction.[53]

Such aspirations gathered pace as the nation spiralled towards a resumption of internecine strife following the recall of the Rump Parliament and the growing conflict between its members and the Army in 1659.[54] By early 1660, it was clear which way the wind was blowing. The mood of the country had swung decisively in favour of a return to the ancient constitution and the principle of kingship, supported by a revitalized Church of England. Religious moderates on both sides, who had witnessed at first hand the slide towards religious anarchy, now petitioned Parliament for the return of the King, and they did so, typically, by invoking the imagery of sick bodies and the power of restorative medicine. Thus, the puritan minister, John Moore, rector of Aller in Somerset, typified the chorus of complaint when he argued that it was impossible to expect that the state, or a sick person, should recover their health if they were surrounded by 'a multitude of Physicians' about the sick bed. He went on to argue that 'if England then would be healed of the falling-sickness, and Convulsion Fits of Division: Let them apply to their stomacks the Leaf of a godly Christianlike Ancient Government, and they shall be healed, or else never'.[55]

The expression of such sentiments linking medicine to politics and promoting an overarching vision of a single polity based on the human body was, then, a consistent theme of puritan thinking in the decades before, during and after the so-called puritan revolution. As in so much else in the puritan mentality, recourse to the imagery of the body politic was founded on biblical precepts, particularly the Pauline injunction for Christians to observe that 'there should be no schism in the body; but that the members should have the same care one for another' for 'if one member suffer, all the members suffer with it' [1 Corinthians 12:25–6]. Here was the basis of the puritan doctrine of callings which, originally intended as a model for the government of the early church, was consistently applied by puritan preachers to the organization of the godly commonwealth.[56] The prime object of government in puritan eyes differed little from that of their royalist and Anglican opponents, despite the propagandistic claims of the latter, who frequently stigmatized all those who had opposed the Caroline church and state as radical incendiaries, anarchists and schismatics. Order, hierarchy and harmony remained the essential building blocks of the new kingdom of Jerusalem for most moderate puritans. Government itself, though it may now have devolved from kings to lesser magistrates, remained essentially divine in origin and charismatic in nature, in keeping with the providentialist nature of puritan religious thinking. Typically, puritan assize sermons in the 1640s and 1650s consistently invoked Psalms 82:6 ['I have said, Ye are gods...'] to bolster the divine calling of the magistrate and thus underpin puritan efforts to implement a godly reformation of society. Typical were the comments of Michael Thomas at the Shropshire assizes in 1659, when he reminded his auditory that '[m]agistrates are called Gods, because they are advanced to do the work of God, for such is the work of Justice'.[57] All these themes—the divine nature of magistracy, the natural harmony of such arrangements, and their place in a theocratic state in which political order rested on a historical contract between rulers and ruled—can be found, for example, in the assize sermon that Zacheus Mountagu preached at the East Grinstead assizes in

Sussex in 1652. Dedicated to the presiding circuit judges, Mountagu condemned the contemporaneous 'levelling humour' and began his sermon by invoking the metaphor of the human body, which like the political, was 'distinguished into superiour and inferiour, into Noble and ignoble parts'. He continued by arguing that 'as that body is a monster which is all head, or where head is too big for the body, so is that which hath no head, or a head too little'. His moderate message was all too clear: 'where all govern there is no government, and where all are chief, there can be no Order'. In every respect this was traditional thinking. Mountagu went on to confirm, for example, that magistracy was divine in origin, citing once again the declaration from Psalms that bestowed divine authority on all who govern and administer justice. He also reiterated age-old arguments, drawn from observing the harmonious operations of nature and the universe, to underpin the view that when 'Government failes in any land, why then such a Land becomes disjointed and convulsed'. Mountagu concluded by describing the contractual origins of modern political arrangements in a way that was fully in keeping with those theories developed by parliamentarian apologists in the 1640s, and without betraying any sense that such ideas were incompatible with harmonist and organicist concepts of the state.[58]

Sin, Sickness and the Body Politic In Puritan England

The puritan preoccupation with the creation and maintenance of a divinely ordained, well-ordered and hierarchical body politic was not simply a heuristic device. It also had practical consequences. Many of the social ills, for example, that beset the Commonwealth and were singled out by puritan preachers for judicial chastisement were those made manifest through the bodies of sinners. Moreover, the sins of sexual incontinency, swearing and excessive drinking contaminated not just the bodies of individual miscreants but also polluted wider society. Sexual promiscuity, of course, like other diseases born of sin, left its distinctive marks on the bodies of the debauched—a further sign, perhaps, of the providential working of God linking individual diseases with wider corruption in the body politic. Puritan moralists were equally quick to denounce those who swore oaths and to describe in lurid detail the punishments that awaited such miscreants at the hands of a vengeful God. Rules for the government of the tongue were thus invoked to correct the failings of this organ for, as one puritan minister recalled: 'No member of the body is subject to so many Moral Diseases, as the Tongue is'.[59] However, of all the sins of the body and body politic that worried puritan and other social commentators in this period, few generated more column inches than that of the perils of drink and drunkenness. Immoderate drinking provided a wealth of opportunities for puritan moralists to expatiate on the political lessons to be learned from such anti-social behaviour. More often than not, these were expressed through the metaphor of the body politic. The drunkard, for example, provided an endless source of didactic sermonizing in which the focus on the transformation of intemperate drinkers into unreasoning 'beasts' had profound implications for social and political order. A distempered drunk, who was not in control of his body, effectively disenfranchised himself from active participation in the day-to-day workings of the body politic. Such scruples applied not only to the common man but also, and indeed in puritan eyes, more specifically to those who wielded power in early modern Britain. This mood is perfectly captured in the reported words of the Elizabethan puritan, Thomas Cartwright, who is alleged to have admonished a recently elected mayor in Warwickshire, renowned for his drunken and dissolute way of living, with the words: 'howe unfit for the office to governe others when he could not rule himselfe'.[60] The physical demeanour of the godly magistrate was thus upheld as exemplary and a pattern for others to follow. His ability to exercise restraint in the use of bodily functions such as the tongue was widely seen in puritan circles as emblematic of the charismatic authority that inhered in the pious magistrate.[61] 'A magistrate must not be drunke', according to the Bristol preacher, Thomas Thompson, for '[w]hat mighty mischiefs are in the ommonwealth by the drunkenness of Magistrates and men of authority'.[62] In the same spirit, the puritan physician, James Hart, proudly declared in 1633 that the godly borough of Northampton included in its constitution a rule forbidding the election of a victualler or innkeeper to the post of bailiff or mayor.[63]

The puritan crusade against drunkenness and illegal alehouses, born from a desire to reform the body politic rather than turn it upside down, was nonetheless a major source of friction between those who supported such a reformation and those who saw it as corrosive of communal solidarity and the old-fashioned social virtues associated with such conviviality.[64] Prior to the outbreak of civil war in 1642, puritan magistrates occasionally launched campaigns to root out what they perceived as the amoral culture of excessive drinking and the alehouse. In godly Dorchester, for example, one recidivist claimed, with some conviction, that the puritan magistrates in the town used the clampdown against drinking and other disorderly behaviour as an excuse to persecute the poor and powerless.[65] As divisive as these tactics may have been, it would be a mistake, however, to conclude that they formed part of a radical programme of political reform, *pace* Walzer and others, designed to overturn the traditional political status quo. The example culled from the Dorchester records and cited above is particularly instructive in this respect as the driving force behind the puritan ruling party in the 1620s and 1630s, the patriarchal figure of John White, subscribed wholeheartedly to a politics founded on the traditional cosmic harmonism represented by a unified, hierarchical and orderly body politic.[66] Excessive drinking continued to evoke the fury of puritan preachers, moralists and magistrates throughout the 1640s and 1650s, and resurfaced as a political issue at the Restoration. In particular, grave concerns were raised by puritan ministers who feared that the return of the King and the old order would unleash a tide of uncontrolled drunkenness that was partially legitimated by the royalist culture of drinking healths to the restored monarch. Francis Walsall, for example, implored Charles II to set an example to others, especially his supporters, by becoming a 'sober prince' and avoiding drunken excess.[67] His colleague Nehemiah Beaton likewise urged his fellow countrymen to demonstrate their loyalty to the new king by avoiding drunken toasts and praying instead for the King's health.[68] The concerns of both men were echoed by the Yarmouth Presbyterian, John Brinsley, who chose the occasion of the King's coronation to chastise those who seemed to think that the only way they might show 'affection to their Soveraign' was 'by drinking and Carouzing of Healths to him'.[69] Alluding to the royal proclamation against excessive drinking issued by Charles shortly after his return to England, Brinsley, like so many of his co-religionists, pinned high hopes on the Restoration and the figure of the King, who was characteristically described as 'the chief Physitian [and] the chief Instrument for the healing' of those 'sad Distractions'. In what can only be described as a bout of wishful thinking, Brinsley went on to eulogize the restored prince as renowned for his 'Sobriety and Temperance' and his 'Moderation and Meekness'. Beguiled by the Declaration of Breda, which had invoked the language of healing, Brinsley applauded Charles for granting... indulgence to consciences truly tender' and for 'endeavouring an accommodation of differences, that there might be... a Christian compliance amongst persons of different perswasions'. The body politic was thus in safe hands, according to Brinsley, for proof of which one need look no further than 'the Zeal which he hath shewen against those Epidemical Sins of Swearing and Drunkenness, which through too much indulgence have been so rife in this Nation'.[70]

The puritan emphasis on sobriety has often been contrasted with the culture of excessive drinking that characterized the cavalier party in post–civil war England and suggests one subtle way in which the puritan conception of the body politic—sober, chaste and polite—differed from that of their Anglican and royalist opponents. There is, of course, a foundation of truth in these stereotypes, though it would be wrong to exaggerate the distance between the two 'parties' on this issue, leastwise in 1660. It is quite conceivable that many moderate puritans were persuaded to support the Restoration because of the various proclamations and protestations emanating from the camp of Charles II in exile that promised a reformation of manners in the body politic. Swearing and drinking, for example, were singled out by the loyal clergyman Anthony Walker as sins worthy of royal displeasure. In a sermon preached in the capital on the day after Charles II's entry into London, Walker blasted those who thought that drinking healths to the King, often in a state of physical collapse, was an appropriate way in which to demonstrate one's loyalty. He particularly despised the implication that to refuse such toasts marked one out as disloyal. In riposte, he argued that the King would not take kindly to such beastly behaviour, citing a speech Charles had made at the Hague to a group of delegates from the London ministers in which he stressed that:

> he would make it his business to bring virtue and sobriety into fashion and repute in England, and though there were a prophane drinking party which would be esteemed his best or only friends, he would make the more haste into England, to let such men know that he was their worst enemy, for they were the Devils party, and none of his.[71]

In the aftermath of the euphoria surrounding the King's return, there was clearly a wide constituency of opinion in favour of a clampdown on immoderate drinking that was not limited to the 'godly party' and transcended former religious and political allegiances. Diehard royalist and Anglican ministers such as Robert Mossom, for example, were equally quick to condemn the practice of drinking healths, admonishing those who over-indulged with the example of the King himself. He thus advised his auditory in a sermon preached to celebrate the imminent restoration in May 1660 that:

> [a]n excess of gladness is allow'd, but not of drunkenness... Wine in a drunken excess, it inflames the heart, intoxicates the brain; and turns all fanatick. You must, you'l say, drink the King's health: But tell me, is it congruous in cups of excess to drink the King's health, when he preserves his health by little drinking?[72]

Despite the wishes of a broad cross section of the religious and political spectrum in the towns and villages of England the message of the divines and moralists went unheeded. As the evidence of the records of countless quarter sessions testifies, disputes over drinking healths and toasts proliferated in the 1660s, helping to create divided communities and provoke bitter controversies that often spilled over into violence and bloodshed.[73] At the same time, growing sexual licentiousness at court, often associated with excessive drinking, threatened to destroy the image of sacred kingship and the desire for moral reform that was promised amidst the euphoria of the early years of the Restoration. The outbreak of a particularly virulent strain of plague in England in the summer of 1665 simply added to many people's convictions that the country was being punished for the carnal sins of those who, as chief members of the body politic, were responsible for setting an example to others over whom they ruled. Disordered bodies thus fomented wider disorder in the body politic and helped to erode yet further faith in an older political order based on organicist and harmonist notions of the state. With each successive crisis in government, culminating in the Exclusion Crisis in the early 1680s, confrontations of the kind described here escalated, and talk of restoring the body politic to health evaporated in a mist of accusation and counteraccusation. The fate of the body politic after the Restoration is exemplified in the case of the Devon nonconformist John Hickes, who, writing in the immediate aftermath of the renewal of religious persecution following the passage of the Second Conventicle Act, continued to voice the hope that 'the Smiles and Favours of Royal Majesty, may be as a Soveraign Balsome, to heal those many Wounds that are now made in our Body Politick, that it may at last be reduced to an Eucrasy, or a Sound, and healthful Constitution'. Should harmony not prevail, Hickes nonetheless desired that 'those who feel the Smart [and] Sigh and Groan under the Anguish of them, may be of a Sedate Spirit, and to be persuaded into a Patient Tolleration thereof; till the Chiefest Physitian by his Infallible and unerring Wisdom... effecteth the Cure'. It is perhaps a token of the failure of Charles II's government, which failed miserably to implement that programme of moral reform foreshadowed in the various declarations issued by the king-in-waiting in 1660, that the magnanimous Hickes was ultimately forced into active resistance against the Stuarts and was executed in the aftermath of Monmouth's Rebellion.[74]

Notes

1. For a good introduction to the traditional role of the body politic in medieval and early modern political thinking, see D. G. Hale, *The Body Politic: A Political Metaphor in Renaissance English Literature* (The Hague & Paris, 1971). The harmonist ideals upon which the concept of the body politic rested are discussed at length in J. Daly, 'Cosmic Harmony and Political Thinking in Early Stuart England', *Transactions of the American Philosophical Society*, 69 (1979), 1–40. Both Hale and Daly, like Walzer, assume the demise of the political resonance of such beliefs by the middle decades of the seventeenth century.
2. M. Walzer, *The Revolution of the Saints: A Study in the Origins of Radical Politics* (London, 1966). Others to follow Walzer's lead include Stephen Collins and David Underdown. Collins, for example, has maintained that puritanism denied 'the traditional idea of order and correspondence', while Underdown argued that the cultural divisions that led to civil war in England were predicated on a dichotomy between two very different principles of political order; S. L. Collins, *From Divine Cosmos to Sovereign State: An Intellectual History of Consciousness and the Idea of Order in Renaissance England* (Oxford, 1989), 6; D. Underdown, *Revel, Riot, and Rebellion: Popular Politics and Culture in England, 1603–1660* (Oxford, 1985), 40–1.
3. K. Sharpe, *Politics and Ideas in Early Stuart England* (London & New York, 1989), 28–31. Sharpe does, however, acknowledge the remissness of historians in investigating how in this period 'the image of the body was subject to varying interpretations and adapted according to circumstances'; ibid., 62. Part of my purpose here is to initiate such a discussion.
4. J. Sawday, *The Body Emblazoned: Dissection and the Human Body in Renaissance Culture* (London & New York,1995), 30, 130. Recent devotees of the line taken by Walzer, Sharpe and Sawday include Michael Schoenfeldt who concurs in seeing the

notion of an organicist state as the product of conservative social, religious and political forces (in this case predominantly Anglican and royalist); see his 'Reading Bodies', in K. Sharpe and S. N. Zwicker (eds), *Reading, Society and Politics in Early Modern England* (Cambridge, 2003), 215–43.

5. D. G. Hale, 'Analogy of the Body Politic', in P. P. Wiener (ed.), *Dictionary of the History of Ideas*, 5 vols (New York, 1973–4), i, 69.
6. Sawday, *Body Emblazoned*, 130. It is not my purpose here to engage fully with this line of enquiry, but it must none the less remain a matter of conjecture as to the extent to which mechanistic conceptions of nature had infiltrated scientific, let alone political, discourse by the middle decades of the seventeenth century.
7. For discussion of the role of the body politic in shaping reactions to the Restoration of Charles II, see my *The Miraculous Conformist: Valentine Greatrakes, the Body Politic, and the Politics of Healing in Restoration Britain* (Oxford, 2013), esp. 111–24.
8. Sharpe, *Politics and Ideas in Early Stuart England*, 40. This is also the view taken by Robert Eccleshall in his *Order and Reason in Politics: Theories of Absolute and Limited Monarchy in Early Modern England* (Oxford, 1978), where he stresses the ability of what others have depicted as the 'monolith' of harmonist thinking to accommodate different political outlooks; ibid., 5.
9. J. Rawlinson, *Vivat Rex. A Sermon Preached at Pauls Crosse on the Day of His Majesties Happie Inauguration* [24 March 1614] (Oxford, 1619), 14. Rawlinson, who delayed publication by five years, courted controversy by taking as his text, 1 Samuel 10:24, and citing the example of the biblical king Saul in what was otherwise a traditional paean to divine right monarchy.
10. Lancashire Record Office, DP 353, fo. 44r.
11. T. Scot, *Vox Dei: Iniustice Cast and Condemned. In a Sermon Preached... at the Assises Holden in St. Edmunds Bury in Suffolke* [20 March 1622/3] (London, 1623), 38–9.
12. T.Sutton, *Jethroes Counsell to Moses: Or, a Direction for Magistrates. A Sermon Preached at St Saviours in Southwarke... Before the Honourable Iudges* [5 March 1621/2] (London, 1631), 3. In similar vein, one Mr Ramsey preached an assize sermon at Thetford in Norfolk in March 1630 where he was reported to have 'touched upon the corruptions of judges and councellors'. Significantly, he did so by recourse to the analogy of the body politic; M. A. E. Green (ed.), *The Diary of John Rous, Incumbent of Santon Downham, Suffolk, from 1625 to 1642* (London, Camden Soc., vol.66, 1856), 50.
13. Puritan respect for the body politic analogy has a long pre-civil war history. In 1584, for example, the eminent Presbyterian preacher, Laurence Chaderton, invoked it in support of his campaign against episcopacy. He also stressed the role of the magistrate in policing callings; [L. Chaderton], *A Fruitfull Sermon, upon the 3, 4, 5, 6, 7, 8 Verses of the 12. Chapiter of the Epistle of S.Paul to the Romanes* (London, 1584), 19–20, 32–3.
14. In an earlier assize sermon preached at Carlisle in 1614, Lancelot Dawes expounded on a similar theme, contrasting the operations of the liver, heart and brain in the body to the work of physicians, divines and magistrates in the body politic. In his politically charged address to the circuit judges, whom he compared to surgeons, Dawes warned that of the triumvirate, 'the brain is subject to most diseases: and... the Magistrate is most obnoxious to falls'. Dawes intention, however, was not to infer criticism of the

king, James I, but rather to warn against corrupt magistrates and lawyers, whom he compares to a swelling in the Spleen: 'as the swelling of the spleen argueth the consumption of other parts: so the inriching of the lawyer, the impoverishing of the client'; L. D[awes], *Two Sermons Preached at the Assises Holden at Carlile, Touching Sundry Corruptions of These Times* (Oxford, 1614), 63, 72–3, 78–80, 140. Dawes (d.1655) would appear to have been a religious moderate, who was nonetheless approved by the House of Commons to sit as a representative in the Westminster Assembly of Divines in the 1640s; see *ODNB*.

15. J. Bentham, *The Societie of the Saints: Or, A Treatise of Goode Fellowes, with Their Good Fellowship: Delivered in the Lecture of Kettering in Northampton-shire, in Foureteene Sermons* (London, 1630), 12.
16. For the medical conservatism of Cotta and Hart, and their opposition to all medical intruders, see P. Elmer, 'Medicine, Religion and the Puritan Revolution', in R. French and A. Wear (eds), *The Medical Revolution of the Seventeenth Century* (Cambridge, 1989), 13–15. For Cotta, it followed as a natural corollary of his belief in the divinely sanctioned vocation of the physician that God had also implanted specific attributes in the *material medica* to match specific remedies and medicines. His opposition to universal panaceas such as *aurum potabile* stemmed from such thinking; see Cotta, *Cotta Contra Antonium* (London, 1623), 5–6. The animus against excessive curiosity consistently informed puritan preaching. In a fast sermon preached before Parliament in 1644, Lazarus Seaman implored his listeners to 'have respect unto our ranke, and station', adding that 'Secret things, high things, other mens matters, needlesse things, and curiosities must be let alone'; L. Seaman, *Solomons Choice, or, a President for Kings and Princes, and All that are in Authority Presented in a Sermon before the Honourable House of Commons... at their Publique Fast* [25 September 1644] (London, 1644), 34.
17. Walzer, *Revolution of the Saints*, 176; D. Cressy, *England on Edge: Crisis and Revolution 1640–1642* (Oxford, 2006), 30–4.
18. S. Marshall, *A Sermon Preached Before the Honourable House of Commons... at their Publike Fast* [17 November 1640] (London, 1641), 48.
19. J. Marston, *A Sermon Preached at St. Margaretts in Westminster... before Many of the Worthy Members of the Honourable House of Commons* [6 February 1642/3] (London, 1643), 5. For suspicions surrounding Marston's commitment to the parliamentary cause, see *Wal. Rev.*, 222. Marston's thinly veiled reference to the execution of Thomas Wentworth, earl of Strafford, echoes the statement of the puritan lawyer and MP, Oliver St John, who, in commenting on the attainder proceedings of Strafford, proclaimed that 'if the body bee distempered, it hath [the] power to open a veine to let out the corrupt blood for curing of it selfe [and] if one member be poysoned or gangrened, it hath [the] power to cut it off for the preservation of the rest'; O. St John, *An Argument of Law Concerning the Bill of Attainder of Thomas, Earl of Strafford* (London, 1641), 72.
20. In December 1644, the puritan minister John Langley echoed Marston's call for the selective application of 'necessary Phlebotomy' to the body politic when he compared the actions of 'good Chirurgions' to those members of the House of Commons who have found that the 'best way to staunch a dangerous bleeding is to make a diversion, and to open a vein in another part of the body'. Elsewhere in this fast sermon preached

before the Commons, Langley applauded Parliament for initiating a campaign of preaching and moral reform in closing theatres and brothels and regulating tippling places, actions which he compared to a form of physic whereby 'the body Pollitick gathers strength upon a seeming kinde of weaknesse'; J. Langley, *Gemitus Colombae: The Mournfull Note of the Dove. A Sermon... Before the Honourable House of Commons, at Their Solemn Fast* [25 December 1644] (London, 1645), unpaginated dedication to the members of the House of Commons; 14, 16, 19, 22.

21. J. Brinsley, *A Parlie with the Sword About a Cessation* [Yarmouth, 28 December 1642] (London, 1643), 21–2. In a series of sermons preached at the beginning of 1642, Brinsley prefigured these comments with a comprehensive and traditional medico-political analysis of the dangers then facing the English body politic. Throughout, he appealed to the rulers of England, including the king in council and Parliament ('that wise and venerable Colledge of State Phisitians'), to act as God's instruments in resolving the political crisis. He even cited as a precedent 'that strange Cure of the Kings Evil', though was careful to stress that the monarch was nothing more than a vehicle of divine agency: 'The King may touch, but it is God must cure'; J. Brinsley, *The Healing of Israels Breaches. Wherein is Set Forth Israels Disease, Cure, Physitian, Danger... As They Were Delivered in Six Sermons at the Weekly Lecture in the Church of Great Yarmouth* [23 February–13 April 1642] (London, 1642), esp. 34, 75 [citation of French physician, Jean Fernel], 77–8, 119–20, 129.
22. J. Bond, *A Doore of Hope, also Holy and Loyall Activity. Two Treatises Delivered in Severall Sermons in Excester* (London, 1641), 97; J. Bond, *Occasus Occidentalis: Or, Job in the West. As it was Laid Forth in Two Severall Sermons at Two Publike Fasts, for the Five Associated Westerne Counties* (London, 1645), 63.
23. A. Tuckney, *The Balme of Gilead, for the Wounds of England: Applied in a Sermon Preached at Westminster, Before the Honourable House of Commons at the Late Solemne Fast* [30 August 1643] (London, 1643), 12.
24. J. Whincop, *Gods Call to Weeping and Mourning. Set out in a Sermon before the House of Commons... Being the Day Before the Treaty (at Uxbridge) Began* [29 January 1644/5] (London, 1645), 48–9.
25. C. Love, *Englands Distemper, Having Division and Error, as Its Cause. Wanting Peace and Truth for Its Cure. Set Forth in a Sermon Preacht at Uxbridge on January 30th being the First Day of the Treaty* (London, 1645), 15–20. Diagnosing the condition of the nation, Love reported: 'Oh how faintly do mens pulses beat as if they were neer death already, some are inclined to malignity, others to Neutrality, the most to formality, selfeishnesse, and unsensiblenesse: Thus by the beating of the Kingdomes pulse you may perceive the poor Land distempered at this day'; ibid., 20.
26. Ibid., esp.20–30, 38. Love's sermon, not surprisingly, caused consternation among members of the 'peace party' at Parliament, as well as in royalist ranks. Some reported that Love was advocating that the King himself should be brought to justice, a radical and largely unheard-of suggestion at this time. Following a complaint from the royalist commissioners, Love was confined to his garrison at Windsor, but was swiftly released following the collapse of the peace negotiations in early March 1645. Love himself was later to achieve notoriety for his role in a Presbyterian plot to reinstate Charles II to the

English throne, for which he was executed on 22 August 1651; *ODNB*, *sub* Love, Christopher.

27. For a particularly good example of a puritan sermon, preached before the Lord Mayor of London at the end of the first civil war, espousing a thoroughgoing version of the role of the body politic in underpinning political order and hierarchical government, see E. Terry, *ΨΕΥΔΕΛΕΥΘΕΡΙΑ. Or, Lawlesse Liberty Set Forth in a Sermon Preached Before the Right Honourable the Lord Mayor of London* [16 August 1646] (London, 1646), 4–5.
28. See, for example, W. Gouge, *The Right Way: Or a Direction for Obtaining Good Successe in a Weighty Enterprise* (London, 1648), 31. The puritan Isaac Ambrose later claimed that fast days were 'soul-feeding days, and soul-curing days; some diseases, some lusts will go out no other ways'; I. Ambrose, *Media: the Middle Things, in Reference to the First and Last Things* (London, 1657), 343. For fasting and puritanism, see especially T. Webster, *Godly Clergy in Early Stuart England: The Caroline Puritan Movement, c.1620–1643* (Cambridge, 1997), 60–74; A. Walsham, *Providence in Early Modern England* (Oxford, 1999), 142–7, 164–6. For the popularity of fasts in pre-civil war England, see N. Mears, 'The Culture of Fasting in Early Stuart Parliaments', *Parliamentary History*, 39 (2020), 423–41.
29. [E. Greaves], *Morbus Epidemicus Anni 1643. Or, The New Disease with the Signes, Causes, Remedies, &c* (Oxford, 1643), 1; J. Sprigge, *Anglia Rediviva Englands Recovery being the History of the Motions, Actions, and Successes of the Army* (London, 1647), 155, cited in R. G. S. Tanes, 'The "New Disease" and the Parliamentary Army at Ottery St Mary November/December 1645', *Devon and Cornwall Notes and Queries*, 34 (1978–81), 110–20.
30. Bond, *Doore of Hope*, 39. The implication of Bond's allusion was clear. The head of the body politic (the King and his advisers), like that of the child suffering from rickets, had grown too large and now threatened the well-being of the rest of the polity.
31. J. Whitaker, *The Christians Great Design on Earth is to Attain Assurance for Heaven... Set forth in a Sermon Preached Before the Right Honourable the Lord Mayor... of London* [8 April 1645] (London, 1645), 20; *idem*, *The Danger of Greatnesse: or Uzziah his Exultation and Destruction Set forth in a Sermon Before the Right Honourable the Lords and Commons Assembled in Parliament* [14 January 1645/6] (London, 1646), 40.
32. W. J. Birken, 'The Dissenting Tradition in English Medicine of the Seventeenth and Eighteenth Centuries', *Medical History*, 39 (1995), 205. This study was largely undertaken under the supervision of the Presbyterian Regius Professor of Medicine at Cambridge, Francis Glisson (for whose religious affiliations, see below 48, 85 n.23). The study of what was initially seen as a peculiarly English disease was earlier the subject of a Leiden medical thesis entitled *De Morbo Puerii Anglorum*, written by the puritan physician and natural philosopher Daniel Whistler (*c*.1619–1684) in 1645.
33. W. Sclater, *A Divine Cordiall for a Devout Soule... In a Sermon Preached at Taunton in the Assize Week* [4 April 1653] (London, 1653), 19–20.
34. J. B[eadle], *The Journal or Diary of a Thankful Christian, Presented in Some Meditations upon Numb[ers] 33:2* (London, 1656), 34; Anon., *ΠΕΡΙΑΜΜΑ ΈΠΙΔΗΜΙΟΝ: Or, Vulgar Errours in Practice Censured* (London, 1659), sigs A5r–v.

35. The royalist cleric turned physician, John Wynell (1606–1670), reiterated these anxieties. Writing in 1659 amidst growing fears of a return to the political and religious chaos associated with the 'good old cause', Wynell declared that it was a self-evident truth that just as 'Africk is never without some new Monster, nor England without some new Disease, as strange & monstrous'; J. Wynell, *Lues Venerea* (London, 1660), 1. Wynell, it should be stressed, was no medical conservative. Elsewhere in this work on the pox, he comes across as very much a modernist, eager to promote new medical thinking (such as the circulation of the blood) and to uphold the virtues of experience and practice over excessive book-learning and respect for medical tradition; ibid., 74–5.
36. D. Border, *ΠΟΛΥΦΑΡΜΑΚΟΣ κάι ΧΥΜΙΣΤΗΣ, or, The English Unparallel'd Physitian and Chyrurgian* (London, 1651). Border (d.1658), who described himself on the titlepage as a 'practitioner in physick', was almost certainly employed as an official compiler of newsletters in the 1650s. In the prefatory dedication to Bradshaw, he describes his work as a 'quintessence' of Hippocrates, Galen and Paracelsus 'and other learned men of these latter times', though he would appear on balance to have favoured Paracelsus over Galen.
37. J. Cook, *Unum Necessarium: or, The Poore Mans Case* (London, 1648), 11–12, 36. Cook was highly critical of the established medical profession. In the same work, he campaigned for a change in the law to allow empirics such as William Trigge (d.1665), who practised *gratis* among the poor, to minister to the sick without molestation from the College of Physicians in London; ibid., 61–3.
38. G. Swinnock, *Men are Gods, or the Dignity of Magistracy, and the Duty of the Magistrate: As it was Presented in a Sermon at the Assize Holden at Hertford* [2 August 1653] (London, 1660), 198, 205, 207, 210, 230, 235–6, 242, 248. Swinnock's medical conservatism, typical of most mainstream puritans, is illustrated by his view that '[e]very calling hath some rule to go by', that of the physician, to be guided by Galen and Hippocrates; ibid., 261–2.
39. W. Thomas, *The Regulating of Law-Suits, Evidences, and Pleadings. An Assize Sermon Preacht at Carmarthen* [16 March 1656/7] (London, 1657), 18. Thomas's tirade against the partiality of jurors and the deceitfulness of witnesses echoes the concerns voiced by the puritan Thomas Scot in various assize sermons preached before the civil war. In 1623, for example, Scot had compared the practice of false swearing to those white witches who masquerade as physicians and 'like the good witch . . . that cures the body peradventure, but wounds the soule'; Scot, *Vox Dei*, 21, 22; cf. *idem*, *God and the King in a Sermon Preached at the Assises Holden at Bury S. Edmonds* [13 June 1631] (Cambridge, 1633), 19.
40. J. Warren, *The Unprofitable Servant: a Sermon Preached at the Assize Holden at Chelmesford* [26 March 1655] (London, 1655), 21; R. Saunders, *Plenary Possession Makes a Lawfull Power: or Subjection to Powers that are in Being Proved to be Lawfull and Necessary, in a Sermon Preached Before the Judges in Exeter* [23 March 1650/1] (London, 1651), 11. Interestingly, the royalist poets Richard Lovelace and John Ogilby compared England under Cromwell to a tyrannical, headless belly; C. H. Wilkinson (ed.), *The Poems of Richard Lovelace* (Oxford, 1930), 155; J. Ogilby, *The Fables of Aesop Paraphras'd in Verse, and Adorn'd with Sculpture* (London, 1651), iii, 13 [image at

sculpture no. 47]. Warren's identification of the stomach as the chief organ in the body might owe something to contemporary interest in the new medical ideas of van Helmont which were becoming widely popularized in the 1650s; see below 73–4.

41. C. Herle, *A Payre of Compasses for Church and State. Delivered in a Sermon Preached at St. Margarets in Westminster, Before the Honourable House of Commons at their Monethly Fast November the Last, 1642* (London, 1642), 7. In this sermon Herle characteristically employed the rhetoric of the body politic to defend Parliament from the accusation that it was opposed to 'all unity and order both in church and state, as if... it meant to make them both, like Pliny's *Acephali*, all body and no head'; ibid., 12. Puritan physicians were equally open to innovative anatomical speculation. As a Leiden student, the Presbyterian Roger Drake (1608–1669) was one of the first to write in defence of Harveian circulation in February 1640 in an exercise dedicated among others to the puritan minister, Francis Cheynell, and John Fiennes, son of the staunchly puritan earl of Saye and Sele. He subsequently published his thesis in 1641, but despite becoming a candidate for membership of the London College of Physicians in 1643 he was unable to elicit the College's official stamp of approval for Harvey's theories as it remained resolutely neutral throughout the dispute. Drake later resigned from the College in 1646 to pursue a clerical career as a prominent spokesman for the Presbyterian movement in England; for Drake, see *ODNB* and below, 47, 84 n.16.
42. H. Wilkinson, *Miranda, Stupenda. Or, The Wonderfull and Astonishing Mercies which the Lord Hath Wrought for England... Presented in a Sermon Preached Before the Honorable House of Commons* [21 July 1646] (London, 1646), 23–4.
43. W. Sclater, *Civil Magistracy by Divine Authority, Asserted, and Laid Forth in a Sermon, Preached at the Assizes Holden at Winchester* [4 March 1652/3] (London, 1653), 29–30. The sermon as a whole is a typical puritan paean to order that invokes the analogy of the microcosm-macrocosm in defence of hierarchy and 'superiority' and as a proof that a 'Politick Inaequality is not against a Spirituall Aequality'; ibid., 10–11, 15. It is also characteristic of mainstream puritan attitudes to chymistry in comparing those who reject ordinances, law-givers and magistrates (i.e. the radical sects) to those 'chymicks, who labour to torture nature, for the extraction of such spirits, as were never inherent in the thing'; ibid., 14. For puritan ambivalence towards 'chymistry', see chapter 3.
44. Hal Cook has suggested that Biggs may have been either Thomas Biggs or his son Henry, both of whom were employed as surgeons in the naval dockyards of Deptford and Woolwich, 'the pseudonym "Noah" stemming from their work environment'. The republican sentiments expressed by Noah Biggs certainly fit with the little that is known of the two surgeons. In 1653, when Thomas Biggs sought to regain his post as naval surgeon at the dockyard, he was able to rely on the support of his well-connected brother-in-law, Rear Admiral Richard Badiley (d.1657), an ardent puritan and Cromwellian; H. Cook, *The Decline of the Old Medical Regime in Stuart London* (Ithaca and London, 1986), 122n; *CSPD, 1652–1653*, 351, 352.
45. In line with their Paracelsian cousins, the Helmontians repeatedly cited the apocryphal text in Ecclesiasticus 38:1, which emphasized the divine nature of the physician's office and the special relationship that existed between God and the true exponents of healing. This extended, in some Helmontians' minds, to the idea that medical knowledge itself was communicated directly to God's chosen *adepti* by a form of direct, ecstatic revelation, or, as Biggs put it, 'from an inward teaching of the mindes

heightening and enlightening by an invisible and yet sensible glorious emanation of light, truth, God, Intellect and Intelligible objects'; N. Biggs, *Matæotechnia Medicinae Praxeωs. The Vanity of the Craft of Physick* (London, 1651), 21, 45, 57, 213 [quote].

46. Ibid., 41, 78. In an aside probably aimed at the Galenists who dominated the London College of Physicians, Biggs made clear his own political allegiance, as well as that of his collegiate opponents, when he disparaged the latter for their failure and 'refractor-inesse' to embrace innovation and the 'Antipathy of their spirits for the most part to this present government'; ibid., 2–3. One of the first to respond to Biggs' work was the College's own chymist William Johnson in his 'Short Animadversions upon the Book Lately Published by one who stiles himselfe NOAH BIGGS, Helmontii Psittacum', appended to Johnson's edition of John Hester's *Three Exact Pieces of Leonard Phioravant* (London, 1652). In describing Biggs as 'the parrot of Helmont', Johnson was probably alluding to the fact that many sections of his work were in fact direct translations lifted from the 1648 Latin edition of van Helmont's works.

47. Ibid., 101–2. In promoting the sacred role of blood and the stomach in the functioning of the human body, Biggs was conflating two important facets of Helmontian teaching that envisaged these two organs as the prime residence of the soul.

48. A. Mendelsohn, 'Alchemy and Politics in England 1649–1665', *Past and Present*, 135 (1992), 48. In refuting the work of Walzer, Mendelsohn alludes to the appropriation of the language of the body politic by rebels and radicals, as well as conservatives, in much the same way as both groups drew on alchemical imagery to promote their particular political aspirations and beliefs. I discuss in more detail some of the issues raised here by Mendelsohn in chapter 4.

49. J. Rogers, *ΔΙΑΠΟΛΙΤΕΙΆ. A Christian Concertation with Mr. Prin, Mr. Baxter, Mr. Harrington, for the True Cause of the Commonwealth* (London, 1659), 92. Rogers, it should be pointed out, was no obscurantist sectary. Clearly *au fait* with recent developments in medical research (he claimed that Harrington's view of government tended 'more to the maintenance of the Diastole then of the Systole of the Commonwealth, i.e. for the promoting then expurging the putrid humours of the Body'), he fled abroad shortly before the Restoration and proceeded MD at Utrecht in 1662; *ODNB*. Interestingly, Rogers' adversary James Harrington may himself have drawn upon strains of neo-platonic thinking, particularly the occult notion of *spiritus*, in re-imagining the harmonious body politic of Oceana; W. C. Diamond, 'Natural Philosophy in Harrington's Political Thought', *Journal of the History of Philosophy*, 16 (1978), 387–98.

50. H. Stubbe, *Malice Rebuked, or A Character of Mr. Richard Baxters Abilities* (London, 1659), 12–13, 21–22, 35, 40, 45, 54–5. Baxter himself, who briefly practised medicine at Kidderminster in the 1640s, was at pains to point out that he did so out of 'necessity' and that he ceased to practise once he had 'procured a godly, diligent physician' to take his place; R. Baxter, *Reliquiae Baxterianae... Faithfully Publish'd... by Matthew Silvester* (London, 1696), i, 83–4, 89. For Baxter's profound debt to medicine which permeated all aspects of his personal life, career, and writing, see T. Cooper, 'Richard Baxter and His Physicians', *Social History of Medicine*, 20 (2007), 1–19.

51. Stubbe, *Malice Rebuked*, 44–5, 47, 52, 53. For background discussion of this case, see J. Winsser, 'Mary Dyer and the "Monster" Story', *Quaker History*, 79 (1990), 20–34. Stubbe, who like John Rogers took up the practice of medicine after 1660 and was

widely considered to have embraced an atheistic materialism, went to great lengths, including consultations with eyewitnesses, to prove that Dyer's monstrous birth was nothing more than an aberration of nature. Citing the medical authority of two physicians, Fortunio Liceti and Jean Riolan, he also rejected the idea that such births were portentous, and roundly concluded that '[i]t is an adulterous generation that asketh a signe; and it is none of the wisest that judgeth thereby'; ibid., 44–5, 54.

52. K. Sharpe, 'An Image Doting Rabble: The Failure of Republican Culture in Seventeenth-Century England', in K. Sharpe and S. N. Zwicker (eds), *Refiguring Revolutions: Aesthetics and Politics from the English Revolution to the Romantic Revolution* (Berkeley and Los Angeles, 1998), 46–7.

53. S. Slater, *The Protector's Protection: Or, The Pious Prince Guarded by a Praying People. A Sermon Preached at St.Edmundsbury in Suffolk... Being a Day Set Apart for Solemn Fasting and Humiliation and Seeking a Blessing upon His Highness the Lord Protector* [13 October 1658] (London, 1659), 38–9; cf. ibid., 43, 49, 53, 56.

54. One manifestation of this growing disaffection with the 'good old cause' was the widespread emergence of a scatological literature that mercilessly punned on the failings of the 'Rump'; see M. S. R. Jenner, 'The Roasting of the Rump: Scatology and the Body Politic in Restoration England', *Past and Present*, 177 (2002), 84–120.

55. J. Moore, *A Leaf Pull'd from the Tree of Life: Medicinall for the Healing of Englands Divisions. Or a Glimpse of the Excellency of a Kingly Government* (London, 1660), 15.

56. It may also have provided a motive and a template for the movement to create county-based 'associations' of ministers in the 1650s which did much to bring together various clergy of a moderate persuasion, including Anglicans, Presbyterians and some Congregationalists. Daniel Cawdrey, for example, repeatedly invoked the example of the body politic when he addressed the Northamptonshire association on the perils of schism and the advantages of church unity in 1657; see D. Cawdrey, *Church-Reformation Promoted in a Sermon on Matth[ew].18. vers[e].15,16,17: Preached at Northampton... Before the Association of Ministers* (London, 1657), 46, 51, 55, 57, 72–3.

57. M. Thomas, *Two Assize Sermons Preached at Bridgnorth... Salop... 1657* (London, 1659), i, 47–8. For the expression of similar sentiments in two sermons preached on the politically charged occasion of the election of the lord mayor of London, in 1644 and 1659, respectively, see Anthony Burges, *The Magistrates Commission from Heaven. Declared in a Sermon Preached in Laurencejury, London* [28 September 1644] (London, 1644), 5–6; P. Nye, *A Sermon Preached to the Honourable Citizens of London* [29 September 1659] (London, 1661), 19.

58. Z. Mountagu, *The Jus Divinum of Government; or Magistracy Proved to be God's Ordinance, and Justice the Magistrates Duty. In a Plain Sermon Preached Before the Judges of Assize at East-Grinsted in the County of Sussex* (London, 1652), 1–2, 7–8, 14, 19.

59. E. Reyner, *Rules for the Government of the Tongue* (London, 1656), sig. A3v. Verbal incontinence was often considered a 'proof' of witchcraft as witches frequently harmed their victims through cursing. For this and related themes, see J. G. Harris, *Foreign Bodies and the Body Politic: Discourses of Social Pathology in Early Modern England* (Cambridge, 1998), 107–40. Those who committed perjury in court were a further threat to the integrity of the commonwealth. In the politicized atmosphere after 1640, they were often thought of as susceptible to, and deserving of, divine judgement.

60. J. Bruce (ed.), *Diary of John Manningham, of the Middle Temple, and of Bradbourne, Kent, Barrister-at-Law, 1602–1603* (London, Camden Soc., vol.99, 1868), 77. The puritan vicar of Dover John Reading, in a sermon extolling the divinely ordained merits of the physician, went on to denounce the abuse of drink and drunkenness which, he claimed, 'transformeth men into variable sortes of beasts'; J. Reading, *A Faire Warning. Declaring the Comfortable Use Both of Sicknesse and Health. Delivered in Several Sermons at Saint Maries in Dover* (London, 1621), 23. He also affirmed that sin, 'that misshapen hagge and feareful Incubus', was the prime cause of all disease, and warned his auditors to avoid the temptation to seek physical comfort from white witches and wizards, the servants of that 'cunning Mountebanke', Satan. The demonological rhetoric here typifies the conventional approach of pre-civil war puritans to medicine, quackery and the allotted role of learned physicians as 'Gods Vice-gerents towards the body'; ibid., 19, 20, 26–7.
61. See, for example, the sermon delivered by the puritan minister of Norwich, John Carter, in June 1650 on the occasion of the mayoral inauguration in that city; J. Carter, 'A Rare Sight, or the Lyon' [18 June 1650] in *The Tomb-stone, or a Rare Sight* (London, 1653), 118, 120.
62. T. Thompson, *A Diet for a Drunkard: Delivered in Two Sermons at Saint Nicholas Church in Bristol... 1608* (London, 1612), 24. Biblical and historical examples of the effects of magisterial inebriation are discussed on pages 24–7. In line with many other puritan preachers, Thompson also visualized drunkenness as a metaphor for excessive intellectual curiosity which was manifest in the contemporary fascination for alchemy, astrology, medical empiricism, cabalism, atheism and other forms of spiritual heresy; ibid., 10.
63. J. Hart, *KAINIKH, or the Diet of the Diseased* (London, 1633), 128–37. In the new charter granted to the godly borough of Colchester in 1635, convicted drunkards, along with adulterers, fornicators and swearers, were excluded from exercising their political rights; J. Walter, *Understanding Popular Violence in the English Revolution: The Colchester Plunderers* (Cambridge, 1999), 162.
64. Divisions over these issues, according to David Underdown, were representative of the wider cultural differences that led to the creation of the two sides that fought the civil war in the 1640s; see his *Revel, Riot and Rebellion*. As will be clear from the preceding analysis, I do not share Prof. Underdown's conviction that these divisions represented an unresolvable dichotomy.
65. The miscreant on this occasion, a glazier named Elias Fry, was later involved in an attempt by the opposition 'party', led by a local butcher Roger Pouncey, to promote a case of witchcraft, which may well have been intended to embarrass the godly ruling group. The case against the suspected witch was rapidly dismissed; D. Underdown, *Fire from Heaven: Life in an English Town in the Seventeenth Century* (London, 1992), 75, 149; Dorset Record Office, B2/8/1, fo. 265v; C. H. Mayo (ed.), *The Municipal Records of the Borough of Dorchester, Dorset* (Exeter, 1908), 423, 665.
66. Underdown, *Fire from Heaven*, 47–8. Underdown refers in particular to an assize sermon that White preached in 1633, but that was not published until the year of his death in 1648, when it was printed, in all probability, in order to embarrass the ageing patriarch and his supporters. By 1648, of course, the country was hopelessly divided,

both politically and religiously, and the ideal of a united body politic was little more than a chimera; J. White, *A Sermon Preached at Dorchester... at the Generall Assizes* [7 March 1633] (London, 1648), esp.7 ('seeing order which is the foundation of peace must needs proceed *ab uno* as well as it tends *ad unum* there must of necessity be one like the head in the body, to command all the members, and direct them in their severall offices and Imployments'), 20, 25, 27; Underdown, *Fire from Heaven*, 210–11.

67. F. Walsall, *The Bowing the Hearts of Subjects to Their Sovereign* [24 May 1660] (London, 1660), 30.
68. N. Beaton, *No Treason to say, Kings Are God's Subjects... In Some Sermons Preached at Lurgarshal in Sussex* (London, 1661), 16.
69. J. Brinsley, *Prayer and Praise. A Two-fold Tribute, to be Payed by All Loyal Subjects to their Supream and Subordinate Soveraign* [23 April 1661] (London, 1661), 11. Brinsley was ejected as town lecturer at Yarmouth in 1662 and died three years later; see *Cal. Rev.*, 75. His son, Robert, practised medicine in the town.
70. Brinsley, *Prayer and Praise*, 12, 13, 17. The Declaration of Breda had begun by asserting that it was now imperative for the people of England to recognize the need to awaken to 'a desire and longing that those wounds which have so many years been kept bleeding may be bound up'; D. C. Douglas (ed.), *English Historical Documents*, 10 vols (London, 1995), vi [1660–1714], 57. Godly clergy like Brinsley undoubtedly drew comfort from proclamations such as those issued by Charles on his return to England in May 1660, when the restored monarch rebuked those 'who spend their Times in Taverns... giving no other Evidence of their Affection to us, but in drinking our Health, and Inveighing against all others, who are not of their own dissolute temper'; Charles II, *A Proclamation Against Vicious, Debauch'd, and Prophane Persons* (London, 30 May 1660).
71. A. Walker, *God Save the King: or Pious and Loyal Joy, the Subjects Duty, for their Soveraign's Safety. Opened in a Sermon at Aldermanbury* [30 May 1660] (London, 1660), 39–40.
72. R. Mossom, *Englands Gratulation for the King and His Subjects Happy Union. First Preach't on the Day of Publique Thanksgiving* [10 May 1660] (London, 1660), 34.
73. See, for example, the detailed depositions taken by Robert Hunt, JP, at Castle Cary in Somerset in January 1661, where one Philip Leigh was accused of refusing to drink a health to the King and the confusion of the Presbyterians and Anabaptists. Leigh, in reply, claimed that his accusers 'had broken the Kings Lawes in drinking a health allready' and added for good measure that he 'would not drink a health to the damnation of any body'; Somerset Heritage Centre, Q/SR/99/23–24.
74. [J. Hickes], *A True and Faithful Narrative, of the Unjust and Illegal Sufferings, and Oppressions of Many Christians... in the County of Devon* (1671), 3–4; *Cal. Rev.*, 260.

3

Providing 'Physick for the Body Politick'

The Politicization of Healers and Healing in England, 1640–1660

Introduction

The concept of the body politic was not an abstract complex of ideas confined to the realm of early modern political theory. On the contrary, it was widely accessible and intelligible, demonstrated a remarkable degree of flexibility, and, above all, appealed to men and women of all backgrounds, regardless of social, religious and political orientation. It therefore provided a rich and convenient language for interpreting the providential will of God with practical applications that extended not just to the world of everyday political conduct, but also to medicine itself as suggested by the example of the puritan preoccupation with 'new diseases' such as rickets. The continuing vitality of the concept of an organic state in the middle decades of the seventeenth century is perhaps most evident in the widespread recourse to medical discourse employed by those actively engaged in the political debates and successive crises that characterized the period. The growing fashion for 'anatomizing' the body politic, including a diagnosis of its ills and prescription for its cure, clearly appealed to a wide cross-section of the population in these troubled times. In this and succeeding chapters, I would like to explore in more detail the relationship between the healing arts and the wider religious and political culture of early modern England, focusing on the role played by medical practitioners in responding to, and participating in, the tumultuous events of the middle decades of the seventeenth century.

While acknowledging that to some extent this is well-trodden historical terrain, what I would like to address here is the largely neglected issue of the extent to which those involved in the day-to-day business of healing were affected by the religious and political upheavals of the mid-century and to assess their contribution to contemporary debates surrounding the ailing body politic. In brief, what I am proposing here is the outline of a historical process that saw the gradual politicization of a large but amorphous group of men and women united by their common endeavour in providing medical help to the lame and sick. Largely ignored in conventional accounts of the religious and political events of this period, medical practitioners were in fact increasingly prominent as advocates for their respective religious and political communities, either as servants of the

Medicine in an Age of Revolution. Peter Elmer, Oxford University Press. © Peter Elmer 2023.
DOI: 10.1093/oso/9780198853985.003.0003

new governments that emerged in the 1650s, or as defenders and activists for the Stuart cause. They were also, of course, simultaneously engaged in the daily business of healing the sick, the organization, theory and practice of which was equally affected by the general collapse of the old order in the years between 1640 and 1660. This is an aspect of the social history of medicine that has received wide coverage in the last thirty odd years or so, with much debate centred on the role played by a revitalized puritanism in shaping the medical, and by extension scientific, agenda of early modern England. Moreover, the legacy of all these developments was to intensify after 1660, when the Restoration, an event imbued with medical connotations, set in motion further protracted debate about the nature of the state and the role of governors and governed in a divided society still recoiling from the horrors of a bitter civil war. This period too witnessed the creation of new organizations for the promotion of scientific innovation, as well as abortive attempts to create new bodies dedicated to the reform of medicine. To appreciate fully, however, the role which the 'puritan revolution' played in these developments, we need first to address a more fundamental issue, namely the extent to which individual medical practitioners responded to, and engaged with, the crisis in church and state engendered by the onset of civil war.

Office-Holding, Puritanism and Medical Practice in Civil War England

In July 1632 an irate patient lying dangerously ill wrote to his physician venting his fury at the latter's inability to provide medical assistance at such a critical moment. The chief source of the patient's anger lay in the fact that his doctor had excused his absence 'in respect of some private meeting at your hall concerning the affaires of your Towne'. The physician in question was none other than William Shakespeare's son-in-law, John Hall (d.1635), who in 1632, after nearly ten years of equivocation, finally took the oath of a burgess in the corporation of his native town of Stratford-upon-Avon. And therein, as his father-in-law may have been tempted to comment, lay the rub, for in becoming a member of the corporation Hall had broken an unwritten rule of early modern English political life that underscored the impropriety of a medical practitioner engaging in the day-to-day business of government. This much is clear from additional comments made by Hall's exasperated patient when he stated, in complete sincerity, that it was 'very strange to me and unheard off that a Physitian should be incorporated of anie Towne or made a member of anie Corporation, not onlie to interrupt his studies [and] hinder his practice, but also to indaunger the life of his patient for want of his presence'.[1]

There is little doubt that Hall's patient was right to point out the rarity of his physician's action, and that his reasons for arguing against political engagement of this kind among medical practitioners were well nigh universal in England before the civil war. Indeed, historians themselves have tended to concur with this analysis, preferring to promote an image of the early modern physician as largely apolitical and unconcerned with the daily affairs of government and the administration of justice. The image of the physician as both temperamentally and professionally disqualified from engaging in such activity has received further confirmation in the work of the medical historian, Margaret Pelling. Noting the unwillingness of medical men, especially physicians, to take on office-bearing roles, she relates this process to her earlier analysis of the gendered nature of the early modern medical 'profession', which she characterizes as problematic, equivocal and peripheral to the broader concerns of male-dominated society, including political life. She concludes that:

> this ambivalence is epitomized in the remarkable degree to which [physicians] were isolated from the normal structures of male authority. They might have been expected to behave like other groups seeking to establish themselves, by seeking and accepting office whenever it was offered. Instead, they seem to have avoided office-bearing at almost every level.[2]

In this and succeeding chapters, I seek to explore this claim in more detail, providing a wealth of evidence to suggest that members of the medical profession, far from excluding themselves from the domain of politics, became increasingly active in the affairs of the body politic as the century wore on. One obvious starting point for such an analysis is that suggested by the example of John Hall and his decision to seek membership of the corporation of Stratford-upon-Avon, one of the hundreds of miniature body politics that dominated political life in early modern England. By the end of the century, as we shall see, it was quite common for medical practitioners, including fully qualified and highly educated physicians, to occupy the various offices of governance within their respective corporations. Despite the demands of their profession, a growing number of medical men, committed to the notion of serving their communities, found time to serve as burgesses, mayors and justices of the peace. Moreover, this process was not confined to the corporate boroughs, but was also evident in the counties, where medical practitioners began to occupy seats on the magisterial bench and even, on occasion, to serve as sheriffs. Some of these men aspired to national office and can also be found representing their communities as MPs at Westminster—a process, like the others described here, which gathered momentum after the Restoration and is discussed more fully in chapter 6.

The impetus to seek office, however, represents only one element in what I describe as the growing politicization of the medical profession in early modern England. Medical practitioners, in growing numbers, served their communities in various capacities, particularly after 1642, when unanimity as to what constituted the true nature of the state gave way to division and controversy. As is well charted, the removal of many of those who traditionally held office at both local and national level in these years created opportunities for new candidates to take their place, some of whom, as we shall see, were increasingly drawn from the ranks of the healing profession. The process was first noted by Gerald Aylmer in his exhaustive study of those who served the republican regime in the 1650s, in which he perceived 'a more than random association between medicine and the puritan-parliamentarian-republican cause'. Aylmer, however, was largely at a loss to explain why this should be so 'unless we are able to suppose that doctors were readier to accept a *de facto* situation, and to serve anybody who offered them employment'.[3] Once again, we are left with an image of the typical early modern physician as largely pragmatic and apolitical in outlook, whose loyalty to the state was unprincipled and lacking in any form of ideological commitment. However, as we shall see, this was far from the case. Those medical practitioners who did serve the state in the years between 1642 and 1660 did so, more often than not, because of a profound attachment to the cause of godly reform and opposition to Stuart absolutism which often extended beyond the mere performance of bureaucratic timeserving. Whether through political and religious pamphleteering or membership of parliamentary or county committees tasked with a variety of financial, military and religious functions, the contribution of medical men to the governance of the body politic in these years was impressive. It is equally important to note, however, that the commitment of a growing number of medics to the puritan-parliamentarian-republican cause was mirrored by the politicization of their medical colleagues from across the religio-political divide who suffered for their loyalty to the Stuarts and the Anglican Church. Excluded from the corridors of power, some chose collusion or neutrality while others engaged in active opposition to the Cromwellian state often exploiting the unique nature of the doctor-patient relationship to assist and foment resistance to what they perceived as an illegal and corrupt regime. In so doing, their actions increased the growing divisions, often bitter, between medical practitioners, which often spilled over into aspects of their everyday medical practice.

So why did medical practitioners of all kinds, physicians, as well as surgeons and apothecaries, become increasingly involved in the daily routine of government and the administration of justice from the 1640s onwards? The answer, to a large extent lies implicit in the case already cited, that of John Hall of Stratford. Hall was a committed puritan, dedicated to the cause of godly reform in church and state who was especially supportive of the efforts of the puritan minister of the town, Thomas Wilson, to achieve these ends. He served as a churchwarden in 1629 and 1633, and consistently opposed attempts to impose ungodly incumbents on his parish of Holy Trinity. Hall's reluctant decision to accept public office in 1632 was almost certainly motivated by a desire to promote the campaign of godly reform in the borough initiated by his friend, Wilson. He soon, however, made himself unpopular, being charged with uttering abusive speeches towards one of the bailiffs, and was ultimately voted off the town council for 'breach of orders' and causing 'continual disturbances at our halls'.[4] Hall was not the first physician to occupy a place in a corporation, or serve office in some other capacity,[5] but his zeal for the cause of godly reform which underpinned his political ambitions was symptomatic of a growing mood of change whereby ever more like-minded, medical colleagues were inspired to seek office after 1642. During the 1630s, these men became increasingly agitated at the direction of church and state under the personal rule of Charles I and witnessed the first stirrings of the politicization of their profession, which took many forms. One of the most noteworthy, and one which cannot have escaped the notice of puritan medics, was the tendency of many of their clerical colleagues, on being deprived of their livings by the Anglican authorities, to take up the practice of medicine. This process—imitated on a much larger scale after the mass ejections of 1662—saw the entry into the profession of a dedicated cadre of refuseniks who rejected the Laudian innovations and provided an inspiration for others equally opposed to the regime of Charles I and his Arminian bishops. They included men of some stature, such as the religious controversialists and staunch Calvinists, John Yates (d.1657),[6] John Burgess (1563–1635) and Alexander Leighton (*c.*1570–1649),[7] as well as men of meaner capacities, sequestrated from rural livings, such as Richard Capel (1586–1656),[8] Walter Jones,[9] John Newton,[10] Randolph Partridge (1579–1658)[11] and Edward Rood (d.1643).[12] To these, we might add the names of those who studied in the 1630s with a clerical career in mind, but who subsequently changed course and opted for medicine as an alternative career. Candidates include Edward Whiston (d.1697), Ahaseurus Regemorter (1615–1650), Roger Drake (1608–1669) and Thomas Coxe (1615–1685).[13] Whiston was licensed to practise medicine by the University of Cambridge in 1639, but subsequently entered the priesthood in 1644 and was ejected in 1662.[14] Regemorter, who was a leading figure in the London College of Physicians in the 1640s, may well have decided to opt for the same career path while studying at Leiden in the 1630s.[15] Similar thinking may have guided his eminent colleague Roger Drake, who gave up his well-established medical practice in 1646 in order to pursue, or perhaps in his mind to resume, an earlier aspiration to follow a career as a Presbyterian minister in post-civil war London.[16]

Another factor that almost certainly assisted the process of politicization outlined here was the impressively close network of familial relationships that underpinned the puritan medical profession in these years. Drake, for example, was the brother-in-law of the physician, Edmund Trench (1608–1669 or 1670), another member of that close coterie of puritan physicians who worked with Glisson on rickets. Other members of the puritan medical establishment in London in the 1640s were closely related through marriage and friendship, either to each other or to their allies in the ministry, and some may have traded on such alliances in seeking positions within the new Presbyterian system of church government then taking shape in the capital. John Clarke (d.1653), for example, who acted as President of the College of Physicians from 1645 to 1650, was appointed as a trier of elders in the first classis of London in August 1645.[17] Such appointments were replicated throughout the country. Jasper Despotine,[18] Roger Goodyer or Goodyear,[19] Ralph Rand (d.1653)[20] and his cousin, Samuel Rand (1588–1654),[21] Tobias Venner (d.1660)[22] and, most striking of all, the eminent physiologist, Francis Glisson (*c.*1599–1677),[23] all served as elders of their respective congregations in the second half of the 1640s.

Dedication to the cause of godly reform was almost certainly the principal spur for other like-minded medical practitioners to enter the service of Parliament, both in civilian and military capacities, after 1642. This is most noticeable in the south-east of England, particularly in those areas where support for the new puritan and parliamentarian regime was strongest. Puritanically inclined medical men served in impressive numbers on a variety of committees that had been established by Parliament to underpin the war effort, raise revenue and govern the areas under its control in the 1640s. Among those active in supervising parliamentary levies of troops and raising money for the war effort were Francis Bannister (Bedford), Gabriel Barber (Hertford and Hertfordshire), Gervase Fullwood the elder (Cambridgeshire, Huntingdonshire and Isle of Ely), Thomas Hubbard (London), John King (St Albans and Hertfordshire), Samuel Reade (Bishop's Stortford), John Saunders (Oxford city and university), Richard Staines (Cambridgeshire, Huntingdonshire and Isle of Ely), John Symcotts (Cambridgeshire, Huntingdonshire and Isle of Ely) and Nathaniel Wright (Herefordshire).[24] The majority of these men were well qualified and highly educated physicians, who would appear to have combined medical practice with service to the state and their local communities. They were also, invariably, committed to the cause of godly reform and often suffered for their dedication to the cause. Gervase Fullwood the elder, for example, working in tandem with his medical business partner, John Symcotts, served the Eastern Association throughout the 1640s. In 1645, his apothecary's shop in Huntingdon was targeted by marauding royalist forces who plundered his house and shop, taking away all his medicinal goods and wares.[25]

In addition to committee work, many of these physicians were noticeably active in the day-to-day government, administration and policing of their respective communities. Extraordinarily for men whose occupations were seen at the time, and since, as largely incompatible with the holding of judicial office, a significant minority served as magistrates on county benches.[26] It is worth examining this sample in a little more detail in order to illustrate the extent to which godly members of the medical profession were becoming attracted to the ideal of serving the body politic in one of its most vital forms. One of the first to take his place on the magisterial bench was the London-based medical practitioner Thomas

Hubbard or Hubbert, who first appears in this capacity in Middlesex in 1645 and remained active until the end of the Commonwealth in 1659.[27] His long and seemingly unbroken service was a reflection of his profound commitment to the Independent or congregational form of church governance, and not surprisingly he used his office to promote and support those who shared his outlook. In 1646, for example, he was approached by a group of Whitechapel Independents in the expectation that he would use his magisterial powers to adjudicate in their favour in an attempt to wrestle control of the parish from Presbyterian authority.[28] A year later, his home in Moorfields was the target of an anti-godly, pro-royalist mob. At the time, rumours abounded as to the motivation of the rioters, some suggesting that it was the work of the London apprentices under instruction from Hubbard's political enemies within the wider puritan camp. Hubbard, however, went to great pains to put the record straight, publishing a detailed account of the events, which saw his house ransacked, in which he firmly placed the blame for this outrage on political subversives opposed to godly reform of any kind.[29] In the months that followed, Hubbard, as JP, was highly active in prosecuting opponents of the parliamentary regime. In May 1648, for example, amid fears of a second civil war, he instigated the prosecution of a mob who had 'tumultuously assembled on the Lords Day in Morefields' and proceeded from there to Charing Cross. In the same month, he was pursuing miscreants for calling Parliament and their committees 'rogues' and uttering invective speeches against them, as well as for threatening to pull down the house of John Williams, a fellow Independent member of the militant Tower Hamlets committee. Hubbard continued as a faithful servant and supporter of the 'good old cause' throughout the 1650s. In May 1651, he examined a group of Ranters based at Whitechapel in the east end of London, and in the years which followed he regularly informed the council of state of his actions in investigating tumults, riots and other forms of political disorder in the volatile neighbourhood of Wapping and his home parish of Moorfields.[30] That Hubbard perceived an intimate link between his work as a physician and his role as a godly magistrate, promoting the healing benefits of a reformed commonwealth, is further apparent by his publication in 1650 of a work in defence of the new regime. Dedicated to the president of the council of state and regicide, John Bradshaw and his fellow JPs in Middlesex, the title of this work, which Hubbard envisaged as a form of 'Gospel Physick', pays eloquent tribute to the growing engagement of medical men with the world of everyday political affairs.[31]

Hubbard was certainly not alone in combining medical and judicial roles during the years of civil war and Interregnum. The career of Gabriel Barber (d.1691) of Hertford, for example, followed a strikingly similar path to that of his London colleague. The son of a prominent local puritan and active opponent of the Caroline regime in the 1630s,[32] Barber graduated MD at Cambridge in 1645 when, as a member of the Eastern Association, he was active as both a JP and commissioner in the county of Hertfordshire.[33] He clearly shared Hubbard's religious and political leanings, acting throughout the 1640s and 1650s as a loyal agent of the government in the town and county of Hertford. In May 1659 an official newsletter reported that Dr Barber was responsible for presenting a petition to Parliament on behalf of the town of Hertford calling for the restoration of all army officers previously displaced so that 'the Militia may be settled in the hands of those that have faithfully adhered to the Good Old Cause, in opposition to Monarchy, Name and Thing'.[34] He continued to worry the authorities after the Restoration, providing security to live peaceably in 1666, and being arrested, but subsequently released, in a general round-up of local dissidents in the wake of the abortive Monmouth Rebellion in 1685.[35] Other physicians to combine the practice of medicine with the duties of magistracy in this period include Bridstock Harford Snr, John Palmer, Richard Staines, John King and Joseph Micklethwaite. Of these five, three were made in the same mould as Hubbard and Barber, providing loyal support to the various regimes of the 1640s and 1650s. Harford, who graduated MD at Oxford in 1639, came from a family of medical practitioners based in the city of Hereford. He served on most of the local assessment commissions in the 1650s and occasionally sat as a JP for the county. His political career ended abruptly at the Restoration.[36] Palmer (1609–1660), the son of a Taunton apothecary, was a zealous puritan and parliamentarian, who not only served as a JP and county committeeman throughout this period but also represented the radical borough of Taunton in the Long Parliament from 1645 to 1653. He stood again for Taunton in 1659 but, despite claiming victory, the result was overturned in the national tide toward moderation.[37] Like many of the medical men noted here, Palmer profited from his political connections. Within the space of two days in April 1648 he was created MD and appointed master of All Souls College, Oxford, in place of the ejected royalist Gilbert Sheldon. The appointment caused outrage in loyalist circles, where it was widely felt that such an office was 'proper only for a Divine'. Just prior to his death, on 4 March 1660, his enemies gained a modicum of revenge when in the general euphoria attendant on the collapse of the republic and the imminent restoration of the Stuarts, the Oxford antiquarian Anthony Wood claimed that large rumps of beef were flung 'at Dr Palmer's window at Allsoles'.[38] Finally, Staines' career followed much the same lines as those of his medical peers described thus far. Like Barber, he graduated MD from Cambridge in 1645, but had been practising medicine for at least eight years prior to this. As a local man, resident in the Isle of Ely, he held close connections with the town of Cambridge and its university, having been appointed by the earl of Manchester to the committee for regulating the universities in 1644. Thereafter, he was a tireless member of the various parliamentary county committees for Cambridgeshire and Huntingdonshire, working alongside fellow physicians such as John Symcotts and Gervase Fullwood (above).[39] He was also active as a JP in the Isle of Ely in the 1640s and 1650s, in which capacity he played a leading role in examining and preparing for trial the cases of several witches identified by the witchfinder Matthew Hopkins.[40] His political advice and judgement was fully respected by those in authority in these years, and in 1656 he was consulted by Major-General Haynes in relation to the impending parliamentary elections in Cambridgeshire and how best to secure the election of the government's candidates.[41] Of the other two doctors noted here, John King (1604–1688) was an assessment commissioner and member of the Eastern Association who graduated MD from Leiden in 1629 and practised at St Albans in Hertfordshire, where he also served on the local bench. Unlike the rest of our sample, however, he would appear to have favoured Presbyterianism.[42] The same is probably true of Joseph Micklethwaite (1594–1658), who served as a commissioner for the East Riding of Yorkshire in 1648 and was later active as a JP for the same jurisdiction. Described as 'well affected' in 1651, the fact that he used his office to protect men with known royalist connections renders it likely that he shared John King's attachment to Presbyterianism.[43]

The Benefits of Office-Holding

The examples cited hitherto of medical men not simply espousing the cause of Parliament in the civil war, but actively engaging in a myriad of ways with the daily governance of the nation in the 1640s and 1650s testifies eloquently to the growing politicization of the medical profession in this period. Though some of their colleagues may have lacked the ideological commitment of the men cited above, participating reluctantly in the military conflicts and civil strife that erupted in 1642, most probably saw these events as an opportunity, not only to promote their medical careers but also to further the cause of godly reform and political change. This was especially true of those who opted to support Parliament, as military success created a whole range of new openings and possibilities. A successful army career as a physician or surgeon, for example, might lead to unexpected offers of promotion or employment by the state, as well as the patronage of powerful generals and political figures. The hypochondriacal parliamentarian general, Sir Thomas Fairfax, was particularly lavish in supporting those medical men who served under him. He thus promoted the award of honorary medical degrees at Oxford to James Ward and Humphrey Whitmore, the latter for medical services rendered to the parliamentary cause in the civil war,[44] as well as extending his influence to include surgeons such as Thomas Allen, Edward Atkinson and Bartholomew Lavender.[45] The purge of loyalist medics from the London hospitals, such as the surgeon Edward Molins, added to the stock of largesse at the disposal of the parliamentarian authorities in the city.[46] Among those to benefit from this process were the puritan physicians Edward Emily, Aaron Gurdon and John Micklethwaite, as well as the surgeon

William King who was the father-in-law of the Digger leader, Gerard Winstanley.[47] Similar opportunities arose in the provinces. Anthony Stephens, for example, surgeon to the parliamentary naval garrison at Portsmouth, used his connections to solicit support for his son, John, a fellow of New College, Oxford, in his attempt to gain the lucrative post of surgeon to the new hospital planned at Portchester Castle on the south coast.[48] On a grander scale, the puritan natural philosopher and physician Daniel Whistler (*c*.1619–1684), who wrote the first published thesis on rickets, was rewarded for his energetic engagement in organizing naval medical services in the 1650s with a fellowship at Merton College, Oxford, as well as the chair of geometry at Gresham College in London. Likewise, Jonathan Goddard (d.1675) and John Bathurst (d.1659), both of whom served as personal physician to Oliver Cromwell in the 1650s and were later rewarded with various administrative and political promotions, owed much of their success to the contribution which they had made to the medical services of the Cromwellian army and navy.[49]

Other medics found lucrative employment in the various organs of the Cromwellian state, often utilizing family connections and kinship networks. Edmund Scroope (1626–1658), for example, the son of the regicide, Adrian Scroope, was awarded the office of keeper of the Privy Seal in Scotland.[50] Loyal physicians were also intruded into public institutions such as the Mint. Here, for example, in the 1650s the two main offices of warden and master were held by practising physicians, whose loyalty to successive parliamentarian and Cromwellian regimes was never in doubt. The post of warden was thus held by Dr John St John, brother of the puritan lawyer and leading parliamentarian, Oliver St John (d.1673), to whom he was undoubtedly indebted for his promotion to this and other military offices (he had earlier served as personal physician to the earl of Essex).[51] St John's deputy at the Mint was another physician, Aaron Gurdon (d.1675), whose medical reputation was made at the Savoy Hospital in London, where he oversaw the treatment of wounded parliamentarian soldiers. So important was his post at the Mint, and such was his reputation in republican circles, that in May 1650 he was put into the commission of the peace in order that 'he may prevent disorders in the Mint, as others have formerly done'.[52]

In the case of a public institution such as the Mint, it is not altogether surprising that senior positions were reserved for members of the medical profession. What is less easy to explain is their prominence in other organs of the state. William Parker (d.1678), for example, who graduated MD at Bourges in 1634 and served as a militia committee man for Westminster in 1647, was later entrusted with the vital role of commissioner for excise in the 1650s.[53] Most illuminating in this respect is the story of Thomas Cummins, who, having been awarded an MD at Oxford in 1653, was effectively head-hunted by the government of the day to act in some capacity as an agent of the newly emerging Cromwellian state. Cummins was a former undergraduate student of Ralph Cudworth at Christ's College, Cambridge, who wrote to Thurloe on his protégé's behalf, recommending him for preferment and a government post. With further testimonials supplied by Sir John Reynolds and Colonel Goffe, Cudworth was simply confirming Cummins' fitness for 'civill employment, he having been bred a scholar'. His remarks, however, are worth citing in full as they give some idea as to what it was that made such men attractive to the movers and shakers within the government. According to Cudworth, though Cummins:

> have the degree and title of doctor of physick, yet he is one, that is farre from being a meer scholar, or one that hath conversed only with books, but hath naturally a singular genius and dexterity *in rebus agendas*, and the management of externall and civill affaires, so his education has been such in travaile abroad, as might not make him onely an accomplisht gentleman, but also afford him much experience of the world, and dispose him for any civill employment.[54]

Political partisanship of the kind suggested here could also, of course, be fostered by the prospect of future prosperity and the potential gains to be made from serving the state, in various functions, in the 1640s and 1650s. The execution of the King and abolition of episcopacy produced a vibrant market in former royal and church lands, which medical supporters of the Commonwealth were not slow to appreciate. On the surface, the scramble to purchase these estates looks decidedly mercenary and opportunistic, and though it would be a mistake to dismiss such motives entirely from the thinking of those who bought crown and church lands, it is also possible to see this process as one driven by an element of ideological commitment to the new regime. Many of the medical practitioners, for example, who did enter this vibrant land market in the 1650s were dedicated supporters of Parliament and the Cromwellian republic. A notable investor in this respect was the eminent physician Thomas Coxe (1615–1685), who invested heavily in former diocesan property in the city of Winchester in the 1650s.[55] In many respects, his career epitomizes so many of the themes previously raised in this chapter. Originally destined for a career in the church, the puritanically inclined Coxe would appear to have shunned this route on graduating MA from puritan Emmanuel College, Cambridge, in 1639, and opted instead for medicine. Following his return from Padua in 1641, where he acquired his MD, he was nominated by the College of Physicians in London to serve in the armies of Parliament on the recommendation of the earl of Essex.[56] Preferments and honours followed the defeat of the royalist forces in 1646. In June of that year, he was made a licentiate of the College of Physicians, becoming a full fellow in 1649 and serving as censor in 1652–3. His growing prominence in intellectual and governing circles is further attested by his close collaboration with Samuel Hartlib, and his association with members of the Boyle circle, including Lady Ranelagh, whose physician he became some time in the late 1640s. Finally, in 1653 he was created master of St Katherine's Hospital in London, a post he was forced to relinquish at the Restoration.[57] Other ideologically committed medics who sought to profit from the purchase of former crown and church lands included John St John,[58] Henry Cleere, father and son,[59] John Dawberne,[60] Thomas Hubbard,[61] Peter Salanova,[62] William Staines,[63] Thomas Symonds,[64] John Troutbeck[65] and the celebrated empiric, William Trigge.[66]

Loyalty to Parliament, and later Cromwell, thus created a range of opportunities for medical men to promote their medical careers as well as to raise their social and political profiles. Some, as we have seen, acquired educational qualifications and academic posts or otherwise secured preferment in their chosen careers. Others invested in the spoils of victory, most notably by securing or otherwise acquiring expropriated royal and episcopal estates on advantageous terms. During the 1650s, all these avenues of self-advancement coalesced in the wake of the Cromwellian conquest of Ireland, when the demand for English physicians, surgeons and other medical personnel created even greater opportunities for those willing to cross the Irish Sea. The importance of Ireland to the careers of a number of medical men, including William Petty, Benjamin Worsley and the Boate brothers, has received widespread attention.[67] They were not alone in their profession, however, in seeing the potential benefits that might accrue as a result of the Cromwellian conquest of Ireland and the expropriation of Catholic lands in the 1650s. Joseph Waterhouse, for example, the brother of Oliver Cromwell's household steward, Nathaniel, was granted an Oxford MD in March 1651 for his services to the armed forces in Ireland. He subsequently claimed, somewhat disingenuously, to have been the only English physician to have accompanied Cromwell to Ireland. Unlike many however, he did opt to remain there, settling in Dublin, and representing Newry in the Irish Convention of March 1660.[68] Other physicians to benefit from service to the army and the administration in Ireland in these years include Charles Goldsmith,[69] Jonathan Edwards[70] and Philip Carteret (d.1672).[71] It was also rumoured in the royalist press that the famous man-midwife and Fifth Monarchist preacher Peter Chamberlen was to escort Cromwell to Ireland in the summer of 1649, there to act in both a medical and political capacity, 'wherein no doubt... the wise doctor may prove of admirable use to the Common-wealth... and prescribe Remedies proper and seasonable'.[72]

The extent to which medical careers in the 1640s and 1650s were indebted to, and shaped by, religious and political allegiance is most readily apparent in the case of the surgeon, Thomas Trapham (d.1683), whose career exemplifies so many of the themes discussed in this chapter. Licensed to practise surgery by the University of Oxford in 1634, he went on to provide loyal service as a parliamentary surgeon throughout the civil war culminating in the decisive victory at

Naseby. His commitment to the cause never wavered. After embalming the body of Charles I in 1649, when he was said to have exclaimed that he had 'sewed on the head of a goose', he was rewarded with the award of a bachelor's degree in medicine at Oxford in May 1649. Further rewards and offices followed in parallel with his continuing devotion to the new regime. In 1651 he attended on Cromwell as his personal surgeon on the Irish and Scottish campaigns, as well as at the battle of Worcester. In return, he was granted oversight of the army's medical services and its treatment of sick and wounded soldiers in London, investing the profits in former crown lands in Lincolnshire.[73] All the while, he remained committed to the cause of godly reformation in church and state, serving as a burgess in his hometown of Abingdon from 1648, as well as sitting on numerous parliamentary committees for Berkshire. As a wholehearted supporter of Cromwell's religious policies, he was responsible for the amalgamation or eradication of parishes known to foster radical dissent or prayer book Anglicanism. He was also an active and energetic commissioner for the ejection of scandalous ministers and played a leading role in the prosecution of heterodox ministers in Berkshire, including the Behmenist mystic John Pordage, whom he threatened to kill with his own sword.[74] Not surprisingly, the Restoration initiated a dramatic reversal of fortune for Trapham. In January 1661 a warrant was issued for the seizure of goods and belongings found in his house at the Savoy that were thought to belong to the late king, Cromwell and other 'convicted persons'. His house was subsequently searched, and property confiscated, on the grounds that he was an 'excepted person'. He now retired to his native Abingdon to practise surgery, but all the while remained under close observation, liable to prosecution as a known dissenter and opponent of the restored regime. In 1660, he was removed from the town council on the grounds that he had been 'unduly elected' in 1648, and in 1671 he and his wife were prosecuted for nonconformity in the local church courts.[75] Trapham's fall from grace and expulsion from the body politic was both swift and devastating, his fate in all likelihood shared by countless other medical practitioners who were equally committed to the programme of social, religious and political reform set in motion by the civil wars of the 1640s. The reaction of such men to the changes brought about by the Restoration differed according to personal and local circumstances. Some opted for diplomatic silence after 1660, seeking solace in a return to medical practice, while others, as we shall see in chapter 5, used medicine as a cover for plotting against the restored regime of Charles II. A lucky few, with the right connections and good fortune, even managed to hold on to offices and privileges won through loyal service in the 1650s. The biggest winners in 1660, of course, were those who had suffered with their deposed monarch, through either loss of estates or forced exile, and it is to the ranks of disaffected royalist and Anglican medical practitioners that we must now turn to appreciate the full impact of the politicization of the medical profession in the two decades prior to 1660.

The Fate of the Loyal: Medical Practitioners and the Defence of Crown And Church

For those on the losing side, defeat in the civil war typically spelled loss of office, penury, and, in extreme cases, exile. Medical practitioners, of course, who opted to fight for King and Church, were not immune from the general backlash aimed at loyalists after 1646. Many would later petition for redress and compensation, citing at length the hardships they had endured, either at home or abroad. Typical was the case of Edward Deantry or Dawtrey, a Cambridge scholar at the outset of the civil war, who was prosecuted by the bailiffs of his native Ipswich for disseminating scandalous verses in the town, as well as spreading rumours that Prince Rupert was invincible, that all Catholics who fought for the King would be granted religious freedom, and that anyone who fought against the King also fought against God.[76] Escaping his gaolers, he soon joined the royalist forces at Oxford and served the cause as sworn physician to Charles I, for which he was rewarded with an Oxford MD. He later claimed that he was imprisoned and ruined for causing the Worcester declaration to be published. Not surprisingly, he petitioned for relief at the Restoration, requesting the office of registrar to the bishop and dean and chapter of Exeter, which he claimed had been promised him by his late uncle and bishop, Ralph Brownrigg (1592–1659). Unsuccessful in this instance, he was however added to the growing list of royal physicians appointed by Charles II in May 1660.[77]

The experiences of men like Deantry were echoed in the stories of dozens of his loyal colleagues in the medical profession. Far from turning a blind eye to the political events of the 1640s and 1650s, large numbers of surgeons, apothecaries and physicians contributed to the Stuart cause, often engaging in espionage and other acts of plotting under the cover of their occupation. Unlike other subjects, surgeons and physicians were often given special dispensation to travel and move around the country. They were also allowed access to prisoners and were thus frequently employed as go-betweens and the agents of fellow conspirators. Surgeons, in particular, excelled in this work, less suspect perhaps because of their lower social and professional status. Many, nonetheless, were arrested and examined by the authorities in the 1650s. John Barton (d.1680), for example, was secured in 1655 on suspicion of purchasing arms.[78] Richard Wiseman (d.1676), who had fought for Charles I in the 1640s and was captured in the aftermath of the battle of Worcester in 1651, was repeatedly arrested on suspicion of engaging in insurrectionary activity in the years that followed. In particular, he was suspected of using his trade, as a surgeon, to communicate sensitive information with royalist prisoners in the Tower of London.[79] John Knight (1622–1680), Humphrey Painter (d.1672) and Richard Pyle, were all similarly implicated.[80] Others, such as Thomas Tudor (*fl.*1654–1660), narrowly escaped capture and punishment.[81] Many of these men had close links to the exiled court, either through previous service to the crown or as a result of their war-time experiences. All were subsequently rewarded at the Restoration with royal appointments.[82] Loyal apothecaries and physicians, too, played their part in promoting the cause of the Stuarts. Many suffered the ignominy of arrest and examination followed by imprisonment. The royal apothecary John Chase, for example, used his role as medical adviser to the King's children as cover to engage in espionage. First arrested in 1643, his house in Westminster was regularly identified as a safe house for royalist intrigue and plotting. He was subsequently rewarded with the post of apothecary to the restored Charles II.[83] Typical of many loyal doctors was the fate of Sir John Hinton (d.1682), who served as physician and accoucheur to Henrietta Maria, and later as personal physician to the King's eldest son, Prince Charles. In 1642, he presented a peace petition to Parliament, for which he suffered arrest, and served the royal family faithfully throughout the civil war. In succeeding years, he was repeatedly arrested and questioned, including on one occasion by Cromwell himself, who, according to Hinton's own account, 'swore by the living God, he would wrack every veine in my heart if I did not discover the designes against him'. He was also able to use his medical expertise to protect fellow royalists from harassment by issuing certificates stressing the dangers to their health that might ensue should they be forced to attend on the council to undergo interrogation.[84] Hinton's sufferings were paralleled by those of several of his medical colleagues, including Peter Barwick (1619–1705),[85] George Bowles,[86] Walter Buchanan,[87] John Consett,[88] Henry Hughes,[89] William Jackson[90] and William Whitewell,[91] many of whom, like the loyal surgeons, were rewarded for their pains by a grateful monarch at the Restoration.[92]

Many, ultimately, opted to join their monarch in exile, where they attempted to eke out a living by attending on fellow courtiers and the royal entourage in the hope of future reward. Samuel Bispham (*c.*1598–1664), for example, who served as physician to Charles I before the civil wars, found service in the diplomatic corps of the royal court in exile.[93] Likewise, Captain Robert Meade (d.1653), who was rewarded with an MD by a grateful monarch in 1646 for negotiating the surrender of Oxford, served as envoy to Sweden on his son's behalf in the 1650s.[94] Some of those driven abroad combined medicine with plotting and were, as a result, closely monitored by the Cromwellian authorities. Dr Tobias Whitaker (d.1664), for example, spent much of the 1650s with the court in exile in Holland, where one government agent described him as 'a very pernitious fellow, whoe acts and speaks all the ill he can of our governors'. Like many of his colleagues, he was rewarded at the Restoration with a position at court as physician to the royal household, a post first promised to him by the King in exile in 1649.[95] Of those former royalist medics who remained in England, some, like Thomas Bayly, Edmund Gayton (1608–1666) and Joseph Martin (*c.*1598–1676), compounded for delinquency and retired into medical practice.[96] Others, such as Samuel Barrow (d.1683),[97] Thomas Clarges (d.1695),[98] Sir John Colladon[99] and John

Windebank (1618–1704)[100] gravitated towards pro-royalist elements within Cromwellian government circles, often working in a variety of posts for the new regime, while all the while preparing the ground for a return to the old order. Some indeed even found a congenial home in institutions such as the College of Physicians in London, where the Presbyterian and increasingly royalist inclined leadership of that body turned a blind eye to their colleagues' former indiscretions and, in some cases, current machinations against the new regime. The eminent anatomist and Harveian Charles Scarburgh (1615–1694) for example, who was made a fellow in 1650, did not retire peacefully to medical practice and research as some of his biographers have assumed. According to his colleague Walter Pope, Scarburgh's house in London became a centre of hospitality, intrigue and scholarship after 1649 for 'distressed Royalists... particularly to the scholars ejected out of either of the Universities for adhering to the King's Cause'.[101] Medicine thus became a refuge for royalist diehards many of whom now found the normal avenues of social advancement blocked by the creation of a republican court and administration. For those who wished to pursue a medical career, three possibilities existed. Firstly, they could choose to practise without any formal education, training, or qualification, an option that would leave them vulnerably placed on the margins of the medical marketplace. Secondly, like many medical students before them, they could travel abroad to study at one of the numerous medical schools on the continent. Or thirdly, they might opt to remain at home and retire to medical study in the recently purged puritan academies of Oxford and Cambridge. All three options had their drawbacks. But just as important, they all afforded ample opportunities to utilize medicine as a convenient vehicle to promote and assist the royal cause. As a result, the politicization of the medical profession, which we have traced so far in respect of those who supported the parliamentarian and puritan cause in the civil war, is equally evident among those of their opponents who entered medicine in the 1640s and 1650s, creating in the process an increasingly divided medical elite whose members were only too aware of the ramifications of religious and political partisanship.

Whatever route these men might take to eke out a career as a medical practitioner in the years of parliamentarian and republican rule, the vast majority rapidly moved to formalize and legitimate their practice after 1660 by seeking official recognition in one form of another. The preferred option of most was to solicit the restored King to use his mandatory powers to grant an MD from either Oxford or Cambridge to deserving supplicants who were only too willing to provide evidence of their loyalty and losses.[102] Typical were physicians like Augustine Caesar (1602–1677), William Crabbe (d.1685), Michael Frere (d.1661) and Edmund Yarborough (1627–1691), who all claimed to have dispensed with the taking of medical degrees in England before 1660 because of their refusal to subscribe to what they considered illegal oaths such as those required by the Engagement of 1650.[103] Others seeking the royal mandate for their deferred

MDs referred in general terms to the recent 'troublesome times',[104] stressed their indomitable loyalty and resulting poverty,[105] or traded on powerful connections within the restored church and state.[106] In addition to the grant of mandated MDs, there were other avenues open to former loyalists who wished to secure official approval for their medical practice. The return of the apparatus of the Anglican Church after 1660, including the system of ecclesiastical licensing, provided one such route. The survival of large numbers of testimonials, often written by fellow sufferers, also attests to an emerging camaraderie and group ethos among those medics who suffered for their loyalty to the Stuart cause. In October 1664, for example, the Norfolk royalist and physician James Windet (d.1664), just a month before his death, penned a glowing testimonial on behalf of fellow medic, Henry Rastall, a candidate for a licence from the archbishop of Canterbury. Both men had suffered for their loyalty, but whereas Windet had been able to afford the cost of repairing abroad to study medicine at Leiden, where he graduated MD in 1655, Rastall had been less fortunate, narrowly escaping execution for his part in royalist plotting in Norfolk in the 1650s and suffering imprisonment and banishment thereafter.[107] In other instances, it is impossible to verify with any degree of certainty the claims of those seeking mandated medical degrees and licences, and the extent to which they had suffered during what many termed the 'years of usurpation'.[108] Enough well documented examples survive, however, to suggest that many medical practitioners did suffer greatly for their unflinching loyalty to the Stuart cause in its darkest hour, and many went on to receive due reward. A remarkable case in point is provided by the early career and exploits of the Cambridge physician Robert Brady (1627–1700), who later succeeded to the post of regius professor of medicine at Cambridge. Brady, who was awarded his MD at Cambridge in 1660 by a grateful monarch, was unstinting in his support for the royalist cause in England and abroad following the execution of Charles I in 1649. In December 1650, prior to completing his medical studies at Cambridge, he was forced to flee the country, having been declared a traitor in the wake of an unsuccessful uprising in Norwich in the aftermath of which his brother Edmund was executed. Following a brief sojourn in the Netherlands, he fetched up at the royal garrison on the Scilly Isles, where, in May 1651, following the surrender of the islands, he obtained articles allowing him to return to the mainland. Taking up residence once again in Cambridge, he finally completed his first medical degree, but was unable to proceed further on account of his continuing support for the cause of Charles Stuart. During the late 1650s he began to practise medicine in his native Norfolk and, like so many other loyal medics, used his practice as a cover for plotting. Acting as an agent for other Norfolk royalists, Brady risked more than his livelihood in continuing to promote the royal cause and suffered at least one spell of imprisonment, for six months, at Great Yarmouth. Rewarded for his pains with the grant of a mandated MD in 1660 and the prestigious mastership of Caius College, Brady was destined to become one of the most outspoken defenders of the restored monarchy in subsequent years, and a prominent figure in the Tory campaign to uphold divine right monarchy and the authority of the Anglican Church in the face of new challenges to church and state in the wake of the Exclusion Crisis.[109]

For those royalists willing to swallow their pride and temporize in the face of the oaths required by the governments of Interregnum England, the medical schools of Oxford and Cambridge offered a safe, temporary haven from the religious and political controversies of the period. Surprisingly perhaps the medical faculties were not dominated in the 1650s by doctrinaire puritans, and many students who later devoted their lives to supporting the restored regime of Charles II found a congenial home there. Martin Llewellyn (1616–1682), for example, who had been ejected from his studentship at Christ Church, Oxford, by the parliamentary visitors in 1648 after serving as a royalist captain in the first civil war, took his MD at Oxford in 1653.[110] He was preceded two year's earlier by another royalist sympathizer, Alan Pennington (1622–1696), who later practised at Chester and was politically active in a circle of ultra-loyal former royalists and devoted Anglicans, committed to supporting the restored government of Charles II.[111] Similar conditions may have prevailed in Cromwellian Cambridge. Among those who graduated MD there in the 1650s was the staunch Anglican Henry Paman (1623–1695), who worked closely with the regius professor, Francis Glisson.[112] Robert Sprackling (d.1670), who was a medical student at Cambridge in the 1650s, later hinted at the degree to which the medical school had become a refuge for loyalists when he observed that the university 'can never forget, that when her Theology and Law lay bleeding and expiring by the Swords of Rebels and Usurpers, Physick alone præserved her perishing fame alive'.[113]

In the case of Interregnum Oxford, medical students who inclined to the Stuart cause and hankered for the re-establishment of the Anglican ministry and its rituals may have found solace in the various informal groups or clubs that met to discuss and research new developments in the field of natural philosophy, including medicine and physiology. One of the chief actors in promoting this activity was the devout Anglican and celebrated physician Thomas Willis (1621–1675), who had served in the royalist armies defending Oxford in the 1640s. Willis, who may have intended to pursue a career in the church, subsequently changed tack and was awarded his bachelor's degree in medicine by a grateful monarch in December 1646. Thereafter, he combined original medical research with a growing practice, all the while using his privileged position in the city to defend and promote High Church Anglicanism. He thus arranged for illegal services using the proscribed Book of Common Prayer to take place in his college rooms, and later continued the same in properties such as Beam Hall, which he acquired in 1657. Related through friendship and marriage to some of the leading clerical defenders of the ceremonies and doctrines of the old church, Willis was belatedly granted his MD by the King in 1660 at the behest of one of his closest friends, Gilbert Sheldon, bishop of London, who shortly after was translated to the see of Canterbury.[114]

As the careers of men like Thomas Willis, James Windet and others suggest, it was probably the case that many like-minded Anglicans and diehard royalists who entered medical study in the 1650s did so as an alternative to studying theology, usually in preparation for a clerical career, in the puritan-dominated faculties of Oxford and Cambridge. Some certainly wasted little time in switching professions after 1660 when the prospect of a new career in the restored Church became a serious option. Typical in this respect was Henry Brunsell (d.1679), the son of a Wiltshire minister, who took up the practice of medicine in the 1650s, but rapidly put it to one side at the Restoration when he was appointed rector of the valuable living of Clayworth in Nottinghamshire. Thereafter, his new career flourished and he acquired numerous preferments in the restored church, mainly through the intercession of his wife's uncle, Matthew Wren, bishop of Ely. In addition to the patronage of Wren, Brunsell's advancement after 1660 probably owed much to the fact that he had been active throughout the 1650s in promoting the royalist cause and plotting on behalf of the future Charles II. Moreover, like other physicians sympathetic to these aims, he probably used his medical practice and connections as a convenient cover for acts of insurgency, and in the process alerted the authorities (who were often aware of such machinations) to the subversive potential of medicine and its practitioners.[115] Others who emulated Brunsell include the son of the Arminian controversialist, Oliver Pocklington (d.1681), who probably practised medicine in Nottingham during the Commonwealth and was awarded a Cambridge MD in 1656 on the recommendation of none other than Oliver Cromwell. He lost little time, however, in switching professions at the Restoration, serving as rector of the parish of Brington in Huntingdonshire from 1663 until his death in May 1681.[116]

The exclusion of loyal Anglicans from the ministry in the 1640s and 1650s may well then have prompted a general influx of new students into the field of medicine and medical practice who might otherwise, under different political circumstances, have trained for the church. Many subsequently claimed to have followed this course. Isaac Barrow (1630–1677), for example, asserted that the reason he chose to study medicine at Cambridge during the Interregnum was because he found 'the times not favourable to men of his opinion in the affairs of Church and State'. In a similar vein, the physician Walter Charleton remarked in 1657 that 'our late Warrs and Schisms, having almost wholly discouraged men from the study of theologie; and brought the Civil Law into contempt: the major part of young Schollers in our Universities addict themselves to Physick'.[117] There can be little doubt that many loyal Anglicans did choose to study medicine rather than theology in the 1640s and 1650s, and then opted to resume their clerical careers following the return of Charles II.[118] Writing in 1663, Edmund Gayton referred to this phenomenon in an attempt to rebut the popular image of the physician as a closet atheist. He thus claimed that '[a] Physician therefore and a Divine you see are not inconsistent, the late Times made many Preachers Physicians, and these Soveraign dayes have made many a Physician Preachers'.

By way of proof, he alluded to the fact that '[m]any able Physicians, my very good friends, are already Divines, and fit for Prebendaries, Deaneries and Bishopricks'.[119]

Gayton, a former student of medicine at Oxford, may have had in mind the career of the physician-cum-cleric, Ralph Bathurst (d.1704). From a staunchly royalist family (six of his brothers were killed fighting for Charles I), Bathurst was originally intended for the priesthood, but took up the practice of medicine instead, it 'being only my refuge in bad times, and not my primitive designe'. In retrospect, he explained that 'I knew no better way than to turn my studies to physick, that so, in spight of the iniquities of the times, I might get a tolerable livelihood, whatever became of me in the university'. A friend and acquaintance of Thomas Willis, Bathurst combined medical practice and research (he graduated MD in June 1654) with support for the Anglican cause in Oxford, assisting as archdeacon to his friend Robert Skinner, the deprived bishop of Oxford, in secretly ordaining those who wished to remain in the Anglican fold. At the Restoration, he promptly gave up the practice of medicine and re-entered the church, acquiring in short order numerous lucrative and influential posts culminating in his appointment as dean of Wells in 1670 and vice chancellor of the University of Oxford in 1673.[120] As these and numerous other examples attest, rather than subscribe to the new order in church and state, many Anglicans, especially those ministers who lost their livelihoods through the forced ejections of the 1640s and 1650s, opted instead for a career in medicine.[121] Others drifted into medicine but, like Bathurst, rapidly switched careers and entered the church at the Restoration.[122] This exodus, moreover, was also noted by their religious and political opponents. As early as 1646, in a fast sermon preached before the House of Commons, the puritan minister Stephen Marshall lamented the number of young students entering law and medicine rather than the church.[123] A few years later, the Helmontian reformer Noah Biggs was scathing in his condemnation of those 'silenc'd ministers', who, 'outed of their benefices, lay hold upon Physick, and commit force and violence to her body... and think their Latin, and their Coat, the grand Charter, to entitle them to the practise in Physick'.[124] In so doing, they set a pattern that was to be imitated by their nonconformist brethren a decade or so later, when the return of the traditional religious and political order heralded another round of mass expulsions from the church and initiated, in the process, a new invasion of the medical profession by clerical interlopers (discussed more fully, below, in chapter 5).

The Puritanism–Science Debate Revisited: The Case of Medicine

One by-product then of the breakdown in religious and political order in England in the 1640s, and the emergence of a new regime in church and state, was the creation of a highly politicized medical profession. How, though, did this effect the organization and practice of medicine in the Interregnum and subsequent years? And more pertinently, how might this process of politicization help to contribute to our better understanding of the relationship between religion and medical change in this period? The debate itself has European-wide dimensions, but within an English context has tended to focus on the role played by puritanism and the 'puritan revolution' in transforming attitudes to science and medicine in the middle decades of the seventeenth century. The ground-breaking work of Charles Webster, in particular, has encouraged historians to view the various proposals for the reform of medicine after 1640 as forming part of a wider programme of social, religious and political change associated with the ascendant puritan party.[125] Much of the ensuing debate has centred on the legitimacy of equating specific attitudes to healing with distinct religious or political orientations, with particular attention given to the applicability of all-encompassing labels like 'puritan' and the search for alternative and more accurate descriptors.[126] One outcome of this debate has suggested a more nuanced reading of what precisely it means to invoke religious labels such as 'puritan' in this period, particularly after 1640, and the growing fragmentation of an earlier broad, but fragile, 'puritan' consensus in the wake of Parliaments' victory in the first civil war. I, for example, have argued elsewhere that the religious disposition of those who most strongly favoured the introduction of chymical medicine, along the lines proposed by medical reformers such as Paracelsus and van Helmont, is best described as non-denominational and 'eirenic' in character.[127] In opposition to Webster, others have pointed to the intrinsic compatibility of the new strains of iatrochemical and alchemical thinking with support for royalism in the middle decades of the seventeenth century.[128] Here, I would like to develop further some of these ideas and suggest in the process a new approach to the questions raised by this debate that is less dependent on over-simplistic categorization and more willing to accede to the possibility that medical practitioners, like those engaged in natural philosophy, opted for what Michael Hunter has referred to as a 'matrix' of competing ideas and positions, both in relation to religious as well as scientific orientation.[129]

If it is possible to detect a distinctively 'puritan' approach to medicine and healing in seventeenth-century England, I would argue that it is most likely be found in the period before rather than after 1640, when the onset of civil war and its contentious aftermath fostered the rapid disintegration of an earlier broad, but fragile, 'puritan' consensus.[130] Before 1640, two distinct phases of puritan interaction with medicine can be identified. In the first instance and concomitant with the emergence of a puritan movement in the early years of the reign of Elizabeth I, it is possible to argue, I think, that many supporters of evangelical Protestantism found many aspects of Paracelsianism and its rejection of the Galenic status quo both congenial and fully consonant with the reformist goals of puritanism. By the end of the sixteenth century, however, the early zeal of puritans for medical change on Paracelsian lines had given way to a more sceptical and critical approach which may in part have reflected growing fears of an upsurge in radical sectarianism and its association with Paracelsus and his followers. As many puritans became more integrated within the Anglican Church, and eager to throw off any association with the Brownists and other separatists, so they became less inclined to promote ideas and attitudes that threatened to undermine social, religious and political conventions or encourage subversive strains of thought such as Paracelsianism and the occult sciences.

Early evidence for puritan interest in the ideas of Paracelsus can be seen in various groups and networks of natural philosophers and physicians many of whom, as religious exiles, had travelled widely on the continent in the mid-sixteenth century. Here, they had first encountered Paracelsianism which they eagerly promoted on their return to England following the Elizabethan settlement of religion after 1558.[131] One particularly important group, based in London, formed around Peter Turner (1542–1614), Thomas Penny (*c.*1530–1589) and Thomas Moffet (1553–1604).[132] All three were passionate advocates of Paracelsus. Turner described him as 'absolutely the most learned chimicall writer and worker that ever wrote' and dismissed his critics as obscurantists. At the same time, as an MP, Turner acted as the spokesman in Parliament for the London Presbyterian movement led by the puritan cleric John Field (d.1588) and proposed the replacement of the Book of Common Prayer with a Genevan style of worship and the introduction of a Presbyterian system of government.[133] Turner's friend and colleague Thomas Penny was equally enthusiastic as a puritan advocate for Paracelsian medical reform. In Penny's case, however, his zeal for religious change may have led him to flirt with more radical elements within the puritan-Presbyterian movement. In his will, made in June 1588, he left bequests to three men—Nicholas Crane (*c.*1522–1588), Giles Wigginton (d.1597) and John Penry (d.1593)—whose careers illustrate the tendency of the early puritan movement to fracture and gravitate towards separatism under the pressure of fast-moving events.[134]

Penny's will is also revealing as it hints at the existence of other networks of puritan medical practitioners that shared the passion of Turner, Penny and Moffet for Paracelsianism. John Banister (d.1599), to whom Penny left a volume of surgical tracts, was an early convert to the merits of iatrochemistry which he advertised in his many writings. He was also well connected in puritan circles.[135] A barber surgeon by training, he nonetheless managed to acquire a licence to practise medicine from the College of Physicians in London in 1594, an extraordinarily rare act of munificence which almost certainly owed a great deal to the intercession of powerful patrons such as the earls of Rutland and Leicester as well as the Queen.[136] In the same year, 1594, Banister's son-in-law Stephen Bradwell or Bredwell, likewise a surgeon with no formal qualification to practise medicine, was granted a licence by the College. He shared his father-in-law's passion for chymistry, describing the art of the chymist as 'the most noble instrument of natural knowledges', and went on to advocate the 'erecting of a laboratorie of an industrious chemist' as the natural adjunct to a botanist's garden from whence all manner of advances might be expected to flow. At the same time, Bradwell occupied a key position in the burgeoning Presbyterian movement in which he acted, in the words of J. M. Corley, as 'the official representative of the London puritans' in their war of words with the Brownists and other separatists.[137]

As puritanism evolved in response to events in the late sixteenth century, there is little doubt that the majority of its adherents who espoused the cause of further reform of the English Church drew back from outright separation amid fears of growing religious anarchy. The collapse of the nascent Presbyterian movement in the aftermath of the Marprelate controversies and the crisis in church and state engendered by the Gunpowder Plot facilitated a growing moderation in puritan circles and grudging accommodation with an episcopal state church that retained, for the most part, its attachment to Calvinism. Increasingly, puritan zealots were now more exercised by the threat of 'papism' rather than committed to exposing the deficiencies of the Anglican Church. In this changing religious environment, most puritan physicians shied away from the heterodox opinions of Paracelsus and grew ever more inclined to promote respect for orthodox medical beliefs. As I have argued elsewhere, puritan physicians before 1640, like their clerical brethren, demonstrated little interest in anything that threatened to undermine the hierarchical nature of the medical profession, a conservative position that reflected, in many respects, the wider puritan preoccupation with order in the body politic as described in the previous chapter. In puritan circles, the vocation of the educated and qualified physician was thus seen as expressive of this deep concern for social order and propriety, and on a par with the respect that was due to the members of other key institutions in the state such as the church and the law. Typical in this respect were the writings of the Northamptonshire puritan and physician, John Cotta, in which he repeatedly argued for the exclusion from practice of all 'ignorant' pretenders to physic, including women, empirics and clergymen, on the grounds that such an intrusion into the medical sphere was proscribed by God, nature and law. In the words of his puritan colleague and successor at Northampton, James Hart (d.1639), who likewise condemned such interlopers, 'God is the God of order, not of confusion, and never did allow of this confused Chaos of callings'.[138] In contrast with their non-puritan colleagues, very few puritan ministers practised medicine while holding a living in pre-civil war England. Only five examples have been found.[139] Most, as we have noted earlier, opted for a medical career after deprivation (see above 47) while others like the puritanically inclined minister Henry Holland (d.1603) defended meddling in medicine on the grounds that he did so only for friendship's sake among family and friends.[140]

The sacrosanct nature of the calling of the physician in puritan eyes was mirrored by the deep respect exhibited by most pre-civil war puritan physicians for the traditional medical wisdom that underpinned their practice.[141] This reverence for the learned foundations of medical study, based primarily on the works of Galen and Hippocrates, was also shared by their clerical colleagues in the pulpit. Here, the alleged atheism of the Greek physician Galen presented a potential stumbling block and congregations were warned to be wary of falling into a trap, 'as Plinie and Galen did', of becoming 'so bewitched with Nature itselfe [that] they forgot *Naturam natura*, the god of Nature'.[142] But with this caveat in mind, puritan approbation of Galen knew few bounds. Edward Corbett, for example, told the House of Commons in 1642 that Galen's relation of the 'making of a Gnat' was all the evidence one needed to prove the wisdom of an omnipotent Creator.[143] Others, such as the puritan divine Thomas Gataker (1574–1654), helped promote Galenism through publishing a posthumous edition of notes on the moral and philosophical aspects of the Greek physician's work by his close friend Theodore Gulston (1575–1632), an eminent member of the London College of Physicians.[144] One of the more notable features of the fast sermons preached before Parliament in the 1640s was the repeated refrain of puritan ministers prescribing the application of Galenic principles, especially the notion of *contraria contrariis* (i.e. the idea that diseases were best cured by the use of medicines whose qualities—hot, cold—were opposite in nature to the disease), to the religious and political problems of the day.[145] Similar sentiments continued to find expression under puritan rule in the 1650s. In 1654, for example, the Presbyterian minister Simon Ford reminded the assize court judges that 'Physitians of the greatest note' were in broad agreement that 'all diseases... are cured by Contraries'. Consciously invoking the analogy of the body politic, he went on to draw the important political lesson that 'the diseases of the body Politick occasioned by remissness, require more rough and churlish Physick to remove them'.[146] In line with mainstream puritan devotion to medical orthodoxy, there is little evidence then in the period immediately before and after the outbreak of civil war to suggest that most puritans, be they physicians of the body or the soul, were anything other than hostile to Galen's nemesis, Paracelsus. In this, they were probably at one with the majority of their Anglican colleagues, who, in the period before and after 1640, consistently linked Paracelsianism with religious schism and radical sectarianism.[147]

Such an association of ideas may well have been founded in fact. The writings of Paracelsus had long exerted a powerful influence upon the religiously heterodox of all confessions and would continue to do so after 1642. It was probably no coincidence, for example, that one of the first to publicize Paracelsian ideas in England was the former Brownist James Forester (*c.*1560–1622?), who, on recanting his former opinions and rejoining the Anglican fold, took over the medical practice of one of the pioneers of Paracelsian medicine in Tudor England, John

Hester (d.1592).[148] A particularly intriguing example of the way in which those inclined to unorthodox religious opinions were also drawn to the ideas of the medical iconoclast, Paracelsus, can also be found in the records of the English Reformed Church in Amsterdam, which functioned as a semi-autonomous congregation modelled on strict Calvinist and puritanical lines. It also served as a refuge for English puritans fleeing persecution in their native homeland. Between 1621 and 1623, a member of the church, Humphrey Bromley, was repeatedly called before the consistory to answer various charges including claims that he had attempted to communicate with angels and professed that all men might be saved, 'both Devills & men'. On being examined, Bromley confessed to having sought the intercourse of good angels, which he was assured on the authority of Paracelsus was both feasible and legitimate.[149] What particularly interested his interrogator, the English minister John Paget, was Bromley's assertion that 'he that had the wiles of philosophie might thereby understand the whole scriptures'. On reading Paracelsus as well as specific biblical texts, Bromley had become convinced that soul, spirit and body were separate entities, and that all souls might be saved. Moreover, these were not mere idle speculations. Bromley, a wax chandler by trade, gave up his original occupation to pursue a medical career based on Paracelsian methods. Most startling of all was his admission that he possessed a box 'wherin was a mans flesh cut from a mans heart on the gallows'. This Paracelsian 'mummia of the ayre' was used by Bromley to heal a female complaint called 'Molla'. He also claimed, in defending the practice, that hangmen in Germany regularly extracted the spirits of dead men which might then be implanted in others to produce medical and spiritual benefits. So confident was Bromley in his abilities as a Paracelsian healer that he set himself up as a mountebank and erected placards on the bourse in Amsterdam, where he advertised his skills as a philosophical alchemist and medical practitioner.[150]

The equation of religious radicalism with medical unorthodoxy in the shape of Paracelsus was widely noted both before and after the outbreak of the civil war. But there is little evidence to suggest that Paracelsianism, or an aversion to the established medical order, was popular in mainstream puritan circles in England in the four decades prior to 1640. Typical of the new conservatism, perhaps, were the views of Francis Herring (d.1628), a puritan fellow of the London College, who not only rejected Paracelsus' doctrine of cure by similars and excoriated his 'frivolous, absurd and ridiculous' medical opinions but also reproved all forms of quackery that threatened to undermine the 'professional' status of the College physicians. Unlike an earlier generation of puritan medics, many of whom cavilled at the monopolistic powers wielded by the College in London, Herring condemned all forms of illegal encroachment. As early as 1599, he commended the work of fellow puritan and physician, Richard Surflet (d.1605), who in a translation of the French doctor Andre du Laurens (1558–1609) had launched a scathing attack on 'the painted crew of seeming Phisitions and prattling practisers bothe men and women, gathering their skill, honestie and most precious secrets, from the rich mines of brazen-faced impudencie and bold blindness'.[151] Three years later, Herring published his own diatribe upon the dangers posed by medical empirics and interlopers and was well positioned thereafter (he held the office of censor in the College on seven separate occasions between 1609 and 1627) to challenge and disarm those who sought to undermine the authority of the College of Physicians. At the same time, Herring, who moved in godly circles, published virulently anti-Catholic verse—evidence no doubt of the altered preoccupations of many early seventeenth-century puritans who now tempered their opposition to the bishops in the wake of a new, more potent, threat in the form of resurgent Roman Catholicism.[152]

While all college fellows had a duty and vested interest in stamping out illicit practice in the capital, some of the most active and vociferous critics of empirics and interlopers were to be found within the puritan ranks of the College. Such a view sits uncomfortably with that put forward by historians such as Hal Cook, who has downplayed the ideological commitment of the fellows in this period, and stressed instead their opportunism and unprincipled willingness to change direction on issues such as medical regulation with each alteration in government.[153] But as the work of scholars such as William Birken has demonstrated, the College was dominated in the 1640s by men fully committed to the cause of religious and political reform, albeit of the kind favoured by the more conservative Presbyterian faction in Parliament and the city of London.[154] Birken, for example, has stressed the commitment of the diehard Presbyterian John Clarke during his period as president (1645–50) to the eradication of the threat posed to the College by the activities of unlicensed empirics. His failure, as Cook admits, had little to do with a lack of nerve but was largely determined by external political events outside the control of Clarke and his like-minded colleagues.[155] In promoting such ends, Clarke's views were not guided by political opportunism but rather represented part of a consistent approach to the problem of medical interlopers that dated back at least to the early years of the seventeenth century. The work begun by fellows such as Herring was frequently taken forward by the next generation of like-minded colleagues. In 1632, for example, with his college friend and co-religionist, Samuel Rand, Clarke had signed a petition to the crown imploring Charles I to act against the intrusive activities of the London apothecaries.[156] Other fellows in the College who shared Clarke's religious principles acted on their qualms. Thus Edward Alston (1597–1669) and Daniel Oxenbridge (1571–1642), who both possessed impeccable puritan credentials, played a prominent role in the College's campaign against two of its most inveterate critics, Gerard Boate (1604–1650) and William Trigge (d.*c.*1665).[157] Such opinions, moreover, were not limited to puritan physicians in the capital. Outside London, puritan colleagues such as Tobias Venner of Bath and James Primrose of Hull authored works lamenting the intrusions of empirics and other unqualified practitioners.[158]

The imperative to police the medical marketplace and exclude unqualified interlopers thus formed part of a wider belief in mainstream puritan circles that social, religious and political order was best served by a strict observation of the hierarchical distinctions in the various organs of church and state. There was little that was 'revolutionary' about these aims, a sentiment most neatly captured in the words of the Northampton puritan and physician, James Hart, in 1633, when he lamented that 'this injury [of medical intrusion] hath heretofore, both out of the pulpit, and by the pen of the learned been spoken against . . . *yet hath all this as yet produced no reformation*'.[159] Nor, it should be stressed, were such goals antipathetic to those of Charles I and his policy of 'thorough' in the years of personal rule (1629–40). While it is undoubtedly true, as Birken points out, that the crown often acted in ways that undermined the authority of the College, it would be wrong to exaggerate the extent to which the regulatory aims of puritan physicians like Clarke, Alston and Oxenbridge were out of step with those favoured by Charles and his chief ministers. In 1635, for example, it was the Laudian Ralph Winterton (1601–1636), Regius Professor of Medicine at Cambridge, who wrote to the president of the College, Simeon Foxe (1569–1642), suggesting that all the various licensing bodies, including the church, should adopt uniform procedures in order to eliminate illicit practice, clerical intruders and general quackery.[160] Though nothing came of this initiative—Winterton's death a few months later probably scuppered the proposal—Charles' government and the College frequently colluded in order to prosecute miscreants. Thus the notorious empiric-cum-cleric, John Evans, whose promotion of the virtues of the antimonial cup upset the royal and collegiate physician, Dr Theodore de Mayerne (1573–1655), was ultimately proceeded against with great vigour in the Court of High Commission by archbishop Laud at the urging of the College. For good measure, Laud was also responsible for proscribing and destroying all extant copies of Evans' book which advertised the virtues of his 'universal medicine'.[161] Moreover, in such cases a declaration of loyalty to church and crown was clearly no defence as the case of William Richardson, vicar of Garthorpe in Leicestershire, suggests. Richardson, too, was prosecuted by Laud in High Commission, where it was alleged that 'his practice of surgery and repairing to his patients in public and scandalous places was no way justifiable'. He was later sequestrated from his living by the puritans in the 1640s, only to be reinstated in 1660.[162]

The decision of most fellows of the College of Physicians to side with Parliament rather than the King in the early 1640s was not therefore, *pace* Cook, one that was dictated by the need to choose between two competing medical policies: 'the preservation of the liberties of patients, practitioners and corporations to make their own medical decisions, or the preservation of the public good through medical policing'. On the contrary, it was the product of a sincere and deeply felt mistrust of royal policy in issues of religious doctrine and practice which had little bearing on medicine or medical matters. In most respects then, it was not attitudes to medical innovation or policing that divided the college fellows in the 1640s, where there was much common ground (antipathy to new therapies and an aversion to unlearned medical interlopers), but rather issues relating to the much broader questions surrounding the future governance of church and state in early modern England. At this point in our story, the process of politicization which I have identified as a central feature of the history of medicine in this period, was in its infancy and was not yet responsible for shaping attitudes to issues such as the provision of medical services or ideas surrounding the cure of sick bodies. Consequently, I find it impossible to concur with the idea implicit in Cook's view of medical politics in this period that Galenism, Laudianism and 'Thorough' were somehow interconnected in an exclusive nexus which alone 'mandated order and obedience for the good of all'. Order, hierarchy and respect for traditional forms of learning and institutions were as much part of the outlook of pre-civil war puritans as they were intrinsic to the social thinking of loyal supporters of the Stuart regime.[163] The real challenge to both—apparent as much in the field of medicine as it was in society generally—was yet to come, the product of a largely unwanted and unforeseen breakdown of religious and political order in the body politic in England after 1640.

In the face of the spread of radical sectarianism and the disintegration of puritan consensus in the 1640s, the London College of Physicians was to prove largely helpless in defending its rights and privileges in relation to the policing of medicine in London. Outside the confines of Amen Corner, the political scene in London was shifting toward a more radical resolution of the nation's problems and the Presbyterian leadership of the College struggled to maintain its authority. Even though the majority of its members were almost certainly unsympathetic to the path that the civil war was taking, there was little they could effectively do to impose medical conformity and order now that power increasingly lay in the hands of men ideologically and temperamentally averse to any policies that seemed to undermine the much vaunted 'liberties of the subject'. In many respects, the writing was on the wall for the College long before 1649, when the execution of the King marked the beginning of a new phase in the English Revolution. It is evident, for example, in the ranks of many of those who had opposed its authority in the 1630s and had been punished for their recalcitrance. Aaron Streater, for example, who was prosecuted by the College in 1639 for setting up handbills advertising his cures, wasted little opportunity in utilizing the freedom of the presses in 1642 to argue that liberty of conscience should be extended to all, including the much-maligned Brownists.[164] Likewise, the Behmenist mystic John Pordage (1607–1681), who was prosecuted in 1637–8 for illicit practice, was already well known in puritan circles for holding a variety of heterodox opinions.[165] It was probably no coincidence that both men were ordained. While mainstream puritan ministers rarely combined the practice of the two vocations of doctoring and preaching, their more radical colleagues, particularly those averse to the idea of state-imposed conformity, often practised both simultaneously.[166] Pordage, it should be noted, was also an associate of the notorious empiric William Trigge, who frequently appeared before the College in the 1630s, including in January 1638, when he was accused of killing a woman with dropsy by 'opening her belly'. In mitigation, he claimed to have done so in the presence, and with the assistance, of Pordage. Trigge, of course, remained a thorn in the flesh of the College for the next two decades, in which period he built up a lucrative practice that was almost certainly protected to some extent by his ideological commitment to the various regimes of the 1650s.[167] In some cases dating from the last days of the Caroline regime, it is even possible to detect collusion between the empirics and some junior fellows within the College, who did not share the conservative religious and political instincts of their superiors. When in July 1640, for example, the apothecary Valentine Fyge was summoned to appear before the *comitia* of the College for practising upon the body of one Mrs Ganocke, he claimed that he did so at the direction of two College physicians, William Staines and Aaron Gurdon. Both men, as previously noted, subsequently served with distinction in various arms of the Cromwellian state.[168]

It is hardly surprising that with the collapse of censorship, the defeat of the King and the failure of the Presbyterians to impose a new form of godly order upon the body politic, monopolistic bodies such as the College of Physicians in London came under ceaseless attack in the 1650s from what we might loosely term the radical wing of the puritan revolution. Not only was its authority to oversee and regulate the medical marketplace in the capital called into question, but its mainly conservative membership, both in religious and medical terms, was forced to witness a new assault on the academic foundations of the medical discipline. Powerless to act otherwise, as Hal Cook and others have shown, the College turned in on itself and emerged re-branded as a corporate institution whose main purpose was to act as a centre of medical research.[169] In the meantime, arguments in favour of a radical overhaul of every aspect of the healing arts were widely disseminated in the free press of the 1650s. This process, epitomized by the various publications and translations undertaken by the radical herbalist Nicholas Culpeper (discussed further below), and a circle of willing collaborators and translators, has been extensively charted by historians of the period and requires no further reiteration here.[170] What is worthy of debate, however, in the context of the present discussion, is the extent to which this 'programme' of medical reform emanated from a specific set of non-medical, i.e. religious and political, beliefs. Was it, as some have argued, primarily the by-product of the 'puritan' obsession with social and intellectual renovation? Or is it possible to provide a more nuanced, and indeed more accurate, account of how non-medical factors may have played a part in turning upside down the early modern understanding of all things medical? In seeking to answer this question, I would like to focus on the fate of one aspect of this medical revolution, though arguably one of the most important, namely the attempt by the reformers to overthrow the authority of Galen and replace it with the new theories of the chymical physicians, particularly those drawn from the writings of Paracelsus and the Flemish iatrochemist, John Baptist van Helmont (1577–1644).

Iatrochemistry and the English Revolution

Prior to 1649, few Englishmen publicly espoused or promoted the new chymical philosophy associated with physicians like Paracelsus. Despite the growing popularity of chymical medicines, and their integration into the traditional pharmacopoeia, there was a widespread reluctance in medical circles to acknowledge the superiority of Paracelsian methods over those used for centuries by physicians trained in the humanist traditions of classical medicine. To some extent, the public ignorance surrounding Paracelsus and the benefits of iatrochemistry was probably due to the absence of vernacular translations of his writings and those of his followers. But it is also noticeable that even some of his most avid English followers were reluctant to put their names to works extolling and commentating on the virtues of a chymical approach to healing, and those that did, such as Robert Fludd (1574–1637), chose to publish their research in Latin and abroad. It might be tempting to conclude from these observations that interest in such ideas was slight before 1649, and restricted to small coteries of *adepti*, whose chymical investigations were largely dependent upon the private patronage of devoted aristocrats and courtiers. The example of men like Bannister and Bromley, cited above, however, suggests that this may be something of an illusion. I suspect, though this is clearly an area where further research is needed, that interest in Paracelsianism and related ideas prior to the English civil wars was much wider than previously thought, but, for a variety of reasons, few felt comfortable making public protestations of support for the new medical ideology. Paracelsus himself was frequently depicted as a dangerous, irreverent and impious iconoclast, a drunk and a lecher, whose attitude to all authority—religious, political and medical—deterred many from sampling his ideas. Though his followers sought to portray a more positive image of the man, there were other elements of his thinking that evoked negative or fearful connotations. Paracelsian chymistry, of course, had its roots in the Renaissance revival of more ancient strands of thought, including medieval alchemy. Alchemy, by its very nature, was a secretive pursuit, clouded in mystery, and frequently associated in the wider culture of early modern England with the fear that excessive curiosity in such matters led men inexorably to the Devil and perdition.

Given these widespread concerns and fears, it is not altogether surprising then that interest in the ideas of the iatrochemists was largely suppressed in pre-civil war England. The real turning point came in about 1649, when private inhibitions were relaxed in the more congenial atmosphere created by the inception of a republic that promised a broad degree of religious and intellectual freedom. Just as religious radicals campaigned for an end to the monopolistic authority wielded by state-sponsored clerics and political radicals urged reform of a legal system widely perceived as oppressive and exclusive, so were the same men inspired to promote a thorough overhaul of the medical profession. One by-product of this process was a massive increase in the publication of medical works in English, ranging from self-help manuals to translations of traditional as well as modern works, including those of Paracelsus and his followers. Many of these works, and the impetus for their production, clearly originated in radical circles dedicated to the ideals of the new commonwealth and the 'good old cause'. William Rowland (*fl.*1651–1669) and William Rand, for example, who were both employed by Culpeper in the 1650s in translating a range of medical texts, demonstrated such credentials. Rowland, a former military surgeon in the Cromwellian army of occupation in Scotland, made clear his commitment to the cause when he petitioned Cromwell in person in the early 1650s, and offered his services to the state in support of the struggle for 'liberty for tender consciences' against the encroachments of Romish 'paganism'.[171] The anti-clerical Rand, on the other hand, who would appear to have dabbled in Socinianism, dedicated the translation of the abridged works of the French physician Jean Riolan (1577–1657) to Henry Lawrence, Lord President of the Council. The dedication, dated 22 December 1656, was replete with religious and political significance as Lawrence was currently embroiled in the controversy surrounding the prosecution of the Quaker James Nayler for blasphemy, whom he bravely defended on the grounds that Nayler's claim to be Christ should be understood in a metaphorical sense, in much the same way that God was present in 'every horse, in every stone, in every creature'.[172] While the translations they produced for Culpeper were largely of conservative medical texts, Rowland and Rand were committed advocates of the merits of the new chymical medicine. In 1661, for example, both men supplied testimonials on behalf of the former Leveller activist-turned-physician, William Walwyn, in a book dedicated to the merits of the use of gentle, purgative medicines prepared along Helmontian lines.[173]

At the same time as Culpeper was busy exploiting the burgeoning market for works in English promoting medical self-help, others were busy preparing new translations of the writings of Paracelsus and his followers. Again, many of these emanated from the pens of radical enthusiasts for the 'good old cause' such as Henry Pinnell, or servants of the state such as William Dugard (1606–1662), John French (*c.*1616–1657) and Ferdinando Parkhurst (*fl.*1621–1674).[174] Likewise, one of the first major works to espouse a new system of chymical medicine, based on the pioneering research and thought of the Flemish iatrochemist, John Baptist van Helmont, Noah Biggs' *Vanity of the Craft of Physick* (1651), was clearly written, as we have seen in chapter 2, by an author committed to the political programme of

Cromwell's Republic.[175] During the course of the 1650s, further medical works either based on, or heavily influenced by, van Helmont's novel chymical theories rapidly appeared with the result that the Flemish doctor threatened to supplant Paracelsus as the prime inspiration of the chymical physicians. Van Helmont's ideas seemed to hold special appeal for those who subscribed to a mystical understanding of the nature of true religion, as for example in the Helmontian insistence upon the role of divine illumination in the acquisition of medical knowledge, a process that seemed fully in accord with the sectarian insistence on the role of the holy spirit in inspiring men to teach and preach the gospels. When van Helmont's works, then, were finally translated into English in 1662, it comes as little surprise to learn that the translator, John Chandler, was a former Ranter turned Quaker, whose adoption of Helmontianism, as I have argued elsewhere, was fully in keeping with the theosophical and pantheistic spirit of radical sectarianism.[176]

And yet, despite all this evidence, it would be a mistake, I believe, to impute the successful spread of Helmontian medical ideas solely to the warm reception afforded such beliefs in radical sectarian circles. Indeed, further exploration of the various milieux in which interest in chymistry in general, and the ideas of van Helmont in particular, flourished in the 1650s suggests that there was no single political or religious ideology which monopolized the promotion of such views. This is most starkly evident from the way in which those supporters of Church and King, defeated in the civil war and demoralized by the abolition of monarchy and episcopacy, were drawn to van Helmont in the period immediately following the execution of Charles I in 1649. Indeed, as I will suggest, the timing may not be coincidental. After 1649, as the medical schools of Oxford and Cambridge filled with former royalists, many became attracted to various aspects of the Helmontian reform programme. This is evident, for example, from the various subjects that prospective medical students sought to debate prior to graduation at Oxford in the 1650s. Ralph Bathurst,[177] Robert Fielding[178] and Richard Kuerden, alias Jackson,[179] men of impeccable loyalist credentials, opted to discuss topics that were redolent of Helmontian concerns such as the role of chemical fermentation in the stomach, the power of the imagination in causing illness, and the feasibility of universal medicines. Others, such as George Thomson, who was to play a leading role after 1660 in promoting the universal benefits of a Helmontian revolution in medicine, may well have encountered the ideas of the Flemish iatrochemist while travelling in Europe in the late 1640s. Having served with the royalist forces in the first civil war, Thomson sought admission to the College of Physicians in London in December 1647 but was denied membership for refusing to pay the requisite fees. Following a brief sojourn at Leiden, where he proceeded MD in 1648, he returned home to practise medicine in and around London and Essex. He later claimed to have adopted the principles of Helmontianism in about 1649.[180]

The dedication of Thomson's Leiden thesis, among others, to one Job Weale, 'medicus' of Kingston upon Thames, is of particular interest as it illustrates numerous themes discussed in this chapter. Weale (1600–1668) was a London apothecary who had become embroiled in a major conflict with the College of Physicians in 1634, when he was accused of prescribing adulterated drugs. Prosecuted by the College authorities, the case itself was probably little more than a smokescreen for an attempt by the College to secure greater regulatory control over the apothecaries. In the light of Weale's subsequent devotion to the royal cause in the 1640s, his actions in 1634 in defending himself and his fellow apothecaries (Weale was treasurer of the Society of Apothecaries) illustrate the pitfalls of correlating specific attitudes to medicine with narrow political and partisan ends. According to the description of the visit to Weale's shop in the official record of the College, where medicines were destroyed and empirics' bills were allegedly found, Weale 'with clamor drewe together such a multitude of people in the streets' that the College's officers were forced to withdraw. Not content with this show of force, Weale then orchestrated the arrest of the president, censors and other members of the College, whom he accused of violating Magna Carta by entering his shop and seizing and destroying his goods. The College responded by soliciting the support of the government, including the Privy Council and Court of Star Chamber, and the dispute threatened to escalate further when two prominent members of the College of Physicians set about creating a rival Society or Company of Distillers in an attempt to undermine the apothecaries.[181] Once tempers cooled, Weale followed the route taken by so many others accused of illicit practice by the College, and retired to Kingston in Surrey, where, outside the reach of the College's jurisdiction and armed with a licence to practise medicine from William Laud, archbishop of Canterbury, he set up practice as a physician.[182] Despite his advocacy of street politics and citation of the rights of the subject enshrined in Magna Carta, Weale was no religious zealot or political incendiary. In 1642, he wrote a short tract, with a suitably inspired medical title, calling for unity in church and state and restoration of order and stability in the wake of the drift to war.[183] And his strong royalist leanings soon became evident when in December of that year he was imprisoned in the Compter at Southwark 'for being refractory to the propositions for raysing of horse, money or plate'. Unperturbed, he continued to play an active role in royalist politics and plotting throughout the 1640s. In May 1648, for example, he attempted to instigate a royalist uprising in Surrey in the hope of securing the King's release from Carisbrook Castle on the Isle of Wight. He was subsequently rumbled, however, by the King's gaoler, Colonel Robert Hammond, who was able to 'perceive by discourse with him, that hee hath beene a great promoter of the Late Surrey petition and an agent of the Malignants there'.[184] In all probability, Weale shared not only Thomson's politics but also his medical interests. In 1666, Thomson alluded to Weale's persecution at the hands of the 'dogmatists' in the 1630s and acknowledged him as his original mentor, who provided him with patients and instructed him 'both in Galenical and Spagyrical Practice'. He died in 1668, but his memory lived on when four years later Thomson praised in print his preparation of *lac sulphuris* and described him as 'a singular physician, and accurate Apothecary'.[185]

The career of Job Weale neatly illustrates an openness to medical change and opposition to the status quo that confounds any simple equation of religious and political sympathies with specific approaches to medical practice and beliefs. Weale's background was distinctly establishment. His father George Weale was the clerk of works to James I and Charles I and was partly responsible for the planning and building of the Banqueting House at Whitehall.[186] But more importantly, Weale was not alone among the apothecaries in combining future loyalty to the Stuarts with concerted opposition to the monopolistic authority wielded by the physicians. In the same year that Weale led the apothecaries' challenge to the College of Physicians, 1634, a group of Weale's like-minded colleagues gave a series of lectures in Apothecaries Hall, steeped in humanist medical learning, that were designed to raise the profile of the apothecary as 'fully-fledged *medicus*'.[187] Two of the four lecturers were devoted to the royalist cause. Thomas Johnson, the celebrated botanist, fled to Oxford shortly after the outbreak of civil war in 1642 and was rewarded for his loyalty with the grant of two medical degrees. He died fighting for the King at the bloody siege of Basing House in 1644.[188] William Broad (d.1642) was equally committed to the Stuarts, acting as physician to the beleaguered forces of Charles I at Berwick upon Tweed during the first Bishops' War. His loyalist credentials are strikingly evident from his will in which he made numerous bequests to local Laudian clergymen as well as the Scottish nobleman Sir Alexander Nesbit (d.1660) who fought for the King in the civil war and lost three sons in the ensuing conflict.[189] Like Weale, Broad had probably left London to follow a career as a physician but remained close to his former colleagues. He named Thomas Johnson as one of the overseers of his will and was closely tied to the 1634 group through a shared interest in botanical research and journeying together through Britain on expeditions designed to catalogue the flora of the country.[190] Dimitri Levitin, who was the first to point to the significance of the lecture series, is surely right to conclude that the aim of the apothecaries was neither economic nor hegemonic but rather that the ensuing debates represent 'a conversation within the same ideological framework'.[191]

Whether these men, if they had survived the civil wars, would have shared the enthusiasm of former colleagues like Weale for Helmontianism is of course unknowable. Other physicians of a royalist bent, however, were attracted to the new medical school of thought. Converts to the doctrines of van Helmont in the 1650s include William Currer (*c.*1617–1668), the loyalist poet and physician John Collop (1625–1697) and John Evelyn's friend, James Thickens or Thickness (d.1666), who was expelled from his fellowship at Balliol College, Oxford, in

1648 and later practised medicine at Maldon in Essex in the 1650s. Currer, a close friend of Elias Ashmole, was a prominent figure in chymical circles in London and Dublin during the 1650s. He fought for the royalist forces in Ireland in the previous decade and compounded in 1651.[192] Collop's poetry, dating from the 1650s, is laced with references to topical medical issues which make clear his disapproval of the evacuative methods favoured by the Galenists and his preference for the milder treatments of the Helmontians. At the same time, his verse attests to a moderate royalism, signified by a disapproval of cavalier excess, and a marked aversion to religious and political controversy. He not only favoured a rapprochement with Cromwell but also promoted a broad-based and tolerant settlement of religious affairs—an aspiration shared by many others attracted to van Helmont.[193] Thickens, who, according to his travelling companion John Evelyn, 'had served his Majestie in the Warrs', later wrote to his friend in 'exile' on the continent, lamenting the sad condition of England, and its religious and political divisions, following the surrender at Oxford. Some time around 1650, however, he gave up rural solitude and from his new base at Maldon in Essex, set up in practice and began an extensive programme of medical research. Samuel Hartlib, on the information of Thickens' friend and fellow chymist Dr Robert Child, reported that he was 'one of the great Helmontians', who had recently compiled an index of van Helmont's writings.[194] Thickens' friendship with Evelyn and Child suggests another conduit for the propagation and dissemination of interest among royalists for the works of van Helmont and the chymical philosophers. Both men were active participants in the scheme of the former royalist Thomas Henshaw (1618–1700) to establish a retreat or 'Model Christian Learned Society' at Kensington in the 1650s, where the participants were expected to live a monk-like existence and dedicate themselves to study in order to 'doe all the good they can to their neighbourhood'. A central feature of this proposed academy was a laboratory for the manufacture of chymical medicines and arcana.[195]

Chymistry, then, undoubtedly appealed to a wide cross-section of religious and political opinion in Interregnum England including disaffected royalists and closet Anglicans. The latter could be found collaborating in organized groups such as that of Henshaw, but they can also be found working together in a variety of different fields and projects. One such, which seems to have escaped the notice of scholars, centred on the dictionary project of Edward Phillips (*fl.*1630–1696), the nephew of the celebrated poet John Milton. In the late 1650s, Phillips brought together a group of experts in a wide range of fields, including medicine, chymistry and various branches of natural philosophy, in order to compile a modern dictionary.[196] A considerable number of those recruited to write entries suggest a tight-knit group of like-minded men with strong royalist credentials who shared a passion for chymistry and its medicinal applications. Among the contributors were the chymical physicians William Currer and Mark Sparck, the Paracelsian translator Robert Turner, the surgeons Edward and William Molins, and as ringleader and head of recruitment, the alchemist Elias Ashmole.[197] Phillips himself was almost certainly drawn into the orbit of royalist chymists through his stepfather Thomas Agar (*c.*1597–1673), clerk of the crown in Chancery, who had married the daughter of the London physician, Thomas Ridgley (*c.*1576–1656), a lifelong devotee of iatrochemistry.[198] Ridgley, who was eventually elected a fellow of the College of Physicians after much opposition, resigned his fellowship on account of his support for the cause of Charles I in 1642 and did not resume it again until 1649. His son Luke (1615–1696) followed in his father's footsteps as an eminent, London-based chymical physician, though like his father he continued to provide medical advice to the gentry and aristocracy of his native Nottinghamshire. Luke also retained the friendship of Thomas Agar, who remembered him in his will of 1673.[199]

Similar clubs or informal networks of men committed to chymical research also seem to have sprung up in the universities, where college heads and officials, under the scrutiny of the puritan authorities, did little to encourage the introduction of such studies into the official curriculum. Courses in chymistry would appear to have been popular with men of all religious and political backgrounds. A particularly intriguing example of this kind can be found at Trinity College, Cambridge, in the late 1640s and early 1650s, where interest in chymical research, as well as natural philosophy, featured strongly among the interests of large numbers of the College's students and fellows.[200] One of the central figures here was a young fellow named Alexander Akehurst (d.1707), of whom Hartlib reported in 1653 that he was 'chymically given' and had employed the German alchemist Johann Hartprecht to construct a furnace in his rooms at Cambridge.[201] Within a year, Akehurst would appear to have suffered some form of nervous breakdown when he was charged with various crimes, including the utterance of 'blasphemous and atheisticall expressions'. The case was referred to a parliamentary committee, which, having heard the evidence, sent the case back to Cambridge for adjudication by the master and fellows of Trinity.[202] While it is impossible to determine the precise nature of Akehurst's indiscretions, it is clear that they were interpreted at the time by the staunch puritan Vice Chancellor of the University, Lazarus Seaman (d.1675), as an assault on the foundations of the godly faith and may have been connected in the minds of men like Seaman with contemporary fears provoked by groups such as the Ranters.[203] One of Akehurst's former students, Oliver Heywood, claimed that he later became a Quaker. Just as important, however, is the fact that he also took up the practice of medicine after the Restoration, presumably incorporating his preoccupation with chymistry into his everyday practice. Akehurst's continuing fascination with scientific novelty is further suggested by the fact that in 1683 his brother-in-law, the ejected minister Daniel Batchelor, bequeathed to him 'all my Philosophicall Transactions in ffoure volumes'.[204]

Akehurst was not alone in Trinity in espousing the virtues of chymical investigations of nature. In 1653, one of his students, Nicholas Hookes (1632–1712), dedicated a collection of poems, written in contemporary 'Cavalier' style, to Akehurst, which included references to him as a modern successor to Paracelsus. They also contain verses in honour of the recently deceased Cambridge apothecary and 'golden Alchymist', John Crane (1571–1652), whom Hookes compared favourably to Galen, Hippocrates and Paracelsus.[205] Crane may in fact have been one of the central figures in promoting alchemical study at Trinity in these years. As a younger man, he had become a close associate of the celebrated adept William Butler (1535–1618), whose alchemical papers and manuscripts he inherited.[206] These in turn, according to Hartlib, passed to his friend Thomas Sclater or Slater (1615–1684), a Cambridge physician with strong connections to Trinity who was ejected as a fellow from the college in the 1640s. Sclater, moreover, shared Crane's deep-seated attachment to monarchical government and the Anglican Church. In 1654 he married the widow of his old friend Dr Thomas Comber (d.1653), former master of Trinity and dean of Carlisle.[207] Trinity may also have been responsible for nurturing the early interest in iatrochemistry of one of the leading figures in post-Restoration Helmontian circles, Daniel Foote (*c.*1630–1700). Foote, who entered the ministry in 1653, only to be ejected in 1662, was a student at Trinity in the early 1650s, where he seems to have come under the spell of another fellow, the physician John Pratt (d.1663), who later bequeathed to him all his medical manuscripts.[208] Like so many of his ejected colleagues, Foote switched to medical practice in the 1660s, proceeding MD at Cambridge in 1664. Some time thereafter, he became a close friend of Francis Mercury van Helmont, the son and heir of the famous physician, whose medical and theological writings he assiduously translated in the 1680s and 1690s.[209]

The varied religious and political backgrounds of this group of Cambridge men, which, as we have seen, replicated the wider phenomenon among the Paracelsian and Helmontian community of Interregnum England, is at first sight bewildering and would appear to obviate any attempt to link support for iatrochemistry with specific religious and political groups. Foote and Pratt were probably inclined toward Presbyterianism, Sclater, Hookes and Crane were closet Anglicans and royalists, while Akehurst drifted toward the Quakers. And yet, despite their differences, all were drawn to the collaborative study of chymistry, which seemed to provide a range of spiritual as much as material benefits to those who laboured in the furnaces. The events of the 1640s, culminating in the execution of a divinely ordained monarch, left many individuals in a profound state of shock. It was widely reported that when the news of the death of Charles I was made public, it 'caused some to die suddenly, some to fall into apoplexy, and others into deep melancholy'. Allowing for a degree of hyperbole, it would nonetheless be wrong to discount the extent to which events such as the regicide traumatized and sickened the nation. The subsequent slide into what many, possibly the majority, perceived as a state of religious anarchy and political instability further accentuated a mood of spiritual crisis in Britain. The growing fascination for chymistry, and related modes of thought such as the mystical writings of Jacob Boehme, should thus be understood within the context of this breakdown in traditional religious and political arrangements. For some, especially those dedicated to memorializing the sacrosanct virtues of monarchical government and alienated by the excesses of the Republic, chymistry provided a source of consolation and escape. The royalist Thomas Henshaw's proposed society of experimentalists at Kensington was to consist of a small group of six like-minded men, 'that will have all in common, dedicating themselves wholly to devotion and studies, and separating themselves from the World, by leading a severe life for diet and apparel'.[210] Others sought refuge in private study and contemplation. In the same year that he published one of the first English translations of the work of van Helmont, the former royal physician Walter Charleton (1620–1707) was reported to have become 'very fantastical', with observers fearing that 'hee will fall madde'. The political nature of the spiritual crisis enveloping Charleton is evident in the work itself, where Charleton, in a manner more reminiscent of the radical sectaries than a former servant of the crown, launched into an assault on that 'dark Lanthorne of Reason', which he concluded:

> 'hath been the onely unhappy cause, to which Religion doth owe all those wide, irreconcilable, and numerous rents and schisms, made by the men of the greatest Logick, and even such, whose intenser flames of Devotion had their mindes the Whitest and most purified from the lees of Temporall interest.[211]

Other royalist converts to Helmontianism in the 1650s like George Thomson laid the blame for the descent into religious anarchy and political rebellion firmly on the shoulders of the 'Dogmatical Galenists', whose 'frequent Sanguimissions' and 'deletory Purgations' vitiated the physical 'Organs or Instruments of the Soul' so that 'the mind possessed with melancholy, black, discontented thoughts… becomes forward, peevish, careless of virtuous Actions, desperately bent to follow for divertissement a voluptuous sensual life, or to continue Innovations, Heresies, Schisms, and factious Rebellions, and what not?'[212] The conversion of men like Charleton, Thomson, Collop and Thickens[213] to Helmontianism in the period around 1649 may also have owed something to the congruity of specific elements of van Helmont's medical thinking with contemporary notions surrounding divinely ordained monarchy. One of the chief tenets of Helmontian medicine was its rejection of the practice of phlebotomy or bloodletting, which of course formed the basis of much traditional Galenic therapy. At the same time, the act of regicide was often described as a politico-medical act, a form of 'cruel phlebotomy' that removed the head from the body politic.[214] In both cases, the act of bloodletting was deemed sacrilegious. In van Helmont's eyes, blood was sacrosanct because it acted as the temporary repository of the soul and as a vehicle for the replenishment of the rest of the body. The blood of a divinely ordained king, such as Charles I, was equally sacrosanct, as his many supporters were only too eager to testify both before and after 1649. In the immediate aftermath of his execution, stories rapidly circulated in royalist circles concerning the miraculous cures wrought by articles of clothing that had been dipped in the blood of the executed monarch.[215] If the blood did act as the receptacle of the soul, as van Helmont alleged, then the spilling of such a precious fluid in the case of a divinely approved monarch must have represented the ultimate act of politico-medical sacrilege. At the same time, it may have induced some loyal physicians to abandon Galenism in favour of a new therapeutical model that proscribed the unnecessary shedding of blood.

The psychological impact of the events of the 1640s, culminating in the execution of the King and the creation of a Republic, was not of course limited to former royalists and Anglicans. From the earliest stages of the political crisis that led to civil war and beyond, men and women exploited the relative freedom of the times to explore and expound new ways of understanding the relationship between man, God and the Creation. Often, such voyages of self-discovery were undertaken in private and within the confines of outward conformity to the official religious and political orders of the day. Others have only come to light, as in the case of Alexander Akehurst, when spiritual crisis triggered mental collapse, and the authorities intervened to relieve the unfortunate victim of their post or rank.[216] In many cases, the alliances formed between men who shared the same intellectual interests and visions were distinctively cross-denominational and ignored religious and political fault-lines. In the case of the iatrochemists, the chymical investigation of the natural world seemed to encourage an antipathy toward religious dogmatism and a preference for theological accommodation and moderation. Such eirenicism was implicit in the chymist's reverence for unravelling divine mysteries through contemplation and experiment and seems to have encouraged mutual forbearance rather than animosity among men of different religious and political backgrounds.[217] Typical in this respect was the work of the royalist John Collop, whom we have already encountered as an early convert to Helmontianism. In 1656 he wrote *Medici Catholicon*, a work that in many respects reads like an updated version of Sir Thomas Browne's *Religio Medici*, and which laments the religious confusion and controversy of the age while arguing for a broad-based and consensual resolution of the nation's problems. It also, at times, echoes the later work of George Thomson in suggesting a medico-physical cause for the religious and political ills afflicting the nation, and in the process provides a rationale for the physician as political commentator and activist. Most striking of all, however, is the degree to which Collop subjects himself and his body to figurative anatomy—a highly introspective self-examination that leads him to conclude that he, like the nation at large, contains all division and devilry, 'a masse of antipathies', that can only be resolved through opening one's mind to medical, and by extension religious and political, experimentation. Collop's work represents a remarkable example of the way in which men of outwardly conformist outlooks were able to break through the constraints of tradition and convention in the wake of civil war and regicide and, in the process, promote intellectual and medical innovation.[218]

In an age of such profound divisions, crises and uncertainty, the chymical investigation of nature, coupled with the aspiration of discovering medicines that might heal the minds and bodies of sufferers, thus provided a real incentive to collaborative research that often transcended narrow sectarian or partisan lines. The politicization of medicine that occurred in England in the wake of the civil war was not then a straightforwardly denominational affair. It often produced strange bedfellows, with Roman Catholics working alongside radical puritans, and elicited comments such as those of the Helmontian, John French, who in 1652 defended the right of Catholics, as well as 'those of any other heterodox judgement whatsoever' to practise their faith in peace according 'to their own light'.[219] The study of chymistry in particular would appear to have fostered these sentiments, creating broad alliances that defied the simple categorization of religious identities used both by contemporaries and subsequent generations of historians. It also helps to explain why, five years after the restoration of the monarchy, the Helmontians were able to mount such a powerful challenge to the authority of the collegiate physicians in London in the shape of the 'Society of Chymical Physitians'.

Notes

1. Shakespeare Birthplace Trust Record Office, ER1/1/94 [Sydrak Davenport to John Hall, July 1632].
2. M. Pelling, 'Politics, Medicine, and Masculinity: Physicians and Office-Bearing in Early Modern England', in M. Pelling and S. Mandelbrote (eds), *The Practice of Reform in Health, Medicine, and Science, 1500–2000: Essays for Charles Webster* (Aldershot, 2005), 85.
3. G. Aylmer, *The State's Servants: The Civil Service of the English Republic 1649–1660* (London and Boston, 1973), 276–7. In fairness to Aylmer, he does suggest possible explanations for the commitment of medical men to the republican cause, most notably where he refers to the fact that many of his sample were educated in Scotland and the Netherlands. I discuss these facets of the problem in more detail in chapter 5, where, if anything, they would seem to have more application in helping to explain the creation of a network of politically active medical practitioners *after* the Restoration.
4. Shakespeare Birthplace Trust Record Office, BRU 2/2, 429; BRU 2/3, 58–60, 69–70, 72–4, 82. For a good account of the background to these events and the divided nature of politics in pre-civil war Stratford, see A. Hughes, 'Religion and Society in Stratford-upon-Avon, 1619–1638', *Midland History*, 19 (1994), 58–84. Joan Lane provides a comprehensive discussion of Hall's medical practice and political career in her biography of Hall in the *ODNB*.

5. Others who sat as aldermen include Francis Bannister (Bedford), Peter Baro (Boston), George Birch (Norwich), George Coldwell (Northampton), William Goodridge (Salisbury), William Leverett (Newark), Robert Pell (New Romney) and Walter Southwell (Canterbury). The list could undoubtedly be extended with further research. Of these, the first five all served as mayor. Bannister and Coldwell were certainly puritans. Baro, mayor of Boston in 1610, was a noted Arminian. He also served as a justice of the peace for Lincolnshire. Other physicians to perform the latter role include the clergyman-practitioner, John Favour, who sat on the bench for the West Riding of Yorkshire, Isaac Barrow (Cambridge), and, in all probability all those named as mayor, above, as the role of JP and mayor were usually conflated in this period.
6. There is no evidence to suggest that Yates was ejected from his Norfolk livings, but he may well have taken out a licence to practise medicine from the University of Cambridge in 1629 as a form of insurance against further threats to his position following his principled opposition to Arminianism throughout the 1620s; see Venn, iv, 488; *ODNB*.
7. For Burgess and Leighton see their respective entries in the *ODNB*.
8. Capel resigned his living at Eastington, Gloucestershire, in 1635 following his refusal to read the recently reissued Book of Sports. He promptly secured a licence from the bishop of Gloucester to practise medicine, but, typically, resumed his ministerial function at the outbreak of the civil war. He was later active in the Westminster Assembly of Divines; *ODNB*.
9. Walter Jones (d.1633) was deprived of the living of Benenden in Kent for nonconformity in 1605. He was subsequently licensed to practise medicine in 1611; Venn, ii, 488; I. Mortimer, 'A Directory of Medical Personnel Qualified and Practising in the Diocese of Canterbury, *c.*1560–1730', *Archaeologia Cantiana*, 126 (2006), 156; P. Lake, *Moderate Puritans and the Elizabethan Church* (Cambridge, 1982), 250.
10. Evidence of Newton's unlicensed medical practice emerged alongside evidence of his nonconformity following a prolonged dispute with one of his parishioners, Richard Ball, and his eventual deprivation from the living of Stock in Essex in 1627; LMA, DL/C/314, fos 130, 150v; cited in T. Webster, *Godly Clergy in Early Stuart England: The Caroline Puritan Movement, c.1620–1643* (Cambridge, 1997), 186.
11. Like Capel, Partridge took out an episcopal licence to practise medicine in the diocese of Canterbury in 1626 following his loss of the curacy of Sutton by Dover in the previous year. He subsequently emigrated to New England in 1637; Venn, iii, 316; Raach, 72.
12. Rood, minister of St Helen's, Abingdon, Berkshire, was deprived of his living in 1629, after which he was reported to have turned to the practice of medicine; G. Gulter, *The Archbishops Crueltie, Made Knowne in a True Story of One Mr. Edward Rood* (London, 1641), A3v. Described by one of his opponents as 'a great disturber of the peace and amitie of the town' who preached against the royal supremacy, Rood was later restored, and, according to his widow, was sent by Parliament to preach in Essex, Kent and Suffolk, where he 'won large sums of money, and multitudes of people to their cause'; M. Brod, 'Dissent and Dissenters in Early Modern Berkshire', D. Phil (Oxford, 2002), 76–7; *CSPD, 1654*, 358; *CSPD, 1655*, 156.
13. For the case of the eminent puritan physician Thomas Coxe, see below note 56.
14. Venn, iv, 384; *Cal. Rev.*, 523–4.

15. The suggestion is made by William Birken in his account of Regemorter in the *ODNB*. Regemorter was the son of the pastor of the London Dutch church, Ambrose Regemorter (d.1639), who was staunchly opposed to the ceremonial innovations of the 1630s. Ahaseurus ultimately graduated MD at Leiden in 1635 and was later a prominent member of that group of puritan physicians, centred on Francis Glisson, who were responsible for carrying out pioneering research into the rickets (for which see above 21–2).
16. Drake, who had graduated MD at Leiden in 1640 and was one of the first Englishmen to defend the notion of Harveian circulation, resigned his post as candidate of the London College of Physicians 'with much profession of humility and thanks' on 4 December 1646. Thereafter, he served the London synod in numerous capacities but was forced to resign all offices at the Restoration, when he retired to Stepney and once again resumed his medical practice; *ODNB*; Innes Smith, 72.
17. W. A. Shaw, *A History of the English Church During the Civil Wars and Under the Commonwealth, 1640–1660*, 2 vols (London, 1900), ii, 400. Clarke married the sister of his friend, Samuel Collins (d.1667), the puritan vicar of Braintree, Essex.
18. The Venetian-born physician Jasper Despotine, of Bury St Edmunds, Suffolk, was named as an elder for the eleventh division of the Presbyterian classis in that county. He would appear to have entered England in the train of William Bedell (1572–1642), a learned minister and later Irish bishop, who visited Venice in the early part of the seventeenth century. He was settled at Bury by about 1610–11 and was described in his grant of denization in November 1630 as 'one of the late King's physicians'. He was twice summoned to appear before the London College of Physicians in 1631–2, on the latter occasion following the death of one of his patients, Lady Walsingham. He escaped with a gentle rebuke; Shaw, *op.cit.*, ii, 428; *ODNB*, sub Bedell, William; *CSPD, 1629–1631*, 391; *CSPD, 1619–1623*, 40; RCPL, Annals, iii, fos 116a, 123b. In a pious will, made in December 1648, he left a number of small bequests to local puritan ministers in Suffolk; WSkRO, IC500/1/107/35 [will of Jasper Despotine, doctor of phisicke, 13 December 1648; pr. 2 July 1650].
19. Goodyer was an elder for the thirteenth division of the Presbyterian classis in Suffolk, which met at his hometown of Lavenham. He was well connected to numerous local puritan clergy and gentry. After Cambridge, he studied for his MD at Leiden (1627–31), where he lodged with his kinsman Hugh Goodyear (d.1661), the long-serving pastor to the puritanical English church in the town. In 1663, he returned to Leiden to put Hugh's affairs in order after his death; Shaw, *op.cit.*, ii, 429; ERO, D/DPb T2/21–23 [1646]; Venn, ii, 240; Innes Smith, 98; A. Veenhoff and M. Smolenaars, 'Hugh Goodyear and His Papers', *Transactions of the Lancashire and Cheshire Antiquarian Society*, 95 (1999), 16, 18.
20. Rand was a member of the classis at Godalming, Surrey, in 1648, where he practised medicine. He graduated MD from Groningen in the Netherlands on the same day as his cousin, Samuel, below, on 18 August 1617; Shaw, *op.cit.*, ii, 433; Innes Smith, 189.
21. Rand was elected an elder in the Presbyterian classis at Stockton, county Durham, in December 1645. Having formerly practised in London, where he seems to have worked closely with his former colleague and friend, John Clarke (above), he was appointed town physician at Newcastle-upon-Tyne in 1637. Removed by the royalists in 1643, he

regained his position in 1652, having in the meantime been appointed by the town council of Newcastle to act as one of the four elders assisting the Presbyterian minister of the parish of All Saints, Richard Prideaux; Shaw, *op.cit.*, ii, 369; *ODNB*, sub Rand, Samuel; Innes Smith, 189.

22. Venner, a prolific author of conventional medical works, served as a Presbyterian elder for the classis of Bath in Wiltshire in 1648; Shaw, *op.cit.*, ii, 415. According to Dr Thomas Guidott, Venner's successor at Bath, the memorial that was erected to his memory in the Abbey was more appropriate for a divine than a physician. He also cast aspersions on his vaunted charity and generosity, implying that Venner was not so great a 'Saint' as the author of the inscription would have one believe; *ODNB*; T.Guidott, *A Discourse of the Bathe... With an Account of the Lives, and Character, of the Physicians of Bathe* (London, 1676), 173 [168–73].
23. Glisson was almost certainly the same as the 'Dr Gliston', who was acting as an elder in the parish of Lexden, Colchester, in 1648. Francis Glisson was certainly living in Colchester at the time of the siege in 1648. He was still there in 1657 when Frederick Clodius, the son-in-law of Samuel Hartlib, wrote to Robert Boyle relating a cure for epilepsy that he had recently received from Glisson at Colchester. Three years later Dr Glisson appears on a list of militia commissioners for Essex (alongside the recorder of Colchester, John Shaw). Evidence of Glisson's attachment to the cause of Presbyterianism is doubly interesting since it underscores yet further the distinctively puritan nature of the research team that set about investigating rickets in the 1640s. It also corrects a widespread view, recently articulated in the entry for Glisson in the *ODNB* by Guido Giglioni, that '[i]n the absence of a direct profession of faith, Glisson's tolerant and conciliatory outlook in matters of thought and scarce interest in the theological questions... pertinent to his medical concerns raise the suspicion of an agnostic attitude and of no identification with particular religious sects'. This may have been true of Glisson's later position around the time he wrote *De Natura Substantiae Energeticae* (1672) but would not appear to reflect his earlier beliefs; Shaw, *op.cit.*, ii, 391; Boyle, *Correspondence*, I, 223 [Clodius to Boyle, 7 July 1657]; Firth & Rait, ii, 1431; *ODNB*, sub Glisson, Francis.
24. For Bannister, see Foster, i, 66; Firth & Rait, i, 169, 227, 620, 635, 960, 1077; ii, 293, 461, 656. In a ship money payment made in February 1637, he was described as 'late mayor of Bedford'; *CSPD, 1636–1637*, 436. A close friend of the county grandee Sir William Boteler (1608–1658), Bannister also served as a sequestration commissioner and continued to sit as an alderman in the borough until shortly before his death in the mid-1650s; TNA, PROB 11/252, fos 385v-386r [will of Francis Bannister, doctor of physick, 26 July 1652, pr. 5 February 1655/6]; BL, Add MS 61,681, fo. 107; G. Parsloe (ed.), *The Minute Book of Bedford Corporation 1647–1664* (Luton, Bedfordshire Rec. Soc., vol. 26, 1949), 1, 3, 17, 33, 36, 71, 92. Reade, who studied medicine at Leiden in the early 1630s without graduating, was a member of the Eastern Association and served as physician to the parliamentary armies in the first civil war. His family's strong puritan credentials are suggested by the marriage of his sister, Elizabeth (1614–1672), to John Winthrop Jnr, Governor-General of Massachusetts. Three other siblings emigrated to America in the 1630s; Innes Smith, 190; Venn, iii, 433; A. Kingston, *East Anglia and the Great Civil War: The Rising of Cromwell's Ironsides in the Associated Counties of*

Cambridge, Huntingdon, Lincoln, Norfolk, Suffolk, Essex, and Hertford (London, 1897), 385; TNA, SP 28/11/II, f.17; 28/143, fo. 82. Saunders (MD Oxford 1628) was chosen as a county commissioner for the university and city of Oxford in 1647 and 1648. He was also provost of Oriel College from 1644 till his death in 1653; Foster, iv, 1315; Firth & Rait, i, 973, 1090. Finally, Wright (MD Bourges, incorporated at Oxford, 1638), the brother of the puritan physician Lawrence Wright, was appointed a commissioner for Herefordshire in June 1647, probably through the influence of his old friend, patient and local puritan grandee, Sir Robert Harley of Brampton Bryan. He later served as a militia commissioner for Shropshire as well as acting as personal physician to Cromwell in Scotland. He most likely remained committed to the godly cause after the Restoration when he listed the ejected minister Francis Tallents (1619–1708) among his most trusted friends; Venn, iv, 475; Foster, iv, 1687; Firth & Rait, i, 967, 1084, 1243; *HMC. Fourteenth Report, Appendix, Part II. MSS of the Duke of Portland, vol.3* (London, 1894), 111, 118, 126, 146; TNA, PROB 11/383, fos 176r–177r [will of Nathaniel Wright, doctor in physic, of Shrewsbury, Shropshire, 22 June 1683, pr. 3 May 1686]. I discuss the careers of Barber, Fullwood, Hubbard, King, Staines and Symcotts in more detail below.

25. J. W., *The Royall Entertainment of the King, by the Royalists of Huntingdon* (London, 1645), 4. There is some confusion surrounding both the occupation and identity of Fullwood, who has often been confused with his son of the same name. I discuss these problems more fully below, particularly in relation to the way in which Fullwood, an apothecary by training and background, was able to utilize his political connections to legitimate his burgeoning status as a physician.
26. In discussing the specific example of physicians serving as justices of the peace, Pelling cites some examples, mainly from the later period, and acknowledges its feasibility, but nonetheless stresses the rarity of the practice; Pelling, 'Politics, Medicine and Masculinity', 91–3.
27. Hubbard's long career on the Middlesex bench can be traced in the frequent references to him in the extant quarter sessions records of that county. He last appears in April 1659, probably falling victim later that year to the backlash against the Rump and other supporters of the 'good old cause'; J. C. Jeaffreson (ed.), *Middlesex County Records*, 4 vols (London, Middlesex County Rec. Soc., 1888–92), iii, 99, 102, 178, 182–6, 257, 279. Nothing is known of Hubbard's medical training or qualifications to practise. He is consistently referred to, however, as a 'doctor in physic' in official documents of the time.
28. K. Lindley, 'Whitechapel Independents and the English Revolution', *The Historical Journal*, 41 (1998), 287–8. Hubbard's long engagement with radical puritanism is further suggested by the fact that in November 1639 he was ordered to be committed if he did not appear to answer unspecified charges before the Court of High Commission; *CSPD, 1639–1640*, 273, 278, 284.
29. Jeaffreson, *op.cit.*, iii, p.99; [Thomas Hubbard], *A Briefe and True Relation of the Great Disorders and Riot Attempted and Committed upon the House and Goods of Thomas Hubbert Esquire... in Moore-fields on the 21 Day of March Last* (London, 1647). Hubbard himself clearly saw the attack on his house as an act of reprisal following his raid, a few days earlier, on a tippling house and his arrest of two of the miscreants.

30. Jeaffreson (ed.), *Middlesex County Records*, iii, 99 and *passim*; Anon., *The Ranters' Creed: Being a True Copie of the Examination of a Blasphemous Sort of People, Commonly Called Ranters… Taken Before Thomas Hubbert Esquire* (London, 1651).
31. T. Hubbard, *Pilula ad Expurgandam Hypocrisin. A Pill to Purge Formality. Wherein is Discovered the Sad and Useful Condition of All Formal Professors of Religion* (London, 1650). As the title suggests, this work was largely an attempt to bolster the commonwealth and undermine the supporters of 'Zion-Colledg-Presbytery'.
32. Gabriel Barber Senior was a leading figure in the movement known as the feoffees for impropriations. He was largely responsible for purchasing the advowson of All Saints, Hertford, in 1626 with the intention of uniting it with the living of St John's and creating a bastion of corporate puritanism. He also played a central role, as a founder member of the Providence Island Company, in promoting puritan emigration to Virginia and the Somers Islands. Like his son, he was active as a JP in the town of Hertford; W. C. Metcalfe (ed.), *Visitations of Hertfordshire… 1572… 1634* (London, Harleian Soc., vol. 22, 1886), 25, 107; I. M. Calder, 'A Seventeenth-Century Attempt to Purify the Anglican Church', *American Historical Review*, 53 (1948), 763; D. R. Ransome, 'Wives for Virginia, 1621', *William and Mary Quarterly*, 48 (1991), 8.
33. Venn, i, 81; Kingston, *East Anglia and the Great Civil War*, 386; W. J. Hardy (ed.), *Hertford County Records. Notes and Extracts from the Sessions Rolls 1581 to 1698* (Hertford, 1905), 85; Firth & Tait, i, 119, 170, 231, 243, 289, 294, 356, 622, 638, 967, 1084, 1238; ii, 1325, 1370, 1371, 1432. In 1643, either he or his father wrote from Hertford to Sir William Lenthall, speaker of the House of Commons, providing information on local malignants; *HMC. Thirteenth Report, Appendix, Part 1. The Manuscripts of… the Duke of Portland. Vol.1* (London, 1891), 139–40.
34. *The Weekly Post* (London, 10–17 May 1659), 15 [13 May 1659]. The petition was also published as *The Humble Petition of Divers Inhabitants of the County of Hertford, who have Faithfully Adhered to the Good Old Cause. Presented to Parliament by Dr. Barber… May 13. 1659* (London, 1659).
35. *CSPD, 1665–1666*, 183; Hardy (ed.), *Hertford County Records*, 352. Barber is not to be confused with the Norfolk physician of the same name, who was in all probability a relation. His career followed a remarkably similar trajectory. He served as a JP, commissioner, and sequestrator in Norfolk throughout the 1640s and was named as a JP in a newly expanded jurisdiction in the city of Norwich, incorporating the precinct of the old bishop's palace, in April 1654; nNkRO, Traf 3286 × 5; Green, *CPCC*, i, 172, 229; Firth & Rait, i, 972, 1089, 1240; ii, 40, 305, 473, 492, 671, 1247; *CSPD, 1654*, 97.
36. Foster, ii, 650; Firth and Rait, ii, 119, 299, 468, 664, 1070, 1325. In November 1649 it was reported that the corporation of Hereford 'have made our Governor, Doctor Harford…free of the city & intend to elect [him a member] of the Common Council'; *HMC, Fourteenth Report, Appendix, Part III. Manuscripts of the Duke of Portland, vol.3* (London, 1894), 171. In 1663, he and his physician son Bridstock, the future MP, were described as 'implacable enemies of the King'. He may, however, have had a change of heart as in 1675, on helping to rebuild the city's hospital, he had erected an inscription that read: 'Fear God, honour the King, relieve the poor: these three are all'; Henning, ii, 492–3. Harford's colleague Roger Bosworth (MD Oxford 1643) also served as a commissioner in the 1650s and represented the city of Hereford in Parliament in 1658–9; Foster, i, 153.

37. D. Underdown, *Somerset in the Civil War and Interregnum* (Newton Abbot, 1973), 125, 131, 157, 185, 189. In addition to sitting on numerous committees in his native Somerset, including those concerned with religious and political deviance, Palmer also acted as an assessment and militia commissioner in Oxfordshire in 1659–60; Firth & Rait, i, 853, 1209, 1243; ii, 42, 307, 476, 974, 1040, 1079, 1331, 1332, 1376, 1378; *The Names of the Iustices of Peace, of England and Wales... 1650* (London, 1650), 48.
38. Foster, iii, 1109; Anon., *The Mystery of the Good Old Cause Briefly Unfolded* (London, 1660), 27; A. Clark (ed.), *The Life and Times of Anthony Wood, Antiquary, at Oxford, 1632–1695*, 5 vols (Oxford, Oxford Hist. Soc., 1891–1900), i (1891), 303. He is probably the John Palmer of Taunton, esquire, who headed the list of Presbyterian elders for his respective Somerset classis in 1648; Shaw, *History of the English Church*, ii, 420.
39. Venn, iv, 143; C. H. Cooper, *Annals of Cambridge*, 5 vols (Cambridge, 1842–53), iii, 372, 459; Firth & Rait, i, 621, 637, 961, 962, 1078, 1079; ii, 294, 462, 658, 1063, 1321, 1431 [where he also appears as Richard Stone, doctor of physic]; Thurloe, *State Papers*, iii, 233–5; *CSPD, 1651*, 54; *CSPD, 1652–1653*, 447.
40. CUL, E[ly] D[iocesan] R[ecords], E12 1647, fos 12–12v, 19–1ªA, 44r–v; EDR, E12 indictments 1646; EDR, E12 1647, fos 21, 23. Staines' role as JP in this affair is noted in M. Gaskill, *Witchfinders: A Seventeenth-Century English Tragedy* (London, 2005), 261, 264–5.
41. Thurloe, *State Papers*, v, 328, 352. Staines, like his younger brother and fellow physician William Staines (*c.*1610–1680), was probably a moderate Congregationalist in religion. William Staines' medical and political career is discussed further below, 92–3.
42. Innes Smith, 133; Firth & Rait, i, 119, 170, 231, 243, 294, 539, 622, 638, 639, 745, 967, 1084; ii, 35, 36, 300, 468, 665, 1070, 1325, 1370, 1432; Thurloe, *State Papers*, iv, 573; *CSPD, 1651*, 185. King's Presbyterian sympathies are inferred from the various letters and papers relating to the case to remove him from the bench in Hertfordshire for speaking against Parliament and abusing his office dated *circa* 1652; Wellcome Library, London, MS 6076. He seems to have moved to London some time after the Restoration, and was buried in the parish of St Andrew Undershaft in 1688.
43. Innes Smith, 158; Firth & Rait, i, 706, 964, 1081, 1141, 1245; ii, 34, 298, 465, 662, 1067, 1068 *CSPD, 1651*, 252, 256; *CSPD, 1657–1658*, 348–9. Micklethwaite was almost certainly related to the London Presbyterian Sir John Micklethwaite, who served as president of the London College of Physicians from 1676 to 1681. For the latter, see below 130, 155 n.37.
44. Ward, originally a graduate of Harvard in 1645, was created B Med by favour of Fairfax in November 1649; Foster, iv, 1569. Whitmore, who was granted his Oxford MD in February 1649 on the recommendation of the general, later claimed to have been active as a physician in Staffordshire and Shropshire during the civil war; ibid., iv, 1622; H. Whitmore, *Febris Anomala or, The New Disease that Now Rageth Throughout England* (London, 1659). Other examples of 'political' promotions at Oxford at this time include Daniel Malden, who, after studying medicine briefly at Leiden in 1648, was made MD in 1649, and the surgeon, Thomas Trapham, created B Med in the same year. Malden was said to have 'engaged himself and shed blood for the Parliament'. I discuss Trapham's colourful career in more detail, above 54–5. For Malden, see Foster, iii, 961; Innes Smith, 151; Wood, *Fasti*, ii, 122.

45. Allen (d.1665) and Lavender (d.1650) both received the imprimatur of Fairfax in seeking the post of surgeon to St Thomas's Hospital in 1649; F. G. Parsons, *The History of St Thomas's Hospital*, 2 vols (London, 1934), ii, 71–6, 264. Allen was finally elected in 1652 and served until his death in 1665. Lavender's career was cut short by his death in 1650. A resident of the radical puritan enclave of St Stephen's, Coleman Street, he was a prominent member of John Goodwin's congregation in that parish and was seemingly well versed in theological matters. In his will, he bequeathed to his brothers a library of printed divinity books as well as 'all my manuscripts of divinity'; TNA, PROB 11/215, fos 98r–v [will of Bartholomew Lavender, 4 May 1650; pr. 28 January 1650/1]. Atkinson's reward for medical services rendered to Fairfax during the civil war was the receipt of a prestigious licence to practise surgery from the University of Oxford in October 1646; Foster, i, 41; Bodl., OUA, Register of Congregation, 1647–1659: NEP/supra/Reg Qa, fos 157r–v. Atkinson continued to serve the state in the 1650s. In 1651, he was surgeon to the garrison at Gloucester. Two years later, he was helping to organize medical services on the east coast of England in 1653, and in 1654 was present in the Scottish campaign. On the latter occasion, he was assisted by a surgeon's mate called Thomas Fairfax; GRO, P154/14 IN 1/1 [parish registers of St Michael's, Gloucester, 1553–1663; see burial of two daughters, 21 June and 15 July 1651]; *CSPD, 1653–1654*, 475, 498, 506, 509; *CSPD, 1655–1656*, 113–14. Some time in the 1650s, Atkinson (d.1665) settled in Aldersgate Street, London, where he entertained an old comrade-in-arms and preacher, John Knowles. Both men were prominent members of the circle of the Socinian John Biddle (d.1662), who was a native of Gloucester; H. J. McLachlan, *Socinianism in Seventeenth-Century England* (Oxford, 1951), 267, 273, 275. Shortly before his death, he received a licence to practise surgery from the archbishop of Canterbury in February 1664. On this occasion, Atkinson was able to count on the support of a number of very well connected and prominent physicians, including Cromwell's muster-master general, William Staines (for whom, see below note 63); LPL, FII/4/2; F1/C, fo. 151v.
46. Molins (d.1663), who had succeeded his father as surgeon to St Thomas' Hospital, Southwark, in 1639, was dismissed by order of the House of Commons in January 1644 'for that he was lately taken in arms at Arundell Castle against the Parliament'. In the early stages of the civil war a large amount of ammunition was discovered together with '2 great pieces of ordnance, one culverin, one great murdering-piece, and four small brass murdering-pieces' at Molins' house in Baldwin's Garden's, near Gray's Inn. Molins himself was reported to be with the King at the time; *ODNB*, sub Molins, Edward; Parsons, *History of St Thomas's Hospital*, ii, 45, 64; *A True and Exact Diurnall of the Proceedings in Parliament* [22–29 August 1642] (London, 1642), 4.
47. Edward Emily (1617–1657) served as physician to the parliamentary forces in the civil war, having previously graduated MD from Leiden in 1640 (incorporated at Oxford 1647). A licentiate of the London College of Physicians, he held the office of senior physician at St Thomas' Hospital, London, from 1652 until his death in 1657. His loyalty to the Cromwellian state was, however, questionable. In 1656, he gave the first Harveian oration at the College, and used it as an opportunity to vent his opposition to the civil and military government of the day; Innes Smith, 79; Foster, ii, 462; *ODNB*, sub Emily, Edward. He may have served in Ireland under the royalist Inchiquin. In August 1649, one Dr Edward Emerly, advocate to the troops in Munster, was paid arrears;

Commons' Journal, vol.6, 282. I discuss the career of Gurdon more fully, below note 52. King (1587–1664?), who enlisted a horse for the army's use in 1642, is first recorded as surgeon at St Bartholomew's Hospital in 1643. He retired due to worsening eyesight in 1656; R. J. Dalton, 'Gerrard Winstanley: The Experience of Fraud 1641', *The Historical Journal*, 34 (1991), 975–6, 977–8, 978–9. Another of King's sons-in-law, Giles Hicks, was recommended to the post of surgeon to St Thomas' Hospital by the parliamentarian general Robert Rich, Lord Warwick, in February 1644; Parsons, *History of St Thomas's Hospital*, ii, 70.

48. *CSPD, 1650*, 102, 575; *CSPD, 1652–1653*, 235, 505.
49. *ODNB*, sub Whistler, Daniel; C. Webster, *The Great Instauration: Science, Medicine and Reform 1626–1660* (London, 1975), 82, 519. Whistler's Leiden MD of 1645 was incorporated at Oxford in 1647; Innes Smith, 247. Goddard served as physician in chief to the parliamentary armies, accompanying Cromwell to Ireland and Scotland in the early 1650s. He was rewarded with the office of warden of Merton College, Oxford, and subsequently sat as MP in the Barebones Parliament of 1653 as well as acting as a member of the Council of State for much of the 1650s. Goddard was also appointed to the professorship in physic at Gresham College; *ODNB*, sub Goddard, John. Bathurst too served in Parliament, representing Richmond in Yorkshire in 1656–8 and 1659; *ODNB*, sub Bathurst, John.
50. Scroope was made a fellow of All Souls College, Oxford, in 1649, and was granted his bachelor's degree in medicine by special dispensation in January 1650; Foster, iv, 1327. Others, such as the unqualified medical practitioner Daniel Border, sought the patronage of powerful men like the regicide, John Bradshaw, to whom he dedicated one of his medical self-help manuals; for Border, see above 23, 37 n.36.
51. St John was awarded an MD from Padua in 1640, having earlier enrolled at Franeker as a medical student in May 1638. He was dead by June 1660, when his brother, Oliver, was ordered to bring to the Treasury commissioners 'the Trial Pieces for gold and silver, lately in the custody of Dr John St John, deceased'; *ODNB*, sub St John, Oliver; Innes Smith, 203; S. J. Fockema Andraea and T. J. Meijer (eds), *Album Studiosorum Academiae Franekerensis (1585–1811, 1816–1844)* (Franeker, 1968), 111; *CSPD, 1644–1645*, 75; *CSPD, 1652–1653*, 9; *Calendar of Treasury Books, 1660–1667* (London, 1904), 2.
52. Originally from Jersey, Gurdon or Gourdain was educated at Cambridge, where he was also awarded a licence to practise medicine in 1632. He would appear to have possessed godly connections as suggested by his appointment to act as tutor to a young Anthony Ashley Cooper. Gurdon gained his MD from Rheims in 1634 and subsequently settled in London, where he came to the attention of the College of Physicians in the early 1640s for illicit practice. He was probably a Helmontian by medical inclination. Gurdon was still in post as Master of the Mint in July 1660, when royalist intriguers were actively seeking his removal. At the time of his original appointment in 1649, he had been the subject of much vilification in the royalist press which had mocked his physical appearance (he had apparently lost an eye) and poked fun at his pretensions to sainthood as a member of Cromwell's inner circle; Venn, ii, 208; K. H. D. Haley, *The First Earl of Shaftesbury* (Oxford, 1968), 12; RCPL, Annals, iii, fos 208a, 217a; *CSPD, 1645–1647*, 343; *CSPD, 1650*, 168; *The Names of the Iustices of Peace… 1650*, 22

[Essex], 26 [Hertfordshire], 29 [Kent], 35 [Middlesex], 55 [Surrey]; Royal Society, B[oyle] P[apers] 25, 153 [entry in Robert Boyle's work diary for 24 September 1655, containing Gurdon's 'specificke' for pleurisy, which in typical Helmontian fashion shunned the classic resort to bloodletting]; Webster, *Great Instauration*, 296–7, 404; *CSPD, 1660–1661*, 138; TNA, E178/6313; Anon., *A Most Learned, Conscientious, and Devout-Exercise; held forth the last Lords-Day, at Sir Peter Temples, in Lincolnes-Inne-Fields; by Lieut-Generall Crumwell. As it was Faithfully Taken Down in Characters by Aaron Guerdon* (London, 1649); *Mercurius Elencticus*, no. 5 [21–18 May 1649], 38–9.

53. Innes Smith, 177; Aylmer, *State's Servants*, 276; Firth & Rait, i, 705, 1011; ii, 20, 87, 422, 471, 668, 823, 1277, 1350, 1353–4, 1417, 1424. Parker's career has often been confused with that of the doctor of the same name who graduated MD from Padua in 1658. Our William Parker was almost certainly another physician-administrator who owed his appointment as excise commissioner and county committeeman for Middlesex and Yorkshire to his radical religious and political associations. His wife was later a Quaker sympathizer; *ODNB*, sub Parker, John; T. Ellwood, *The History of the Life of Thomas Ellwood... The Second Edition* (London, 1714), 248–50.

54. Foster, i, 363; Innes Smith, 60; Thurloe, *State Papers*, iii, 614–15. The most notable feature of this testimonial, is, I think, Cudworth's reference to the benefits of foreign travel, which imbued the young traveller with a greater understanding of European culture and politics. Cummins had in fact spent time at Padua and Leiden in 1646–7 and was reported to have only recently returned 'from forrain parts' in 1655. As Aylmer noted, the possession of an overseas medical degree was a common denominator among a large number of those medics he identified as active in government in the 1650s. My much larger sample discussed in this chapter would appear to confirm this observation; Aylmer, *State's Servants*, 276–7.

55. Bodl., Rawlinson MS B 239, nos 527, 567. Coxe's connections in Hampshire extended to the fact that his younger brother, Henry, held the living of Bishopstoke in that county from which he was ejected in 1660. Coxe was also proposed by Hartlib as a suitable professor for a new college at Winchester to be funded by the parliamentarian general, Sir William Waller; Birken, 'Dissenting Tradition', 207; *Cal. Rev.*, 139; SUL, HP 47/9/33A–B [undated].

56. *ODNB*. Coxe's early attraction to puritanism and a career in the church have previously evaded his biographers. In 1639, the Lord Mayor of London, Sir Morris Abbott, certified that he had taken Coxe's oath of allegiance and supremacy to the crown. At the same time, the master and eight fellows of Emmanuel College, Cambridge, provided a certificate of his good behaviour, describing him as an MA who, 'during the seven years of his residence there... gave such diligent attention to good letters as to make them hope that his studies would turn to the glory of God and the welfare of the Church'; *CSPD, 1638–1639*, 525, 529. That Coxe had intended to follow a different career path is also suggested by the comment of one of his patients in 1662, the former Independent, John Ellis (d.1681), who affirmed that he was 'designed formerly for another study [but] rather chose the power of herbs to know, And that good Art, whence health to man doth grow'; J. Ellis, *S. Austin Imitated: Or Retractions and Repentings in Reference unto the Late Civil and Ecclesiastical Changes in the Nation... in II Books* (London, 1662), 364.

57. Munk, i, 247; *ODNB*. Though his army career is not thought to have begun until 1643, he is probably the Dr Coxe mentioned in a pro-parliamentary letter from Warwick, dated 27 October 1642, in which he is said to have witnessed the battle of Edge Hill four days earlier; Anon., *Speciall Newes from the Army at Warwicke since the Fight: Sent from a Minister of Good Note, to an Alderman Here in London* (London, 1642), A2r. Among other achievements, Coxe is said to have been instrumental in persuading his army colleague and puritan friend, Thomas Sydenham, to take up medicine. Sydenham, like Coxe, utilized his religious and political connections in the 1650s in the search for preferment. From 1655 until 1660, he served as comptroller of the pipe in the Upper Exchequer. He also sought, unsuccessfully, to obtain a seat in Parliament in 1658 and 1659.
58. Innes Smith, 203 [and note 51 above]. St John invested with a consortium in the purchase of land at Belchamp St Paul's, Essex, formerly in the possession of St Paul's Cathedral.
59. Henry Cleere Snr and Jnr both held the rank of captain in the parliamentary armies, serving as surgeons in various campaigns. In 1651, when they were living at Islington in Middlesex, they purchased former crown estates in Buckinghamshire, Cumberland and Surrey. They subsequently retired to Hampton Wick after the Restoration, when both men, their families and servants were frequently prosecuted for attending Presbyterian conventicles at nearby Kingston upon Thames; I. Gentles, 'The Debentures Market and Military Purchases of Crown Land, 1649–1660', Ph. D. (London, 1969), 267; Kingston Museum and Heritage Service, Kingston, KE2/7/5; 2/7/12/1; 2/7/15/7. One Henry Cleere, of Hampton, Middlesex, was licensed to practise surgery in the dioceses of London and Winchester in 1635; LPL, Laud, 1, fo. 228.
60. Like the Cleeres, Dawberne served as a surgeon in the civil war. In the 1650s, he was described as 'esquire' and living at Walton, Surrey. According to Gentles, he acted as one of the agents in the purchases made by Colonel Okey's regiment, in which he had formerly served. In 1652, he received, with Okey, 123 acres of a former royal estate in Bedfordshire, and the following year bought Dorney House in Surrey from the officers of Colonel Ingoldby's regiment for £182; Gentles, 'Debentures Market', 273.
61. Hubbard, who as we have already seen was ideologically committed to the cause of godly reform in church and state (above 48–9), was appointed one of the thirteen trustees to implement the Act for the Sale of Crown Lands in 1649. He subsequently bought a small parcel of Theobald's Park in Hertfordshire for £200, which he later re-sold to John Spencer and Major Edmund Rolfe; Gentles, 'Debentures Market', 56n, 169; *Commons' Journal*, vi, 246, 259.
62. Peter Salanova (Sallenove, Sellaneuve), of Weymouth, Dorset, served as a surgeon in the garrisons of Weymouth and Melcombe Regis. He had previously operated as an apothecary in the service of the western forces. He purchased crown lands in the 1650s in partnership with two other men, William Murford and Daniel Henchman, but later sold out to Murford; Gentles, 'Debentures Market', 274.
63. Staines (d.1680), like Thomas Coxe, was a student at puritan Emmanuel College, Cambridge, where he graduated MD in 1639. After briefly falling foul of the College authorities in London, he was admitted as a candidate in December 1639 and was elected a fellow in October 1641. During the civil war, he served as commissary general

of musters in the northern army, a position to which he was re-appointed in July 1659. In 1652, he purchased the former royal manor of St Florence, Pembroke, for £689, as well as estates in his native Essex. Despite falling under a brief cloud in 1650, when officers in the army were asked to confer with the government 'concerning Dr Stane', whose loyalty and affection to the government was a cause for concern, he would appear to have retained the confidence of those in power. In 1653, he was ordered to sort through the Scottish records in the Tower of London (presumably in connection with the Cromwellian annexation of Scotland), and in 1658 wore mourning at Cromwell's funeral. A year later he was elected MP for Thetford in Norfolk. An Independent in religion, he donated £200 to the London dissenters' subscription to the crown in 1670. He remained committed to the nonconformist cause until the end of his life. In his will, he asked that provision be made for poor ministers that 'labour in the Word and Gospell' and made individual bequests to Dr John Owen (1616–1683) and his Leadenhall Street meeting as well as fellow Congregationalists George Griffiths and John Collins; Venn, iv, 143; Munk, i, 231–2; Gentles, 'Debentures Market', 339; *CSPD, 1650*, 171; *CSPD, 1653–1654*, 194; *CSPD, 1658–1659*, 131; *CSPD, 1659–1660*, 57; G. S. de Krey, *London and the Restoration 1659–1683* (Cambridge, 2005), 410; TNA, PROB 11/362, fo. 323v [will of William Stane, doctor of physic of the College of Physitians London, 2 February 1679/80, pr. 24 March 1679/80]. For Staines' brother, Richard, who shared his religious and political sympathies, see above 50–51.

64. Symonds served as surgeon to the earl of Essex's regiment of horse, as well as the regiments of Colonel Sheffield and Colonel Harrison, in the civil war. He is probably the same as the Thomas Symon who was nominated as surgeon to Colonel Alured's regiment of horse in September 1659, and confirmed as appointed in the following month following the army's expulsion of the Rump; Gentles, 'Debentures Market', 342; *CSPD, 1659–1660*, 202, 243. As a civilian after the Restoration, he maintained close links with former colleagues. The parliamentary surgeon Edward Atkinson, for example (see note 45 above), described him as a 'loving friend' and named him as one of the executors of his will, entrusting the education and upbringing of his only son, Thomas, to Symonds (then of Friday Street, London) in 1664; TNA, PROB 11/317, fos 103r–v [will of Edward Atkinson, surgeon, of Aldersgate Street, St Botolph Aldersgate, London, 27 December 1664; pr. 13 July 1665].

65. Troutbeck, who defected to his old friend Monck in 1659, claimed compensation at the Restoration for crown lands in Yorkshire which he had purchased from Adam Baynes and Adam and Joseph Eyre in 1653; Gentles, 'Debentures Market', 237, 346. For Troutbeck's career and radical medical and religious beliefs, See Appendix 1 (a).

66. Trigge (d.1665), who had been a persistent thorn in the side of the London medical authorities in the 1630s and 1640s, seems to have made a fortune selling his remedies and nostrums. Large amounts were re-invested in the purchase of former crown lands in Theobalds Park, Hertfordshire, all of which was lost at the Restoration. The Restoration cleric and chymical physician, John Ward, claimed that Trigge had told him that he had lost between four and six thousand pounds in this adventure. A resident of Tower Hamlets, his radical political leanings are further suggested by his appointment in July 1659, along with Sir Henry Vane and others, to the militia committee of his local neighbourhood; RCPL, Annals, iii, fos 103b, 106a, 110a–b, 135a,

150a, 169b, 173b, 189a, 189b, 207b, 208a; *CSPD, 1637–1638*, 2; Gentles, 'Debentures Market', 168, 346; FSL, V.a.292, f.21v; iii, 565; *CSPD, 1651–1652*, 550; *The Weekly Post*, no. 11 (12–19 July 1659), 94; Firth & Rait, ii, 1308; R. Barker, *Consilium Anti-Pestilentiale* (London, 1665), 5.

67. For a succinct summary of the medical situation in Ireland in the 1650s, and the role of men like Petty, Worsley and the Boates, see T. Barnard, *Cromwellian Ireland: English Government and Reform in Ireland 1649–1660* (Oxford, 1975), 240–2. All four were prominent members of the circle of Samuel Hartlib. Others with medical interests or qualifications, similarly indebted or linked to Hartlib and Ireland, include Robert Wood and Sir Anthony Morgan; ibid., 224, 236 and *passim*. To this list we might also add Robert Whitehall (d.1685), who was awarded his bachelor's degree in medicine at Oxford following support from Richard Cromwell in 1657. At the same time, he was also recommended to his brother, Henry, who was asked to find him suitable work in Ireland. Whitehall subsequently taught school at Limerick; Foster, iv, 1619; P. Toon (ed.), *The Correspondence of John Owen (1616–1683)* (Cambridge & London, 1970), 100; BL, Lansdowne MS 822, fo. 166.
68. Foster, iv, 1579 [who mistakenly refers to him as John]; BL, Lansdowne MS 823, fos 58, 282, 284, 285; *CSPD, 1651*, 182; A. Clarke, *Prelude to Restoration in Ireland: The End of the Commonwealth, 1659–1660* (Cambridge, 1999), 178 and n.
69. Goldsmith, who held a B Med from Cambridge, was twice cited before the College of Physicians in London in the 1630s for illicit practice. During the civil war, he served the parliamentary garrison at Plymouth, before enlisting to serve in Ireland in January 1652; Venn, ii, 230; RCPL, Annals, iii, fos 133b, 200a; R. N. Worth, 'The Siege Accounts of Plymouth, *Transactions of the Devonshire Association*, 17 (1885), 227; *CSPD, 1651–1652*, 114, 132.
70. Edwards would appear to have been an unqualified practitioner, who combined a career in medicine (he was physician to the precinct of Trim in 1655) with both legal and clerical duties. Among other things, he served as a master in the Irish Court of Chancery as well as officiating as a minister at Navan in 1658. In April 1653 he was rewarded for his service to the Commonwealth government with a grant of lands in the precinct of Tredagh; Barnard, *Cromwellian Ireland*, 288; Representative Church Body Library, Dublin, GS 2/7/3/20, 53, 57, 65, 77, 95, 100, 106, 121; National Library of Ireland, Dublin, MS 11,959, 224.
71. Carteret possessed a Leiden MD (1645) and served in the administration of Ireland throughout much of the 1650s. There, he was on friendly terms with numerous radicals as well as John Thurloe in England. Henry Cromwell, however, would appear to have been suspicious of his radical leanings, describing him in March 1658 as an 'Anabaptist'. He was in fact a Baptist and the son-in-law of Colonel Richard Lawrence (d.1684). At the Restoration, Cartaret returned to England with a commendation from Cromwell and would appear to have settled into medical practice at Southampton. He is not to be confused with Sir Philip Carteret, FRS; PROB 11/341, fo. 338v [will of Philip Carteret, doctor of physic, of Southampton, Hampshire, 30 September 1671; pr. 24 April 1673]; Innes Smith, 42; National Library of Ireland, MS 11,961, 190–1; Green, *CPCC*, iii, 1910–1911; Thurloe, *State Papers*, iii, 141; iv, 349; v, 45; vi, 552; vii, 21, 639; Clarke, *Prelude*, 105.

72. *Mercurius Elencticus*, nos 10 [25 June–2 July 1649], 74; 11 [2–9 July 1649], 88; 12 [9–16 July 1649], 93. The same newspaper reported that Cromwell was also to be accompanied by Dr Jonathan Goddard (d.1675), 'the Holborne mountebank', who was subjected to similar ridicule. However, on this occasion, the correspondent would appear to have confused Jonathan Goddard with the chymical physician William Goddard, who was a resident of the parish of St Andrew Holborn. For Jonathan Goddard, see above, note 49. For William Goddard, see Appendix 1 (a). Whether Chamberlen did embark for Ireland is not recorded. However, he certainly possessed connections there and visited the country on at least two occasions in the 1660s. In 1666, he was lodging with 'one of the heads of the Dutch church' in Dublin, and two years later his return from Ireland, via Chester, was recorded by a government agent in the city; *CSPD, 1665–1666*, 332; *CSPD, 1668–1669*, 497, 498.
73. Foster, iv, 1503; *CSPD, 1644–1645*, 25; *CSPD, 1652–1653*, 320; *CSPD, 1657–1658*, 269; *CSPD, 1658–1659*, 41, 319; Gentles, 'Debentures Market', 346. Trapham held the post of surgeon to the Savoy Hospital in London. In his capacity as surgeon there, he was thanked by Thomas Wharton, who described him as 'chirurgo expertissimo', for his contribution to that physician's ground-breaking work on the glands, *Adenographia: sive, Glandularum Totius Corporis Descriptio* (London, 1656).
74. J. Pordage, *Innocencie Appearing, Through the Dark Mists of Pretended Guilt. Or, A Full and True Narration of the Unjust and Illegal Proceedings of the Commissioners of Berks... against John Pordage of Bradfield* (London, 1655), 20, 94, 103; Trapham's role as a 'strong and aggressive Presbyterian' on various county committees is discussed more fully in M. Brod, *Abingdon Area Archaeological and Historical Society Newsletter* (Spring 2005), 6–7 and *idem*, 'Dissent and Dissenters in Early Modern Berkshire', 87, 94.
75. *CSPD, 1660–1661*, 382, 481; WSA, D1/54/5, fo. 1r; G. C. Peachey, 'Thomas Trapham—Cromwell's Surgeon—and Others', *Proceedings of the Royal Society of Medicine*, 24 (1931), 1448. Trapham lived in the parish of St Helen's, Abingdon, which was also home to another former Cromwellian medic, Dr Tobias Garbrand (d.1689). He was ejected as principal of Gloucester Hall, Oxford, at the Restoration when he turned to the practice of medicine. Like Trapham, he and his wife were also harried by the authorities for refusing to attend their local parish church; Foster, ii, 546; *Cal. Rev.*, 217; WSA, D1/54/5, fo. 1v.
76. *HMC. Thirteenth Report, Appendix, Part 1. MSS of the Duke of Portland. Vol. 1*, 76; CUL, MS Mm.I.45 [Baker MS 35], 44–5; Venn, ii, 22; Another Cambridge medical student to share Deantry's loyalism was Thomas Shawberry (d.1643), who in March 1642 was called to the bar of the House of Commons to answer accusations that he had called the parliamentary leader 'King Pym' and had threatened to 'cut him in pieces if he had him'. Fined and briefly imprisoned, order was given to write to the University to bar his admission to a degree. At the outbreak of the civil war, he departed for the royalist headquarters at Oxford, where he died the following year; *Commons' Journal*, ii, 478; V. F. Snow and A. S. Young (eds), *Private Journals of the Long Parliament*, 3 vols (New Haven and London, 1982–92), ii (7 March–1 June 1642) 39, 42, 43; Cooper, *Annals of Cambridge*, iii, 319–20; Oxfordshire RO, PAR 213/1/R1/1 [parish registers of St Peter's in the East, Oxford, 1559–1653; burial, 22 November 1643].

77. For Deantry's various attempts to secure preferment and reward at the Restoration, see *CSPD, 1660–1661*, 23, 221, 393, 425, 563. In addition to his appointment as a royal physician, Deantry was made an honorary fellow of the London College of Physicians and later claimed the title of royal physician to the Tower of London; TNA, LC3/25, fo. 51; LC3/26, fo. 141v; Munk, i, 332; LPL, VX 1A/10/40. He served in London during the plague, producing a graphic picture of the hopeless state of contemporary medical services in a work which he co-authored with fellow physician, Nicholas Davis, entitled *The Resolution of Those Physitians Presented by the Colledge to the Right Honourable the Lord Mayor and Court of Aldermen...for the Prevention and Cure of the Plague* (London, 1665).
78. Thurloe, *State Papers*, iii, 662. Barton was later prosecuted for recusancy in 1681; Jeaffreson (ed.), *Middlesex County Records*, iv, 151.
79. Thurloe, *State Papers*, iii, 243–4, 322–4, 407–9. The interrogations reveal that the authorities were clearly of the opinion that Wiseman's intercepted letters contained evidence of medical cant, i.e. the use of medical terminology to disguise ulterior political motives. They also suggest another feature of the increasingly politicized nature of medical practice at this time, namely Wiseman's fear that if he should reveal his sources 'it would cleere mee, but ruine my reputation amongst those of the royall partie, in whom my livelihood consisted'. For an overview of Wiseman's career, see *ODNB*.
80. For Knight, see *ODNB*, which refers to his serving the court in exile where he mixed 'light espionage with medical duties'. Painter was described in 1655 as one of a number of 'intelligencers', who sent weekly newsletters to exiled royalists; *CSPD, 1655*, 193. Richard Pyle was denounced as 'the agent for the King in the West' in 1655. He almost certainly used his family connections in Hampshire in 1651, and again in 1655, to foment support for royalist uprisings, and was again implicated in abortive attempts to stir up a royalist insurrection in Sussex and Kent in 1658; *HMC. Thirteenth Report, Appendix, Part 1: MSS of the Duke of Portland, vol. 1*, 583; Thurloe, *State Papers*, iii, 344–5, 429; vii, 98.
81. Tudor, who was reported to have been involved in royalist conspiracies in France in early 1654, narrowly escaped capture at Norwich later the same year, only to be seized at Shimpling Hall. He was engaged at the time in collecting money from royalist sympathizers in the county. Committed to custody for having a hand in recent plotting, he subsequently escaped; Thurloe, *State Papers*, ii, 353, 508.
82. Barton, Tudor and Wiseman obtained posts as surgeon to the king; TNA, LC 3/24, fo. 24; LC 3/26, fo. 144. Knight, Painter and Pyle were all rewarded in February 1661 with the most prestigious office for a royal surgeon, that of sergeant surgeon to the king; TNA, LC 3/24, fo. 16. Any collegial goodwill generated by the men's shared commitment to the royal cause in the 1650s soon evaporated, however, at the Restoration. The state papers recount in some detail the unseemly squabbling between these men over primacy of place at the court of Charles II; see for example *CSPD, 1660–1661*, 556; *CSPD, 1661–1662*, 484–5. In addition to these men, we might add John Watson, who petitioned for the post of sergeant surgeon in 1660 on the grounds that his father had previously held this post, and for his own sufferings in the civil war, when he was

'almost ruined by imprisonment, plundering, sequestering, and decimating'. He was appointed surgeon in ordinary supernumerary, without fee, in July 1660; *CSPD, 1660–1661*, 210; TNA, LC 3/26, fo. 144.

83. J. F. Merritt, *Westminster 1640–60: A Royal City in a Time of Revolution* (Manchester & New York, 2013), 151; E. L. Furdell, *The Royal Doctors, 1485–1714: Medical Personnel at the Tudor and Stuart Courts* (Rochester, NY, 2001), 182–3.
84. *ODNB*; HLRO, HL/PO/JO/10/1/122; *CSPD, 1655*, 250 [Hinton's certificate on behalf of John Spencer, previously in arms for the late King, but now compounded]. In the popular press, Hinton was accused in 1642 of drawing up a petition 'in the behalfe of the bishops' as well as 'carrying the same up and downe to the Innes of Court, and other places, to get hands to it'; *Diurnall Occurrences in Parliament* [3–10 January 1642] (London, 1642), 4; ibid., [10–17 January 1642] (London, 1642), Ar. The tactic of using sympathetic co-religionist doctors to provide one with medical certificates as well as passes to leave the country on health grounds was widely used by Roman Catholics in England before the civil wars, and again during periods of intermittent crisis such as those generated by the Popish Plot. Hinton's kinsman Anthony Hinton (1617–1678), a London apothecary, acted as postmaster for royalist spies. He was captured, imprisoned and confessed in 1656; N. Akkerman, *Invisible Agents: Women and Espionage in Seventeenth-Century Britain* (Oxford, 2018), 100–2.
85. For Barwick, an indefatigable supporter of Anglicanism in the 1650s whose patients seem to have been drawn exclusively from the upper echelons of royalist and Anglican circles, see my entry in *ODNB*.
86. Bowles, who practised at Oundle in Northamptonshire, was a medical graduate of Leiden (MD 1641). His impeccable Anglican credentials are neatly advertised in the story told of him that he cured a parliamentary captain suffering from dysentery by administering the torn leaves of the Book of Common Prayer boiled in milk. After the Restoration, he also remembered those who suffered with him and tried where possible to provide assistance. In 1660, for example, he supplied a testimonial on behalf of Henry Frere, B Med, who was seeking a vacant fellowship at Cambridge. Frere was the son of Thomas Frere, rector of Whitwell, Rutland, who had suffered imprisonment alongside Bowles before the Restoration; Innes Smith, 2; R. T. Gunther, *Early Science in Cambridge* (Oxford, 1937), 267; *CSPD, 1660–1661*, 349.
87. Buchanan, the son of a clergyman, was a London apothecary who described himself as doctor of physic. He was reported in government newspapers in August 1659 as having been arrested in a house near Lincoln's Inn on suspicion of involvement in a recent royalist insurrection at the spa town of Tunbridge in Kent; *The Loyall Scout* (London, 1659) [5–12 August 1659], 124; *The Weekly Post* (London, 1659) [9–16 August 1659], 122. For spas as a suitable site for insurgency and plotting, providing yet further evidence of the growing politicization of medicine at this time, see below 193–4.
88. Consett (d.1673), variously described as practitioner and doctor of physic, suffered sequestration for delinquency and being in arms against Parliament in 1649. At the Restoration, he published two volumes of mediocre verse extolling the return of King and Church while lamenting the miserable depredations suffered by the nation in the

1640s and 1650s. He subsequently served as vicar of Bossall, Yorkshire, from 1666 until his death in 1673; Green, *CPCC*, iii, p.2048; J. Consett, *The Olive Branch, or The Miraculous Restauration of Peace, both to Church and State in Great Britain and Ireland* (London, 1660); *idem*, *The Rod of Recompence* (London, 1660); Venn, i, 380.

89. For the picaresque adventures of the physician and cavalier poet, Henry Hughes, which included attempts to infiltrate the inner circles of the exiled court to offer his services as a spy, see *ODNB*.
90. Jackson, who was said by Anthony Wood to have been 'in the old king's service at Colchester, and in the service of this king' (presumably in exile), was made an MD at Oxford by decree in 1661; Foster, ii, 796; Wood, *Fasti*, ii, 255. He practised at Nantwich in Cheshire after the Restoration.
91. Whitewell, who practised at Salisbury in Wiltshire, was implicated in the planning of Penruddock's rising in 1655. One witness, who was present at Penruddock's house a few days before the insurgency, claimed to have overheard Whitewell and his fellow conspirators 'talke of what sport they should have on Monday, and... of what they would dow with the [assize] judges'; Thurloe, *State Papers*, iii, 295. Among those implicated with Whitewell was the Salisbury apothecary, Edmund Mackes (d.1675). Like Jackson, Whitewell was rewarded for his pains at the Restoration with a mandated degree from Cambridge. Testimonials vouching for his deserving loyalty were signed, among others, by the prebend of Salisbury Humphrey Henchman; Venn, iv, 397; *CSPD, 1660–1661*, 147. For Henchman's role in promoting the cause of the Society of Chemical Physicians in 1665, see below 127–9.
92. As noted above, Jackson and Whitewell were granted MDs, while Barwick and Bowles were both made physicians in ordinary supernumerary to Charles II in June 1660; TNA, LC 3/2, fo. 23v; LC 3/25, fo. 51; LC 3/26, fo. 141.
93. Bispham (MD Leiden 1628), who claimed in 1660 to be the last surviving physician to Charles II's father, petitioned in that year for the post of chancellor of the diocese of Chester, which he claimed had been originally promised to him by the King on reversion in 1635. The death of the last incumbent in 1647, and the 'distractions of the times', precluded his appointment. Despite his frequent protestations, he does not appear to have succeeded in any of his aims, including re-appointment as a royal physician; Innes Smith, 22; Foster, i, 131; *CSPD, 1659–1660*, 84, 423.
94. Foster, iii, 997; Wood, *Ath. Ox.*, iii, 342; Wood, *Fasti*, ii, 98. There is no evidence that Meade actually practised medicine.
95. *ODNB*, sub Whitaker, Tobias; Innes Smith, 247; Thurloe, *State Papers*, ii, 434; vii, 247; *CSPD, 1653–1654*, 96; TNA, LC 3/24, fo. 16. Whitaker, who practised at Norwich, Ipswich, and London before the civil war, possessed an MD from Leiden (1624). Unlike some of his royalist colleagues, he was indefatigably opposed to the innovations of van Helmont, whom he castigated as 'mad' and whose medical philosophy he saw as a product of the late fashion for sectarianism in religion and learning. He was equally dismissive of 'our Universities' which he likened to 'an Amsterdam of Opinators'; T. Whitaker, *An Elenchus of Opinions Concerning the Cure of the Small Pox* (London, 1661), 4.

96. For Bayly, see Foster, i, 92; Wood, *Fasti*, ii, 48; Green, *CPCC*, i, 320. Gayton claimed to have attended the duke of York at the surrender of Oxford and Uxbridge (1646). He served as Esquire Bedel of Arts and Medicine from 1636 to 1648 prior to taking his B Med and acquiring a licence to practise medicine from Oxford University in the latter year; *ODNB*; Foster, ii, 554; E. Gayton, *The Religion of a Physician, or Divine Meditations upon the Grand and Lesser Festivals, Commanded to be Observed in the Church of England* (London, 1663), epistle dedicatory to James, duke of York. Martin, a surgeon by training, held several royal commissions, including the post of vice admiral of Devon and Cornwall. He was also chancellor of the diocese of Exeter in 1638; *DCNQ*, 14 (1926), 55–6; *CSPD, 1660–1661*, 84.
97. Ejected from Trinity College, Cambridge, according to Sir Thomas Clarges (below), because of 'his affection to his Majesty', Barrow was appointed physician to the armies in Scotland in 1654 and became judge-advocate of the army in December 1659. Like Clarges, a friend of Monck, the two men played a critical role in persuading Monck to dissolve the Rump and hold free elections, thus freeing the way for the Restoration. Barrow subsequently accompanied Clarges to Breda, but unlike the latter, he was not knighted, possibly because of lingering suspicions about his relationship with Cromwell. He was nonetheless appointed physician in ordinary supernumerary by a grateful monarch in June 1660; R. Baker, *A Chronicle of the Kings of England* (London, 1684), 651; A. L. Wyman, 'Samuel Barrow, MD, Physician to Charles II and Admirer of John Milton', *Medical History*, 18 (1974), 335–48; TNA, LC3/2, fo. 23v; LC3/25, fo. 51; LC3/26, fo. 141.
98. Clarges trained as an apothecary before the civil war, but, out of necessity, served the royalist forces around Oxford in 1643 in various capacities as physician, surgeon and apothecary. He sat as an MP for various Scottish seats between 1656 and 1660, and acted as the eyes and ears of his brother-in-law, General Monck, for much of this period, pushing the latter towards the restoration of the monarchy; *ODNB*; M. Brod, 'Thomas Clarges', *Abingdon Area Archaeological and Historical Society Newsletter* (2005); T. D. Whittet, 'Sir Thomas Clarges, Apothecary and Envoy', *Journal of the Royal Society of Medicine*, 81 (1988), 464–7.
99. Colladon, a Huguenot and protégé of Sir Theodore Mayerne, would appear to have acted as physician to the royal household in the 1640s, with responsibility for the king's children. His duties frequently took him to France, and he may have acted as a government spy, or more likely as a double agent, in the 1650s. He was appointed physician in ordinary supernumerary by a grateful master, Charles II, in 1661, and was knighted three years later; Venn, i, 371; HLRO, HL/PO/JO/10/1/149, 201, 207; *CSPD, 1645–1647*, 247; *CSPD, 1650*, 333; *CSPD, 1651–1652*, 415 [where Colladon refers to having been busy with 'the good man, who causes us great fear', presumably a reference to Charles Stuart]; *CSPD, 1653–1654*, 430; Thurloe, *State Papers*, vii, 51; TNA, LC 3/24, fo. 17.
100. Windebank was apparently a marked man in 1650, when the authorities granted him excusal, because of his occupation as a physician, 'to go further from his house the limits expressed in the late Act for confinement of delinquents'. In June 1654, however, he was granted his MD at Cambridge by letters patent signed by

Cromwell, probably as a reward for assistance rendered to the state's medical services in the first Anglo-Dutch War; Foster, iv, 1659; *CSPD, 1650*, 125, 537; *CSPD, 1652–1653*, 598. After the Restoration he retired to private practice at Guildford, Surrey, where he joined the growing ranks of committed royalist medics who accepted public office—in his case as a local county commissioner and JP for Surrey. His loyalty was later rewarded with his appointment as physician in ordinary to Charles II in March 1677; *Calendar of Treasury Books, 1660–1667*, 176; *CSPD, 1672*, 72; *CSPD, 1677–1678*, 12, 13–14; TNA, LC3/28, fo. 26.

101. W. Pope, *The Life of the Right Reverend Father in God Seth, Lord Bishop of Salisbury* (London, 1697), 18–19. Other committed royalists, who nonetheless continued as members of the London College in these years, include William Rant, Thomas Winston and Francis Prujean. Rant (d.1653), despite contributing money to the royal cause, remained active in the College throughout the 1640s, serving as censor in 1640, 1645, 1647 and 1650. Winston (*c.*1575–1655), described by one of his colleagues as one of the last of the College's 'dogmatical Galenists', had a long and distinguished medical career. He was almost certainly a royalist by inclination, suffering sequestration of his estates and assets in the late 1640s, though questions have been raised about his dalliance with the powers that be after 1649. Finally, the case of Francis Prujean (1597–1666) offers perhaps the best evidence for the remarkable pliability of the College in this period in accommodating men of varied religious and political affiliations. Despite being dogged by persistent claims that he was a closet Catholic, Prujean served the College faithfully throughout this period, culminating in his period of office as president in the critical years from 1650 to 1653. For the careers of all three men, see their respective entries in the *ODNB*.

102. The vast majority of mandated medical degrees were granted at Cambridge, possibly on account of the university's greater need to 'demonstrate its loyalty to the restored regime' as compared to 'loyalist' Oxford; J. Gascoigne, *Cambridge in the Age of the Enlightenment: Science, Religion and Politics from the Restoration to the French Revolution* (Cambridge, 1989), 27.

103. For Caesar (MD Oxford, 1660), who practised medicine at Rochester in Kent, see Foster, i, 229; *CSPD, 1660–1661*, 163. Crabbe (MD Cambridge, 1661), who was licensed to practise medicine by the University of Cambridge in 1654, claimed to have deferred taking his MD for twelve years on account of his refusal to swear 'unlawful oaths imposed by the usurpers'; Venn, i, 410; *CSPD, 1660–1661*, p165. Frere (MD Cambridge, 1660) was ejected from his physic fellowship at Queen's College, Cambridge, for refusing the Engagement in 1650. Shortly before his death in 1661 he signed letters testimonial on behalf of fellow sufferer, Robert Tyringham, ejected from Peterhouse, who was seeking a licence to practise medicine from the archbishop of Canterbury. Tyringham's application was counter-signed by another ultra-royalist medic, Peter Barwick; Venn, ii, 179; *Wal. Rev.*, 39; *CSPD, 1660–1661*, 148; LPL, FII/3/267. Yarborough (MD Cambridge, 1665), who was similarly ejected from his fellowship at Jesus College, Cambridge, in 1650 for refusing the Engagement, subsequently practised medicine at Doncaster in Yorkshire, where in 1672 he agreed to join an association of graduate physicians whose principal aim was to suppress the activities of dangerous empirics and other illicit practitioners; Venn, iv, 486; *Wal. Rev.*, 37; *CSPD, 1664–1665*, 313; BL, Sloane MS 1393, fos 14, 17.

104. Nicholas Edwards (MD Cambridge, 1663), for example, claimed that 'owing to the troublesome times', he was unable to 'graduate in the ordinary way'; Venn, ii, 89. Others in this category include John Davenant (MD Cambridge, 1661) and Edward Gelsthorpe (MD Cambridge, 1663). For Davenant, see Venn, ii, 13. Charles II declared that Gelsthorpe (d.1677) should be awarded his MD, dispensing with the normal statutes, 'in consideration of his loyalty and sufferings during the usurpation'; Venn, ii, 206; *CSPD, 1663–1664*, 288–9, 301.
105. Richard Robinson (MD Cambridge, 1681), for example, sought exemption from the normal requirements on the grounds, substantiated by the College of Physicians in London, that his father was unable to support his medical studies as he had been ruined by his loyalty in the late civil wars; Venn, iii, 473; *CSPD, 1679–1680*, 534–5. Others advertised their fierce devotion to the Stuarts by citing their willingness to take up arms for Charles I in the conflict. Samuel Jackson (d.1675), for example, the son of an Oxford apothecary, who fought for the King in the first civil war, was awarded his MD by royal mandate in 1671, despite the murmurings of Convocation which feared the growing resort by the crown to the use of such means. On this occasion, however, Jackson's friend, Dr Peter Mews (appointed bishop of Bath and Wells in 1672), was able to allay the fears of the Oxford masters, for 'having informed them how much he had merited of the King, that he might have received the same favour at our first return, that Lord Arlington had a very particular favour for him, and how much the University owed to his kindness in keeping off mandates, they were very well satisfied'. Mews concluded that 'I am not a little pleased that my fellow soldier [i.e. Jackson] is thus gratified'; Foster, ii, 796; *CSPD, 1671*, 330, 334–5. In similar fashion, Thomas Fettyplace (d.1670) successfully petitioned the King for the grant of his Cambridge MD in 1663 in part by claiming to have participated in Booth's uprising in Cheshire in 1659; Venn, ii, 135; *CSPD, 1663–1664*, 182. Finally, Richard Lister (MD Cambridge, 1678), who quit university as a young man to fight for Charles I, subsequently claimed 'all along [to have] applied himself to the study of Physic but has been prevented from taking any degree because of his loyalty and . . . by reason of his foreign employments [on royal service in Guinea]'; Venn, iii, 90; *CSPD, 1678*, 237.
106. Robert Crawley (1619–1695) probably owed his mandated Cambridge MD, awarded in 1660, to the fact that he was the son of Francis Crawley, Justice of the Common Pleas under Charles I, who suffered greatly for his loyalty. Crawley practised at Luton in Bedfordshire and was made an extra-licentiate of the London College of Physicians in July 1656; Venn, i, 415; *ODNB*, sub Crawley, Francis; Munk, i, 274. Richard Stokes (MD Cambridge, 1663), who was made a royal physician in 1665, almost certainly owed such patronage, in part at least, to the deep-seated loyalty of his clergyman father, Dr David Stokes (d.1669); Venn, iv, 167; *ODNB*, sub Stokes, David; *CSPD, 1663–1664*, 182; TNA, LC3/26, fo. 143; LC3/27, fo. 47v. Likewise, Arthur Walpole (MD Cambridge, 1661), ejected as a fellow at Queen's College, Cambridge, in 1644, may have owed royal support for his MD to his brother, John (d.1672), who acted as standard bearer to both Charles I and Charles II; Venn, iv, 324. For William Whitewell (MD Cambridge, 1661), see above note 91.
107. Innes Smith, 251; *ODNB*; LPL, FII/5/103; F1/C, fo. 167. A friend of the Norwich physician Sir Thomas Browne, Windet was the author of two poems published at the Restoration, one lamenting the execution of Charles I, the other celebrating the return

of his son. Anthony Wood later claimed that Windet was 'rather shaped for the faculty of divinity than for that faculty he professed', an insight which, as I explain below, may have applied to many other royalist sympathizers who turned to a career in medicine in the 1650s; J. Windet, *Ad Majestatem Caroli Secundi Sylvae Duae* (London, 1660); Wood, *Fasti*, ii, 193.

108. It is also worth pointing out that not all those who sought the royal mandate were successful. In 1660, for example, the medical student Thomas Cock petitioned for an MD, 'being of doctor's standing'. Despite the fact that he claimed to have been taken prisoner at the battle of Worcester in 1651 'on suspicion of being the King', he does not appear to have received royal approval; *CSPD, 1660–1661*, 164. He was probably the medical practitioner of the same name who produced a series of medical self-help manuals in 1665 in which he defended Galen and Galenic remedies from the aspersions of the chymists.

109. For Brady's early career, see especially the article in the *ODNB* by Patrick Wallis. In early 1671, Brady petitioned for the reversion of the regius professorship in physic at Cambridge. In so doing, he reprised his sufferings in the 1650s, alluding to Cromwell's role in obstructing his MD, his frequent periods of imprisonment, and his role in paving the way for the restoration of Charles II; *CSPD, 1673–1675*, 135. The reversion was finally granted in February 1674, and Brady subsequently served as regius professor from 1677 until his death in 1700. Though historians have tended to focus on Brady's political and literary achievements (discussed in more detail below, in chapter 6), his contribution to contemporary medicine was not negligible. An early admirer of Harvey who worked closely with his predecessor as regius professor, Francis Glisson, his clinical interests extended to pioneering the use of quinine and corresponding with Sydenham on the treatment of rheumatism; Venn, i, 203; *CSPD, 1671*, 78; *CSPD, 1673–1675*, 135; R. G. Frank Jnr, 'The Physician as Virtuoso in Seventeenth-Century England', in B. Shapiro and R. G. Frank (eds), *English Scientific Virtuosi in the Sixteenth and Seventeenth Centuries* (Los Angeles, 1979), 74; Gascoigne, *Cambridge in the Age of the Enlightenment*, 61.

110. At Christ Church, Llewellyn belonged to a group of wits, poets and writers centred on their patron, Brian Duppa (1588–1662), dean of the college and chaplain to archbishop Laud. In 1646, he published *Men-Miracles*, which satirized the Presbyterian and Parliamentarian cause, and was probably responsible for authoring the last Cavalier play to be performed at Oxford prior to its surrender. In the year he was awarded his MD, he appended commendatory verses to William Harvey's *Anatomical Exercitations* (London, 1653). At the Restoration, he was rewarded with the post of principal of St Mary's Hall, Oxford, which he held until 1664. In that year, he moved to High Wycombe in Buckinghamshire, where he played a prominent role in the corporation defending the Anglican and Stuart cause (discussed in more detail below, 184 and n); Foster, iii, 921; *ODNB*, sub Lluelyn, Martin.

111. Foster, iii, 1142; Bodl., OUA, Register of Congregation, 1647–1659: NEP/supra/Reg Qa, fo. 73 [where he claimed to have studied medicine for twelve years prior to the award of his B Med and MD in 1651], 150v. For his connections among the Anglican community in Chester, see below 153 n.25.

112. Venn, iii, 302; Foster, iii, 1112; *ODNB* [which disputes some of the dates of awards and offices given in Venn and Foster]. Paman's career bears comparison with that of another royalist medical student, William Quatremaine (d.1667), who, having deferred his medical education to serve the royal interest, was awarded his MD at Oxford in 1657. On the evidence of the medical *quaestiones* that he chose for disputation prior to graduation, Quatremaine, like Paman, shared an interest in the work of Francis Glisson, more specifically the latter's view that a nutritive fluid passed through the nerves rather than the lymph ducts; Foster, iii, 1225; Bodl., OUA, Register of Congregation, 1647–1659 [NEP/supra/Reg Qa], fo. 153v. After the Restoration, Quatremaine was rewarded for his earlier loyalty, having served as a doctor in the armies of Charles I during the civil war and later as an informant in royalist circles in Sussex in the 1650s. In June 1660 he was appointed physician to Charles II and shortly after was elected MP for Shoreham, where he served the Admiralty interest; Henning, iii, 308–9; *CSPD, 1657–1658*, 358; *CSPD, 1658–1659*, 110; TNA, LC3/24, fo. 16.
113. R. Sprackling, *Medela Ignorantiae: Or a Just and Plain Vindication of Hippocrates and Galen from the Groundless Imputations of M[archamont] N[edham]* (London, 1665), A2v. According to Anthony Wood, Sprackling later converted to Roman Catholicism and practised among his co-religionists at Preston in Lancashire before becoming reconciled to the Church of England shortly before his death; Venn, iv, 1400; Wood, *Ath. Ox.*, ii, 368.
114. For an excellent overview of the life and career of Willis, see the article in the *ODNB* by Robert Martensen, who demonstrates how Willis's later neurological research complemented 'the theological task of the high-church divines with whom he prayed'. These themes are developed more fully in the same author's *The Brain Takes Shape: An Early History* (Oxford, 2004). Less convincing is the depiction by Michael Hawkins of the young Willis as a penniless empiric and 'piss prophet' in his 'Piss Profits: Thomas Willis, His *Diatribae Duae* and the Formation of His Professional Identity', *History of Science*, 49 (2011), 1–24.
115. Foster, i, 200; Venn, i, 243; Wood, *Fasti*, ii, 133; *CSPD, 1658–1659*, 352; C. S. L. Davies, 'Conspiracy, Kinship, and Preferment in the Interregnum and Restoration: the Brunsells and Holders of Nottinghamshire', *Midland History*, 31 (2006), 5–7. Brunsell had two brothers, the eldest of whom, Samuel, briefly studied medicine at Leiden in 1640, before entering the church as a 'moderate episcopalian'. A younger brother Oliver (B Med Cambridge, 1658) practised at Mansfield in Nottinghamshire.
116. Foster, iii, 1173; Venn, iii, 375; Toon (ed.), *The Correspondence of John Owen*, 92. As a restored clergyman Pocklington was an active persecutor of local Quakers; see Besse, i, 266.
117. A. Napier (ed.), *The Theological Works of Isaac Barrow, D. D.*, 9 vols (Cambridge, 1859), i, xli; W. Charleton, *The Immortality of the Human Soul, Demonstrated by the Light of Nature. In Two Dialogues* (London, 1657), 50. Both examples are cited in Gascoigne, *Cambridge in the Age of Enlightenment*, 60, 62. Gascoigne rightly stresses the innovative nature of medical research at Cambridge both before and after the Restoration.
118. Among those who would appear to fall into this category we might include William Quarles (d.1672). Quarles took up the study of medicine following ejection from his

fellowship at Pembroke College, Cambridge in 1644, but subsequently entered clerical orders in 1663 serving as rector of Elmesthorpe in Leicestershire; Venn, iii, 412; CUL, CUA, Grace Book H (1645–1668), 146.

119. Gayton, *The Religion of a Physician*, (b)1v, (b)2r.

120. T. Warton, *The Life and Literary Remains of Ralph Bathurst, MD, Dean of Wells, and President of Trinity College in Oxford* (London, 1761), 35, 204; *ODNB*. Bathurst was another Anglican royalist with wide scientific interests, including chymistry. In the 1650s, he attended the lectures of the chymist Peter Stahl, who had been invited to Oxford by Robert Boyle. In 1651 and 1654, his choice of medical *quaestiones* to debate as part of his MD degree showed a clear bias toward the new physiology as well as Helmontianism; Webster, *Great Instauration*, 139; Bodl., UOA, Register of Congregation, 1647–1659: NEP/supra/Reg Qa, fos 150v, 152v.

121. Other loyalist clerics, not mentioned elsewhere in this chapter, who opted to study and/or practise medicine in the 1640s and 1650s include: James Arderne (d.1681), John Arnway (d.1653), Christopher Baitson, David Barton, Nicholas Battersby, John Collins (d.1684), John Consett (d.1673), Thomas Cookson, Thomas Daffy (d.1680), Michael Dolling, Samuel Dries, Francis Fotherby, John Longworth (d.1678), William Morgan (d.1662), William Page (d.1663), John Peckham (d.1645), Joseph Soane (d.1683), Benjamin Spencer, William Stamp, Jonas Stile (d.1663), Thomas Thexton, Rowland Watkyns (d.1664), John White (d.1671), John Wynell, William Withers (1568–1647) and Edmund Yalden. This list, which is by no means exhaustive, is largely compiled from biographical information gleaned from the *ODNB*, *Wal. Rev.*, Venn and Foster, and Innes Smith. While little is known about the kind of medicine practised by most of these clerics, the surviving evidence suggests that many adopted a progressive approach to medical theory and practice. Page, a client of archbishop Laud before the civil war, was a keen student of Harvey in the 1650s who probably graduated to iatrochemistry; *HMC. Eleventh Report, Appendix, Part VII* (London, 1888), 186 and *passim*; Bodl., UOA, Register of Congregation, 1647–59: NEP/supra/Reg Qa, fo. 151v; Webster, *Great Instauration*, 139n; TNA, SP 29/66/27. Likewise Yalden, who following his ejection as rector of Compton in Surrey in the 1640s, took up medicine thereafter probably under the tutelage of his uncle, the celebrated botanist and medical practitioner, John Goodyer (1592–1664). Reinstated at the Restoration, he later supplied the empiric William Salmon and the iatrochemical publisher William Cooper with Helmontian medical receipts. Yalden's source was the Helmontian physician Richard Pratt; *Wal. Rev.*, 187; *ODNB*, sub Goodyer, John; W. Salmon, *Doron Medicum* (London, 1683), 523; W. Cooper, *Collectanea Chymica* (London, 1684), 68–9. For royalist and Anglican interest in iatrochemistry, see chapter 4.

122. Examples include John Walton (licensed to practise medicine in the diocese of Chester, 1662); Hamnet Ward (MD Anjou, 1646), John Ward, Stephen Warman (B Med Cambridge, 1660), George Welstead (extra-licentiate, College of Physicians, London, 1652), Richard Whitelocke, William Williams (licensed to practise medicine by the University of Cambridge, 1657) and Thomas Wren (MD Oxford, 1660).

123. S. Marshall, *The Right Understanding of the Times: Opened in a Sermon Preached to the... House of Commons* [30 December 1646] (London, 1647), 40.

124. N. Biggs, *Matæotechnia Medicinae Praxeως. The Vanity of the Craft of Physick* (London, 1651), 25. For Biggs, see above 24–5.
125. Webster, *Great Instauration*, 246–323. For an earlier attempt to locate support for medical reform in this period within the wider 'puritan' reform movement, see J. E. C. Hill, 'The Medical Profession and Its Critics', in *idem, Change and Continuity in Seventeenth-Century England* (London, 1974), 157–78.
126. The controversy surrounding the use of the term 'puritan' has a long history, and one, of course, not limited to its application to scientific and medical issues. For a valuable introduction to the state of scholarship with respect to puritanism, see the various essays in J. Coffey and P. C. H. Lim (eds), *The Cambridge Companion to Puritanism* (Cambridge, 2008). Equally helpful is the overview of the various debates surrounding puritanism, including the thorny issue of definitions, in J. Spurr, *English Puritanism, 1603–1689* (Houndmills, 1998). With specific reference to puritanism's relationship to science and medicine, see I. B. Cohen (ed.), *Puritanism and the Rise of Modern Science: The Merton Thesis* (New Brunswick, NJ, 1990), which includes a chapter by Hal Cook devoted to an assessment of the contribution of Charles Webster to this debate. Webster himself has defended his original position with regard to puritanism and medicine in the introduction to the second edition of *The Great Instauration* (Bern, 2002).
127. P. Elmer, 'Medicine, Religion and the Puritan Revolution', in R. French and A. Wear (eds), *The Medical Revolution of the Seventeenth Century* (Cambridge, 1989), 10–45, especially 34–45.
128. J. A. Mendelsohn, 'Alchemy and Politics in England 1649–1665', *Past and Present*, 135 (1992), 30–78. There is much to commend Mendelsohn's broad argument in favour of alchemy as essentially compatible with royalist modes of thinking, particularly with respect to the frequency with which alchemical writers and practitioners invoked royal imagery in their work. Some, however, have been quick to criticize the very wide definition of 'alchemy' adopted by Mendelsohn, and the manner in which he conflates related but different bodies of thought such as mystical Behmenism with alchemy; see for example N. Smith, *Literature and Revolution in England, 1640–1660* (New Haven & London, 1994), 395n.
129. M. Hunter, 'Introduction. Fifteen Essays and a New Theory of Intellectual Change', in *idem*, Science *and the Shape of Orthodoxy: Intellectual Change in Late Seventeenth-Century Britain* (Woodbridge, 1995), 11–18.
130. Historians continue to debate the extent to which it is possible to talk of a distinctive puritan movement, both before and after 1640. Central to this debate is the problem of the relationship of the radical sects, which emerged most fully after 1640, to the puritan mainstream, which commentators such as Patrick Collinson have depicted as overwhelmingly conservative in outlook. For an illuminating and insightful attempt to depict a more nuanced relationship between 'mainstream' puritanism and its radical and subversive fringe, the latter sharing certain characteristics and habits of thought with the former; see D. R. Como, *Blown by the Spirit: Puritanism and the Emergence of an Antinomian Underground in Pre-Civil-War England* (Stanford, CA, 2004), 1–32. Notwithstanding the clarity of Como's arguments, any attempt to construct a single, seamless 'puritanism' after 1640 remains deeply problematic.

131. See especially C. Webster, 'Alchemical and Paracelsian Medicine', in *Health, Medicine and Mortality in the Sixteenth Century*, ed. C. Webster (Cambridge, 1979), 328–32.
132. All three were part of a larger network of naturalists and experimenters centred on Lime Street in London. For an illuminating re-evaluation of the importance of such movements in late Tudor England, see D. E. Harkness, *The Jewel House: Elizabethan London and the Scientific Revolution* (New Haven & London, 2007), esp. chapter 1.
133. *ODNB*, sub Turner, Peter; P. Turner, *The Opinion of Peter Turner... Concerning Amulets or Plague Cakes* (London, 1603), 8–9. Interestingly, Turner was not alone in the House of Commons as an advocate of Paracelsus. Other MPs who shared his passion for the Swiss medical reformer included Richard Bostocke (MP Bletchingly 1571, 1584, 1589) and his friend and colleague, Thomas Moffet (MP Wilton 1597). For Bostocke, who authored the first pro-Paracelsian text in English where he compared Paracelsus' pioneering role in medicine to that of Luther in religion, see R. B[ostocke], The Difference Betwene the Auncient Phisicke... and the Latter Phisicke (London, 1585); D. Harley, 'Rychard Bostok of Tandridge, Surrey (c.1530–1605), M.P., Paracelsian Propagandist and Friend of John Dee', Ambix, 47 (2000), 29–34.
134. TNA, PROB 11/73, fos 145v–146r [will of Thomas Penny, doctor in physick, 4 June 1588, pr. 23 January 1588/9]. For Penny, see *ODNB*. Crane, a separatist, was arrested in October 1587 and sent to Newgate where he died the following year. Wigginton, a radical puritan, became an associate of the 'prophet' William Hacket who was executed in 1591. Penry, who was a Presbyterian in 1588, became disillusioned with the movement. He subsequently assisted in clandestine publications attacking episcopacy and was executed as a separatist in 1593. All three men have entries in the *ODNB*.
135. Banister was a close friend of the London barber surgeon Thomas Banks (d.1598) whose daughter Katherine (d.1633) married as her second husband the leading East Anglian puritan Sir Thomas Barnardiston (d.1610). She became a leading patron of puritanism; TNA, PROB 11/91, fos 372r–374r [will of Thomas Bancks, citizen and barber surgeon, of London, 15 October 1595 and 25 March 1598, pr. 17 May 1598]; *ODNB*, sub Barnardiston, Katherine.
136. For Banister, see *ODNB*. Banister, who practised at Nottingham in the 1570s, used his connections with the godly in Newark to promote the early career of his son-in-law, Stephen Bradwell. In particular, he sought the support of his friend Dr William Leverett (d.1579), an alderman of Newark who had played a critical role in establishing godly rule in the town in the early years of the Reformation; Nottinghamshire Archives, Newark Borough Extracts 40; C. Brown, *History of Newark-upon-Trent*, 2 vols (Newark, 1907), ii, 2, 4, 5, 13, 28, 30, 32, 263. Interestingly, the evidence of medical links between Newark and London persisted into the seventeenth century. Another beneficiary of Penny's will was the Newark physician, Anthony Hunton (d.1624). He, too, was a puritan, but probably sympathetic to Galenic humoralism (Penny left him a copy of the works of the staunch Galenist Donato Antonio Altomare, 1506–1562). In 1616, the puritan minister and educationalist John Brinsley (1566–1624) thanked Hunton profusely for curing him of a debilitating bout of melancholy earlier in his career; J. Brinsley, *The First Booke of Tullies Offices Translated Gramatically* (London, 1616), fos A2v–A3r. Hunton provided

commendatory verses to John Gerard's *Herbal* (1597) and a prefatory letter and verse to Banister's *Compendius Chirurgerie* (London, 1585).

137. Munk, i, 107; J. Gerard, *Herbal* (London, 1597), preface; S. Bradwell, *A Detection of Ed. Glovers Hereticall Confection* (London, 1585); *idem*, *The Rasing of the Foundations of Brownisme* (London, 1588); J. M. Corley, 'Some Elizabethan Controversies about the Church and the Ministry', D. Phil (Durham, 1959), 408–58. Corley is almost certainly correct in identifying Bradwell's religious mentor as the leading Presbyterian John Field (he is simply refered to as 'F' in the writings of Bradwell's adversary Robert Browne). Bradwell witnessed Field's will in 1588; TNA, PROB 11/72, f.330v [will of John Field, preacher and minister, of London, 16 February 1587/8, pr. 1 June 1588].

138. Elmer, 'Medicine, Religion and the Puritan Revolution', 13–16. In addition to the evidence cited there for Cotta's puritanism, see also my recent article on Cotta in the *ODNB*. Hart was a contemporary of Cotta, and was living in the parish of All Saints, Northampton, in 1614, when he was presented before the church courts for not receiving communion at Easter. In 1631, he served as one of the trustees of the will of the puritan clergyman and schoolmaster Simon Wastell (d.1632) of Northampton. In 1638, the puritan lawyer, Robert Woodford, described Hart as a participant in godly debates in the town over issues such as kneeling for the sacrament, bowing before the altar, and the thorny issue of the extent to which the elect should socialize with known profane persons; NRO, Peterborough Diocesan Records, CB 44, 41, 63; *ODNB*, *sub* Wastell, Simon; New College, Oxford, MS 9502 [diary of Robert Woodford, 1637–1641], *sub* 17 March 1637/8.

139. Thomas Bosse, Henry Holland, John Newton, Walter Wells and John Yates. Bosse, a clergyman in Leicestershire who was ejected in 1662, was licensed to practise medicine in the archdeaconry of Leicester in 1639; *Cal. Rev.*, 65; LRRO, 1D 41/34/1, fo. 30v. John Newton (d.1647) was deprived of the living of Stock in Essex in 1627, partly because of his medical practice. He subsequently took out an episcopal licence; LMA, DL/C/314, fos 130, 150v; DL/C/343, fos 214v, 225v; T. Webster, *Godly Clergy in Early Stuart England: The Caroline Puritan Movement, c.1620–1643* (Cambridge, 1997), 186. Walter Wells graduated MD at Leiden in 1616 and was licensed to preach by archbishop Abbot in 1628. As lecturer at Godmanchester, Wells was on close terms with Oliver Cromwell (he was party to the marriage settlement of his daughter Elizabeth in 1646) and corresponded with Samuel Hartlib and John Dury in the early 1630s; Innes Smith, 245; NRO, F(M)Charter/2147; J. Morrill, *The Nature of the English Revolution. Essays by John Morrill* (London & New York, 1993), 137–9. John Yates (d.1657), a Cambridge BD, was licensed to practise medicine by the university in 1629. A powerful preacher and controversialist, he held numerous livings in Norfolk; *ODNB*, sub Yates, John. For Holland, see below and *ODNB*, sub Holland, John.

140. RCPL, Annals, ii, 115; *ODNB*, sub Holland, Henry. The celebrated puritan preacher Richard Baxter (1615–1691) defended his brief career as a practising cleric in the 1640s on the grounds of 'necessity'. As soon as he 'could endure it no longer', he 'procured a godly, diligent physician to come and live [in Kidderminster] and never meddled with it more'; J. M. Lloyd Thomas (ed.), *The Autobiography of Richard Baxter, Being the Reliquiae Baxterianae Abridged from the Folio (1696)* (London, 1925), 78.

141. Elmer, 'Medicine, Religion and the Puritan Revolution', 16–19.
142. Lancashire Record Office, DP 353, fo. 24r.
143. E. Corbett, *Gods Providence. A Sermon Preached Before the Honourable House of Commons, at their Late Solemne Fast* [28 December 1642] (London, 1642), 10. For earlier examples of the puritans' respect for Galen and Hippocrates, see T. Granger, *The Application of Scripture or The Maner How to Use the Word to Most Edifying* (London, 1616), 5 and *passim*; R. Bolton, *Two Sermons Preached at Northampton at Two Severall Assises There... 1621... 1629* (London, 1639), 57. In the latter example, Bolton compared the wisdom required of a magistrate to that of a physician: 'If a Physitian should fall to practice, before he be skilled in Hypocrates and Galen, in the natures, causes, signes, symptoms, prognosticks, and remedies of diseases, he is like enough to kill all before him'. In the same sermon, he devoted a large section to defending the disparaged name of 'puritan'; ibid., 79–84.
144. *ODNB*, sub Goulston, Theodore. Oddly, given Gataker's pronounced puritanical views, he dedicated this edition to William Laud, archbishop of Canterbury. Presumably the two men shared a similar faith in the intellectual merits of Galenism and medical orthodoxy in an ordered commonwealth. Gulston, a member of the Virginia Company, would appear to have possessed strong links with numerous puritan clerics in London. In his will of 1632, he gave money for commemorative rings to Gataker as well as three other eminent figures in the puritan movement in the capital, namely Dr William Gouge (1575–1653), William Foxley and Nathaniel Shute (d.1638); TNA, PROB 11/161, fos 509r–v [will of Theodore Gulston, doctor in phisick, of St Martin's Ludgate, London, 26 April 1632; pr. 1 June 1632].
145. B. Pickering, *A Firebrand Pluckt Out of the Burning. A Sermon Preached... Before the Honourable House of Commons, at their Late Solemne Fast* [27 November 1644] (London, 1645), 6. See also: O. Sedgwick, *England's Preservation or, a Sermon Discovering the Onely Way to Prevent Destroying Judgements: Preached to the Honourable House of Commons at their Late Solemne Fast* [25 May 1642] (London, 1642), 31; R. Vines, *The Impostures of Seducing Teachers Discovered; in a Sermon Before the Right Honorable the Lord Mayor and Aldermen of the City of London* [23 April 1644] (London, 1644), 39.
146. S. Ford, *Primitiae Regiminis Davidici. Or, the First Fruits of David's Government... Represented in a Sermon at the Assises held at Reading* [28 February 1654] (London, 1654), 10. In what was undoubtedly a hard-hitting sermon even by the standards of the day, Ford commented on various diseases of the body politic that currently plagued Reading and the county of Berkshire, alluding in general to radical sectarianism, anabaptism and familism, and singling out for special condemnation a fellow clergyman, a blasphemer, 'in whose house... the Devil is visibly as familiar, as any one of the family'. The allusion is a thinly veiled reference to John Pordage, rector of Bradfield, who was subsequently ejected on various charges including devil worship and providing hospitality to a host of radical enthusiasts. Pordage himself had trained as a physician, and had provided medical services to the parliamentary armies in the early stages of the civil war. As a Behmenist, he was almost certainly attracted to the medical teachings of Paracelsus. For Pordage, see above 70 and below note 112.

147. See, for example, J. D[oughty], *A Discourse Concerning the Abstrusenesse of Divine Mysteries... Another Touching Church-Schismes* (Oxford, 1628), ii, 22–3. In 1647 the supporters of Parliament were compared to 'states Paracelsians who with their desperate drugges or dregges, have occasioned the disease of a Nation'; *Treasons Anatomie or the Duty of the Loyall Subject* (1647), 8–9. Much the same language was deployed in a royalist newssheet of 1649 to stigmatize 'those State-doctors' such as Fairfax, 'who are like Paracelsus and with their desperate drugs kill all that comes in their lawlesse hands'; *Mercurius Pragmaticus*, no. 7 [29 May–5 June 1649], unpaginated.
148. *ODNB*, sub Forester, James. Forester was responsible for the posthumous publication of Hester's *The Pearle of Practise, or, Practisers Pearl for Physick and Chirurgerie* (London, 1594), which appeared just one year after he officially recanted and disassociated himself from his former friends and followers of the separatists, Henry Barrow and John Greenwood. Rejoining the Anglican fold, he subsequently became rector of Mavis Enderby in Lincolnshire in 1606 and was later appointed chaplain to Queen Anne of Denmark.
149. Gemeente Archief, Amsterdam, 318/2 [Notulen van het Consistory or Book of Discipline, 1621–1627], 2, 11. Bromley also invoked the authority of 'Dr Heurnius' in citing Paracelsus' judgement with respect to the morality of communicating with angels. Johannes (1543–1601) and Otto Heurnius (1577–1652) were highly respected members of the Dutch medical elite, who both lectured in medicine and anatomy at the University of Leiden.
150. Ibid., 11–12, 36. Throughout these long-drawn-out proceedings, it is clear that what most irked the church authorities was not Bromley's subscription to Paracelsianism, but rather the confidence and faith that he demonstrated in his ability to read and interpret the scriptures for himself; see also A. C. Carter, *The English Reformed Church in Amsterdam in the Seventeenth Century* (Amsterdam, 1964), 61–64, especially 63.
151. F. Herring, *A Modest Defence of the Caveat Given to Wearers of Impoisoned Amulets* (London, 1604), 21, 31–3; A. Du Laurens, *A Discourse of the Preservation of the Sight: of Melancholike Diseases; of Rheumes, and of Old Age... Translated... by... Richard Surphlet* (London, 1599), A3r, B2v. For Surflet, see M. A. L. Cooke, 'Richard Surflet, translator and practitioner in physic', *Medical History*, 25 (1981), 41–56. Surflet was extraordinarily well connected to the contemporary puritan scene. In his revealing will and inventory, made shortly before embarking as physician-cum-preacher aboard the second East India Company expedition, he left bequests to those giants of the puritan movement, Walter Travers (d.1635), Stephen Egerton (d.1622) and Eusebius Paget (d.1617). Surflet's translation of Du Laurens also contained epistolary poems by the Calvinist theologian Gabriel Powell (1576–1611) and future heresiographer Ephraim Paget (1574–1646), son of Eusebius; TNA, PROB 11/107, fos 349r–v [will of Richard Surflet, 1 March 1603/4, pr. 26 June 1606]; Du Laurens, *Discourse*, B3r.
152. J. Oberndorffer, *Anatomyes of the True Physition and Counterfeit Mounte-Banke... Translated into English by F[rancis] H[erring]... Hereunto is Annexed: A Short Discourse or Discovery of Certaine Stratagems* (London, 1602); the latter republished as *Beware of Pick-purses* (London, 1605); *ODNB*, sub Herring, Francis; A. James, *Poets, Players and Preachers: Remembering the Gunpowder Plot in Seventeenth-Century England* (Toronto, 2016), 130–1.

153. H. J. Cook, *The Decline of the Old Medical Regime in Stuart London* (Ithaca, NY, & London, 1986), 94–132.
154. W. J. Birken, 'The Royal College of Physicians of London and Its Support of the Parliamentary Cause in the English Civil War', *Journal of British Studies*, 23 (1983), 47–62.
155. For Clarke, see above and Birken's article in the *ODNB*; cf. Cook, *Decline of the Old Medical Regime*, 105–6, 113, where he errs in describing Clarke as a 'strong Independent'.
156. For Rand and Clarke, see *ODNB*. The Presbyterianism of Rand is discussed above note 21.
157. RCPL, Annals, iii, fos 173b, 188b. For the puritan backgrounds of Alston and Oxenbridge, see *ODNB*. Oxenbridge's distaste for Laudianism is evident in the fact that in 1639 he stood bail for the puritan canon of Durham Cathedral, Peter Smart; *CSPD, 1638–1639*, 457. The trials and tribulations of Boate, who, like Evans, was forced to appear before the Court of High Commission, and Trigge are summarized in their respective entries in the *ODNB*. For Trigge see also note 66 above.
158. For Venner, see above note 22 and *ODNB*. Primrose (d.1659), like Venner, a medical conservative, was the author in 1638 of a Latin treatise condemning the practices of a wide range of medical 'quacks' and intruders. It was translated into English in 1651 by his colleague Robert Wittie (1613–1684), a staunch parliamentarian and Presbyterian who shared Primrose's devotion to Galenism; Elmer, 'Medicine, Religion and the Puritan Revolution', 30–1 and n. The assumption that Primrose was a Catholic, based on the fact that he was prosecuted under the recusancy laws in the late 1630s, is clearly erroneous.
159. J. Hart, *KAINIKH, or the Diet of the Diseased* (London, 1633), 13 (my emphasis).
160. RCPL, Annals, iii, fos 157b–158b [Winterton to Foxe, 25 August 1635]. Winterton was a protégé of Laud to whom he dedicated his celebrated edition of the *Aphorisms* of Hippocrates (Cambridge, 1635), as well as his *Poetae Minores Graeci* (Cambridge, 1633). He owed the grant of his Cambridge MD of 1633 to the personal intervention of his patron; *ODNB*, sub Winterton, Ralph. Foxe, who was president of the College of Physicians from 1634 to 1641, was the younger son of the martyrologist John Foxe (d.1587). William Birken has recently argued that Foxe's aversion to the Arminianism and ceremonialism of the Laudian church was evident in his authorship of a brief life of his father, appended to the 1641 edition of the *Acts and Monuments*. If so, then I would also concur with Birken's suggestion that this represented an expression of mainstream puritan distaste for the 'Romish' innovations associated with Laud and Charles I, rather than evidence of a 'hidden revolutionary side'; *ODNB*, sub Simeon Foxe.
161. RCPL, Annals, iii, fos 155b, 156b. Evans was a minister who famously made and sold an 'antimonial cup' that was said to cure all ills. It was practising ministers such as Evans, with their 'universal cures', that so incensed puritan physicians like Cotta and Hart and provoked them to publish scathing denunciations of such medical intruders and their equally dangerous panaceas; Elmer, 'Medicine, Religion and the Puritan Revolution', 13–15. For a brief account of Evans' career, see the article by Bernard Capp in *ODNB*.

162. *CSPD, 1635*, 188, 193, 211; *CSPD, 1638–1639*, 114–15; *Wal. Rev.*, 243. Richardson was also prosecuted for non-residence in his parish and frequenting alehouses. For a further example of the diligence of the Laudian authorities in prosecuting unruly vagabonds masquerading as mountebanks, see the case of Nicholas Slater of Royden in Essex, who was prosecuted in High Commission in 1638 for various offences, including wandering the countryside and practising medicine without a licence. Imprisoned in Newgate, he was forbidden visitors on the pretext that he was prescribing physic; *CSPD, 1638–1639*, 75.
163. H. Cook, 'Policing the Health of London: The College of Physicians and the Early Stuart Monarchy', *Social History of Medicine*, 2 (1989), 29–30, 30–1. While I am indebted in much of the preceding commentary to the valuable research undertaken by William Birken in uncovering the puritan roots of so many members of the College of Physicians at this date, I do dissent from his work in one important respect, namely in rejecting his depiction of these puritan physicians as part of a wider movement dedicated to a radical and revolutionary programme of reform. I cannot concur with his view, therefore, that the College on the brink of civil war was 'a far more genuinely revolutionary body... than has ever been imagined'. Recent historical work has been slow to recognize the profoundly conservative nature of mainstream, pre-civil war puritanism, and the reluctance of many of its adherents to take up arms against their king, but for a good example of a puritan physician who exhibited these traits in both his medical and political careers, see the account of the life of John Bastwick in F. M. Condick, 'The Life and Works of Dr John Bastwick (1595–1654)', Ph. D. (London, 1983). Among other things, Condick fully explodes the myth of Bastwick as the 'headstrong radical', preferring instead to promote an image of the man as a 'cautious conservative', who became the reluctant and misunderstood victim of circumstances beyond his control; ibid., 9–10. For an abridged version of this account, see Condick's entry on Bastwick in the *ODNB*.
164. RCPL, Annals, iii, fo. 202b; A. S[treater], *A Letter Sent to My Lord Mayor* (London, 1642). In a pamphlet published a year earlier, Streater, who signed himself 'Physitian of Arts in Oxford approved by Authority: the Kings Majesties Servant in Ordinary', claimed to be able to cure all forms of agues. In typical 'puritan' fashion, he also condemned those who resorted to white witches, sorcerers and seventh sons for cure, emphasizing the importance of seeking lawful means for the cure of all ailments; A. Streater, *An Ague, which Hitherto Amongst All Sorts Hath Beene Accounted the Physitians Shame* (London, 1641). His published work was dismissed as 'very absurd' by the College's censors in December 1641, and he himself was dubbed 'a mad and stupid quack'; RCPL, Annals, iii, fo. 212b. Streater, a native of Lewes in Sussex, was ordained there in 1634. He had earlier studied briefly at Oxford, but was dead by 1654; WSxRO, Ep.II/1/1, f.31r; Foster, iv, 1435; SUL, HP 29/4/20B. Streater's brother John was a well-known political pamphleteer and advocate of classical republicanism in the 1650s. He also had plans, never completed, to publish the whole corpus of Boehme's writings in English; *ODNB*, sub Streater, John; N. Smith, 'Popular Republicanism in the 1650s: John Streater's *Heroic Mechanicks*', in Q. Skinner and D. Armitage (eds), *Milton and Republicanism* (Cambridge, 1995), 137–55.

165. RCPL, Annals, iii, fos 188b, 189b, 209a, 209b–210a, 210b. As early as 1634, Samuel Hartlib reported that 'one Pordage broches new-fangled opinions concerning the signes, that no Man can trie himself by them, but was to stay for an over-powring light'. The intelligencer also noted that the puritan vicar of St Stephen's, Coleman Street, John Davenport, 'hase preacht against him [and] much taken against his tenents'; SUL, HP 29/2/40B. Davenport's hackles may well have been raised by Pordage's close relationship with the eminent puritan patrons, Sir Horace and Lady Vere, to whom he acted as private chaplain. His role as preacher in the Vere household was also cited by the College of Physicians as grounds to refuse his request for a licence, despite the recent award of a Leiden MD in 1639 (incorporated at Cambridge in October 1640); Innes Smith, 185. Pordage's later career as army physician and mystical theologian is discussed further above 70.
166. The eccentric Jacobean preacher Henoch Clapham (d.1637) was another who integrated medical practice into his ministry. So too did the leader of the early English Baptist movement John Smyth (d.1612) who, prior to breaking with the Church of England in 1607, was fined and suspended by the diocesan authorities in Lincoln for practising physic without a licence. Ensconced in Amsterdam, where he established his own congregation, he subsequently subsisted through medical practice; *ODNB*; S. Wright, *The Early English Baptists 1603–1649* (Woodbridge, 2006), 17–18, 28. For Clapham, who made the outrageous claim that the plague was not infectious and that those who died from it did so through a lack of faith, see *ODNB*, sub Clapham, Henoch. He finally settled in Kent, where he obtained a licence to practise medicine from the archbishop of Canterbury in 1618, and was buried at Eastry, Kent, on 2 May 1637; LPL, Abbot 1, fo. 231; CCAL, U3/267 [parish registers of Eastry, Kent, 1559–1736].
167. RCPL, Annals, iii, fos 207b, 208a. For a summary of Trigge's subsequent career, see above note 66. Trigge was also in trouble with the College authorities in September 1640, when he was ordered to appear with two other men, Emery and Hubbart. It is tempting to speculate that the latter was Thomas Hubbard, who, like Trigge, was active on behalf of the republican cause in Tower Hamlets. For Hubbard's support for Independency and the 'good old cause', see above, 48–9.
168. Staines, a candidate for membership at this stage, was not in fact made a fellow of the College until October 1641. He had been cited to appear before the College in April 1639 and to show by what authority he practised in London; Annals, iii, fo. 197b. Fyge, who lived in the parish of St Bride's, Fleet Street, was to play an important role as a Presbyterian activist in the religious and political life of the capital in the 1640s and 1650s. Between 1655 and 1660 he served as a ruling elder in the fifth classis of the London province, as well as a member of the Grand Committee of the Provincial Assembly in 1655; Sion College, MS Acc L4012/E17; M. Mahony, 'Presbyterianism in the City of London, 1645–1647', *The Historical Journal*, 22 (1979), 105, 108, 109; J. R. Woodhead, *The Rulers of London 1660–1689: A Biographical Record of the Aldermen and Common Councilmen of the City of London* (London, 1965), 74. Fyge did possess an archiepiscopal licence to practise medicine, issued in 1635, but this extended only as far as the dioceses of Chichester and Lincoln; LPL, Laud 1,

fos 232v–233. He was prosecuted on three separate occasions by the College in 1632, 1640 and 1641–2 for illicit practice but stubbornly refused to acknowledge the College's legal authority; RCPL, Annals, iii, fos 123b, 207a, 211a, 213a, 213b, 214a. For the chymical interests and political concerns of his son, Thomas, see below 137, 162 n.82.

169. Cook, *Decline of the Old Medical Regime*, 115–20. For an earlier treatment of this theme, see C. Webster, 'The College of Physicians: "Solomon's House" in Commonwealth England', *Bulletin of the History of Medicine*, 41 (1967), 393–412; *idem*, *Great Instauration*, 315–23.

170. For a useful summary, see Webster, *Great Instauration*, 264–73; B. Woolley, *The Herbalist: Nicholas Culpeper and the Fight for Medical Freedom* (London, 2004), 288–326. The relationship between the book trade and medicine is explored more fully in E. L. Furdell, *Publishing and Medicine in Early Modern England* (Rochester, NY, and Woodbridge, 2002).

171. *CSPD, 1652–1653*, 69. Rowland was responsible, along with Abdias Cole and Culpepper himself, for translating the works of the French physician Lazarus Riverius (1585–1655) into English.

172. J. Riolan, *A Sure Guide; or, the Best and Nearest Way to Physick and Chyrurgery... in Six Books... Englished by Nich. Culpeper, Gent., and W. R. Doctor of the Liberal Arts, and of Physick* (London, 1657), Br–B2r [epistle dedicatory signed by William Rand]; J. T. Rutt (ed.), *Diary of Thomas Burton, Esq., Member in the Parliaments of Oliver and Richard Cromwell from 1656 to 1659*, 4 vols (London, 1828), i, p.62. Rand, a member of the Hartlib circle, wrote numerous letters to fellow Socinian sympathizer and iatrochemist, Benjamin Worsley, in which he offered trenchant criticism of the excessive power and authority of the clergy, referring in one letter to the 'Sorcery of the reverend Clergie'. His pronounced anticlericalism has been suggested as the source of his admiration for the writings of Thomas Hobbes, whom he wished to convert to the cause of the nascent Republic; see J. R. Collins, *The Allegiance of Thomas Hobbes* (Oxford, 2005), 191–2. It is possible that Rand's particular brand of radical speculation may have led him into trouble with the authorities. In October 1653, order was made to arrest one William Rand, of St Bride's, London, to bring him before the Council for questioning, and to search his house for scandalous papers; *CSPD, 1653–1654*, 437.

173. W. W[alwyn], *Health's New Store-House Opened* (London, 1661), 26 [Rand] and postscript [Rowland]. Rowland's preference for chymical medicines is further suggested by his translation and publication of Johann Schroeder's, *The Compleat Chymical Dispensatory in Five Books* (London, 1669) in which he promoted the use and sale of his 'Pilulae Rulandinae Universales'; ibid., Av–A2r. Rand was converted to the merits of Helmontian iatrochemistry while travelling in the Low Countries in the late 1640s and early 1650s, where he met the *adeptus* Johann Moriaen. He was subsequently active within the Hartlib circle as an advocate of a Graduate College of Physicians that would have preserved the medical profession from the intrusion of unlearned quacks, while at the same time undermining the excessive regulatory and elitist authority of the London College of Physicians. For Rand, see especially Webster, *Great Instauration*, 304–8 and below, note 175.

174. I discuss Pinnell and French in my 'Medicine, Religion and the Puritan Revolution', 25, 26–30, 36–7, 39, 42. Dugard was responsible for translating *Paracelsus His*

Dispensatory and Chirurgery (London, 1656). Initially a staunch royalist, he changed sides in 1650, and was responsible for publishing the anti-trinitarian *Racovian Cathechism* (London, 1652), which was condemned by a parliamentary committee as 'blasphemous and scandalous'. He nonetheless retained his commission as an official printer to the government of the Interregnum, possibly through the friendship of republican radicals such as John Milton and John Harrington; *ODNB*, sub Dugard, William. Parkhurst was responsible for the translation and publication of the Paracelsian *Medicina Diastatica or Sympathetical Mumie* (London, 1653), in which he advertised his intention to publish further works of a similar mystical nature, including treatises on the tree of life, a cabalistical concordance and 'many other Pieces both Philosophicall and Mathematicall'. In 1656 he was appointed registrar to the Commissioners for Discoveries, a post he seems to have retained after the Restoration; *ODNB*.

175. Charles Webster has argued convincingly for the identification of W. R., 'Mystica-Physophilos', who supplied an epistolary poem to Biggs' work, with William Rand, above; Webster, *Great Instauration*, 191, 263n. One might go further and speculate that Rand, utilizing his Dutch connections, acted as an agent in providing Biggs with some of the raw materials—the original writings of van Helmont—which were so clearly paraphrased in Biggs' final work. Whatever the case, Rand was subsequently an enthusiastic advocate of van Helmont, and in a letter to Hartlib written in February 1653 communicated plans for a new and improved edition of the collected works of the Flemish iatrochemist; SUL, HP 42/17 [Rand to Hartlib, 14 February 1652/3].
176. For the Quakers' predilection for chymical forms of medicine, see my 'Medicine, Science and the Quakers: the "Puritanism-Science" Debate Reconsidered', *Journal of the Friends Historical Society*, 54 (1981), 265–86. I have since discovered a vast array of new evidence, which I hope to publish in due course, providing overwhelming evidence of the Friends' promotion of iatrochemical methods and practice.
177. Bodl., OUA, Register of Congregation, 1647–1659: NEP/supra/Reg Qa, fo. 150v. Bathurst's devotion to Anglicanism and his role in preserving its rituals in Interregnum Oxford is discussed below 170. He was also one of the first to enrol in the private chymistry lectures given by Peter Stahl (d.1674) at Oxford in the 1650s.
178. Bodl., OUA, Register of Congregation, 1647–1659: NEP/supra/Reg Qa, fo. 152v. Fielding was the son of the Gloucestershire minister Roger Fielding, who was sequestrated from his living in 1644 for being absent at Bristol as a malignant. Robert was ejected from his fellowship at Balliol College in 1648; *Wal. Rev.*, 23, 173; Foster, ii, 490. I discuss Fielding's later medical and political career in Gloucester after the Restoration in chapter 6 below.
179. Bodl., OUA, Register of Congregation, 1647–1659: NEP/supra/Reg Qa, fo. 151r. For Kuerden, alias Jackson, see Foster, ii, 795; Wood, *Fasti*, ii, 94, 275; *ODNB*, sub Jackson, Richard; W. D. Shannon, *Seventeenth-Century Lancashire Restored: The Life and Work of Dr Richard Kuerdon, Antiquary and Topographer, 1623–1702* (Manchester, Chetham Soc., vol.54, 2020). After the Restoration, Kuerden settled at Preston, where he neglected his medical practice in favour of antiquarian research (for which, see below 281). The influence of van Helmont on the medical disputations of all three

men has been noted by Charles Webster, though he fails to note the royalist sympathies of Fielding and Kuerden; Webster, *Great Instauration*, 139–40.

180. RCPL, Annals, iv, fos 11a, 12a; Innes Smith, 232; G. Thomson, *A Letter Sent to Mr Henry Stubbe* (London, 1672), 4–5. For a summary of Thomson's life and career, see Appendix 1 (a).

181. RCPL, Annals, iii, fos 138b, 140a–b. The background to these events is described in some detail in Cook, 'Policing the Health of London', 20–2. Weale's collaborator in this struggle, Richard Edwards was also a royalist sympathizer who suffered at the hands of the sequestrators; see *CSPD, 1637–1638*, 370, 399; *CSPD, 1639–1640*, 414; Green, *CPCC*, iii, 2344–6.

182. LPL, Laud 1, fo. 279. As we shall see in the next chapter, the support of the ecclesiastical authorities in granting such licences was to prove a potent weapon against the College in the heightened atmosphere of the 1660s, when genuine suspicions of the religious motives of the leadership of the College of Physicians in London, combined with widespread support at court and among leading church dignitaries for the goals of the chymists, threatened to destroy the College's monopoly.

183. J. Weale, *A Preparative for the Fast; or, a Sovereigne Balsome for the Cure of the Distemper of the Times* (London, 1642).

184. *HMC, Thirteenth Report, Appendix, Part IV* (London, 1892), 385. His incarceration in 1642 is confirmed by a certificate, dated 5 October 1653, in which various citizens of Kingston confirmed that Weale had subscribed for lands in the Irish adventure in 1642, but had been prevented from completing his purchases due to imprisonment, lawsuits and 'great charge of children'. He was in fact a large investor in Irish lands (he subscribed for £600 but paid only £374 8s.) and eventually drew estates in the barony of Slane in county Meath; *CSP Adventurers*, 275, 345; J. P. Prendergast, *The Cromwellian Settlement of Ireland* (Dublin, 1922), 410. Weale's involvement in the Irish adventure also provides a cautionary tale for those historians who have seen this process as dominated by committed puritans and parliamentarians.

185. George Thomson, *ΛΟΙΜΟΤΟΜΙΑ or The Pest Anatomized* (London, 1666), 176; Thomson, Letter Sent to Mr Henry Stubbe, 5, 26. Weale himself was enrolled at Leiden in December 1640, but he does not appear to have graduated; Innes Smith, 244. In his will, made in 1668, he alluded to 'the great losses I have sustained by the late troubles' but makes no reference to medical colleagues or associates; TNA, PROB 11/327, fos 260r–262r [will of Job Weale, physitian, of Kingston upon Thames, Surrey, 25 February 1667/8; pr. 25 June 1668].

186. For his will, which contains a Calvinist preamble, see TNA, PROB 11/167, fos 33r–v [will of George Weale, clerk of his majesties works of whitehall and St James, 1 July 1633, pr. 9 January 1634/5].

187. D. Levitin, '"Made Up from Many Experimentall Notions": The Society of Apothecaries, Medical Humanism, and the Rhetoric of Experience in 1630s London', *Journal of Medical History and Allied Sciences*, 70 (2015), 549–87. The original lectures can be found in the Folger Shakespeare Library, Washington DC, MS E.a.5.

188. For Johnson, reviser of Gerard's *Herbal*, see *ODNB*.

189. Broad may have been a native of Berwick to which he returned shortly after 1634; see *CSPD, 1639*, 507; Durham University Library, DPRI/1/1642/B7/1–6 [will of William

Broad, doctor of physic, of Berwick upon Tweed, Northumberland, undated, pr. 24 December 1642; inventory dated 29 December 1642]. The clergymen Gilbert Dury (who received a copy of Bartholinus' *Anatomy*), George Sydserfe and Henry Valentine (d.1643) were all unswervingly loyal to Charles I.

190. The four lecturers of 1634—Thomas Johnson, William Broad, James Clarke and John Buggs—were part of a wider coterie of apothecary-physicians that included Job Weale and whose contribution to Johnson's revised edition of Gerard's *Herbal* is acknowledged throughout the 1633 edition of that work.
191. Levitin, '"Made Up from Many Experimental Notions"', 582.
192. Green, *CPCC*, iv, 2780. Currer later signed the petition of the chymists seeking to secure a patent for a Society of Chemical Physicians in London in 1665; for a brief biography of Currer, that supplements the account in the *ODNB*, see Appendix 1 (a). For Currer, Ashmole and the dictionary project of Edward Phillips, see above 77–8.
193. Very little is known of Collop's life, nor the source of his MD. In addition to the brief entry in the *ODNB*, see F. N. L. Poynter, 'An Unnoticed Contemporary English Poem in Praise of Harvey and Its Author', *Journal of the History of Medicine and Allied Sciences*, 11 (1956), 374–83; C. Hilberry, 'Medical Poems from John Collop's *Poesis Rediviva* (1656)', *Journal of the History of Medicine and Allied Sciences*, 11 (1956), 384–411. At the Restoration, he appealed for arrears, withheld for his loyalty, and was awarded £80. He was also the author of an anthology of loyalist verse published as *Itur Satyricum: In Loyall Stanzas* (London, 1660). His interest in medical innovation would appear to have survived the Restoration. In 1665 he signed, along with fellow iatrochemists Jeremiah Astel and Richard Barker (both supporters of the Society of Chemical Physicians, for whom see Appendix 1 (a)), a testimonial on behalf of one John Dabbs, MA, an applicant for a medical licence from the bishop of London; Bloom and James, 45.
194. BL, Add. MS 78,311, fos 1–31 [letters of Thickens to Evelyn, 1640–1661]; Foster, iv, 1469; E. S. de Beer (ed.), *The Diary of John Evelyn*, 6 vols (Oxford, 1955), ii, 470; SUL, HP 28/2/30A–B, 46A. Thickens or Thickness was falsely reported by Hartlib to have died in 1652. He was still alive, though very ill, in 1661, when there was a brief exchange of letters between him and Evelyn; BL, Add. MS 78,311, fo. 31 [Thickens to Evelyn, 2 September 1661]; BL, Add. MS 78,298, fo. 113r [Evelyn to Thickens, 5 September 1661].
195. SUL, HP 28/1/65A [Ephemerides, June-September 1650]. At about the same time, Dr Child also reported that Henshaw and others, including Thomas Vaughan, were 'endeavouring to forme a Chymical Club' to promote this particular branch of learning; ibid., HP 28/1/61B. Henshaw had joined the royal forces at York at the outbreak of civil war in 1642. Shortly after he was arrested in London, and on his release, secured a pass to travel overseas in the company of, among others, John Evelyn and James Thickens; *ODNB*, sub Henshaw, Thomas; BL, Add. MS 78,311, fo. 9v [Thickens to Evelyn, 16 November 1644]; fos 32–40 [letters of Henshaw to Evelyn, from various addresses in Italy]. Other members of Henshaw's circle included the alchemist Thomas Vaughan (1621–1666), the antiquarian Elias Ashmole (1617–1692) and Sir Robert Paston (1631–1683), who sponsored Henshaw's chymical research. All three were committed royalists. For Henshaw's relationship with Paston, see especially D. R. Dickson, 'Thomas Henshaw and Sir Robert Paston's Pursuit of the

Red Elixir: An Early Collaboration Between Fellows of the Royal Society', *Notes and Records of the Royal Society of London*, 51 (1997), 57–76. Evelyn, it should be noted, was also on familiar terms with the Helmontian Dr William Rand, whom we have already encountered as a key figure in the medical reform movements of the 1650s. In 1657, Rand dedicated his recent translation of the life of Peiresc to Evelyn who shared his passion for chymistry. For correspondence between the two, see BL, Add. MS 78,298, fos 68r [Evelyn to Rand, 4 March 1656], 78r–v [same to same, 9 April 1657], 180v [same to same, 20 March 1659].

196. For a recent re-appraisal of the project which attempts to rescue Phillips from the charge of plagiarism and deceit, particularly in employing fictional consultants, see J. Considine, 'In Praise of Edward Phillips', *Studia Linguistica Universitatis Iagellonicae Cracoviensis*, 132 (2015), 211–28. I would like to thank Prof. Jonathan Barry for alerting me to the existence of this article.
197. E.Phillips, *The New World of English Words: Or, A General Dictionary* (London, 1658), a2r. For Currer, a close friend of Ashmole, and Turner, see Appendix 1 (b). Peter Mark Sparck or Spark (d.1676), a native of the duchy of Holstein, was described on his monument in the church of Bishop's Stortford, Hertfordshire, as one 'most expert in the art of chymistry'. He was rejected for naturalization in 1657, but was granted the same in 1662. In the same year, he was made physician in extraordinary to Charles II and in 1663 was granted an archiepiscopal licence to practise medicine *gratis* on account of his friendship with Sir Edward Turnour (1617–1686), Speaker of the House of Commons; Sir H. Chauncy, *The Historical Antiquities of Hertfordshire* (London, 1720), reprinted London, 1826, i, 329; W. A. Shaw (ed.), *Letters of Denization and Acts of Naturalization for Aliens in England and Ireland, 1603–1700* (Lymington, Huguenot Society, vol.18, 1911), 72, 73, 74, 81; TNA, LC3/26, fo. 143; LPL, FII/4/158; F1/C, fo. 136v; ERO, D/ABW 68/33 [will of Peter Mark Sparke, doctor in physic, of Bishop's Stortford, Hertfordshire, 24 February 1675/6, pr. 3 May 1676]. For Edward Molins, see note 46 above. For his brother William (1617–1691), see *ODNB*, sub Molins, William. His recipes for a 'salivating pills for the pox' and 'powder for an old sore' were collected by the chymical physician Augustus Kuffeler; CUL, MS Ll v 8, 392. Another contributor was the geometer and astrological physician John Wyberd (MD Franeker, 1644, incorporated Oxford 1654), who, like Currer, served as a physician in Ireland in the early 1650s; B. S. Capp, *Astrology and the Popular Press: English Almanacs 1500–1800* (London & Boston, 1979), 340.
198. For Agar and Phillips, see especially J. T. Shawcross, *The Arms of the Family: The Significance of John Milton's Relatives and Associates* (Lexington, KY, 2004), 47–72 [Agar], 73–94 [Phillips].
199. TNA, PROB 11/343, ff.185r–186r [will of Thomas Agar, gentleman, of London, 10 June 1671 & 27 October 1673; pr. 5 November 1673]. The patronage networks of the Ridgleys, father and son, which included the earls of Rutland and Sir Gervase Clifton, are worthy of a study in their own right. Thomas Ridgley practised at the start of his career in Newark, Nottinghamshire, which as we have seen featured prominently in earlier discussions of Paracelsianism. His son Luke perpetuated the connection. In 1675, he certified the practice of Matthew Jenison, apothecary, of Newark, who was seeking an archiepiscopal licence to practise medicine; LPL, VX 1A/10/75/1–3.

200. For a good introduction to the role of Interregnum Trinity College in the promotion of the new science, including chymistry, see R. Serjeantson, 'The Education of Francis Willughby' and A. M. Roos, 'The Chymistry of Francis Willughby (1635–72): The Trinity College, Cambridge Community', in T. Birkhead (ed.), *Virtuoso by Nature: The Scientific Worlds of Francis Willughby FRS (1635–1672)* (Leiden, 2016), 44–98; 99–121.
201. Venn, i, 11; SUL, HP 28/2/53A.
202. The proceedings against Akehurst are calendared in *CSPD, 1654*, 246–7; *CSPD, 1655*, 58; Thurloe, *State Papers*, ii, 463; Rutt (ed.), *Diary of Thomas Burton*, i, 130.
203. Among various suggestions of eccentric behaviour on Akehurst's part, on one occasion in 1654 he was alleged to have addressed the unruly students at supper in the College Hall by telling them that 'in Heaven they should have a Tennis-Court, and Bowling-greenes & cry spiritually Rub, rub, rub'; V. Morgan, *A History of the University of Cambridge*, 4 vols (Cambridge, 1989–2004), ii [1546–1750], 139. It is possible that the case against Akehurst was instigated as part of a backlash orchestrated by Lazarus Seaman against the supporters of Charles Hotham (1615–1672). In 1651, Hotham, a fellow of Peterhouse, who had previously been reprimanded for preaching against the Engagement, petitioned the parliamentary committee for the reform of the universities, complaining of the dictatorial behaviour of Seaman, the master of Peterhouse. He was subsequently deprived of his fellowship when he published private transcripts of the parliamentary committee's proceedings. Hotham responded by securing the signatures of thirty-three colleagues, including Akehurst and John Pratt (for whom, see below note 208). Akehurst and Hotham shared common intellectual interests. Like Akehurst, Hotham constructed a laboratory in his rooms at Peterhouse. His chymical studies formed part of a wider theosophical enterprise, focused on the writings of the Silesian mystic Jacob Boehme, whose works he helped to translate and publish in English; *ODNB*, sub Hotham, Charles; C. Hotham, *A True State of the Case of Mr Hotham* (London, 1651), 14–15.
204. Rev. J. Hunter, *The Rise of the Old Dissent, Exemplified in the Life of Oliver Heywood... 1630–1702* (London, 1842), 44–5; TNA, PROB 11/375, fos 11r–v [will of Daniel Batcheler, Master of Arts, late of Stepney, now of Leatherhead, Surrey, 12 October 1683; pr. 10 January 1683/4]. In 1666, Alexander Akehurst, was living at Leatherhead in Surrey where he was practising medicine with a licence issued by the archbishop of Canterbury the previous year; TNA, PROB 11/322, fos 1v–2r [will of Raphe Akehurst, haberdasher, of Cliffe near Lewes, Sussex, now residing in Dublin, 27 August 1666; pr. 5 October 1666]; T. C. Wales and C. P. Hartley (eds), *The Visitation of London Begun in 1687*, 2 vols (London, Harleian Society, vols 16 and 17, 2004), i, 331, 333n; LPL, VG 1/1, fo. 183; Sheldon, fo. 203.
205. N. H[ookes], *Amanda, A Sacrifice to an Unknown Goddesse, or, A Free-Will Offering of a Loving Heart to a Sweet-Heart* (London, 1653), 93–6, 109–10, 133–4. For Hookes, see the brief biography in the *ODNB*. Further evidence of the passion for chymistry and informal instruction in that art is suggested by payments made by the College in 1658 to the Greek chymist Constantine Rhodocanaces (*fl.*1658–1678). In 1660, while visiting Oxford, Rhodocanaces published a poem in praise of the Restoration. He was

subsequently employed by Charles II as a royal chymist; Trinity College Library, Cambridge, Senior Bursar's Audit Book, 1658, fo. 330r; C. Rhodocanaces, *Carmina Graeca Rythmica Gratulatoria de reditu Serenissimi Sacratissimi & Theophylactou Principis Caroli II* (Oxford, 1660); TNA, LC 3/26, fo.142; LC3/24, fo.26; *CSPD Addenda, 1660–1685*, 496. Rhodocanaces's *Alexicacus, or Spirit of the True Salt* (first extant edition 1664) went through seven editions. I am very grateful to Richard Serjeantson for sharing with me his knowledge of Rhodocanaces and the Trinity College archives.

206. For Crane and his friendship with Butler, see L. Martin, 'John Crane (1571–1652): The Cambridge Apothecary and Philanthropist', *Medical History*, 24 (1980), 432–46. Crane specifically requested to be buried next to his 'worthy and honoured good friend' Dr Butler in the church of St Mary's, Cambridge, in his will of 1651; TNA, PROB 11/222, fo. 169v [will of John Crane, esquire, of Cambridge, 26 June 1651, 21 April 1652; pr. 23 June 1652].

207. SUL, HP 29/8/7B; Foster, iv, 1324; Venn, iv, 88; *Wal. Rev.*, 41, 350; Martin, 'John Crane', 434; W. M. Palmer, 'The Reformation of the Corporation of Cambridge, July 1662', *Proceedings of the Cambridgeshire Antiquarian Society*, 17 (1912–13), 124–7. Crane was seemingly at the centre of a complex web of senior Anglican clerics and royalist sympathizers that included former bishops such as Matthew Wren, Ralph Brownrigg and Theophilus Buckworth as well as physicians such as Sclater, William Rant (d.1653) and Thomas Buckenham (d.1682), all of whom were generously remembered in his will. Sclater was elected MP for Cambridge University in 1659 and was created a baronet at the Restoration. He later served as a loyal and trusted servant of the state in various capacities in and around Cambridge until his death in 1684. I discuss this aspect of his career more fully in chapter 6.

208. *Cal. Rev.*, 204, 398. Pratt, who proceeded MD in 1645 and was licensed to practise medicine by the University in 1649, acted as examiner (along with Francis Glisson) for candidates seeking similar licences from the University in 1652; CUL, CUA, Grace Book H (1645–1668), 80–1. His medical case book and other papers are preserved in the Sloane MSS in the BL, as are those of his student, Foote. Pratt suffered a similar fate to Foote at the Restoration, being ejected from his fellowship at Trinity in 1660. Thereafter, the two men seem to have sought refuge in Sion College, where they were both residing at the time of Pratt's death in 1663; *Cal. Rev.*, p.398. Pratt and Glisson were both remembered in the will of John Crane, who left money to fund a house in Cambridge for the regius professor of medicine; TNA, PROB 11/222, fos 169v–175r.

209. In 1682, Foote was acting as amanuensis to van Helmont. He is almost certainly the 'D. F. D. P.' [i.e. Daniel Foote Doctor of Physick], who translated C. P., *A Dissertation Concerning the Pre-Existency of Souls* (London, 1684) 'upon the recommendation of F. M. H. [i.e. Francis Mercury van Helmont] their Friend'. Among other works, Foote was also responsible for translating the work of the Dutch physician John Conrad Amman on teaching the deaf entitled *The Talking Deaf Man* (London, 1694), which included an advert referring to the imminent publication of a related work by van Helmont entitled *The Alphabet of Nature*, as well as the same authors *The Divine Being and Its Attributes.* Both works were almost certainly prepared for publication by Foote. For a recent re-evaluation of Foote's manuscript and published works,

including discussion of his fascination with 'chymistry' and the Quakers, see D. Thorley, 'Daniel Foote, M. D., of Cambridge: The Evidence in Print and from the Sloane Collection', *eBritish Library Journal* (2013), article 15.

210. *CSPD, 1651*, 31; SUL, HP 28/1/61B; 28/1/65A.

211. SUL, HP 28/1/58A–B; J. B. van Helmont, *A Ternary of Paradoxes... Translated, Illustrated, and Ampliated by Walter Charleton, Doctor in Physick, and Physician to the Late King* (London, 1650), 2v; J. B. van Helmont, *Deliramenta Catarrhi: Or, The Incongruities, Impossibilities, and Absurdities Couched Under the Vulgar Opinion of Defluxions. The Author that Great Philosopher, by Fire, Joh. Bapt. Van Helmont... The Translator and Paraphrast Dr. Charleton* (London, 1650). Charleton suffered from life-long depression and later wrote about the condition in his *Natural History of the Passions* (London, 1674). His collapse of faith in 1650 may have induced a decline into immorality. In the 1690s, it was widely reported in dissenting circles that old Dr Charleton was a debauchee given to 'lewd and filthy discourse'. The nonconformist physician Henry Sampson, who noted these indiscretions, nonetheless admired his earliest writings, particularly his translation of van Helmont's *De Lithiasi* (1650); BL, Add. MS 4460, fos 69v–70r.

212. G. Thomson, *Μισοχυμίας ἘλεΓχθ: or, A Check Given to the Insolent Garrulity of Henry Stubbe* (London, 1671), 43–4.

213. In the context of the present discussion, it is perhaps worth noting the frequency with which Thickens referred to his own politically induced state of melancholy in the 1640s. In October 1646, for example, following the defeat of the King in the first civil war, he wrote to Evelyn describing himself as 'a Country melancholy fellow' who had no political news to relate, except to note that 'now is the Fall of the Leafe & of honest men'; BL, Add. MS 78,311, fo. 21v [Thickens to Evelyn, 6 October 1646]; cf. fo. 16 [same to same, 26 January 1646], where he refers to a recent bout of melancholy. The correspondence breaks off suddenly after 1650, when Thickens would appear to have moved to the borough of Maldon where he became actively engaged in Helmontian research.

214. The phrase was employed by the Presbyterian Edward Willan in a sermon preached on parliamentary election day in Suffolk in March 1661; E. Willan, *Beatitas Britanniae: Or, King Charles the Second, Englands Beatitude, as Preached to the Incorporation of Eye, in the County of Suffolk, March 31 1661* (London, 1661), 27. Willan subsequently conformed. Likewise, some royalist preachers, who disdained the unnatural bloodletting of the civil wars, dismissed phlebotomy as 'not cure, but mischief'; B. Holyday, *Against Disloyalty, Fower Sermons Preach'd in the Times of the Late Troubles* (Oxford, 1661), 83; cf. the sentiments of the loyalist Edward Stanley who celebrated the fact that the Restoration had been a bloodless coup and that those 'physicians' responsible, aware of previous excesses, 'have wrought this Cure upon a sick State without any Phlebotomies at all'; E. Stanley, *Three Sermons Preached in the Cathedral Church of Winchester* [19 August 1660] (London, 1662), 29.

215. In 1649, for example, shortly after the execution of Charles I, numerous reports circulated in England recounting the miraculous cures of several women suffering from a range of ailments associated with scrofula. In one case, that of a fourteen-year-old girl from Deptford, who had been blind of the king's evil for eight years, it was

reported that she had recovered her sight 'by using a cloth that was dipped in the king's blood 3 times a day and at the end of the 18th day she could see'; *Mercurius Pragmaticus*, no. 9 [12–19 June 1649], unpaginated; Bodl., Ashmole MS 826, fo. 125; Isle of Wight Record Office, OG/CC/77 [Anne Lennard to her father, Sir John Oglander, 3 August 1649]. Stories of the miraculous cures, both of the king's evil and other diseases, performed by Charles I while imprisoned on the Isle of Wight continued to circulate in Restoration England. They are alluded to, for example, by the loyalist cleric Meric Casaubon in his *Of Credulity and Incredulity in Things Natural, Civil, and Divine* (London, 1668), 293–4.

216. The best source for Akehurst's mental breakdown is found in a letter which one of his students, James Jolly, wrote to Cromwell in 1654, in which he attempted to excuse his teacher's idiosyncratic behaviour as the result of a temporary relapse, and asserted his otherwise godly ways and thoughts; Thurloe, *State Papers*, ii, 464. Jolly was the son of Major James Jolly (1610–1666) of Chester, a committed Independent, who fought for Parliament in the civil war. Two other sons became nonconformist ministers after the Restoration. Like Akehurst, Jolly was drawn to the early Quakers. Though he would appear to have stopped short of joining the sect, he went so far as to renounce the profits of his fellowship and to denounce the function of the university as a seminary for preachers. Jolly also followed Akehurst into medicine. In 1665, he signed the Helmontians' petition in favour of the creation of a Society of Chemical Physicians; see Appendix 1 (a).

217. For more detailed discussion of the cross-denominational and eirenic character of the iatrochemical movement in England in the seventeenth century, see my 'Medicine, Religion and the Puritan Revolution', 24–43.

218. Whereas Thomson established a causal link between bad medicine and the propagation of immorality and irreligiosity, his Helmontian colleague John Collop sought to explain what he called 'this morris dance of religions' by a reverse process that stressed the negative impact of the 'irreligious disputes of... mysticall religion' upon physical health. Religious disputes thus drew blood from the heart to the head, leaving the former 'destitute of zeal to God' and filled with choler. This in turn produced 'that phrantick zeal which discomposes the world... stuffing them with phlegm which lulls them into a Lethargy of indifferency in religion; or raising those melancholy vapors which cause these Epileptic paroxismes in quaking enthusiasts'; J. C[ollop], *Medici Catholicon* (London, 1656), A2r–v.

219. J. French, *The Yorkshire Spaw, or a Treatise of Four Famous Medicinal Wells* (London, 1652), 123. Chymically inclined Catholics included the physician John Fryer and the aristocratic enthusiast Sir Kenelm Digby, both of whom later supported the chymists in 1665; see Appendix 1 (a).

4

'By Virtue of our Hermetick Physick, the Head, Heart, and Hands of Hierophants might be Purified'

The Society of Chymical Physicians and Medical Reform in Restoration England

Introduction

1665 was a tumultuous year in the medical history of London. The onset of bubonic plague in the late summer, which led to the deaths of tens of thousands of men and women over the course of the following year, affected all aspects of life in the capital. Social and economic activity in the city was paralysed and a religious and political vacuum was created by the mass exodus of the rich and powerful to country retreats and other places of refuge. The ensuing medical crisis, one which London's citizens and governors had faced on numerous occasions in the past, was largely placed in the care of a handful of brave men and women who soldiered on, against the odds, in providing a modicum of services that included the oversight of pesthouses, the imposition of quarantine procedures, and a desperate struggle to cope with the removal and burial of ever-expanding numbers of victims of the plague. The medical establishment, in the form of the College of Physicians, was largely powerless to intervene. Most of its members fled the city along with their wealthy patients, but in so doing they also created an opportunity for other practitioners to take their place and in the process to stake a claim to medical legitimacy unhindered by the lapsed authority of the College. The largest beneficiaries of this medical vacuum were the chymical physicians.

In the previous year, a group of iatrochemists, largely inspired by the writings of the Flemish physician Jan Baptist van Helmont, had taken the first steps in laying down a new challenge to the monopolistic authority of the College of Physicians. The Society of Chymical Physicians, as the group styled themselves, agitated throughout 1665 to undermine and supplant the College as the principal medical body in the capital. The appearance of the plague, seen by many, if not most, as a rebuke to the sins of the nation also provided a useful narrative for the iatrochemists in their controversy with the collegiate physicians. Here was a

Medicine in an Age of Revolution. Peter Elmer, Oxford University Press. © Peter Elmer 2023.
DOI: 10.1093/oso/9780198853985.003.0004

heaven-sent opportunity to prove the value and worth of Helmontian medicine. The ensuing struggle for supremacy, the outcome determined as much by religious and political factors as medical ones, was to prove a critical moment in the history of medicine in Restoration England. In the event, the chymists failed to overthrow the traditional apparatus of medical authority in London and to discredit the humoral methods that underpinned the practice of the majority of collegiate physicians. The conflict nonetheless continued to shape medical thinking for much of the rest of the century. In what follows, I hope to demonstrate how the origins, aims and demise of the Society of Chymical Physicians is best understood within the context of the wider religious and political debates that characterized the early years of the Restoration, a period that witnessed a resumption of conflict and debate within the body politic as a result of the failure of successive governments to heal the wounds of civil war.

The Society of Chymical Physicians: Politics, Religion and the Struggle for Medical Change in Restoration London

The story of the attempt by the Society of Chymical Physicians to overhaul the practice of medicine in the capital has often been told.[1] Historians, however, have disagreed as to the principal factors that lay behind the attempt to build a new medical society on iatrochemical lines. Some have interpreted the iatrochemists' assault on the privileges of the Galenic physicians as an extension of the earlier quarrel between learned medical practitioners and their lower status rivals, the apothecaries, who were keen to legitimate their incursion into the medical marketplace.[2] Others have detected continuity in the arguments of the Society's spokesmen with their chymical predecessors in Interregnum England, particularly those physicians, natural philosophers and reformers who formed the core of the intellectual coterie surrounding Samuel Hartlib.[3] More recently, Hal Cook has proposed that the origins of the Society, its initial successes, and ultimate failure reside in broad political factors, especially those relating to the intricacies of court patronage.[4] None of these explanations are mutually exclusive, and all contain important insights. Here, however, I would like to develop some of the themes and ideas first propounded by Cook to illustrate the central theme of this book, namely the growing politicization of the practice of medicine in late Stuart England. The argument that follows thus supports much of Cook's emphasis on the role of patronage in medicine, a theme subsequently developed by historians of medicine in a variety of related contexts,[5] while at the same time seeking to expand understanding of the impact of religious and political debate upon the world of Restoration medicine.

In April 1664, the House of Commons refused to ratify the new royal charter for the London College of Physicians, leaving it, in the words of Hal Cook, in 'a frail institutional and legal condition'. Within days of this decision, Thomas O'Dowde, a groom of the bedchamber to Charles II and one of the prime movers behind the attempt to establish a 'Society of Chymical Physitians', was actively canvassing the King in the hope of obtaining royal patronage for an alternative medical institution for London.[6] Mobilizing support from within the highest echelons of the court and government circles, O'Dowde's lobbying tactics finally paid off when a year later he and his chymical associates were granted an audience with the King in Council in order to put forward their proposals. No account of this meeting survives, and the efforts of the chymists finally came to nothing. Many, in fact, died bravely attempting to provide succour to those poorer citizens who remained in the capital throughout the plague epidemic. Others among the group published spirited defences of chymical medicine and attacks aimed at exposing the deficiencies of their adversaries, the college doctors (the vast majority of whom were assumed to be Galenic in orientation), but all to no avail. Their opponents rallied and amidst a fusillade of apologias, the chymists were defeated, their cause fatally undermined by divisions within their own ranks and the ability of their opponents to exploit the widely held view that the Society was little more than a front for religious and political subversives who had managed to inveigle their way into courtly and aristocratic circles.

What this story of bravado and ultimate failure does not accurately reflect is the extent to which the origins of the Society, and its ultimate demise, were shaped by broader religious and political concerns that increasingly affected discussion of all aspects of the healing arts in the second half of the seventeenth century. These are hinted at in Cook's work but, as I argue here, ran much deeper than his account suggests. This is numerous ways. It is apparent, for example, in the remarkable extent to which Charles II was willing to encourage and reward, in myriad ways, those chymists and iatrochemical practitioners who flocked to his court after 1660. Though Charles' amateur passion for chymical experiments and demonstrations has frequently attracted comment (usually to depict him as little more than a dilettante), little attempt has been made to uncover the full extent of his preoccupation with medical innovation and his promotion of those who publicized the benefits of 'alternative' cures, including Helmontian physic. Charles was not alone, however, at court in supporting such men and ideas. Many of his closest aristocratic advisers were similarly drawn to the study of chymistry and used their substantial reservoirs of courtly patronage to both protect and promote the interests of a range of empirics and healers, many of whom laboured in the 'pyrotechnical arts'.[7] Above all, however, the chymical physicians probably owed their greatest debt to the leading churchman in England, Gilbert Sheldon, archbishop of Canterbury. Sheldon not only offered support and protection to various iatrochemical practitioners, but, as I suggest below, he may well have actively promoted the chymists' cause by utilizing the ecclesiastical licensing system in order to counter what he saw as the pernicious influence of a puritan medical establishment, the London College, which he believed was providing a refuge for nonconformist physicians in the capital as well as institutional support to their fellow practitioners throughout the rest of the kingdom.[8]

In 1660, shortly after the Restoration, it was reported to Samuel Hartlib that the new king was reputed to be a 'Teutonicus and lover of chymistry'. Hartlib's death in 1662 robbed him of the chance to witness at first hand the extraordinary devotion of Charles II, and other members of his entourage, to chymistry and related studies which, ironically, found greater favour at the restored court of the Stuarts than it did at that of Hartlib's preferred Maecenas, Oliver Cromwell. With a laboratory at St James' Palace, staffed by a regular professor of chymistry and laboratory assistants, Charles was frequently to be found observing and participating in the latest experiments devised by his servants or others recommended to his service.[9] Among those rumoured to have performed their chymical operations in private before the King were the celebrated German iatrochemist Albertus Otto Faber (1612–1684), the London empirics Lionel Lockyer (d.1672) and William Trigge (d.1665), Richard Barker (later knighted by the King), and the Helmontian physician George Starkey, reputedly under the guise of the pseudonymous *adeptus*, Eirenaeus Philalethes.[10] Like many of his subjects, Charles was also a great believer in self-medication. In 1676, for example, he was reported by the earl of Bath to have employed 'Monsieur Rabell's water' on a wound which, the following morning, 'took away the swelling and payne'. Three days later, Charles claimed to be perfectly recovered, and so 'adds great fame to this new remedy, especially being now experimented by the King himselfe, to the great displeasure of our doctors and surgeons'.[11]

Charles' love of chymistry may have gone hand in hand with his disapproval of the methods of the Galenic physicians. This was certainly the opinion of one anonymous Restoration critic of the medical establishment who claimed in 1678 that the King was known to have favoured the methods of the chymical doctors over and above those of the Galenists.[12] If his patronage and appointment of medical practitioners to the royal household is a guide, then there seems little doubt that Charles was keen to promote chymical medicine. At least eight of those who signed the petition of the chymist's Society were the recipients of this form of royal patronage.[13] Three others were awarded mandated Cambridge MDs at the behest of Charles.[14] Moreover, Charles' passion for all things chymical, including alchemical speculation, was shared by other high-profile members of his court. His cousin Prince Rupert, for example, was known to dabble in such pursuits.[15] It is also noteworthy how many of the signatories to the chymists' petition were linked in some way to the household of the King's brother, James, duke of York. The French physician Pierre Massonet, for example, had served as a tutor to the young prince in the 1640s. Acting as a double agent in the following decade, he re-entered the royal household at the Restoration, when he claimed to be acting as physician in ordinary to the duke. Unlike some of his colleagues at court, however,

Massonet does not seem to have prospered. He consistently sued for the payment of arrears for various posts, some of which he claimed to have held for over thirty years, and at one stage added the detail that his wife was forced to work as a washer woman in the royal employ. He was finally rewarded for his indefatigable services to the Stuart cause in 1672, when he was created physician in ordinary to the King, though it is highly unlikely that Massonet benefited financially from the appointment.[16]

Of equal significance for the chymical physicians was the support of numerous high-ranking aristocrats at the court of Charles II, many of whom demonstrated a genuine interest in promoting iatrochemistry and related projects. Foremost among this group was George Villiers, duke of Buckingham, a passionate devotee of experimental chymistry who possessed his own laboratory at Wallingford House. Buckingham, not surprisingly, was the subject of numerous epistolary dedications by grateful chymical physicians, who eulogized his achievements and, in some cases, predicted great things of the duke. Edward Bolnest, for example, praised him for his 'acute genius' in discovering 'the Vanity of the Galenick way'. His colleague Marchamont Nedham went so far as to suggest that the duke was 'a Prince by Merit, as well as Title, for whether you take him in the Chymical, or in his Politick capacity, he appears no less in either'. Here was a man of whom much was expected, one who 'can be greater, if he please, because with so rare a Wit and other Abilities of mind, seated in a comely Body, I know not what he may effect in Philosophy and Politie, by plying his Laboratory at Home, and another at Court'.[17] Moreover, Buckingham's interest in chymistry would appear to have continued into the 1670s, at a time when he was becoming increasingly involved in political machinations aimed at undermining the 'absolutist' policies of the crown. In 1673, the Helmontian physician Thomas Sherley dedicated his *Philosophical Essay* to Buckingham, in which he lauded the duke as 'a great experimental philosopher', whose insights into the natural world were 'acquired by a constant, and curious, Anatomizing of all sort of Concrets in your Laboratory'.[18] In 1677, he was the subject of yet another fulsome dedication in a work published by the prolific Helmontian William Simpson.[19] One practical by-product of the duke's interest in chymistry was the construction of a successful glass-making factory at Vauxhall, a project that drew in other chymically minded dependants and business partners such as the former royalist, Thomas Paulden, and the duke's secretary, Martin Clifford.[20]

Another powerful figure at court and supporter of the chymists, who would appear to have shared Buckingham's enthusiasm for a medical alternative to Galenic orthodoxy, was the Irish peer, James Butler, first duke of Ormond.[21] At least two of his personal physicians exhibited a marked preference for iatrochemistry and alchemical speculation. In 1652 William Fogarty, an Irish Catholic employed by the duke, was said, on the authority of Samuel Hartlib's son-in-law Frederick Clodius, to have recently come into possession of the medical and alchemical papers once owned by the celebrated *adeptus* Dr William Butler (1535–1618) of Cambridge. Fogarty supposedly promised to give them to Clodius 'upon condition that he should explain the doubtful and enigmaticall passages unto him'.[22] At the Restoration, Ormond employed another chymical physician and former associate of Hartlib, William Currer, as his personal physician. A royalist, Currer had served the parliamentary forces in Ireland in the early 1640s, but subsequently lost his post, presumably because of his political affiliations. He was re-appointed in 1660, probably at the instigation of his patron, Ormond, the most senior figure in the restored government of Ireland, and seven years later was named as one of the founder members of the Irish College of Physicians, a body that was largely incorporated at the prompting of the duke.[23] Like the King, Ormond also used his substantial powers as lord lieutenant and chancellor of Trinity College, Dublin, to recommend suitable candidates for medical degrees. His support for John Archer in 1664 once again appears to confirm the duke as a favourer of chymical medicine. Archer, who claimed to have studied and practised physic in Dublin for seven years and to have been obstructed by unnamed rivals from obtaining his degree, was subsequently awarded his MD following a petition to the duke. Ormond may even have promoted Archer's career in England for in 1670 he was appointed chymical physician in ordinary to Charles II, and thus joined a growing band of iatrochemists who found favour at the Restoration court.[24]

Despite the menial and plebeian associations of laboratory work, aristocrats like the duke of Buckingham were not averse to following the example of the King and engaging in chymical operations and manual experiments. Other nobles and courtiers who signed up to O'Dowde's petition in 1665 and were equally at home in the laboratory as in the court included Philip Herbert, fifth earl of Pembroke, Sir John Mennes and Sir Kenelm Digby. Pembroke's chief interest, according to John Aubrey, lay in chymistry and the compounding of medicines, while Mennes, who probably practised medicine in the 1650s as a cover for plotting, was skilled in physic and chymistry, and claimed a special skill in the cure of venereal disease. Sir Kenelm Digby's engagement with chymistry predated the civil war. During the Interregnum he was actively engaged in a number of projects of an iatrochemical nature and was a leading advocate of a scheme to establish a Chemical Council.[25] He also employed a number of chymical operatives, including Dr Richard Farrar or Ferrar, well known to Hartlib and Boyle in the 1650s, who would appear to have later found employ with the King in his ever-expanding medical household.[26]

The patronage of such eminent courtiers was clearly invaluable for the chymists. However, the most practical source of support for the nascent Society, and one glossed over in previous accounts of the origins of the Society of Chymical Physicians, was provided by two of the most powerful clergymen in England: Gilbert Sheldon, archbishop of Canterbury, and Humphrey Henchman, bishop of

London. Both men, in their respective offices, wielded important powers of medical patronage. Sheldon, for example, as archbishop of Canterbury (1663–1677) was able to grant licences to medical practitioners throughout the province of Canterbury, as well as award Lambeth medical degrees. In the case of the diocese of London, held by the two men from 1660 to 1675, the bishop was able to grant similar licences, a practice that potentially undermined the ability of the College of Physicians to enforce its own monopoly of medical practice in and around the city of London. Given the support of Sheldon and Henchman for the Society of Chymical Physicians in 1665, it is perhaps unsurprising that the licensing system over which they presided was consistently used to legitimate the practices of iatrochemists and other empirics, much to the irritation, one imagines, of the College. Many of the signatories of the chymists' petition were either licensed in this way (and thus granted immunity from prosecution by the College) or supplied testimonials for fellow chymists and like-minded practitioners.[27] Typical was the case of Robert Turner, a prolific translator of occult and Paracelsian texts, who was licensed by Sheldon, as bishop of London, in 1661. He subsequently provided testimonials for four new candidates between 1661 and 1666 and, in all probability, acknowledged his gratitude to the authorities by dedicating one of his last published works, *The Brittish Physician* (1664), to Sir Richard Chaworth (d.1672), vicar general of the province of Canterbury and chancellor of the diocese of London, whose job it was to oversee the licensing process in his respective jurisdictions.[28] Turner's example also illustrates how the chymical physicians used the ecclesiastical licensing system to promote their beliefs and practices throughout the rest of the kingdom. In 1662 Turner was one of six men who supplied medical testimonials on behalf of William Bruton (d.1680) of Alwington, Devon, who was seeking a licence to practise medicine from the bishop of Exeter. At least three of the other signatories were fellow London chymists, all of whom would later sign the engagement of the Society of Chymical Physicians in 1665.[29]

The tendency of chymical physicians like Turner and his colleagues to legitimate their London practices through the ecclesiastical licensing process may well have been encouraged by senior churchmen like Sheldon and Henchman as both men demonstrated more than a passing interest in the new medicine. Sheldon, for example, was reported as early as 1654 to be conversant with an unnamed chymist responsible for manufacturing a red powder that was widely believed to act as a cure-all.[30] After the Restoration, he was responsible for granting a Lambeth medical degree to the surgeon and experimental chymist, Edmund King (1630–1709), and probably continued to promote his career at court thereafter.[31] Effusive dedications to the archbishop on the part of O'Dowde and Thomson in their pamphlet campaign against the Galenists in 1665 suggest yet further evidence of a genuine sympathy on the part of Sheldon for the aspirations of the chymists. Thomson strongly hinted at Sheldon's passion for chymistry, describing him as one 'who hath been pleased to express very much kindness and love for this Noble Art, to the no small encouragement of the Professours thereof'. Such encouragement, in all probability, extended to Sheldon's employment of the services of the Helmontians. One of their leading spokesmen in Restoration England, Albertus Otto Faber, provided a detailed account of his treatment of the archbishop in his last illness in which he prescribed his celebrated *aurum potabile*.[32] Moreover, Sheldon's colleague Henchman may have shared the archbishop's preference for alternative therapies as suggested by his patronage of the iatrochemist, Major John Choke or Chalk. In July 1667 Choke was appointed chymist in ordinary to the King and was granted a licence to practise medicine throughout the diocese of London by Henchman, who personally attested to 'having known of the wonderful cures, which he has wrought on many desperate cases'.[33] Choke was no ordinary empiric. In 1670, in conversation with Roger Boyle, earl of Orrery, whom he was treating with a Helmontian receipt, he claimed to be Jan Baptist van Helmont's son-in-law, having married his widowed daughter.[34] He was subsequently forced to recant, for in 1684 it was reported that Prince Rupert had once tried to introduce Choke to his putative brother-in-law, the celebrated chymist and mystical philosopher Francis Mercury van Helmont (1614–1698). According to an unnamed informant, Choke was forced to excuse himself, 'and withal declared, that what was reported of him was a mistake, and that it was not his Sister, but a Servant of the House whom he had married'.[35]

The support of senior churchmen such as Sheldon and Henchman for the chymists is thus partly explicable on medical grounds. It seems equally likely, however, particularly in regard to the militant Sheldon, that the patronage of such leading clerics was also informed by a marked antipathy to the perceived 'puritanism' of the London College of Physicians which acted as an important refuge for nonconformist medical practitioners in the early years of the Restoration.[36] Nowhere was this more apparent than in the support which the College gave to many ejected ministers, or the sons of the same, who had been attracted to the study and practice of medicine in the face of the legal and institutional proscription of dissent after 1660. This was most effectively done through the College's grant of the title of extra-licentiate, which allowed the holder to practise medicine anywhere in England. No oaths were required, and only the briefest of examinations by the College's censors or president was sufficient for the award to be granted. Given that the office of censor, like that of president, was dominated for much of the 1660s and 1670s by former Presbyterians and nonconformist sympathizers, this route to professional legitimation proved a highly popular one in the dissenting community. It is unlikely, however, that this practice was smiled upon by archbishop Sheldon, who was dedicated to the task of stamping out dissent and imposing a rigid conformity on the restored Church.[37]

Of the seventy-one men who were granted extra licentiate status between 1660 and 1688, thirty-three (about 46 per cent) were either former ministers (thirteen), the sons of ejected ministers (eight), or otherwise active in dissenting circles (twelve).[38] A typical beneficiary of the College's sympathetic approach to the plight of former ministers who had lost their livings and college fellowships between 1660 and 1662 was the Congregationalist, John Hutchinson. Ejected from his fellowship at Trinity College, Cambridge, at the Restoration, he subsequently travelled abroad where, among other things, he attended anatomical dissections in France. On his return home (probably in early 1662), he was invited to become a fellow of the College of Physicians, but refused the offer, and was content instead to submit to an examination by the College's censor Dr John Micklethwaite 'upon which he was approv'd, and had a Licence to practise as a Physician *per totam Angliam*'.[39] Micklethwaite's period of office, coinciding as it did with a mass exodus of ministers from the Anglican Church in the wake of the imposition of the Act of Uniformity on St Bartholomew's Day (24 August 1662), proved fortunate for other former ministers who now sought a new career in medicine. On 10 November 1662, for example, the College censors licensed two more ejected ministers, John Pringle and Edward Richardson. Pringle, like many of his former clerical colleagues who took up the practice of medicine, combined the cure of bodies with the cure of souls, and acted as pastor to a dissenting congregation in Newcastle-upon-Tyne.[40] Richardson's subsequent career as a plotter and fugitive from justice can only have exacerbated Sheldon's antipathy for the College. Within a few months of acquiring the status of an extra-licentiate in the College, Richardson played a leading role in the Farnley Wood Plot of 1663 for which he was arrested and imprisoned at York. Managing to escape, he fled to Holland, where he proceeded MD at Leiden in 1664, and spent the next ten years or more ministering to the English churches at Haarlem (1665–70) and Leiden (1670–75), as well as providing spiritual and material succour to exiled dissenters and fellow conspirators who sought refuge in Holland.[41] The example of Richardson may represent an extreme case as most ejected ministers would appear to have eschewed overt opposition to the new regime. However, he was certainly not alone among his extra-licentiate colleagues in pursuing such ends. The two brothers Ichabod and Isaac Chauncy, for example, were both engaged in active resistance to the restored Stuarts. Ichabod was repeatedly accused of fomenting opposition in Bristol after the Restoration, while Isaac was prosecuted for seditious behaviour in 1669, the year in which he was approved for practice by the College in London. Like many of their dissenting brethren, the two men undoubtedly owed much to the network of sympathetic nonconformist colleagues both within and outside the College in receiving their licences. Ichabod, for example, was approved for practice by four members of the College (the president Edward Alston, George Ent, William Staines and John Micklethwaite), all of whom were prominent in, or attached to, dissenting circles.[42] Indeed, such was the fear surrounding the political activities of these men that some of their Anglican opponents genuinely believed that they were using medicine and their connections within the College to subvert the entire religious settlement. In 1671, for example, amid growing concerns among dissenters regarding the growth of persecution, the Somerset cleric John Beale reported that ministers' sons were being sent from America to England as physicians where, with the consent of the London College, they were being encouraged to set up in practice throughout the realm. His informant was himself a nonconformist physician practising in Bristol who was adamant that the phenomenon was part of a plot 'to convert our confused church' to the 'narrowe way' of New England.[43]

It was no doubt the activities of men like Richardson and the Chauncys, who were determined to overthrow the Restoration settlement, which aroused fear and opposition in Anglican circles to the College, and may in the process have fatally prejudiced the College's attempt to seek a renewal of its charter in parliament in 1664.[44] In December of that year, in the face of parliamentary opposition to its attempt to renegotiate its charter and reaffirm its authority to police the practice of medicine in London and its environs, the College acted by extending its membership to a new class of physician, the honorary fellow. Seventy-three new fellows were inducted into the College, the vast majority former royalists or those who had suffered for their loyalty during the 1640s and 1650s.[45] There can be little doubt that this strategy was partly dictated by political considerations, a belated attempt as it were to convince Parliament and the King that the College was a loyal and conformable institution. However, the inclusion of a minority of men whose religious and political loyalties were at best debatable, and at worst antithetical to the Restoration, probably did little to assuage implacable opponents of the College such as Sheldon. Among those who paid the requisite fee for honorary admission were Nicholas Barbon or Barebon,[46] Henry Glisson,[47] Richard Griffiths,[48] Aaron Gurdon, Nicholas Lamprière or Lemprière,[49] Walter Needham,[50] William Parker, Thomas Tymme,[51] Thomas Trapham, Timothy van Vleteren,[52] Humphrey Whitmore and John Yardley,[53] all of whom were tainted by their former allegiance to the governments of Interregnum England.[54]

The perceived infiltration of the medical profession in this way by religious and political dissidents clearly jarred with men like archbishop Sheldon, who just seven months later instituted a comprehensive audit of the medical licensing system in the province of Canterbury as part of a clampdown on nonconformity. Sheldon accordingly requested that his bishops, through their subordinate officers and surrogates, supply him with 'the names, surnames, degrees and qualities of all practisers of physic within their respective dioceses... whether licensed, and by whom, and how they appear affected to his majesty's government, and the doctrine and discipline of the Church of England'.[55] The timing of this process was surely significant, occurring as it did at the height of renewed fears surrounding the onset of plague and the willingness of nonconformist preachers and physicians alike to exploit the opportunities that arose in the wake of plague-related disorder and dislocation. It is little wonder that some in the College of

Physicians, most of whose members fled London at the commencement of the plague, linked the archbishop's support for the chymical physicians with what they perceived as an attempt by the leadership of the Anglican Church to revitalize its regulatory medical powers at the expense of the College's authority in such matters.[56]

If these fears receded following the collapse of the projected Society of Chymical Physicians towards the end of 1665 (discussed more fully below), then they never entirely disappeared for the remainder of Charles II's reign. Indeed, the revival of the chymists' aspirations in the mid-1670s once more raised the spectre of a challenge to the authority of the College, and again it was the aging archbishop that the chymists looked to for protection and support. This time, however, Sheldon's motive for supporting the chymists was transparent. The new campaign against the College was spearheaded by a former Dublin apothecary, Adrian Huyberts, who was prosecuted by the College for illicit practice in 1675.[57] Before the case was heard in King's Bench, however, Huyberts pre-empted the College's charge by publishing a vindication of his stance. In *A Corner-Stone Laid Towards the Building of a New Colledge... in London*, he rehearsed the familiar legal arguments against the College's power to prosecute unlicensed healers, disparaged the collegiate physicians for their failure to advance medicine, and promoted the benefits of chymistry, 'the Queen of Arts' and 'Mother of Physick'. Just as importantly, however, he acknowledged the patronage of archbishop Sheldon 'under whose protection it hath been my happiness to practise and do the like services for several of his Majestyes, and the Duke of York's servants here at White-Hall and St James's'. Huyberts was in fact licensed by the archbishop in the same year as his prosecution, further fuelling speculation that he was indeed acting as Sheldon's mouthpiece.[58] Certainly, it is not difficult in Huyberts' work to discern the aspirations of his powerful patron, as, for example, when he pleaded:

> what a happiness it be, if the reverend Church-men would consider these things, and what Authority hath been intrusted in them only by the Law, for the approvement of Physicians, and the prevention of that Tyranny which the more idle and formal speculators of Physick, have hitherto exercised over the industrious practical Physicians, under pretence of Law... For it is still to be presumed, the reverend Bishops are the only Trustees in the Law concerning this matter.[59]

As if to emphasize the point, Huyberts indulged in some very effective mudslinging, reviving earlier speculation that the College was little better than a refuge for dissenting clerics, who were queueing up to be 'herded' into the College. He reserved his particular ire for those former schoolmasters or preachers, who went abroad to 'to be made doctors at Leyden, and the like places beyond-Sea; and by reading a few Books and prating intrude into a Calling, which is not to be acquired but by years of labour and studie of Experimental, not School-philosophy'. These men, he claimed, were increasingly infiltrating the London College:

> to which they have been, and are admitted upon producing a Diploma . . . and the answering of a few questions about Doctrine and Method; and because Leyden in Holland hath been a fruitful Mother of such English Brats, (too many of which are now domineering among us) they are by our own University-men in scorn called Leaden Doctors.[60]

The suspicion that Huyberts was voicing the views of his patron and other powerful figures at court is reinforced by the fact that earlier the same year, in February 1675, Charles II had written to the College of Physicians warning it to desist from the practice of bestowing honorary fellowships upon any physicians who had 'graduated in Universityes beyond the Seas', a form of code for the Dutch universities in general, and Leiden and Utrecht in particular. Consequently, the King insisted that such offices should only be offered in future to those who had either studied at Oxford or Cambridge, or had their foreign degrees incorporated at the same, having sworn the requisite oaths of loyalty to the crown.[61]

Huyberts' concerns were not then simply rhetorical but were genuine and reflected a growing belief that medicine, like society in general, was being torn apart by the religious and political divisions set in motion by the Restoration settlement. As for the chymists, they continued to batter at the door of the London College, but all to no avail. Within a short time, they had lost some of their most powerful supporters (Henchman died in 1675, soon followed by Sheldon in 1677) and issues of political patronage became increasingly subsumed in the larger conflicts being fought out in the wake of the Popish Plot and the Exclusion Crisis. Before we look more closely at these developments, however, I would like to return briefly to events surrounding the demise of the Society of Chymical Physicians focusing particularly on the religious and political divisions that played such an important part in its ultimate downfall.

Accounting for Failure: Religious Radicalism and Medical Reform in Restoration England

Traditional explanations for the failure of the projected Society have focused on various factors, including the plague-related deaths of many of its leading protagonists as well as the success of the collegiate physicians in countering many of the more extreme claims of the chymists. The College's apologists, for example, repeatedly sought to steal the chymists' thunder by arguing that many of its members were themselves practising chymists who commonly integrated chymical medicines into their armoury of cures and therapies. However, the principal cause of failure, acknowledged by the chymists' themselves, was internal dissension, a fact that their opponents were quick to exploit. As earlier commentators have noted, the Society of Chymical Physicians was a somewhat amorphous group, incorporating disaffected university-educated physicians alongside those that their opponents liked to stigmatize as unlearned empirics and unqualified quacks. It also contained men of mixed religious and political persuasions, both in its core membership, as well as among its aristocratic and court support. To some extent, these problems were not insuperable or necessarily fatal within the context of the early years of the Restoration. Men of differing religious and political opinions were often able to put aside their differences in order to accomplish a greater good. It none the less remained difficult to counter the accusations of opponents who insisted on drawing a link between the activities of medical 'enthusiasts' with the actions of those who sought to undermine the established order in church and state. The point was well made by William Johnson, the College of Physicians' own chymist, who repeatedly associated the medical 'enthusiasm' or fanaticism of the chymists with the religious 'enthusiasm' displayed by 'our Fanaticks'. Their aim, he claimed, was nothing less than the destruction of all learning, which itself was envisaged as a prelude to social and political anarchy. In order to expose the fraudulent nature of the Society's plans, it was therefore crucial for Johnson and his colleagues to highlight at every opportunity the divisions within the ranks of the chymists and to stigmatize 'those Fanaticks in Physick' as little better than unlearned empirics, 'Foot-Men, Gun-Smiths, Heel-Makers, and Botchers', who are only 'made Doctors in the Opinion of the Vulgar'.[62]

Johnson was only too aware of the growing divisions in the ranks of the chymists, alluding on more than one occasion to George Thomson's despair at the antics of some of his erstwhile colleagues.[63] And, as the following example attests, Johnson was doing no more than reporting the truth. In the early stages of the plague, the chymists achieved a major propaganda victory when one of their number, Edward Bolnest, was chosen by them, on the King's command, to act as physician to the strategically important town and port of Southampton.[64] Bolnest, however, much to the irritation of Thomson, failed to take up his post, preferring instead to haggle with the government over the terms of his contract. Thomson indignantly reported of his former colleague that he 'could not rest himself satisfied with the Kings [sic] royal word and pleasure (which would have been reward enough to a truly ingenuous man) but he must stand upon stipulation, upon a contract and mercenary terms, with the most potent prince in Christendome, to the great prejudice and disgrace of this noble Art, and the disrepute of the Learned professors thereof'. He therefore had no alternative but 'utterly to disowne' Bolnest, and to:

> openly protest that it was done without my consent or knowledge, having not been at the Convention this half a year. For I am resolved never to joyne with some men that carry an Enterprise to bring a black cloud upon learning, and a vile estimation upon schools of sound Education; and shall always defend Decency, Eutaxie, and good Government in the Church and State.[65]

Bolnest, a client of the duke of Buckingham, was almost certainly representative of what one might loosely term the radical or dissident wing of the iatrochemical movement in Restoration London. Rumoured to have been a soldier under Cromwell in Ireland, his behaviour in ungraciously insisting upon a written contract with the crown prior to departing for Southampton no doubt helped to confirm the worst fears of the chymists' critics and the anarchic and 'levelling' consequences of a totally unregulated medical marketplace.[66] Thomson himself had heavily intimated that Bolnest was a member of a chymical 'convention' or club, whose principles were anathema to his own, based as they were on a dutiful respect for the Stuarts and the Anglican Church. It would be fascinating to know more about this radical medical underground that operated in London in the 1660s and 1670s. Rarely discerned, it is possible to catch glimpses of it from a variety of sources, most of which strongly suggest that interest in chymistry and medical innovation in this period continued to prosper in radical religious and political circles. One such opening on to this secretive world is provided by the correspondence of the Independent minister John Allin who, following his ejection from Rye in Sussex in 1662, moved to London in order, like so many former colleagues in the Cromwellian church, to follow a new career in medicine.

Allin's life in London in the early years of the Restoration, and his attempt to start a new career as a chymical physician, can be constructed from the voluminous surviving correspondence that he held with his former friends and associates in Rye, more especially with fellow physician and iatrochemist, Philip Frith (d.1670).[67] Allin corresponded regularly, providing detailed accounts of his new life in London and his struggle to attain financial solvency through the establishment of a successful medical practice. At the same time, he seems to have acted as an agent for various Rye merchants and sailors, as well as sending books, chymical equipment and almanacs to his friends in the port town who included the dissenting astrologer Samuel Jeake the elder (1623–1690).[68] Allin himself, it would appear, was closely involved in the preparation, publication and dissemination of almanacs, claiming on one occasion to be a close friend of the celebrated astrologer John Booker (1602–1667).[69] Allin's keenness to become a doctor is attested by his regular attendance at anatomies at the Barber Surgeons' Hall, as well as his membership of chymical clubs. The latter, at which like-minded physicians gathered to help and support each other in the free exchange of information relating to their occupation, also acted as a focal point for the discussion and publication of iatrochemical works and translations.[70] Allin was almost certainly a Helmontian by orientation. He was on friendly terms with the New England adept, George Starkey, whose medicines he manufactured and administered to his patients, but was not averse to chide him for his arrogance in seeking to anatomize the bodies of plague victims.[71] Allin, too, like Starkey and other chymical colleagues, harboured pretensions to write and publish. In September 1665, fearful that he might perish in the plague, he advised his friend Frith to take care of a book he had written entitled *Liber Veritatis or the True Use of Elixir Magnum... Given to a Friend by a True Master of the Arte.*[72] Despite visiting a potential publisher, the work was not forthcoming. Likewise, in July 1670, in his last letter to Frith, who died the following month, Allin claimed to be engaged in translating the works of the French Paracelsian Bernard Penot and invited Frith to send him one of his manuscripts so that he might publish it alongside his own work.[73] In the event, neither saw the light of day, though an edition of Penot's writings did appear much later in 1692 under the initials B.P.[74] It is tempting to speculate that the author was Allin's friend and chymical colleague Benedict Porter, who belonged to the same club as Allin, many of whose members, as noted above, were actively engaged in promoting the publication of works of this nature.[75]

Other members of this club, frequently mentioned in Allin's letters, included his friends Robert Pratt and John Stacy. Pratt was a prominent figure in iatrochemical circles. In 1665 he was appointed as Bolnest's replacement as chymical physician to the plague-ridden town of Southampton.[76] He was also highly active, along with other club members, in supporting fellow chymists who wished to secure episcopal licences to practise medicine.[77] It has not been possible to substantiate Pratt's radical credentials. Many of his chymical friends, however, who were either the recipients of licences or provided testimonials for others, were clearly connected to an underground network of radical dissidents that was seeking to exploit the licensing system in order to acquire medical (and perhaps social) respectability. In 1669, for example, Pratt, along with Allin's friends, Benedict Porter and John Stacy, supplied testimonials on behalf of Charles Wilcox, a candidate for a licence from the bishop of London.[78] Wilcox claimed to have served as master of the pesthouse in Tower Hamlets during the plague as well as surgeon to the royal garrison in the Tower of London, and was duly granted his licence. However, Wilcox's profession of conformity to the restored Anglican Church (all candidates were expected to subscribe to the Thirty-Nine Articles) may not have been sincere. Throughout the 1670s he fought a long campaign for reimbursement of moneys expended in his role as physician to the Tower during the plague but was blocked at every stage by the intervention of the ultra-royalist lieutenant of the Tower, Sir John Robinson. Though the official documents do not state the specific nature of Robinson's objections, they were almost certainly related to Wilcox's radical religious predilections. Allin himself had described Wilcox as an 'Anabaptist' in 1666, and there is little doubt that many of his chymical colleagues harboured similar heterodox beliefs. It was probably no coincidence, for example, that another of Wilcox's referees in 1669 was none other than that well-known purveyor of chymical pills, Lionel Lockyer, who had exhibited Ranter sympathies during the Interregnum.[79]

In all probability, Lockyer played a pivotal role in supporting and possibly coordinating the chymists' campaign to infiltrate the medical profession in and around London in the early years of the Restoration. His name appears as a referee on numerous applications for episcopal and archiepiscopal licences, and he may well have been a member of Allin's chymical club.[80] Moreover, his reputation as a self-taught practitioner, together with his radical past, was bound to attract the attention of the chymists' enemies as well as some of their more politically conservative supporters.[81] In Lockyer's case, moreover, it is quite possible that he continued to associate with former radical colleagues who subscribed to a form of religiosity that was at variance with all orthodox forms after the Restoration. Among those fellow chemists who received testimonials from Lockyer, for example, were Thomas Fyge and Abiezer Coppe who both shared their mentor's unconventional religious interests. Fyge (d.1705) was a wealthy apothecary with extensive connections in London dissenting circles. Like his father, Valentine (d.1685), who had been prosecuted by the College on various occasions before the civil war, he became active in city politics. He also shared Lockyer's antinomian leanings and in 1666 dedicated a work advocating a quietist approach to religion to his friend Lockyer in the hope that it might act like 'the Medicine of the Soul' and 'be as effectual for the purifying and healing of the minds of men, as your Universal Pill hath been successful in the cure of their Bodies'. According to one associate, Fyge was one of only two men that Lockyer trusted with the preparation and sale of his famous pills and he eventually succeeded to his mentor's business in partnership with Lockyer's heir Thomas Watts.[82] Coppe (d.1672), who practised under the alias of Higham, likewise shared Lockyer's preference for chymically prepared remedies and recommended other empirics' pills.[83] His attempt to secure an ecclesiastical licence, moreover, received the imprimatur of William Russell, another leading figure in iatrochemical circles in London after the Restoration.[84] Russell, who was appointed chymist in ordinary to Charles II in November 1683, was a life-long devotee of the virtues of iatrochemical methods and remedies. In 1684, he published a defence of the chymists in which he castigated the approach of 'Book-Doctors' and promoted in its stead the virtues of experimentation as practised by true physicians such as Paracelsus and van Helmont.[85] He may also have shared Coppe's radical sympathies. In December 1684, he appointed the surgeon and Quaker sympathizer John Walraven as executor of his will.[86]

Further evidence for the radical associations of the iatrochemical movement in Restoration London is evident in the career and networks of another popular vendor of chymical nostrums in this period, Richard Matthews. Matthews' pill became the focus of a heated controversy in iatrochemical circles following the chymist's death in 1661 as various former associates disputed who in fact was responsible for the original invention. The Helmontian George Starkey was adamant that he was the first to make the celebrated pill, a point vigorously disputed by Matthews' widow, Anne.[87] The dispute over priority was typical of so many similar disputes that broke out between rival operators at this time. Of particular interest here, though, is the possibility that the main combatants divided along religio-political lines. Starkey, who initiated the controversy, was a Presbyterian who gave a warm and public welcome to the restoration of Charles II in 1660. The majority, however, were men with distinctly murky pasts.[88] Matthews, for example, was probably a Baptist or former Baptist, who was clearly very familiar with the radical scene in London at this time, and whose supporters and colleagues included other Baptists such as Paul Hobson (1616–1666), Ahaseurus Fromanteel (1607–1693)[89] and George Kendall.[90] In the first edition of his *The Unlearned Alchymist*, published in 1660, Matthews went out of his way to distance himself from former associates who had fallen into antinomianism and Ranterism, alluding in the process to the activities of prominent figures in radical circles such as Joseph Salmon and Abiezer Coppe. This digression, which was prompted by Matthews' urgent need to prevent the use of his pill for sinful purposes, especially in curing those suffering from venereal diseases, suggests once more a close link between radical freethinking and interest in iatrochemistry in Interregnum England.[91] It also provided useful ammunition for the chymists' opponents both within and outside the College who wished to stigmatize the whole iatrochemical movement as essentially antithetical to the social, intellectual and religious conventions of Restoration society.[92]

In addition to Lionel Lockyer, the former Ranter Coppe was able to call on the support of another well-connected London physician with radical associations, Humphrey Brooke (1618–1693), who attested to Coppe's medical knowledge and skills in 1667. Brooke was the son-in-law and champion of the former Leveller leader William Walwyn (1600–1681) who, as a young man at least, would appear to have shared his father-in-law's radical, political aspirations. In all probability, he also shared his preference for chymically prepared medicines.[93] After receiving his MD from Oxford in 1660, he was made a candidate of the London College of Physicians, and seems to have played a double-handed game thereafter, providing numerous testimonials for a host of medical practitioners, many of whom would have been classed by his colleagues as little better than illiterate interlopers.[94] Later, the poacher may have turned gamekeeper, as he was elected on five separate occasions to act as a censor for the College. Unfortunately, we know little about Brooke's response to the religious and political debates engendered by the Restoration. His radical past may well account for the fact that it took fourteen years for him to become a full fellow of the London College. In addition to his association with radical politics, he may also have suffered as a result of the role that he played, with his father-in-law, in regulating the distribution of crown lands and adjudicating any disputes that arose as a result of the sale of these estates to their new owners in the 1650s.[95] It is also possible to detect an element of the old 'levelling' commitment to egalitarianism and social justice in the advice that he proffered to his children in 1681 with regard to future careers. Medicine, he argued, was the ideal choice of occupation as it lay 'in the middle region, not too high for the converse of the meanest, not too low for the respect of the greatest'. And if they could not become physicians, he advised that they should at least avoid 'being engaged in any thing that is vexatious to the people, [for] I had rather you should be Coblers, than Excise-men, Sergeants, Promoters, Projectors, or any other professions that depends not upon honest business'.[96]

Finally, evidence of the close ties of former radicals with the Restoration iatrochemical fraternity is suggested by the careers of William Rand and John Troutbeck. Rand (d.1663) was a professed admirer of Walwyn's medical practice, based as it was on Helmontian precepts, and was happy to promote the careers of fellow chymists. In April 1662, he, along with Brooke, supplied testimonials on behalf of the Oxfordshire medic (and in all probability, iatrochemist), Edward Harris.[97] Rand, who promoted his own scheme to undermine the monopolistic powers of the London College in the 1650s, held distinctly radical religious opinions that bordered on outright Socinianism. Ironically, given his signature to Harris's application for an episcopal licence, he was also an outspoken critic of the excessive power and authority wielded by the clergy. Rand's pronounced anticlericalism is also apparent in the enthusiastic reception that he afforded to the publication of the works of Thomas Hobbes in the 1650s. Despite what he saw as Hobbes' unhealthy obsession with royal government, Rand was convinced that Hobbes would make a useful recruit to the republican cause, which he consistently upheld.[98] Rand's anti-clericalism was also shared by another prominent Restoration iatrochemist, John Troutbeck (d.1684). Troutbeck, who signed the chymists' petition in 1665, was a former army surgeon who had served under Monck in Scotland. In 1659, he was responsible for sponsoring a translation of Thomas Erastus's *The Nullity of Church Censures*, a work probably undertaken by Troutbeck's nephew, Edmund Hickeringill (1631–1708). In the preface, Hickeringill praised his uncle and patron for his piety, virtue, and reason, declaring that in religious matters '[y]ou never Churched it, nor Kirked it [nor] professt a Sect or Sectling'. Twenty-five years later, Hickeringill, who was by now a conformable minister of the Church of England, albeit one with deep reservations about the power of the bishops and the legality of the church courts, gleefully referred to the fact that his uncle had altered the terms of his will 'lest any of the lawn-sleeves should lay their fingers on't'.[99]

As this mass of evidence suggests, the opponents of the chymists in 1665 were without doubt painting an accurate picture of Restoration iatrochemistry when they depicted many of its devotees as 'fanatically inclined', a form of shorthand in the early 1660s intended to denote anyone who opposed the idea of a settled and unified Church of England under episcopal rule. The fact that so many of these men utilized the licensing powers of the restored church to promote their own and others medical opinions and to undermine the authority of the London College may simply reflect a pragmatic approach to life in the face of the changed political circumstances and uncertainties of the early years of the Restoration. However, quite why the ecclesiastical authorities chose to collude with sections of the London radical underground in this way is open to question.[100] What seems beyond doubt, however, is that the exposure of such collaboration almost certainly dealt a fatal blow to the aspirations of the chymists and their supporters at court leaving leaders like George Thomson to lick their wounds and re-assess the situation.

It cannot be a coincidence that in his later published works, in which he continued to extol the virtues of chymically prepared medicines, Thomson pronounced on the advantages that might accrue to the established church and state if Helmontian medicine was adopted nationwide. In what must have seemed like music to the ears of men like Sheldon, Thomson now argued vociferously for a thoroughgoing overhaul of contemporary medicine not just on medical grounds, but also for the benefits that it might bring to society as a whole. The seeds of such an approach were evident in some of the earliest pamphlets that Thomson wrote. In 1665, for example, in a dedication to the archbishop, he made explicit the link between rebellion, sin and disease, when he argued that the application of Helmontian therapies would not only cure sick bodies but also improve the spiritual, moral and religious well-being of the people.[101] And while he proved willing to forgive associates like Nedham for 'what he did amiss in Olivers dayes', he was less indulgent towards the Galenists of the College who 'accuse Loyal Subjects of Rebellion, when they have been, and still are in their hearts'.[102] Stung, however, by the repeated accusations of critics who implied that Thomson and his 'impudent Crew' were really fomenting rebelliousness and fanaticism, the staunchly loyal chymical doctor astutely withdrew from associating with known radicals and began to argue instead for a medical restoration that was more in keeping with his own vision of a conformable religious and political Restoration. Indicative of this new approach was his response in 1671 to renewed criticism of the chymists by the College's spokesman, Henry Stubbe, in which he deplored the latter's attempt to 'defend their Good Old Cause' and went on to blame the Galenists for the moral, as well as physical, decline of the nation. In particular, he directly blamed the religious divisions of the age upon the methods used by atheistical Galenists, arguing, in typical Helmontian fashion, that the bodily disorders that ensued from the use of such methods lead inevitably to corruption of the 'Organs or Instruments of the Soul', and thus by degrees:

> The mind possessed with Melancholy, black, discontented thoughts, incapable to receive truth, becomes forward, peevish, careless of virtuous Actions, desperately bent to follow for divertissement, a voluptuous sensual life, or to continue Innovations, Heresies, Schisms, and factious Rebellions, and what not?[103]

In 1675, when a renewed attempt was made by the chymists to obtain incorporation and oust the collegiate physicians from their pedestal, Thomson published his last work advocating medical reform. Once again, he made a plea to the King to erect 'a Learned Chymical Society, which may be a President to Foreign nations to imitate', while at the same time distancing himself from both the unlearned pseudo-chymist and the dogmatical Galenist. On this occasion, however, he attempted to tar both with the brush of nonconformity for although they were 'really of no Religion, yet sometimes [the pseudo-chymist], as well as the Galenist, will profest to be of some Congregational Church, or of some Fanatical Conventicle, to the end... he may set a specious gloss of piety upon his fraudulent ways, thereby gaining more reputation amongst the Brethren, [so that] he may cozen his patients more plausibly'.[104] The work itself was nothing less than a manifesto for the complete transformation of society, albeit one designed on markedly traditional lines. The 'Benefits accruing to mankind by this Heroic Enterprize of a Chymical Colledge' were duly listed, pride of place being given to the religious, moral, and political advantages that Thomson believed would follow the adoption of Helmontian medicine. If the body were properly fortified in this way, Thomson argued, then men's souls might likewise be sustained while all thoughts of atheism, hypocrisy, prophaneness and debauchery would be 'lessened, quailed and restrained'. He concluded that:

> by virtue of our Hermetick Physick, the Head, Heart, and Hands of the Hierophants, might be purified: Their Exemplary Dumb and Deaf Preaching up of Vice throughout all the World, be corrected: Circumstances and Punctilio's in Religion lovingly, calmly proposed, debated and Accepted. And those fierce Eager Altercations about Adiaphora laid aside... Quakers, Catabaptists, Independents, Separatists, Schismaticks, and multitudes of Phanaticks, might be brought to more Integrity of mind in Religion [and] be reclaimed far better than by any rigid Persecuting Course whatsoever.[105]

Indeed, Thomson's vision was little short of revolutionary. There was no area of society that would remain untouched by the introduction of learned chymical medicine. The administration of the law, government and personal morality were all expected to improve. Stronger and fitter subjects would be better equipped to fight wars and help colonize the globe. In short, 'the whole Kingdome will by degrees be brought into a far more flourishing condition than formerly'.[106]

The Fate of Helmontianism in Later Stuart England

By the mid-1670s, the reform-minded chymists were irredeemably divided as to how best to promote the medical beliefs and practices of their heroes, men like Paracelsus and van Helmont. Earlier efforts to achieve a consensus, and to bury religious and political differences, had ultimately floundered in the face of a concerted opposition that repeatedly, and with some justice, invoked the radical and subversive character of the iatrochemical reform movement in Restoration England. But this, as we have seen, was only part of the picture. The attempt to create a Society of Chymical Physicians in Restoration England, attracting as it did men from a wide range of backgrounds, gives the lie to those who have seen the origins of medical reform in seventeenth-century England as the exclusive prerogative of mid-century 'puritans'. Support for the new medicine could be found throughout the social, religious, and political spectrum. One is tempted to conclude then that its failure had more to do with the public manner in which these issues were debated, rather than with any irreconcilable differences between proponents of the two medical systems, based, as some have assumed, on established religio-political fault-lines. The history of the reception of iatrochemistry in England, from its earliest days to the middle decades of the seventeenth century, provides countless examples of its appeal to physicians and patients across the religious and political divide. In private at least, it may even have helped individuals of different persuasions to overcome their mutual antipathies and to have established some common ground upon which new alliances and networks might be forged. The eirenic possibilities of the new medical theories were certainly not lost on those devotees who coalesced around Samuel Hartlib in the 1640s and 1650s, many of whom were attracted to iatrochemistry precisely because it promised an end to religious conflict and the dissolution of theological internecine warfare. This mindset is best summed up in the words of the Restoration Helmontian Robert Godfrey (d.1674), who shortly before his death declared himself 'one of those who doubt whether or no the most holy God minds a name or a form so much as the Heart of a Person'. He concluded that:

> it will not be said in the last day, come hither, yee Episcopalians, that is as such an associated people, or ye Papists, or yee Presbiterians... Independents... Anabaptists, or ye Quakers (which are all but Nicknames) and enjoy the Kingdom Prepared you.... But rather; Come hither yee that served me with an upright Heart in Self-Denial... That imbrued not your hands in the Blood of the Innocent.[107]

Whereas prior to 1640 diplomacy dictated that the proponents of chymical medicine, alongside their Galenic detractors, rarely found the need to openly acknowledge their innermost religious beliefs, the events of the 1640s and 1650s made it virtually impossible for medical practitioners of whatever background to avoid discussion of such issues. Medicine and healing, like other areas of public discourse, had become unavoidably drawn into the wider debates raging in Interregnum England over how best to resolve the unprecedented divisions unleashed by civil war and the ensuing years of religious and political instability. Under the circumstances, it was inevitable that the taint of religious heterodoxy that attached itself to the new schools of iatrochemical thought—ideas that had been granted wide publicity in the 1650s through the publication of a multiplicity of new translations and original works—would now return to haunt it after 1660. The failure of the Society of Chymical Physicians lay not so much in the novelty of the medical beliefs and practices propagated by its spokesmen, which were widely admired in Restoration society, but rather in the inability of its proponents to overcome the stigma of social and intellectual subversion that clung to iatrochemistry for much of this period. The Helmontians, in short, were both the beneficiaries, and ultimately the victims, of a process of politicization that was gradually infecting all aspects of medical practice in the second half of the seventeenth century.

It would be a mistake, however, to conclude that the failure of the chymists to challenge the authority of the College of Physicians and acquire official recognition through incorporation represented a defeat for Helmontianism and related ideas. In many respects, the chymists continued to prosper at the expense of medical traditionalism, a trend that was most obvious at the court of Charles II. If anything, the failure of men like O'Dowde and Thomson and their powerful backers at court simply spurred them on to seek other routes to promote their practices and beliefs. And in Charles II they found a remarkably willing ally. In 1667, the King initiated a concerted campaign to promote chymistry and chymical medicine at court, appointing numerous practitioners of the new medicine to positions of prominence within the royal household. In 1667, for example, he inaugurated a new office, that of chymist in ordinary, many of the holders of which were to prove outspoken proponents of Helmontian medical values. One of the first to be appointed to this new post, George Acton, was to prove every bit as combative as his colleagues who failed a few years earlier to topple the collegiate physicians. Wisely dedicating his published works to his patron Charles II, whom he addressed as one well versed in hermetical and chymical medicine, Acton repeatedly lambasted 'Gallenical Physitians' for their excessive dependence on blood-letting and advocacy of humoralism, and praised the Helmontians for promoting 'gentle' chymical and herbal cures that sought to pacify the *archeus* and treat diseases otherwise given over as incurable.[108] Others appointed to labour in the royal laboratories proved equally committed to the Helmontian project. John Choke (1667), Albertus Otto Faber (1674) and William Russell (1683), were, as we have seen, committed advocates of the new medicine.[109] They were joined by men who shared the King's passion for chymical investigation, but who frequently lacked any formal medical qualifications other than the possession of a licence granted by the ecclesiastical authorities.[110] The chymists at court were further boosted by the King's decision in the late 1660s to create another new post, that of chymical physician to the person of the King, which again was dominated by Helmontians. The key appointment here was that of Thomas Williams (*c.*1621–1712), who had played a leading role behind the scenes in promoting the aims of the Society of Chymical Physicians in 1665. Initially appointed to the rank of physician in ordinary supernumerary in 1667, two years later Williams was promoted to the more substantial office of chymical physician to the King on a salary of twenty marks a year. The warrant for his appointment specifically refers to the King's wish to 'encourage so important an art' as chymistry while acknowledging Williams' 'extraordinary learning and skill which he shows in compounding and inventing medicines, some of which have been prepared in the royal presence'. He was thus granted the right 'to make experiments in all his Majesty's laboratories'.[111] Williams rapidly consolidated his position at court. By 1674, when he was raised to the knighthood, he was spending over £1,000 a year on laboratory equipment. At the same time, he was actively pursuing political office, culminating in his election as MP for the constituency of Weobley in his native Herefordshire in 1675.[112]

Williams' meteoric rise to a central position in the entourage of chymically inclined medical practitioners at court was paralleled by the extension of royal patronage to a host of like-minded physicians, surgeons and apothecaries who were promoted to various positions within the ever-expanding medical retinue of Charles II. In addition to Williams and Bolnest, seven of those who signed the chymists' petition in 1665 were either already affiliated, or were later appointed, to positions at court.[113] Other appointments reinforce the image of Charles II as a favourer of medical innovation and chymical experimentation. William Clarke,[114] Luke Eales,[115] Gabriel Hubbard,[116] Nathaniel Slade,[117] Peter Mark Sparck[118] and Thomas Waldron,[119] for example, were, in all probability, granted the status of royal physicians because of their preference for chymical physic. Thomas Sherley (above, 126) and Edmund Dickinson (1624–1707), on the other hand, may, like Williams and Bolnest, have owed their promotions to the chymical interests of aristocratic supporters at Whitehall. Sherley, for example, a kinsman of Sir Thomas Williams, identified himself with the duke of Buckingham's entourage, while Dickinson was brought to the attention of the King in 1677 following his successful cure of the lord chamberlain, Henry Bennet, earl of Arlington (1618–1685). Dickinson subsequently set up an alchemical laboratory under the royal bedchamber, accessible by a private staircase, where he performed experiments before the King and the duke of Buckingham.[120]

The court thus offered, as recent studies have demonstrated, an ideal environment in which to promote intellectual and scientific innovation. Iatrochemistry and alchemy flourished within the walls of the early modern court, and that of

Charles II was no exception.[121] But it was not the only outlet for the promotion of such ideas and practices. Other organs of the state also feature prominently in the spread of iatrochemical ideas and methods. The medical services attached to the armed forces proved particularly fertile ground in this respect, a reflection in all probability of the greater freedom enjoyed by medical practitioners serving in the army and navy to experiment and innovate. In particular, surgeons seem to have benefited in this way. In civilian practice, they were normally expected to observe strict boundaries as to what they may or may not do in treating sick bodies, with particular emphasis placed upon the notion that treatment of internal maladies was reserved to trained and qualified physicians. The exigencies of war, however, undermined this principle and encouraged multi-tasking among the corps of surgeons that dominated the medical services of both the army and the navy. It is probably no coincidence, therefore, that a number of those practitioners who supported the Helmontian reform movement in the 1660s had either served in the armed forces or had close connections with them. William Currer and John Troutbeck, for example, had long and distinguished careers within the medical services of the army and navy. Currer had served in Ireland in the 1640s and was rewarded for his loyalty to the Stuart cause in 1660 through his appointment to the senior post of physician general to the army in Ireland, a position he held until his death in 1668. Troutbeck, on the other hand, who served the armies of the Commonwealth in various capacities in the 1650s and was a close confidante of General Monck in Scotland, later served as a naval surgeon in the Second Anglo Dutch War.[122] Troutbeck's naval associations are particularly interesting given the support for the chymists exhibited by many aristocrats and courtly patrons with connections to the administration of the royal navy in the middle years of the 1660s. Prince Rupert and the duke of York, who both featured prominently in naval circles at this time, shared the King's passion for chymistry. Likewise Sir John Mennes (1599–1671) and Sir John Ernle (d.1697), both signatories to the chymists' petition in 1665, were prominent figures in the administration of the Restoration navy. Mennes was appointed comptroller of the navy in 1661, while Ernle began a long and illustrious career in the admiralty around 1664.[123] It may well have been connections such as these that encouraged the King in 1664 to authorize another member of the Society of Chymical Physicians, the iatrochemist Thomas Smart, to conduct trials of his chymical pill, *aurum purgans*, among the naval surgeons.[124] While the outcome of these trials is not recorded, the navy continued to employ chymical physicians to prepare medicines in later years. Among those paid for their services in supplying the garrison at Tangier with medicines in 1680 was the Helmontian physician William Bacon, a protégé of those two leading lights of the chymists' Society, George Starkey and George Thomson.[125]

Service in military circles may, in fact, have provided many enthusiasts for chymical medicine with their first taste of Paracelsian and Helmontian therapies and ideas. The battlegrounds of the civil war provided ample opportunity for medical practitioners on both sides of the political divide to experiment with new methods of cure. In the ensuing decade, the campaigns in Ireland and Scotland, coupled with conflict in mainland Europe and the Caribbean, provided further opportunities for chymically inclined physicians and surgeons to ply their trade unimpeded by peace-time constraints. Military hospitals, both at home and in the field, may also have provided chymical physicians with large numbers of patients for clinical trials like those proposed by Smart in the Restoration navy. Ralph Bathurst (d.1704), John French (*c.*1616–1657) and Aaron Gurdon (d.1675), all of whom were employed by the state to treat military casualties, may have utilized such appointments in order to experiment in this way.[126] Other iatrochemists who are known to have practised medicine and surgery in the armies of the civil war include Roger Dixon, Benedict Porter and John Pratt.[127] Foreign travel and enforced exile—the lot of many royalists—may also have encouraged others, especially those seeking employment as mercenaries, to dabble in chymistry. The leading Scottish courtier, Sir Robert Moray (d.1673), who worked alongside Charles II in his newly established laboratory at Whitehall in the early 1660s, first encountered chymistry while an exile in Holland in the previous decade.[128] In 1681, Colonel William Doughty, a former royalist soldier, petitioned the crown, in the course of which he described in detail his lengthy wanderings through France and attempts to establish himself as a chymist and physician at Montpellier, Toulouse and Montauban. Like fellow royalist combatant and iatrochemist Dud Dudley (*c.*1600–1684), a prominent figure in the Hartlib circle in the 1650s, Doughty was a schemer and visionary. Among other things, he claimed to have invented a new method of tanning leather, and in appealing to Charles II for help, must have been aware of the King's sympathy for men of his interests and loyal background.[129]

Popular at court and welcomed in aristocratic and military circles, chymical medicine also experienced something of a boom among the populace at large in the second half of the seventeenth century. Utilizing the commercial appeal of the printing press, the chymical physicians in general, and Helmontians in particular, were adept at advertising and marketing their new remedies, as well as providing a modicum of intellectual as well as empirical evidence to support their radical claims. By the end of the century, most market towns in England had access to chymical remedies, either through those supplied to local shopkeepers (usually apothecaries) by London-based practitioners or those made and sold locally by provincial-based physicians. Chymical physicians routinely publicized these outlets in cheap broadsides or pamphlets. They also formed close bonds with fellow chymists, swapping recipes and sharing details of the success and failure of the various nostrums on the market.[130] Lay interest in Helmontian remedies and chymical medicine had even penetrated Wales.[131] Networking took many forms. In the capital, chymical clubs flourished after the Restoration. Established chymical physicians also provided vital assistance in supplying colleagues applying for ecclesiastical licences with testimonials. Detailed study of the licensing system, and the records of those who supplied such testimonials, provides countless examples of this kind of mutual self-help. It also suggests that some accounts of the number of chymical physicians operating in England in Restoration England have severely under-estimated the extent to which iatrochemistry had penetrated the medical marketplace.[132] By the end of the seventeenth century, far from witnessing the demise of the Helmontian Revolution (as suggested by Andrew Wear), most evidence would seem to point to a flourishing trade in chymically prepared medicines. Typical in many respects were the self-styled Helmontians John Lamport (or Lampard) and John Yarwood, who established regular circuits and surgeries in the market towns of Hampshire, Sussex and Leicestershire. Like many of their London-based colleagues, they too sought to advertise and legitimate their practices in print. They also attempted to distance themselves from the charge of their opponents that they were little better than quacks and empirics by providing evidence of the philosophical basis of their procedures and cures. Both Lamport and Yarwood invoked the technical language of Helmontianism, referring to the role of the *archeus* and gases in the origin and treatment of diseases, while Lamport demonstrated a familiarity with the early pioneers of English Helmontianism, citing the writings of George Thomson ('an ancient, ingenious, industrious Artist'), George Starkey and Noah Biggs.[133]

The failure of the chymists to achieve incorporation in 1665 then should not be understood as evidence of the failure of the Helmontians to influence the debate over medicine in the second half of the seventeenth century. On the contrary, they played a vital role in stimulating new approaches to healing, and its wider role in the body politic, in this period. Indeed, it could be argued that their success in this respect ultimately undermined any prospect of subverting the legal authority of their opponents as the latter increasingly took on the mantle of their critics. Nowhere is this more apparent than in the reaction of the College of Physicians to later attempts by the chymists to undermine the monopolistic powers wielded by the collegiate physicians in London. Thus in 1675–6, in the face of a renewal of hostilities between the two camps, prompted as we have seen by the archbishop of Canterbury, Gilbert Sheldon, the defence of the College was placed in the hands of a young physician with impeccable iatrochemical credentials, Charles Goodall (*c*.1642–1712).[134] Goodall was almost certainly hand-picked for the job. Crucially for the College's detractors, he possessed court connections—he had been appointed to the growing ranks of the royal chymists and chymical physicians in 1671—as well as links to some of the leading natural philosophers and chymists of the age, including Robert Boyle.[135] His own standing as a chymical physician thus gave added bite to his denunciation of the empiric Huyberts and his ilk and underpinned the College's attempt to resist any further encroachments on its authority. This brief episode, which helped make Goodall's name and reputation, marked another significant stage on the College's road to embracing reform. And despite the fact, as Goodall himself pointed out, that there was nothing intrinsically new in the fact that many of the College's members were chymically inclined, there is little doubt that the College as an organization was proving increasingly receptive to innovation. In the same year as Huyberts' renewed attack, for example, the College's officers proposed that its members should dispense free advice to the poor—a measure designed in part to answer those critics, including the chymists, who depicted the collegiates as greedy, selfish, and uncaring. In the 1690s, the College would erect a dispensary at Amen Corner. In the meantime, however, several of its members utilized the College's laboratories to further their own or collaborative research projects. In 1683, Dr Tancred Robinson reported visiting the College where he found several members engaged in experiments on the properties of mineral waters 'for by chance yesterday I went into the elaboratory there, where I observ'd all their furnaces and instruments at work upon those tryalls'. Unable to 'learn the design', he suspected that the 'cheife undertakers' were Drs Goodall and Edward Tyson.[136]

Though tensions between conservatives and reformers no doubt continued to exist, and occasionally surface, within the College after 1675, the choice of the chymist Goodall rather than the Galenist Henry Stubbe to defend its honour and privileges signified an important break with the past. At the same time, as others have noted, Helmontianism became subsumed within a new form of chymical practice and philosophy that owed more to Boyle than van Helmont.[137] And while this process was never clear-cut or simple, there seems little doubt that part of the attraction of men like Goodall for Boyle's corpuscularianism resided in its self-conscious avoidance of the twin dangers of 'enthusiasm' and quackery. Above all, it allowed Goodall and his colleagues to espouse the many virtues of chymically prepared medicines and the new natural philosophy while at the same time defending the privileged status of the learned physician. By the end of the seventeenth century, chymistry had evolved into a respectable science and chymical medicines were routinely prescribed and administered by physicians operating across the religious and political spectrum. Courses in chymistry were widely available, offered by private individuals or, increasingly, through established organizations and learned bodies such as the universities or Society of Apothecaries. While much of the credit for this transformation must be attributed to men like Boyle, who laboured tirelessly to promote a reformed medicine based on chymical lines, it would be a mistake, nonetheless, to under-estimate the contribution that the followers of Paracelsus and van Helmont made to the reform of medical practice in Britain in the second half of the seventeenth century.

Notes

1. It was first brought to light by Sir Henry Thomas with his chance discovery of a stray broadside advertising the aims of the chymists; see his 'The Society of Chymical Physitians. An Echo of the Great Plague at London, 1665', in E. A. Underwood (ed.), *Science, Medicine and History*, 2 vols (London, 1953), ii, 56–71. For a useful summary of scholarly understanding concerning the origins of the Society, and the rise and decline of Helmontianism in Restoration England, see A. Wear, *Knowledge and Practice in English Medicine, 1550–1680* (Cambridge, 2000), 356–8 and *passim*. For my reservations with regard to some of Wear's conclusions, see below, note 132.
2. P. Rattansi, 'The Helmontian-Galenist Controversy in Restoration England', *Ambix*, 12 (1964), 1–23.
3. This is the central thrust of Charles Webster's discussion of the origins of the reform movement of 1665; see his 'English Medical Reformers of the Puritan Revolution: A Background to the "Society of Chemical Physitians"', *Ambix*, 14 (1967), 16–41. Webster argues that an important precedent here was the scheme devised in the mid 1650s by William Rand to create a 'College of Graduate Physicians' in London.
4. H. J. Cook, 'The Society of Chemical Physicians, the New Philosophy, and the Restoration Court', *Bulletin of the History of Medicine*, 61 (1987), 61–77.
5. See, for example, the essays in V. Nutton (ed.), *Medicine at the Courts of Europe, 1500–1837* (London and New York, 1990); B. T. Moran, *The Alchemical World of the German Court: Occult Philosophy and Chemical Medicine in the Circle of Moritz of Hessen (1572–1632)* (Stuttgart, 1991); F. Dawbarn, 'Patronage and Power: The College of Physicians and the Jacobean Court', *British Journal for the History of Science*, 31 (1998), 1–19. For a case study of the role of patronage in the career of an English Paracelsian physician, see *idem*, 'New Light on Dr Thomas Moffet: The Triple Roles of an Early Modern Physician, Client and Patronage Broker', *Medical History*, 47 (2003), 3–22.
6. According to one of the Society's founder members, William Goddard, the group first began to meet regularly to pursue the goal of incorporation in May 1664, just one month after the London College of Physicians had been rebuffed by Parliament. To expedite its aims, the Society's members (Goddard, writing in October 1666, lists among those still living Marchamont Nedham, Edward Bolnest, Thomas Williams, Richard Barker, Robert Bathurst, Edward Coke, George Thomson and William Barkley) employed one Thomas Dangerfield, an attorney in the Court of King's Bench, 'for the drawing of severall petitions & other writeings for the modelling of a draught of a Charter or Warrant for his Majestie' as well as to perform other duties relating to these negotiations. Following the collapse of the Society, Dangerfield threatened to sue Goddard for unpaid fees, which the latter sought to recoup from his former colleagues by initiating a suit in the Court of Chancery; see TNA, C 10/477/110.
7. It should be stressed that powerful figures at the English court, including the monarch, had long used their authority and connections to protect illicit and unconventional healers from the monopolistic powers wielded by the College of Physicians. For countless examples in the century before 1640, see especially M. Pelling, *Medical*

Conflicts in Early Modern London: Patronage, Physicians, and Irregular Practitioners 1550–1640 (Oxford, 2003), *passim.*

8. In what follows, I reject Robert Martensen's view that Sheldon's support for the chymists in 1665 was half-hearted and temporary and that it represented a form of lip service to the king's interest in such matters; R. L. Martensen, *The Brain Takes Shape: An Early History* (Oxford & New York, 2004), 111.
9. *The Diary and Correspondence of Dr John Worthington*, ed. J.Crossley, 3 vols (Manchester, Chetham Soc., vols 13, 36, 114, 1847–1886), i, 195 [Worthington to Hartlib, 4 June 1660]. The Restoration cleric-cum-physician John Ward, who was intimately acquainted with the fringe medical scene in London in the early 1660s, reported that the King 'delights much in chymistry', employing a chymist and two operators in a laboratory at St James' Palace; FSL, V.a.292, fo.6v. Nicholas Le Févre (d.1669) was appointed apothecary and operator in chymistry to Charles II on 20 June 1660; TNA, LC3/24, fo. 16. In addition to healing those sick of the plague in London in 1665, he signed the chymists' petition in the same year; for further details of his career, see Appendix 1 (a).
10. Faber professed to have emigrated to England by personal invitation of the King shortly after the Restoration. He later claimed to have held the appointment of physician in ordinary to Charles II, for which there is no extant evidence. He was, however, created chymist without fee to the royal person in 1674 (renewed 1676), having earlier received £50 for unspecified services to the restored Stuarts; *CSPD Addenda 1660–1685*, 489; TNA, LC3/27, fo. 48; *Calendar of Treasury Books, 1660–1667*, 276. Lockyer was reported to have performed chymical experiments before the King at Whitehall on 13 June 1664; *Aut Helmont, Aut Asinus: Or, St. George Untrust Being a Full Answer to His Smart Scourge* (London, 1665), A3r. Trigge was rumoured to have been knighted shortly before his death (in early 1665) by a grateful monarch 'for ye good service hee did in ye Recovering ye Queen'; FSL, V.a.293, fo. 129v. Barker, who probably inherited Trigge's practice, was knighted by Charles II. He was also appointed physician in ordinary (probably without fee) to the king on 31 December 1673; see Appendix 1 (a). For Starkey as Eirenaeus Philalethes, see J. Ferguson, *Bibliotheca Chemica*, 2 vols (Glasgow, 1906), ii, p.488.
11. *HMC. Eleventh Report, Appendix, Part VII* (London, 1888), 12.
12. S. W., *Medela Medicorum, or, an Enquiry into the Reasons & Grounds of the Contempt of Physicians* (London, 1678), A4v, A5r–v.
13. Richard Barker (physician in ordinary, 1673); Edward Bolnest (chymical physician in ordinary, 1670); Pierre Massonet (physician in ordinary, 1672); Thomas Norton (physician in extraordinary, 1668); John Spranger (physician in extraordinary, 1661); John Troutbeck, (surgeon in ordinary supernumerary, 1660); Edward Warner (physician in ordinary supernumerary, 1660); and Thomas Williams (chymical physician in ordinary supernumerary, 1667). An eighth candidate, William Boreman, claimed the title of 'royal physician' in 1684, but no record of his appointment survives; LPL, VX 1A/10/212/1–4. It is possible, however, that he may have been appointed by the Board of Greencloth in 1665. John Pordage (d.1688), the son of the mystical Behmenist of the same name (1607–1681), who was a close friend of Boreman, was appointed in this way. Testimonials taken in 1669 confirmed that Pordage Jnr was appointed to 'take

care of such as should have the sickness in his Majestyes household' as well as to 'administer physicke to his Majesty's Life Guard of Foot'. One of the testimonials was signed by the royal physician and iatrochemist, Edward Warner; LPL, VX 1A/10/243; VG 1/6, fo. 64v; Sancroft, fos 265r–v.

14. Thomas Horsington (1663), John Troutbeck (1661) and Thomas Williams (1669). Horsington was promoted on the recommendation of one of the leading spokesmen for the Society of Chymical Physicians, George Thomson. Other signatories attesting to his fitness for an MD included fellow chymical physicians Joseph Dey and John Fryer. Troutbeck was a protégé of George Monck, earl of Albemarle, and probably received his medical degree as a reward for the role he played in assisting his patron's efforts in bringing about the Restoration. Williams was a familiar figure at court, where he already held the post of chymical physician to the King and regularly practised his skills in the royal presence; for further details of all those cited here, see Appendix 1 (a).
15. The chymical physician and signatory Everard Maynwaring dedicated the second edition of his *Tutela Sanitatis. Sive Vita Protracta. The Protection of Long Life, and Detection of Its Brevity* (London, 1664) to Prince Rupert. Likewise, George Thomson's manifesto for a wholesale reform of society based on Helmontian principles was addressed to the Prince in 1675. According to Thomson, he had heard it said 'What a Philomathes and Philalethes, Sincere Lover and Defender you were of Essential Truths and Ingenious Arts in General, especially Mechanical Pyrotechnical Operations, an Assertor of Experimental, Optical and Sensible Effects, Fruits and Products of things, and that for this reason you had an extraordinary kindness for our most Excellent Philosopher Van Helmont, your Country-man'; G. Thomson, *Ορθο-μιθοδος ἰατω-χυμνεή: Or The Direct Method of Curing Chymically* (London, 1675), A3v.
16. For Massonet, see Appendix 1 (a). Other signatories who would appear to have retained close links with the duke of York's household include Sir John Ernle, Sir John Werden and Robert Werden; see Appendix 1 (b).
17. E. Bolnest, *Medicina Instaurata, or, a Brief Account of the True Grounds and Principles of the Art of Physick* (London, 1665), A2v–A3r, A4v [epistolary discourse by Nedham]. Similar praise was lavished on the duke by the chymical physician Everard Maynwaring (for whom, see Appendix 1 (a)) in the preface to his *Solamen Ægrorum, sive Ternarius Medicamentorum Chymicorum* (London, 1665). Bolnest would appear to have retained his links with Buckingham after the collapse of the chymist's projected society in 1665. In 1672, he penned another obsequious dedication to the duke in which he alluded to the latter's continuing interest in all things chymical; E. Bolnest, *Aurora Chymica. Or a Rational Way of Preparing Animals, Vegetables, and Minerals, for a Physicall Use* (London, 1672).
18. T. Sherley, *A Philosophical Essay: Declaring the Probable Causes, whence Stones are Produced in the Greater World* (London, 1673), A2v, A3r. Sherley (1638–1678) was a former pupil and friend of Henry Oldenburg, who may have introduced him to the natural philosopher Robert Boyle. Sherley paid homage to van Helmont and Boyle, his principal mentors, in his *Philosophical Essay*. In 1667 Oldenburg reported to Boyle that Sherley, a former soldier, was in possession of a box, given to him by a mutual friend who had recently attended the peace treaty at Breda, which may have contained the

recipe for 'the *ludus* of van Helmont'. He was now resolved, according to Oldenburg, 'to fall to his practice of Physick in good earnest'. Within a short time, he seems to have attracted the attention of the King (possibly through the intervention of his kinsman and fellow chymist, Thomas Williams), and in 1672 he joined a long list of fellow iatrochemists who were rewarded with a royal appointment as physician in ordinary supernumerary. In 1675, he obtained further promotion when he was made physician to the person of the King; Boyle, *Correspondence*, i, 96–9; iii, 330 [Oldenburg to Boyle, 3 September 1667]; *CSPD, 1673–1675*, 605; TNA, LC 3/24, fo. 17; 3/25, fo. 51; 3/26, fo. 141; 3/28, fo. 26.

19. W. Simpson, *Philosophical Dialogues Concerning the Principle of Natural Bodies* (London, 1677), A2v–A3r. Simpson (d.1680) was a chymical physician based at York and the author of a treatise on the plague. He later became involved in a heated pamphlet debate with his local Galenic rival, Robert Wittie, over the merits of the spa waters at Scarborough.
20. For Clifford and Paulden, see Appendix 1 (b). Another signatory of the chymists' petition who later supported the duke in Parliament was the naval commander Sir Frescheville Holles (d.1672). Holles shared the duke's conviction of the need to construct a church settlement informed by a broad-based religious tolerance; see Appendix 1 (b).
21. I discuss Ormond's role as a sponsor of medical innovation in Ireland, and his support for loyalist iatrochemists such as Peter Belon, in my 'Promoting Medical Change in Restoration Ireland: The Chemical Revolution and the Patronage of James Butler, duke of Ormond (1610–88)' in J. Cunningham (ed.), *Early Modern Ireland and the World of Medicine: Practitioners, Collectors and Contexts* (Manchester, 2019), 84–101.
22. SUL, HP 28/2/27B–28A, 29A. The papers were given to Fogarty by fellow Catholic and physician, Daniel Higgins. Both militant supporters of the Irish Catholic Federation in the 1640s, Higgins was executed in 1652 following the fall of Limerick. Since both men were accused of manufacturing gunpowder for the Catholic forces, it seems likely that Fogarty was reprieved by the intervention of Ormond. The latter's interest in these manuscripts may itself have arisen from the duke's fascination for such arcane matters and the possibility that Ormond considered Butler a distant kinsman. For Higgins, see D. F. Cregan, 'The Confederate Catholics of Ireland: The Personnel of the Confederation, 1642–9', *Irish Historical Studies*, 29 (1995), 505; SUL, HP 15/5/18B. Fogarty (MD Angers, 1644), who was later implicated in the Popish Plot, died in prison in 1678. Following a dispute over the possession of his papers and writings, they were ordered to be released to Sir James Butler, council at law, another kinsman of the duke; *CSPD, 1678*, 426, 431; TNA, PC 2/67, 131.
23. For Currer's career, see Appendix 1 (a).
24. For Archer's career as writer and physician, which omits reference to his Dublin MD, see *ODNB*. Despite royal patronage (Archer claimed to specialize in the cure of venereal diseases at court), he was considered as little better than an empiric by the College of Physicians in London, who repeatedly prosecuted him in the 1680s. Despite attempts to prohibit his practice, Archer continued unabashed. In 1685, for example, he advertised his services in an almanac, where he described himself as 'one of his majesties Sworn Physicians' and resident at Knightsbridge, where 'melancholy, Consumptive and

Distracted Persons are cured with the greatest care and speed'; L. Coelson, *Speculum Perspicuum Uranicum... 1685* (London, 1685). For Archer's appointment as chymical physician in ordinary to Charles II, see TNA, LC 3/26, fo. 142.

25. For all three, see Appendix 1 (b). To this list one might speculatively add the name of Sir Geoffrey Shakerley, the governor of Chester Castle, who was involved in 1670 in a scheme to extract silver from lead ore in north Wales. His partner in this enterprise was his brother-in-law Alan Pennington (1622–1696), a local physician, who like Shakerley, acted as a loyal government correspondent in the 1660s. Another enthusiastic aristocrat and prominent courtier, Henry Pierrepont, marquess of Dorchester (1607–1680), owned his own laboratory and acted as patron, among others, to the chymist Thomas Smart (see Appendix 1 (a)). Surprisingly, he did not append his name to the Society of Chymists petition in 1665.
26. W. R. Newman, *Gehennical Fire: The Lives of George Starkey, an American Alchemist in the Scientific Revolution* (Cambridge, MA, 1994), 67, 74–5, 300n; Boyle, *Correspondence*, i, 99 (where Starkey describes Farrar as 'the earl's parasite'); Royal Society Library, Boyle Papers 25, 156, 180; RB/1/29/8; Bodl., Ashmole MS 419, vol. 2, fo. 1. For Farrar as physician to Charles II, see the undated petition of his widow Elizabeth; *CSPD, 1670, with Addenda 1660–1670*, 616. Farrar's ultra-traditional Anglican credentials are suggested by the fact that he was the brother of Nicholas Farrar or Ferrar (1593–1637), scion of the godly Arminian household or 'nunnery' established at Little Gidding in the 1630s; J. Glanvill, *Saducismus Triumphatus: Or, Full and Plain Evidence Concerning Witches and Apparitions* (London, 1681), ii, 230–1.
27. Jeremiah Astel (1663), Richard Barker (1663), John Troutbeck (1678) and Robert Turner (1661) were all licensed in the diocese of London. William Barkley (1665) was licensed by Sheldon as archbishop of Canterbury, while Robert Bathurst (1664), Thomas O'Dowde (1665) and Thomas Tillison (1666) were all licensed to practise in the neighbouring diocese of Winchester. For details, see Appendix 1 (a). It is possible that George Morley, bishop of Winchester (1662–84), shared the sympathy of his friend, Gilbert Sheldon, for Helmontian physic (discussed further below). It has been suggested, for example, that the royalist poet and physician John Collop (for whom, see above 76–7, 81–2) was the 'J.C., M.D.', who defended Morley, as bishop of Worcester, in his controversy with Richard Baxter in the early years of the Restoration; F. Bussby, 'George Morley, Bishop of Worcester, 1660–62', *Transactions of the Worcestershire Archaeological Society*, 37 (1960), 20.
28. R. Turner, *BOTANOΛOΓIA, or, The Brittish Physician* (London, 1664), A3r. Turner was licensed on 23 March 1661. A few months later, he supplied a testimonial on behalf of Thomas Stockton, of All Hallows', London; Bloom and James, 29, 70, 71, 82–3; Wellcome Library, London, MS 5337, *sub* Minors, Thomas.
29. DRO, PR 518, sub Allington [*sic*]. The three signatories were Edward Bolnest, William Boreman and Robert Bathurst. The other medical signatories were Isaac Playford and Dr Peter Salmon. Playford (d.1667), who was living in Spitalfields at the time of his death, may have been related to Samuel Playford of Southwark, licensed by the bishop of Winchester in July 1665 (among those who signed letters testimonial were the chymical physicians Edward Bolnest and Robert Turner); LMA, P93/DUN/279 [parish registers of St Dunstan's, Stepney, Middlesex, 1666–1684]; A. R. Bax, 'Marriage and

Other Licences in the Commissary Court of Surrey', *Surrey Archaeological Collections*, 11 (1893). One Samuel Playford served as a captain in the parliamentary armies in the first civil war and Ireland; Green, *CPCC*, iii, 1802. Salmon (d.1675), a fellow of the London College of Physicians, was appointed physician in ordinary supernumerary to Charles II in September 1662; Munk, i, 223; TNA, LC 3/25, fo. 51; 3/26, fo. 141. The tendency of the chymical physicians to provide certificates of medical competence to like-minded friends and colleagues provides yet further evidence for the importance of collaborative networks and cooperation among early modern medical practitioners, as suggested, among others, by Patrick Wallis in his recent critique of the notion of the individualistic and competitive medical marketplace; see P. Wallis, 'Competition and Cooperation in the Early Modern Medical Economy', in M. S. R. Jenner and P. Wallis (eds), *Medicine and the Market in England and Its Colonies*, 47–68.

30. *Conway Letters: The Correspondence of Anne, Viscountess Conway, Henry More, and Their Friends, 1642–1684*, ed. M. H. Nicholson (New Haven, 1930; rev. ed., S. Hutton, Oxford, 1992), 106 [Henry More to Lady Conway, 19 September 1654]. Sheldon may also have used his powers as archbishop to licence medical books favourable to the chymists' cause. Everard Maynwaring's *Morbus Polyrhizos et Polymorphaeus* (London, 1665), an iatrochemical analysis of the scurvy that includes references to the work of van Helmont and his English followers, including George Thomson and Marchamont Nedham, carries the imprimatur of the archbishop's secretary at Lambeth House.
31. King was the son of the Northampton physician, Edmund King (d.1651). He was awarded his B Med by Sheldon on 12 May 1663. Less than three weeks later, he was granted a licence by the archbishop allowing him to practice medicine anywhere in England. Under Sheldon's patronage (Robert Martenson in the *ODNB* plausibly suggests that King may have been introduced to Sheldon by fellow Anglican Thomas Willis), King's career took off. In 1666 he was elected a fellow of the Royal Society and was involved in many of that group's most ground-breaking work, including research into blood transfusions and respiration. In 1671, his Lambeth degree was upgraded to a Cambridge MD, awarded at the prompting of the King, and in January 1675 he was appointed one of the royal physicians. In the light of the discussion to follow, however, one of the most significant events in King's career took place in 1677 when the King recommended him to the London College of Physicians for an honorary fellowship. Against all protocol, the College refused to accede to the royal request. It may well be that the College resented the fact that King was a mere surgeon by training, but it is just as likely that their refusal to admit King was an act of defiance aimed at his patron, Sheldon; *ODNB*, sub King, Edmund; LPL, FII/4/58; F1/C, fos 121v, 126v; Venn, iii, 18; TNA, LC 3/28, fo. 26; *CSPD, 1676–1677*, 505; RCPL, Annals, iv, fos 120a–121b.
32. T. O'Dowde, *The Poor Man's Physician... The Third Edition* (London, 1665), A2r–A3r; G. Thomson, *Galeno-pale: Or, A Chymical Trial of the Galenists* (London, 1665), A2r–A4r [quote at A2r]; A. O. Faber, *De Auro Potabile Medicinali, ad Potentissimum Principem, Carolum II* (London, 1677), appendix entitled 'Of some Cures more, done since the former were published', 5–8. Faber treated Sheldon continuously throughout the period from the 8 to 25 October 1677 and claimed, on the authority of a witness, Dr. R., that he was then cured. He died on 9 November 1677. Even the chymists' opponent and College apologist, Nathaniel Hodges, acknowledged the archbishop's

approval of chymistry 'as the most probable means to discover a sensible Philosophy, and to furnish noble Medicines for the benefit of Mankind'; N. Hodges, *Vindiciae Medicinae & Medicorum: Or An Apology for the Profession and Professors of Physick in Answer to the Several Pleas of Illegal Practitioners* (London, 1665), A4v.

33. Choke was appointed chymist in ordinary without fee to the King on the same day that he was granted his Lambeth licence, 11 July 1667; TNA, LC 3/26, fo. 142; Bloom and James, 43; *CSPD, 1667*, 285, 352.
34. *CSP Ireland, 1669–1670; Addenda, 1625–1670*, 18, 85, 89, 103, 653. Among others that Choke claimed to have cured 'when all physicians had left him' was the chymists' patron, the duke of Buckingham. In addition to various medical receipts which Choke claimed to have received from van Helmont for cure of the gout, stone, scurvy, and dropsy, he was also widely acclaimed for perfecting a teething necklace, 'no heavier than a nutmeg', which was approved, among others, by Choke's chymical colleague, Edward Warner; R. Porter, *Quacks: Fakers & Charlatans in English Medicine* (Stroud, 2000), 105, 116; *CSPD, 1675–1676*, 300.
35. F. M. van Helmont, *The Paradoxal Discourses of F. M. van Helmont Concerning the Macrocosm and Microcosm, or the Greater and Lesser World and Their Union* (London, 1685), unpaginated 'Preface to the Reader' by J. B., dated 5 October 1684. The events recounted here must have taken place before the death of Prince Rupert in 1682. Described variously as major or lieutenant colonel, it is possible that Helmont's 'son-in-law' may have been the same as the Captain Choke who was arrested in 1663 for plotting; TNA, SP 29/62/16.
36. In what follows, I expand upon the analysis first laid out by William Birken in his 'The Dissenting Tradition in English Medicine of the Seventeenth and Eighteenth Centuries', *Medical History*, 39 (1995), 197–218.
37. Between 1660 and 1682, the presidency of the College was dominated by former puritans, dissenters and nonconformist sympathizers. For brief biographies of these men, which emphasize their puritan roots and support for their co-religionists after 1660 (Edward Alston, 1655–66; Francis Glisson, 1667–9; George Ent, 1670–5 and 1681; John Micklethwaite, 1676–80 and Thomas Coxe, 1682), see ibid., 201–5 and respective articles in the *ODNB*. Of the fourteen men who held the post of censor between 1660 and 1670, eight (George Ent, Jonathan Goddard, Sir John Baber, Daniel Whistler, John Micklethwaite, William Staines, Thomas Coxe and Nathan Paget) were either nonconformists or sympathetic to Dissent. Of the other six, only two (Charles Scarburgh and Thomas Croyden) were demonstrably opposed to Dissent and wholehearted in their support for restored Anglicanism. These figures are based on the lists compiled by Hal Cook from the Annals of the College, for which see Cook, *The Decline of the Old Medical Regime*, Appendix 1, 267.
38. Ejected ministers and licentiates: William Bagley (1676), Jeremiah Butt (1679), Ichabod Chauncy (1666), Isaac Chauncy (1669), Henry Godman (1664), John Hutchinson (1662), Richard Inglett (1661), John Manship (1663), John Peachey (1683), John Pringle (1662), Edward Richardson (1662), Andrew Tristram (1667) and Edward Warren (1667). Sons of ejected ministers and licentiates: John Carte (1674), Nathaniel Firmin (1676), Edward Harding (1661), Clopton Havers (1684), Samuel Haworth (1680), John Martyn (1683), Charles Nichols (1687) and Edward Oakes

(1661). Other licentiates, either dissenters or sympathetic to dissent: Gabriel Barber (1678), Richard Clampe (1661), Jan Coughen (1672), Richard Edwards (1662), John Griffith (1670), Oliver Horsman (1682), William Jacob (1660), Thomas Marshall (1674), Joshua Palmer (1683), Arthur Parsons (1684), Benjamin Temple (1677) and Robert Whitaker (1669). It is highly probable that these numbers represent an underestimate of the strength of dissent among the extra licentiates. John Feake (1676), for example, was the son of the infamous fifth monarchist Christopher Feake. Moreover, the College continued to extend its patronage to dissenters after 1688. Both Matthew Toogood (29 November 1694) and Joseph Warder (29 December 1691) combined a medical practice with their duties as pastors of Independent congregations in Somerset and Surrey, respectively. The careers of many of these men are discussed in more detail in the next chapter.

39. *Cal. Rev.*, 287; Venn, ii, 440. Hutchinson subsequently settled at Hitchin in Hertfordshire, where he practised physic for thirty years before moving back to London and setting up a successful practice at Clapham in Surrey.
40. Munk, i, 307; *Cal. Rev.*, 400; Venn, iii, 400. Imprisoned at Newcastle in 1665, Pringle seems to have worked closely with another dissenting minister-cum-physician, Richard Gilpin. In November 1668, for example, both men were reported to be preaching at the Barber Surgeons' Hall in the town; *CSPD, 1668–1669*, 73.
41. Munk, i, 307; *Cal. Rev.*, 410–11; Venn, iii, 451 [though Venn confuses Richardson with another man of that name]. Richardson's involvement in the Yorkshire plot is based on a close reading of the official state papers for this period by Richard Greaves; see his *Deliver Us From Evil: The Radical Underground in Britain, 1660–1663* (Oxford and New York, 1986), 177–80 and *passim*. However, Greaves' subsequent claim that Richardson 'shunned radical schemes after fleeing to the Netherlands' is not borne out by the surviving evidence. For example, in the late 1660s and early 1670s, an English informant living in Haarlem claimed that the dissident spy Colonel John Scott frequently lodged with Richardson. Others testified that Richardson was often in the company of radical exiles and plotters such as the regicide Colonel Thomas Wogan; R. L. Greaves, *Enemies Under His Feet: Radicals and Nonconformists in Britain, 1664–1677* (Stanford, CA, 1990), 199; Bodl., Rawlinson MS A 176, fos 21, 32v; Rawlinson MS A 188, fo. 317. Intriguingly, both Richardson and Scott would appear to have shared a strong interest in chymistry and Helmontianism (discussed more fully, below 200). Richardson may also have acted as mentor to the Quaker apostate Jan Coughen, the son of an Anglo-Dutch merchant, who, on Richardson's advice, studied medicine at Leiden and became an extra licentiate of the London College in 1672; see below 199–200.
42. For Ichabod, see Munk, i, 354; RCPL, Annals, iv, fo. 90a and below 204, 205. For Isaac, see Munk, i, 415–16; *Cal. Rev.*, 112 and *ODNB*. For Isaac Chauncy's pronounced interest in all matters iatrochemical, see especially the correspondence between him and his American brother-in-law Gershom Bulkeley cited in T. W. Jodziewicz, 'A Stranger in the Land: Gershom Bulkeley of Connecticut', *Transactions of the American Philosophical Society*, 78 (1988), 23. Isaac also subscribed to the publication of Christopher Packe's edition of the *Works* of the celebrated Dutch chymist Johann Rudolph Glauber in 1689. For the appeal of chymistry to New England's early puritans,

see W. Woodward, *Prospero's America: John Winthrop Jr, Alchemy, and the Creation of New England Culture, 1606–1676* (Chapel Hill, NC, 2010). I hope to address the interplay of North American and British engagement with chymistry in due course.

43. BL, Add. MS 78,313, fo. 60r [John Beale to John Evelyn, 21 June 1671]. Beale's informant may well have been Ichabod Chauncy, educated in New England, who was practising in Bristol at this time and retained strong links with puritan leaders on the other side of the Atlantic.
44. The debate surrounding the new charter is discussed in Cook, *Decline of the Old Medical Regime*, 137–45.
45. Among those who can be safely identified as wholehearted in their support for the restored monarchy and church were: Samuel Argell or Argall, Matthew Bacon, Peter Balle, John Bidgood, Nicholas Carter, Walter Charleton, Sir John Colladon, Robert Fielding, Edward Gelsthorpe, Lancelot Harrison, Sir John Hinton, Edmund Meara, John Christopher Moesler, Henry Paman, Nicholas Stanley, Henry Titchborne, Sir Theodore Vaux, William Waldegrave, Thomas Willis, John Windebank, Thomas Witherley and Henry Wyvill. Argell, Bacon, Meara, Titchborne and Waldegrave were all Roman Catholics or crypto-Catholics.
46. Barbon (MD Utrecht, 1661) was the son of the fiery Cromwellian radical and MP, Praisegod Barbon. Though he would appear to have shunned medical practice in favour of a career as a property speculator and all-round entrepreneur, he did use his medical qualifications to support the candidacy of men seeking medical licences from the church in London, including the notorious empiric Thomas Saffold (d.1691); *ODNB*; Munk, i, 345; Bloom and James, 67–8 [Saffold, 1674]; LPL, VX 1A/10/60 [John Langford, 1674].
47. Glisson (MD Cambridge, 1639) was the brother of the more celebrated physician and Presbyterian elder Francis Glisson. Henry served as physician-general to the parliamentary forces in the first civil war. He, too, later used his authority as an extra-licentiate to sponsor the archiepiscopal licence applications of seven aspiring physicians, including John Pordage Jnr (d.1688), the son of the radical Behmenist; Venn, ii, 223; Munk, i, 343; Webster, *Great Instauration*, 55; LPL, VX 1A/10/23 [Thomas Clarke Jnr of Okehampton, Devon, 1670]; 1A/10/26 [Francis Hann of Loxbeare, Devon, 1670]; 1A/10/37/1–2 [Samuel Leigh, 1671]; 1A/10/186 [Robert Sparke of Newington, Surrey, 1682]; 1A/10/187 [Samuel Wall of St Martins in the Fields, Middlesex, 1682]; 1A/10/225/1–2 [Samuel Smith of Southwark, 1685]; 1A/10/243 [John Pordage of St Andrew's, Holborn, Middlesex, 1687].
48. Griffiths (d.1691), a fellow of University College, Oxford, in the 1650s, was destined for a career in the church but at the Restoration, 'being not minded to conform', opted instead for medicine, proceeding MD at Caen in 1664. He practised at Richmond, Surrey, and in 1681 published a sustained critique of the contemporary fashion for what he deemed the excessive use of phlebotomy, a practice which he blamed on the English infatuation for all things French. He later became a full fellow of the College in 1687, serving as censor and registrar in 1690–1; *ODNB*; Foster, ii, 612; Munk, i, 471; Wood, *Fasti*, ii, 198, 224; R. Griffiths, *A-la-mode Phlebotomy No Good Fashion, or, The Copy of a Letter to Dr Hungerford* (London, 1681).

49. Nicholas Lamprière or Lemprière (MD Caen, 1639) was originally from Jersey. During the 1650s, he served the Cromwellian state in various capacities, including as a commissioner for assessment and JP in the county of Surrey. He was the brother of Michael Lemprière, a staunch Cromwellian and Baptist who was one of the chief supporters of the Interregnum regimes on the island of Jersey throughout the 1650s. Nicholas may have shared his brother's radical religious leanings; Venn, iii, 74; Munk, i, 337; *Commons' Journal, 1651–1660*, 845; Green, *CPCC*, iii, 2230; Bodl., Tanner MS 55, fo. 132; H. Jenkinson and D. L. Powell (eds), *Surrey Quarter Sessions Records... 1659–1661* (Frome & London, Surrey Rec. Soc., vol.13, 1934), 13; T. Aston, *Satan in Samuels Mantle, or the Cruelty of Germany Acted in Jersey* (London, 1659), 25; *ODNB*, sub Lemprière, Michel.
50. Walter Needham (1632–1691) was a product of Interregnum Cambridge. He graduated MD there in 1664, and rapidly gained a reputation as an anatomist culminating in the publication of his highly original research on the foetus. Dissenting sympathies and connections are suggested by his close friendship with the ejected minister and physician John Reynolds, with whom he collaborated over the case of the abstinent Martha Taylor. In addition, in 1657 Needham, along with the radical surgeon Thomas Trapham, signed a codicil to the will of Aaron Gurdon. Trapham and Gurdon were also 'political' beneficiaries of the College's decision to create honorary fellows in 1664; *ODNB*; Munk, i, 472; J. Reynolds, *A Discourse upon Prodigious Abstinence* (London, 1669), A3r and *passim*; TNA, PROB 11/347/583 [will of Aaron Geurdain, doctor in phisick, of Bevis Markes, London 16 July 1657; pr. 22 July 1675].
51. Thomas Tymme (1618–1687) was the son of the alchemist-clergyman of the same name (d.1620) who was responsible, among other things, for publishing a translation of the works of the French Paracelsian Joseph Duchesne (Quercetanus) in 1605. Tymme Jnr was a medical student at Cambridge in the 1640s, when he would appear to have served as physician to the armies of the Eastern Association. At the same time, he played a prominent role in the removal of the Laudian rector of his native parish of Hasketon in Suffolk. In 1649, he was appointed to act as a medical examiner by the University of Cambridge and to assist the regius professor, Francis Glisson, in examing licentiates. His daughter Mary married Benjamin Calamy (d.1686), the son of the celebrated puritan clergyman Edmund Calamy (d.1666). In later years, Tymme was on close terms with the Whig plotter and exclusionist Roger Whitley, whom he met on numerous occasions in opposition clubs in London to discuss political events in the wake of the abortive Rye House Plot; Venn, iv, p.281; Munk, i, p.334; *ODNB*, sub Tymme, Thomas [which fails to mention his alchemical interests or translations]; TNA, SP 28/21/I, fo. 86; 28/24/IV, fo. 419; C. Holmes (ed.), *The Suffolk Committees for Scandalous Ministers, 1644–1646* (Ipswich, Suffolk Rec. Soc., vol. 12, 1970), 77–8; CUL, CUA, Grace Book H (1645–1668), 49; Bodl., MS. Eng. Hist. c.711, fos 27r–57v.
52. Timothy van Vleteren (d.1665), who gained a medical degree from Caen in 1664, was the son-in-law of the radical preacher and prophet William Sedgwick, who left him £300 in his will; Munk, i, 344; Venn, iv, 294; TNA, PROB 11/313, fo. 168v [will of William Sedgwick the elder, 28 November 1663; pr. 26 February 1663/4].
53. John Yardley (d.1697) was the son of the Presbyterian minister John Yardley (d.1679), who was ejected at Cranham in Essex in 1662. He was educated at Cambridge in the

1650s, and after a short spell at Leiden graduated MD at Padua in 1662. He subsequently settled at Bishop's Stortford, where he practised medicine and served as a JP for Hertfordshire in 1685 and again from 1695 until his death in 1697; *Cal. Rev.*, 550; Venn, iv, 487; Innes Smith, 255; Munk, i, 350–1; W. Le Hardy (ed.), *Hertfordshire County Records. Calendar to the Sessions Books and Sessions Minute Books... 1658 to 1700* (Hertford, 1930), 526; W. J. Hardy (ed.), *Hertford County Records. Notes and Extracts from the Sessions Rolls 1581 to 1698* (Hertford, 1905), 361–3, 366, 378, 428–9.

54. The religious and political affiliations of Gurdon, Parker, Trapham and Whitmore are discussed more fully in chapter 3 above.
55. Bodl., MS Add. C.308, fos 33r–v. I dissent from Birken's view that this charge represented little more than a routine procedure 'little different from that issued by his predecessors in compliance with the medical licensing laws'; Birken, 'The Dissenting Tradition in English Medicine', 199. On the contrary, the exceptional nature of the request is evident in the surviving returns and frenzied activity in dioceses like Exeter and Worcester where the archbishop's orders were clearly expedited with care and urgency. For Devon, see DRO, PR 362-4/33/1-29. For detailed investigations into the medical credentials claimed by one professed surgeon in the diocese of Worcester following receipt of the archbishop's orders in the summer of 1665, see WRO, 795.02/ BA 2302/11, nos 2476, 2478.
56. It may not have been coincidental that the physician delegated by the College to compose the first response to the charges made against it by the chymists and their aristocratic supporters was Nathaniel Hodges (1629–1688). Hodges, a mere 'candidate' for admission to the College, devoted a chapter of his book, dedicated to Sheldon (note 32 above), to a critique of the existing episcopal licensing system and the way in which it encouraged unlearned empirics. Hodges, moreover, was himself a nonconformist sympathizer, whose father Thomas (d.1672) was a celebrated puritan preacher in the 1640s (albeit one who subsequently conformed); N. Hodges, *Vindiciae Medicinae & Medicorum*, 72–85. For the Hodges', father and son, see *ODNB*, sub Hodges, Nathaniel and Thomas.
57. The legal background to this case and its indefinite conclusion is discussed in Cook, *Decline of the Old Medical Regime*, 188–90. Educated at Trinity College, Dublin, Huyberts trained as an apothecary under Jacob Rickman in Dublin. During the 1650s, he would appear to have settled in Holland, where he ministered to the medical needs of the émigré royalist community. Huyberts moved to England some time after 1669 and settled at Kensington; A. Huyberts, *A Corner-Stone Laid Towards the Building of a New Colledge... in London* (London, 1675), 32–8. Huyberts was probably the son of the Dublin apothecary Hubert Adrian, who was knighted in 1660; T. Barnard, *Cromwellian Ireland: English Government and Reform in Ireland 1649–1660* (Oxford, 1975), 86n.
58. Huyberts, *A Corner-Stone Laid*, 38, 19; In addition to the support of Sheldon, Huyberts may have been dependant on the court connections of his friend, the royal surgeon and fellow Dutch exile, Richard Wiseman (d.1676), who, in a testimonial supporting Huyberts' application for an episcopal licence, described him as 'very long knowne to me both beyond sea and here in England'. His licence was granted on 5 February 1675; ibid., p.32; LPL, VX 1A/10/74/1–4; VG 1/1, f.269; Sheldon, f.255v.

59. Huyberts, *A Corner-Stone Laid*, 12–13.
60. Ibid., 19, 30.
61. BL, Sloane MS 3299, fo. 73.
62. W. Johnson, *Ἀγυρτο-Μάστιξ: Or, Some Brief Animadversions upon Two Late Treatises* (London, 1665), 5, 18, 37, 41–3, 68–9, 86. Johnson, like many of his opponents, fell victim to the plague some time in 1665. For similar attacks by defenders of the College equating the chymists' medical 'enthusiasm' with the religious extremism of the radical sectaries, see R. Sprackling, *Medela Ignorantiae: or a Just and Plain Vindication of Hippocrates and Galen from the Groundless Imputations of M. N.* (London, 1665), 157–8, 158–9, 161–2; G. Castle, *The Chymical Galenist: A Treatise wherein the Practise of the Ancients is Reconcil'd to the New Discoveries in the Theory of Physick* (London, 1667), A6r. Nathaniel Hodges went once step further. In a brazen attempt to curry favour with Sheldon, he sought to compare the College's beleaguered members with the sufferings undergone by loyal, Anglican clerics during the Interregnum; Hodges, *Vindiciae Medicinae & Medicorum*, A3r–v.
63. Note, for example, his observation that 'there is now a great falling out among themselves, as I perceive by Master Thomson's bitter inveighing against the Dropping Doctor, against Mr Odowde, and some others'. Johnson alleged that in a conversation with Thomson, 'in the heat of his railing, he told me, they especially were the persons that obstructed their business and disenabled them from achieving' their ends; Johnson, *Some Brief Animadversions*, 95, 109. Johnson's work carries an imprimatur dated 10 May 1665.
64. T. O'Dowde, *Two Letters Concerning the Cure of the Plague. The One to Thomas Eliot Esq.... The Other the Mayor of the Town of Southampton* (London, 1665).
65. G. Thomson, *Loimologia. A Consolatory Advice, and Some Brief Observations Concerning the Present Pest* (London, 1665), 15. Bolnest's name is strikingly absent from the list of chymical doctors, students and practitioners which Thomson appended to this work in support of the Society's aim of incorporation.
66. For Bolnest's radical past, see Appendix 1 (a).
67. Excerpts from a small fraction of the total correspondence of nearly two hundred letters were published in W. D. Cooper, 'Notices of the Last Great Plague, 1665–6', *Archaeologia*, 37 (1857), 1–22. The original collection today forms part of the Frewen MSS in the East Sussex Record Office at Brighton.
68. Jeake's son, also Samuel, seems to have inherited his father's interest in distillation and chymical medicines; see M. Hunter and A. Gregory (eds), *An Astrological Diary of the Seventeenth Century: Samuel Jeake of Rye 1652–1699* (Oxford, 1988), 56–7.
69. ESxRO, FRE 5548 [Allin to Frith, 27 October 1666].
70. See, for example, ESxRO, FRE 5611 [Allin to Frith, 14 November 1668], 5623 [same to same, 10 February 1670], 5625 [same to same, 17 March 1670].
71. ESxRO, FRE 5608 [Allin to Frith, 3 October 1668], 5466 [Allin to Frith, 14 September 1665]. In the latter, Allin refers to the recent death of Starkey as well as six unnamed chymical physicians, who succumbed to the disease following what he perceived as their arrogant attempt to anatomize the cadavers of plague victims. Allin concluded, after noting the deaths of at least 140 other doctors, surgeons and apothecaries in the

city, that 'God is resolved to shame the pride of all glory [for] there is no boasting before him, much lesse against him'.

72. ESxRO, FRE 5465 [Allin to Frith, 7 September 1665]. Frith was clearly a beneficiary of this interchange of ideas and writings. In 1666 he made a copy of Albertus Otto Faber's *Some Kindling Sparks in Matter of Physick*, which was not published until 1668. Frith's source was almost certainly Allin, and further copies of the manuscript were made by their mutual friend Samuel Jeake the younger; ESxRO, Frewen MS 606, fos 135–40; M. Hunter, G. Mandelbrote, R. Ovenden and N. Smith (eds), *A Radical's Books: The Library Catalogue of Samuel Jeake of Rye, 1623–90* (Woodbridge, 1999), xxii–xxiii.
73. ESxRO, FRE 5628 [Allin to Frith, 28 July 1670].
74. B. Penot, *Penotus Παλίμξθ: or The Alchymists Enchiridion. In Two Parts... Faithfully Englished... by B. P. Philalethes* (London, 1692). Penotus was an eminent French Paracelsian; see A. G. Debus, *The French Paracelsians: The Chemical Challenge to Medical and Scientific Tradition in Early Modern France* (Cambridge, 1991), 36, 38.
75. Dr Porter and his chymical cures are frequently mentioned in Allin's surviving correspondence with Frith; see, for example, ESxRO, FRE 5599 [Allin to Frith, 9 June 1668]; FRE 5601 [same to same, 22 June 1668]; FRE 5604 [same to same, 15 August 1668]. Like so many of the chymists, Porter's practice was underwritten by a licence from the bishop of London, granted by Richard Chaworth in 1667. Testimonials claimed that Porter, who was originally licensed by the bishop of St David's in 1634, had served as physician and surgeon under the royalist Colonel Thomas Cardiff in south Wales during the civil wars; Bloom and James, 64–5; Wellcome Library, MS 5338, *sub* Porter, Benedict.
76. For Allin's friendship with Dr Pratt, with whom he collaborated closely on various alchemical and medical projects, see ESxRO, FRE 5618 [Allin to Frith, 24 July 1669], FRE 5627 [same to same, 31 March 1670]. That it was Pratt, and not Bolnest, who went to Southampton in 1665 is confirmed by the protracted legal battle that Dr Robert Pratt subsequently waged against the corporation of Southampton for the recovery of his costs and fees in treating plague victims in the town; see Southampton City Archives, SC2/1/8, fos 223v, 238v, 251r. I strongly suspect that it was Pratt who confirmed Allin's story, recounted to Frith, of the recent appearance of the devil at the mayoral election at Southampton in 1665, it being related to him 'by a friend lately in those parts'; ESxRO, FRE 5505 [Allin to Frith, 6 February 1666]. The close relationship between Allin, Pratt and Stacy is confirmed in a letter written by Allin to Samuel Jeake the elder in 1670 in which he passed on the respects of his two friends. Jeake may well have received medical advice from Stacy as in 1679 he recorded payment for a 'Letter from Dr Stacy'; ESxRO, FRE 5629 [Allin to Jeake the elder, 13 October 1670]; Hunter and Gregory (eds), *Astrological Diary*, 57n. Stacy probably shared Allin's nonconformist principles. In 1684, John Stacy, 'professor of medicine', of St Olave, Southwark, was named in a mass presentment of dissenters at the Surrey Quarter Sessions; SHC, QR 2/5/Epiphany 1684, 113–24.
77. In addition to Charles Wilcox (discussed below), Pratt signed testimonials on behalf of Nicholas Rookes of Shadwell in 1670 and Charles Wheatly of Sussex in 1679; Bloom and James, 66; LPL, FII/20/104. He too possessed a licence to practise in the diocese of London, dated 5 December 1664; LMA, MS 09540/1, fo. 29v.

78. Guildhall Library, MS 10,116/6; Bloom and James, 73 [which gives the date in error as 1699]. Other signatories included George Pope of Whitechapel, 'practitioner in physick' and the former radical Lionel Lockyer (discussed below). In 1688, Pope was prosecuted by the College of Physicians for failing to pay a fine of £35 imposed for practising without due authority; RCPL, LEGAC/ENV98. Wilcox may be the man of the same name, described as a 'glassman', of Ratcliffe, who was buried at St Dunstan's, Stepney, on 4 April 1703. He was certainly living in the same parish in November 1666 when Wilcox, described as a physician, buried an infant son at Stepney; LMA, P93/DUN/128 and 278 [parish registers of St Dunstan's, Stepney, Middlesex, 1702–1709; 1622–1666].
79. Wilcox petitioned the Privy Council for reimbursement in 1671 and 1679. On the latter occasion, he claimed to have served as physician at the Tower until September 1667, when he was presumably removed. His case was finally referred for arbitration to Sir William Wild, a former judge of the Court of King's Bench, though no outcome is recorded. He was still petitioning for relief out of the estate of his deceased former master, Sir John Robinson, in 1681; TNA, PC 2/62, 381; 2/68, 241; 2/69, 393; ESxRO, FRE 5508 [Allin to Frith, 13 February 1666].
80. Lockyer provided testimonials for Thomas Fyge, alias Frye (1661), John Hall (1667), Abiezer Coppe (1667), Charles Wilcox (1669), and John Booth (1670).
81. William Johnson, for example, specifically named Lockyer alongside O'Dowde 'and the rest of those Fanaticks in Physick' in his diatribe aimed at undermining the chymists; Johnson, *Some Brief Animadversions*, 5; see also 127–8. For Lockyer and his radical past, see my 'Medicine, Religion and the Puritan Revolution', in R. French and A. Wear (eds), *The Medical Revolution of the Seventeenth Century* (Cambridge, 1989), 23–4.
82. Fyge's religious moderation is also suggested by the fact that in 1680 he attempted to intercede with the authorities on behalf of the prominent Quaker George Whitehead; Bloom and James, 50; J. R. Woodhead, *The Rulers of London 1660–1689: A Biographical Record of the Aldermen and Common Councilmen of the City of London* (London, London & Middlesex Archaeological Soc., 1965), 74; T. F[ydge], *The Citizens Sacred Entertainment: Being an Essay to Ingratiate the Practice of Vertue, to Consummate the Happiness of Humane Nature, and to Gratifie Ingenuous and Religious Spirits* (London, 1666), A2r–A4r and *passim*; L. Coelson, *Speculum Perspicuum Uranicum, or, An Almanack for the Year... 1680* (London, 1680); TNA, PROB 11/481, fos 33v–35r [will of Thomas Fyge, apothecary, of St Botolph Bishopgate, London, 22 December 1704; pr. 26 March 1705]; Besse, i, 507. Valentine Fyge (see above 71 and n), who retired to his native Staffordshire to practise medicine, probably shared his son's chymical interests. In 1663 the nonconformist William Westmacott (d.1721) moved to Stafford in the hope of succeeding to Fyge's practice. Westmacott had himself briefly trained under the tutelage of the London iatrochemist Abraham Hargrave, who later published a full-scale attack on the monopolistic powers wielded by the College of Physicians in 1676; FSL, MS V.a.441, 16; A. Hargrave, *Reason in Season: or, a Word on the Behalf of the Non-Collegiate Physicians and of the Right of the People in the Choice of Their Physicians* (London, 1676). Hargrave, like so many of his chymically inclined colleagues, received a licence to practise from the bishop of London, supported, among others, by Robert Turner of the Society of Chymical Physicians; Bloom and James, 54.

83. Describing himself as a resident of the city of London, Coppe was granted a licence to practice medicine and surgery in one of the archbishop's peculiars on 13 February 1667; LPL, VH 28/5; VH 1/1, 5. According to Anthony Wood, Coppe changed his name at the Restoration to Higham and practised medicine at Barnelms (Barnes) in Surrey. If so, then he is almost certainly the same as the 'Mr Higham of Barnelms', whom the empiric Bromfield, who also lived at Barnes, described as visiting his house on 19 February 1671. Bromfield claimed that Higham 'had been an eminent practitioner in Physic near 30 years' who had prescribed Bromfield's pills to his own patients, declaring that 'I have not met with any medicine, either in England, or my foreign Travels comparable to your Pills, for the cure of Diseases in general'; M. Bromfield, *A Brief Discovery of the True Causes, Symptoms, and Effects of that Most Reigning Disease, the Scurvy. Whereunto is added a Short Account of those Incomparable and Most Highly Approved Pills, called Pillulae in Omnes Morbos* (London, 1675), 10 [the testimonial, with others, was removed from later editions of this work].
84. Russell has frequently been confused with the Baptist of the same name who died in 1702. Both men were ardent advocates of iatrochemistry. Coppe's referee was appointed chymist to Charles II and was brother of the prolific alchemical translator Richard Russell. Like so many of his chymically inclined colleagues, Russell suffered repeated harassment at the hands of the College's officers. He died some time between 29 December 1684 and 10 February 1685; *ODNB*, sub Russell, William [which fails to note the date of Russell's royal appointment, prosecution by the College of Physicians or date of will]; Annals, iv, fo. 143a; RCPL, LEGAC/ENV 100; TNA, PROB 11/379, fos 208v–209v [will of William Russell, doctor in physic, of London, 29 December 1684; pr. 10 February 1684/5].
85. TNA, LC 3/28, fo. 28; W. Russell, *A Physical Treatise, Grounded Not Upon Tradition, nor Phancy, but Experience* (London, 1684), A5r; 39, 45–6, 50–1. According to the Paracelsian John Headrich, Charles II frequently used Russell's 'royal tincture' and valued him so greatly 'that he was often in his Conversation, upon such grounds as his Royal prudence thought reasonable'; J. Headrich, *Arcana Philosophia, or Chymical Secrets Containing the Noted and Useful Chymical Medicines of Dr Wil[lliam] and Rich [ard] Russel Chymists* (London, 1697), A5r.
86. TNA, PROB 11/379, fos 208v–209v; SHC, QR2/5/Michaelmas 1683, 277. Walraven almost certainly shared Russell's passion for chymistry. In 1689 he subscribed to Christopher Packe's edition of the *Works* of Glauber.
87. For a brief discussion of this dispute, focused on Starkey's desire to defend his professional integrity as a chymist, see W. R. Newman and L. M. Principe, *Alchemy Tried in the Fire: Starkey, Boyle, and the Fate of Helmontian Chemistry* (Chicago & London, 2002), 153–4.
88. For Starkey's Presbyterianism, see above 138.
89. Anne Matthews, 'A Precious Pearl', appended to R. Matthews, *The Unlearned Alchymist* (3rd ed., London, 1663), 1–2 [separately paginated]. Hobson's active involvement in plotting against the crown in the early 1660s is discussed more fully in the following chapter. For Fromanteel, a clockmaker by trade who fled to Holland after 1667 to avoid religious persecution, see *ODNB*. He was named as one of the joint executors of Matthews' will; Matthews, *Unlearned Alchymist*, 10; TNA, PROB 11/307,

fos 60v–61r [will of Richard Mathew, chymist, of the Tower of London, 7 October 1660; pr. 16 January 1661/2].

90. Kendall (d.1666) was the author of *An Appendix to the Unlearned Alchimist* (London, 1663?) in which he upheld Starkey's claim to be the inventor of the original recipe. He was clearly writing with the support of Matthews' executors and former colleagues, including Fromanteel, Jonathan Loddington and his own grandfather Ambrose Andrewes, who was described as one of Matthews' original operatives in manufacturing the pill; ibid., 24, 48; TNA, PROB 11/321, ff.68v–69r [will of George Kendall, of Stepney, Middlesex, 29 May 1666; pr. 7 June 1666]. His career was a chequered one. Kendall, who described himself as MA, was probably the graduate of New Inn Hall, Oxford, who took up a clerical living in his native Northamptonshire in the late 1630s before sliding into hererodoxy. Thomas Edwards refers to his presence in the Isle of Ely as a 'great sectary' in the early 1640s (his will refers to lands at Whittlesea in the Isle). Shortly thereafter, he became vicar of Hemel Hempstead in Hertfordshire, where it was reported that he had converted the parish to anabaptism and was 'the chief promoter of all the distractions there'. Little is heard of him thereafter, but there are grounds for supposing that he is the same as the George Kendall, MA, who took up a post in the naval dockyards at Deptford and Woolwich in the mid 1650s and was the author of a work that sought to undermine one of his colleagues, Edward Hayward, clerk of the survey at nearby Chatham (a Mr Kendall of Chatham was listed as one of the outlets of Matthews' pill in 1660). Hayward hinted at a radical and disreputable past, questioning Kendall's MA and moral probity, and describing him as a 'high pretender' to religion. Kendall the chymist died some time between 29 May and 7 June 1666. A former associate John Allin described him as 'long since dead' in October of that year; Foster, ii, 843; H. I. Longden (ed.), *Northamptonshire and Rutland Clergy*, 16 vols (Northampton, 1938–52), viii, 73; T. Edwards, *Gangraena* (London, 1646), iii, 79–80; S. Wright, *The Early English Baptists 1603–1649* (Woodbridge, 2006), 128; G. Kendall, *The Clerk of the Surveigh Surveighed and His Rigging Cast* (1656); E. Hayward, *The Answer of Edward Hayward... to a Most Abusive and Scandalous Pamphlet... by George Kendall, MA* (London, 1656), A2r; 6, 7; ESxRO, FRE 5447 [Allin to Frith, 12 October 1666].

91. R. Matthews, *The Unlearned Alchymist* (1st ed., London, 1660), 46–63. That the 'giddy professor of religion' whom Matthews had known for twenty years, and who asked him if he 'seriously' read the scriptures, was Joseph Salmon is strongly suggested by Matthews' comment that he had once tried to seduce the wife of a merchant in Barbados; ibid., 58–9 [Salmon emigrated to Barbados in about 1655; see *ODNB*]. Coppe is almost certainly alluded to as the author of a recent work 'wherein he doth avow there is no hell but what is in a mans self'; ibid., 60.

92. Iatrochemical links to the radical seeker communities of Interregnum England are also suggested by the early association of Richard Barker, one of the most prominent spokesmen for the chymists after the Restoration, with Captain William Rainsborough of Stepney, brother of the murdered parliamentarian officer. Some time around 1650, Laurence Clarkson (1615–1667) claimed the two men formed part of a Ranter gathering at Ilford in Essex. A decade later, Barker, now established as a successful empiric in London despite frequent attempts by the College of Physicians to

proscribe his practice, provided surety for Rainsborough, who was accused of selling arms in his charge to civilians; L. Clarkson, *The Lost Sheep Found* (London, 1660), 27, 30; *CSPD, 1660–1661*, 505; A. L. Morton, *The World of the Ranters* (London, 1970), 98, 103, 107, 133, 135.

93. For William Walwyn's debt to Helmontianism, see Wear, *Knowledge and Practice in English Medicine*, 353–4, 387–90, 391–4 and *passim*. Brooke, whose medical expertise and learning were praised by his father-in-law, may have harboured alchemical interests of his own. In October 1650, one Dr Brooks consulted with the astrologer Elias Ashmole to determine whether he 'shall get any of Dr Currer's skill in transmutation of metal or not'; C. H. Josten (ed.), *Elias Ashmole (1617–1672): His Autobiographical and Historical Notes, His Correspondence, and Other Contemporary Sources Relating to His Life and Work*, 5 vols (Oxford, 1966), ii, 551. By 1654, he was assisting his father-in-law's early medical endeavours by allowing his *vitae* and aromatic spirits to be purchased from his house in Duke's Place, Aldgate. There is also a hint of Helmontianism in Brooke's advice to plague victims in 1665 that they should avoid excessive fearfulness in the face of the epidemic as this was the chief cause of the contagion; *ODNB*, sub Brooke, Humphrey; [H. Brooke], *Cautionary Rules for Preventing the Sickness* (London, 1665), 7–8.
94. Brooke was particularly active in the 1660s, when he supported the licence applications of Edward Harris of Chipping Norton, Oxfordshire (1662), John Lane of Ascot under Wychwood, Oxfordshire (1662), George Sainthill of Exeter (1664), Thomas Newman (1667) and Coppe (1667). In 1682, as a full fellow of the College, he wrote a letter in support of Fulk Baker, citizen and apothecary of London, who was seeking a licence from the archbishop of Canterbury; LPL, FII/3/110; FII/2/120; FII/5/108a-c; VX 1A/10/10; VH 28/5; VX 1A/10/173/2. Brooke, moreover, was not alone as a member of the College of Physicians in signing such testimonials. That for Lane, for example, was also signed by Nathan Paget and Jonathan Goddard, two members with distinctly radical political pedigrees; see *ODNB*, sub Paget, Nathaniel, and Goddard, Jonathan.
95. I. Gentles, 'The Debentures Market and Military Purchases of Crown Land, 1649–1660', Ph. D. (London, 1969), 166. Along with other physicians such as Benjamin Worsley and William Petty who supported the change of regime in 1649, Brooke also served as an army physician in Ireland in 1651; *CSPD, 1651*, 541.
96. H. B[rooke], *The Durable Legacy* (London, 1681), 156.
97. LPL, FII/3/110. Rand testified to the efficacy of Walwyn's chymical remedies in the latter's *Health's New Store-House Opened* (London, 1661), 26.
98. For Rand's radical religious, political and medical associations, see above 113 nn.172, 173, 114 n.175, 117 n.195, 139. Jeffrey Collins has suggested that as a physician of republican political leanings and unorthodox religious views, Rand's interests 'closely paralleled' those of another member of the Hartlib circle, William Petty; J. R. Collins, *The Allegiance of Thomas Hobbes* (Oxford, 2005), 192–4.
99. T. Erastus, *The Nullity of Church Censures* (London, 1659), unpaginated dedication to John Troutbeck of Hope, 'late Chyrurgion-Generall in the Northern Army'; E. Hickeringill, *Works*, 3 vols (London, 1716), iii, 117. For a synopsis of Troutbeck's life and career, see Appendix 1 (a). For Hickeringill's highly unorthodox views and resulting conflict with the ecclesiastical authorities in Restoration England, see *ODNB*

and J. T. I. Champion and L. McNulty, 'Making Orthodoxy in Late Restoration England: The Trials of Edmund Hickeringill, 1662–1710', in M. J. Braddick and J. Walter (eds), *Negotiating Power in Early Modern Society: Order, Hierarchy and Subordination in Britain and Ireland* (Cambridge, 2001), 227–48.

100. One possible explanation is that the ecclesiastical authorities in London and elsewhere were more interested in clamping down on mainstream dissent, which they understandably perceived as a much greater threat to its authority. Alternatively, many former radicals may have conformed or gone through the motions of outwardly submitting to the Church. Lionel Lockyer, for instance, was sufficiently respected in his home parish of St Saviour's, Southwark, to receive burial there and have a magnificent monument erected in the church eulogizing his achievements and the merits of his pill. It was recorded for posterity by John Aubrey and survives today; see TNA, PROB 11/339, fos 64v–67r [will of Lionell Lockyer, physician, of St Thomas', Southwark, Surrey, 4 March 1671/2; pr. 18 May 1672]; J. Aubrey, *The Natural History and Antiquities of Surrey*, 5 vols (London, 1729), v, 205–6.

101. 'And were this course followed, and generally countenanced, those rebellious and enormous Vices of the Minde, too grassant at this day among us, which in great part arise from the Feral, Anomalous, unheard of Prodigious, and untractable Diseases of the Body, might in some measure be reformed'; G. Thomson, *Galeno-pale*, A3r. Nedham, likewise, linked the viciousness of the times with the emergence of new, more complex, diseases, which accordingly required different and more effective (i.e. iatrochemical) forms of treatment; M. N[edham], *Medela Medicinae: A Plea for the Free Profession, and a Renovation of the Art of Physick* (London, 1665), 29–55. In subsequent chapters, Nedham expatiated at length on the way in which modern diseases had mutated, focusing especially upon pox, plague and scurvy.

102. G. Thomson, *ΠΛΑ'ΝΟ-ΠΝΙΓΜΟ'Σ. Or, A Gag for Johnson* (London, 1665), 15–16, 17, 18.

103. G. Thomson, *Μιωχυμίας 'ΕλϵΓχθς: or, A Check Given to the Insolent Garrulity of Henry Stubbe* (London, 1671), 43–4. Thomson's insinuation that the 'Dogmatical Galenists' were closet atheists, 'their Moral Actions being sutable to their Physical Tenents' (43), was particularly apposite given the dubious reputation of his antagonist, Stubbe.

104. Thomson, *Direct Method of Curing Chymically*, 171–2, 186. There was some truth to Thomson's insinuation that nonconformist sects encouraged their members to consult physicians of the same denomination. I discuss this further in chapter 5.

105. Ibid., 186–7. While there is little reason to doubt Thomson's loyalty and commitment to the restored Church, there is some evidence for religious moderation and even-handedness in his religious outlook as suggested by the fact that in his will he made equal bequests of £10 to both those 'Poore that are non-Conformists' as well as 'such of the poore distressed Loyalists' in his home parish of St Mary le Bow; TNA, PROB 11/353, fos 271v–272v [will of George Thomson, doctor in physic, of London, 30 December 1676; pr. 16 March 1676/7].

106. Ibid., *Direct Method of Curing Chymically*, 188–99.

107. R. Godfrey, *Various Injuries and Abuses in Chymical and Galenical Physick* (London, 1674), 136–8. Godfrey was almost certainly a Quaker or Quaker sympathizer. In his

published work, he explains how he underwent an apprenticeship in the art of chymistry at the direction of 'a true hearted Chymical Physitian', now dead, whose practice had been inherited by a son of the same name. Godfrey's will, made in 1674, makes it clear that the two men concerned were the Quakers Thomas Bourne the elder (d.1672) and younger (d.1690), who practised medicine in Bristol. Godfrey left bequests to Thomas' widow and son as well as giving £10 to 'the poore amongst the people called Quakers which inhabitt within the Citty of London'; ibid., A5r–A6v; 160; TNA, PROB 11/344, fos 54v–55r [will of Robert Godfrey, physician, of the city of London, 17 January 1673/4; pr. 21 January 1673/4]. For the Bournes, see R. Mortimer (ed.), *Minute Book of the Men's Meeting of the Society of Friends in Bristol 1686–1704* (Bristol, Bristol Rec. Soc., vol. 30, 1977), 235; Besse, i, 58. I discuss more fully the eirenic associations of the English iatrochemical movement in my 'Medicine, Religion and the Puritan Revolution', 34–45.

108. G. Acton, *Physical Reflections upon a Letter Written by J.Denis... to Monsieur de Montmor... Concerning a New Way of Curing Sundry Diseases by Transfusion of Blood* (London, 1668), epistle dedicatory to Charles II and 4–5; *idem*, *A Letter in Answer to Certain Quaeries and Objections Made by a Learned Galenist, Against the Theorie and Practice of Chymical Physick* (London, 1670). In the latter, Acton described himself as a 'doctor of physick' living in Silver Street, near Bloomsbury market. He was appointed chymist in ordinary without fee, on 1 August 1667; TNA, LC 3/26, fo. 142.

109. TNA, LC 3/26, fo. 142 [Choke]; 3/27, fo. 48 [Faber]; 3/28, fo. 28 [Russell]. For Choke and Russell, see above 129, 137. For Faber, see 150 n.10, 183.

110. The other chymists in ordinary were Anthony Bruser (1667), Anthony Colley (1670), William Jones (1667), William Morden (1669), Edward Pattison (1682), Constantine Rhodocanaces (1670; and chymist to the King in 1674) and William Savage (1667); TNA, LC 3/24, fo. 26 [Rhodocanaces]; 3/26, fo. 142 [Bruser, Colley, Morden, Rhodocanaces and Savage]; 3/28, fo. 28 [Pattison]. Though appointed as chymists, all were practising physicians, many of whom acquired immunity from prosecution through the aegis of an episcopal or archiepiscopal licence. Choke, Colley, Jones and Savage were all approved in this fashion; Bloom and James, 34, 43, 68; LPL, VG 1/3, fos 103v–104; Sheldon, fo. 219. Extraordinarily, Morden, who received the normal testimonials, was ultimately refused a licence by the bishop of London 'by reason of the Parties insufficiencie'; Bloom and James, 61. Savage had been hauled before the College of Physicians in November 1656, when he promised to 'bid farewell [to] medicine'; RCPL, Annals, iv, fo. 65b.

111. TNA, LC 3/26, fo. 14; *CSPD, 1668–1669*, 315. The warrant for Williams' appointment was issued on 7 May 1669. Two months earlier, Charles had paved the way for his elevation to the royal household when he requested that Cambridge University grant Williams an MD by royal mandate. The official request specifically refers to his attendance on the royal person 'for some time past', as well as his 'singular knowledge in compounding medicines'; ibid., 224; Venn, iv, 418. The official record in the state papers would appear to contradict the date of Williams' appointment given elsewhere as 1667; cf. TNA, LC 3/24, fo. 16; 3/30, fo. 42. For a synopsis of Williams' career, see Appendix 1 (a).

112. *Calendar of Treasury Books*, vol.3 (1669–72), 938. For Williams' political career, which I discuss within the context of the wider political and religious concerns of the chymical community at Charles' court, see Henning, iii, 726–7 and Appendix 1 (a). Williams' rise to prominence at court, like that of so many of his chymical colleagues, was almost certainly indebted in large part to the support and patronage of the duke of Buckingham. Edward Bolnest, for example, whom we have already encountered as a protégé of the duke and signatory of the chymists' petition in 1665, was, like Williams, created chymical physician to the King in 1670; TNA, LC 3/26, fo. 142 [Edward Boldnesse].
113. Physicians in ordinary: Sir Richard Barker (1673), Pierre Massonet (1672), Edward Warner (1660). Physicians in extraordinary: Thomas Norton (1668), John Spranger (1661). Apothecary and operator in chymistry: Nicholas Le Févre (1660). Surgeon in ordinary: John Troutbeck (1660).
114. Clarke (d.1684) was appointed physician in ordinary to Charles II on 3 February 1672 and practised medicine at Bath and Stepney in Middlesex. He served as sheriff of Middlesex in 1666. His passion for chymistry led him to publish *The Natural History of Nitre: or, a Philosophical Discourse of... Nitre, with Its Vertues and Uses* (London, 1670). He may also be the same as 'Clerke chemist' who wrote a short letter, no longer extant, to Robert Boyle in November 1680; TNA, LC 3/27, fos 46v, 47v; Foster, i, 285; *CSPD, 1666–1667*, 15; Boyle, *Correspondence*, v, 226.
115. Venn refers to Eales (1634–1710) as a royal physician in receipt of a grant of arms in 1670; Venn, ii, 93. His name, however, does not appear in Robert Bucholz's electronic database of court officers, 1660–1837; www.luc.edu/history/fac_resources/bucholz/DCO/DCO.html. Eales was nonetheless awarded his MD at Cambridge by royal mandate in 1660; *CSPD, 1660–1661*, 147. The Helmontian Christopher Packe reprinted two letters of Eales, dated June and August 1695 from Welwyn in Hertfordshire, in which he recounted the successful administration of Packe's *sal solutivium* in the case of a fifteen-year-old boy suffering from epileptic fits and hypochondriachal melancholy; C. Packe, *Medela Chymica or, an Account of the Vertues and Uses of a Select Number of Chymical Medicines* (London, 1708), 84–5. His iatrochemical credentials are also suggested by his subscription to the English edition of works of the Dutch chymist Johann Glauber, printed by Packe in 1689. Eales was on friendly terms with the ejected nonconformist physician John Hutchinson, whom he lavishly praised for his learning. He may well, therefore, have been related to another former minister, Nathaniel Eales or Eeles, who was ejected from his living at nearby Harpenden in 1660; *Cal. Rev.*, 287, 180–1.
116. TNA, LC 3/26, fo. 141v. Hubbard (d.1716 or 1717) was the subject of an effusive dedication by the Paracelsian John Headrich, a former assistant to Richard Russell, brother of the royal physician and chymist, William Russell (see 137, 167 n.109). In the epistle dedicatory to his *Arcana Philosophia or, Chymical Secrets* (London, 1697), Headrich claimed that he had been persuaded to publish this compilation of chymical remedies, based on the cures of Richard and William Russell, by a former physician to Charles II, presumably Hubbard (A4v). Hubbard, like so many of his chymical colleagues, was licensed by the bishop of London in October 1667, but later

prosecuted by the College of Physicians in 1682. He, too, subscribed to the *Works* of Glauber, published by Packe in 1689; Bloom and James, 56; RCPL, LEGAC/ENV 81.

117. TNA, LC 3/28, fo. 25v. Slade, who possessed a Leiden MD (1667), was yet another royal physician to support Packe's project to publish Glauber's works in English (where he signs himself as MD, of Wrexham). For his nonconformist background in Exeter, see below, 197, 237n.

118. For Sparck or Spark, see chapter 3, note 197.

119. TNA, LC 3/24, fo. 16; 3/25, fo. 51; 3/26, fo. 141; 3/25, fo. 50v. Waldron (d.1677), who proceeded MD at Oxford in 1653, defended in the same year the decidedly Helmontian proposition that the opening of the stomach was the seat of the soul; Foster, iv, 1555; Bodl., UOA, NEP/supra/Reg Qa: Register of Congregation, 1647–1659, fo. 151v. If his practice was influenced by Helmontianism it might explain why he had to wait ten years as a candidate before being admitted as a fellow of the College of Physicians in London; Munk, i, 351–2. His iatrochemical credentials are further suggested by the fact that he supplied a testimonial in 1672 for one Thomas Wall, a pupil of the Helmontian and former Oxford medical graduate, Robert Fielding (see 271).

120. Dickinson's appointment to the royal household on 10 February 1677 continued after Charles' death in 1685. The post became vacant following the deposition of James II in 1688; TNA, LC 3/24, fo. 16; 3/56, 11. For Dickinson, and his pronounced interest in transmutational alchemy, see the entry by Lawrence Principe in the *ODNB*. Royal and aristocratic patronage of the kind described here extended beyond the physicians.

121. The seminal work here in directing historians of science to the court as one of the main foci of scientific activity in this period is M. Biagioli, *Galileo, Courtier: The Practice of Science in the Age of Absolutism* (Chicago, 1993). In line with others, however, Biagioli has suggested that the 'weakness' of the English crown, in contrast to more powerful absolutist regimes such as those of the Medici in Florence or the Bourbons in France, led English natural philosophers to cultivate institutions other than the court for the promotion of their studies; *idem*, 'Etiquette, Interdependence, and Sociability in Seventeenth-Century Science', *Critical Inquiry*, 22 (1996), 230. For an attempt to depict the restored court of Charles II as conducive to the propagation of medical innovation, see S. Werrett, 'Healing the Nation's Wounds: Royal Ritual and Experimental Philosophy in Restoration England', *History of Science*, 38 (2000), 377–99.

122. For Currer and Troutbeck, see Appendix 1 (a). It should also be noted that one of the earliest proponents of Helmontianism in England, Noah Biggs, has been speculatively identified as a naval surgeon in the Cromwellian dockyards of Kent. If so, he may have been an associate of George Kendall; see above 39 n.44, 164 n.90.

123. For the iatrochemical interests and connections of Prince Rupert and the duke of York, see above, 125. For Mennes and Ernle, see Appendix 1 (b). The duke of York's commitment to chymical medicine is suggested by his confirmation, as newly crowned king in 1685, of many of those iatrochemists whom his brother had appointed to medical posts at court, as well as his patronage of 'empirics' such as the anti-Galenical, Samuel Haworth (for whom, see below, 218).

124. Hampshire Record Office, 18M51/636/22. This item consists of a small, printed pamphlet addressed to Sir John Lawson (d.1665), commander in chief of the royal navy and 'the Gentlemen the Chirurgeons bound to sea on his Majesties Service'. It was almost certainly privately printed, that in the Hampshire Record Office being the only surviving copy. In the work itself, Smart claimed to be writing to Lawson on the personal instructions of the King. In order to promote and publicise the benefits of his pill, Smart appended a list of several cures performed with his nostrum in and around London, dating from 1657. The work itself was signed, in ink, by Smart, and dated 10 February 1663/4 from Dorchester House, the home of his patron the marquis of Dorchester. For Smart, see Appendix 1 (a). Less than ten years later, when England was once again engaged in naval warfare with the Dutch, Charles was eager to trial and promote the use of the 'royal stiptique' in the royal navy; Werrett, 'Healing the Nation's Wounds', 390, 392. Hal Cook, moreover, has observed that the navy of William and Mary also encouraged medical experimentation and the trials of Helmontian 'empirics' such as John Colbatch (1666–1729); see his 'Practical Medicine and the British Armed Forces after the "Glorious Revolution"', *Medical History*, 34 (1990), 1–26.
125. TNA, PC 2/69, 76; W. Bacon, *A Key to Helmont, or, a Short Introduction to the Better Understanding of the Theory and Method of the Most Profound Chymical Physicians* (London, 1682), 31–2. Bacon (1633–1690), who hailed from North Petherton in Somerset, was licensed to practise medicine by the archbishop of Canterbury in December 1675. Among those who supplied testimonials was the chymical physician Edmund Dickinson, whose early support Bacon acknowledged in the work cited above. For Bacon's 'gentle' origins, to which he also alludes in *A Key to Helmont*, see G. D. Squibb (ed.), *The Visitation of Somerset and the City of Bristol 1672* (London, Harleian Soc., vol. 11, 1992), 88–9; TNA, PROB 11/400, fos 69v–71v [will of William Bacon, gent, of Maunsell, North Petherton, Somerset, 10 January 1687/8; pr. 1 July 1690].
126. Along with other royalist sympathizers, Bathurst, who diverted from the church to medicine while at Oxford in the 1650s, demonstrated an early interest in Helmontianism (above 74, 104 n.120). In 1653 he interrupted his studies in order to assist Daniel Whistler in treating sick and wounded sailors at Harwich and Ipswich; *CSPD, 1653–1654*, 104, 507; ESkRO, HD 36/A/213. Bathurst's signature, which is attached to the latter document authorizing payment to a surgeon at Ipswich, 25 September 1653, proves conclusively that it was Ralph and not John Bathurst (d.1659) who was serving on the medical staff on the east coast at this time. John French began his medical career as a physician treating the parliamentarian wounded at the Savoy Hospital in London in the 1640s. Rewarded with an Oxford MD in 1648, he subsequently devoted himself to translating the works of the continental chymists, Ercker, Agricola and Glauber, some of which were published in the following decade. He died in 1657 while serving as physician to the expeditionary forces in northern France. As a firm believer in the medical benefits of spa water, on which he published, he was one of the first to advocate their use in the treatment and recovery of wounded and maimed soldiers; *ODNB*; SUL, HP 28/2/42B. For the career of the Helmontian

Gurdon, who helped French pioneer the use of spa water treatment at the Savoy, see *CSPD, 1652–1653*, 307, 332 and above 52, 90 n.52.

127. For Dixon, see above 234 n.105. For Porter, see note 75 above. Pratt, who acted as mentor at Cambridge to the Helmontian Daniel Foote, served as an officer and physician to the parliamentary armies in the first civil war. While serving under Sir William Waller in 1644, Pratt's surgeon was court martialled for calling him a 'fool, ass and cox-comb' in a dispute over the bleeding of a patient; TNA, SP 28/35/III, fo. 380; J. Adair, 'The Court Martial Papers of Sir William Waller's Army', *Journal of the Society for Army Historical Research*, 44 (1966), 210–11 and Appendix 2 (a).
128. A former soldier, Moray later became one of the founder members of the Royal Society and a leading adviser to the crown on royal policy in Scotland. In the light of earlier discussion highlighting the eirenic associations of iatrochemistry, it may be significant that Moray's most recent biographer has suggested that his counsel to the king was 'marked by consistent and principled moderation'; *ODNB*, sub Moray, Sir Robert.
129. *CSPD, 1680–1681*, 566. Dudley, best known for his pioneering attempts to smelt iron ore with coal, was a seasoned soldier who had seen service in Scotland in 1640 and fought continuously for the royal cause until his capture at Worcester in 1651. Impoverished through his loyalty, he was forced to turn to the practice of medicine after the Restoration. Initially licensed by the bishop of Worcester, he eventually secured an archiepiscopal licence in 1679, mainly on the strength of a testimonial submitted by his close friend and fellow royalist Elias Ashmole, and countersigned by three high-ranking physicians, including the iatrochemist Edward Warner (for whom, see Appendix 1 (a)). Dudley was well known to Hartlib and possessed a millennial zeal for chymistry typical of the Hartlibians. In 1665, for example, he declared, in what may have been an allusion to the activities of the Helmontians at the court of Charles II, that God was 'about to reveal many of his secrets, unto his Israel in this latter Age'. He was also known to the Helmontian George Starkey. In October 1655 Starkey gave evidence to a court in Bristol in a case involving Dudley and a commercial dispute over rights to mining in the Forest of Dean; *ODNB*, sub Dudley, Dud [which makes no mention of the work of Charles Webster, nor refers to Dudley's later career as a physician]; Webster, *Great Instauration*, 394, 397, 399–401; LPL, CX 1A/10/126/1–3; Sancroft, fo.221; D. Dudley, *Metallum Martis* (London, 1665), unpaginated epistle dedicatory to Parliament; P. McGrath (ed.), *Merchants and Merchandise in Seventeenth-Century Bristol* (Bristol, Bristol Record Soc., vol. 19, 1955), 114–15.
130. Many of these letters were re-published in the works of later Helmontian physicians such as Christopher Packe. Other unpublished letters testify to the widespread interest in communicating this kind of information, including among physicians previously unconnected with iatrochemistry. Thus Benjamin White (1632–1713), who practised at Lewes in Sussex after the Restoration, wrote to the royal accoucheur Hugh Chamberlen the elder in 1674, providing details of preparations of pills, including Matthews' pill, and expressing the hope that the two men might continue a correspondence based on their mutual interest in such remedies; Wellcome Library, London, MS 7671/6 [White to Chamberlen the elder, 18 February 1673/4]. The chymical physician Samuel Haworth wrote approvingly of White's practice in 1683,

describing him as 'eminent... learned... ingenious... [and] a Person of excellent Skill and Success'; S. Haworth, *The True Method of Curing Consumptions* (London, 1683), 104–5, 114–15, 177. For White, a medical graduate of Leiden (1655), see Foster, iv, 1616; Innes Smith, 247.

131. A. Withey, 'Unhealthy Neglect? The Medicine and Medical Historiography of Early Modern Wales', *Social History of Medicine*, 21 (2008), 168. For a case study of the Monmouthshire yeoman, John Gwin, who was an avid reader of Helmontian literature, including the works of George Starkey, see *idem*, 'Medicine and Mortality in Early Modern Monmouthshire: The Commonplace Book of John Gwin', *Welsh History Review*, 23 (2006), 48–73.
132. Andrew Wear, for example, has claimed that 'Helmontian medicine... had largely disappeared from view' by the end of the seventeenth century, and that '[i]ts following was never very large'; Wear, *Knowledge and Practice in English Medicine*, 366. These conclusions are not borne out by my own research, which suggests that the thirty-five physicians who signed the chymists' petition in 1665 represented the tip of a very large iceberg.
133. J. Lamport, *A Direct Method of Ordering and Curing... the Smallpox* (London, 1685), 8–9, 10–11, 13; J. Yarwood, *Physick Refin'd: Or, A Little Stream of Medicinal Marrow, Flowing from the Bones of Nature* (London, 1683), 37, 58, 62, 66, 109. Lamport, who dated his conversion to Helmontianism to about 1665, was another chymist to receive official sanction through an episcopal medical licence, on this occasion granted by the bishop of Chichester. In the body of his book, he cites numerous examples of cures performed in the Portsmouth-Chichester area and advises prospective patients either to repair to his house at Havant or to visit one of his regular surgeries at the George Inn in Chichester and Half Moon in Petersfield. Like Thomson in 1665, he ends the work by issuing a challenge to his detractors to engage in a healing contest; Lamport, *Direct Method*, 16 and *passim*; WSxRO, Ep I/3/1, fos 18r (license to practice surgery, 1666), 23v (licence to practice medicine, 1672 or 1673). Yarwood, who was based at Shepshed in Leicestershire, conducted a surgery at nearby Loughborough on market days, where he dispensed free advice and medicines to the sick poor. Interestingly, both men recommended Matthews' pill which they affirmed was truly the invention of George Starkey; Lamport, *A Direct Method*, 10–11; Yarwood, *Physick Refin'd*, 17, 25.
134. C. Goodall, *The Colledge of Physicians Vindicated, and the True State of Physick in this Nation Faithfully Represented* (London, 1676). The work, which relied heavily on legal argument, was dedicated to Sir Francis North, Lord Chief Justice of the Common Pleas. In addition to the works of Huyberts and Hargrave (above), an anonymous group styling themselves 'the Chymists of London' published a new manifesto in 1676 aiming to rebut the calumnies issuing from the College of Physicians, 'being by them Publickly struck at, as men illiterate and insufficient for the Practice of Physick'; *The Principles of the Chymists of London Stated, with the Reasons of Their Dissent from the Colledge of Physicians; As They were Unanimously Agreed on by Them, at a Meeting in London... In Two Parts* (London?, 1676), A2v.
135. TNA, LC 3/26, fo. 58v. Goodall, who graduated MD at Leiden in 1670, had earlier demonstrated an avid interest in chymical nostrums such as Delaune's pill and a

'grand Arcanum' which cured epileptic, hysteric and convulsive fits when he wrote to Robert Boyle recommending their use and further investigation. He asked Boyle to respond by sending chymical receipts recently recommended by their Helmontian colleague, Daniel Coxe, in his book against the apothecaries; Boyle, *Correspondence*, iv, 118–24 [Goodall to Boyle, 29 November 1668]. Goodall himself was probably sympathetic to Dissent. For his friendship with fellow chymist and whig John Locke, see below 211–12.

136. Cook, *Decline of the Old Medical Regime*, 233; Bodl., Lister MS 35, fo. 89 [Tancred Robinson to Martin Lister, 15 March 1682/3]. Tyson (1651–1708) probably shared Goodall's whig and nonconformist proclivities. His father Edward was a loyal Cromwellian, who served as lord mayor of Bristol in 1659–60, and may have fought in Ireland in the early 1640s. In London, Tyson lived with his brother-in-law Richard Morton (1637–1698), a leading figure in dissenting circles who took up medicine after the Restoration following his ejection from the living of Kinver in Staffordshire; *ODNB*, sub Tyson, Edward, and Morton, Richard; M. F. Ashley Montagu, *Edward Tyson, MD, FRS, 1650–1708 and the Rise of Human and Comparative Anatomy in England* (Philadelphia, Memoirs of the American Philosophical Society, vol. 20, 1943), 5–10; Thurloe, *State Papers*, iv, 353, 379.

137. See, for example, A. Clericuzio, 'From Van Helmont to Boyle. A Study of the Transmission of Helmontian Chemical and Medical Theories in Seventeenth-Century England', *British Journal for the History of Science*, 16 (1993), 303–34.

5
Healers and Healing in the First Age of Party
Medicine, Politics and Dissent

Introduction

In 1674 Marchamont Nedham composed a final, spirited attempt to persuade the nobility, gentry, and magistracy of England to implement a thorough-going reform of the practice of medicine. Lamenting the earlier failure of the Society of Chymical Physicians, of which he had been an important and vocal member, Nedham added, in passing, an important observation about the significance of religious attachments among medical practitioners in an age of growing inter-denominational conflict. Of healers in general, he wrote:

> Some are for the Church of England, some for the Church of Rome, some for the Presbyterian; some for the Independent, some among the Baptised; some for the Fifth Monarchists; some for the Quakers; every man for himself, and God for all: And so the World is very luckily divided; every Party taking its own Proselyte to be the Ablest, and the most conscientious Doctor. Is this not a short Cut (think ye) to get Custom . . . after which, the few Men of no Party, whatever their Industry and Art be, are left to be turn'd to grass upon the cold Common of Integrity.[1]

Putting to one side any feelings of sympathy one might feel for Nedham, who, during a long career as a political journalist demonstrated a remarkable aptitude for trimming and shifts of allegiance, we ought, I feel, to take seriously the central tenet of his complaint, namely, that by the final quarter of the seventeenth-century medicine and healing had fallen prey to religious and political partisanship. If Nedham was right, then the decades following the Restoration must have witnessed an acceleration of that process of politicization among the practitioners of the healing arts which, I have argued earlier, originated with the breakdown of religious and political consensus in the early 1640s. In this and the following chapter, I seek to explore this process, which, I suggest, reached its apogee in the late 1670s and early 1680s and continued to shape the lives of healers for decades to come during the so-called 'age of party'. Broadly speaking, I suggest that it is

Medicine in an Age of Revolution. Peter Elmer, Oxford University Press. © Peter Elmer 2023.
DOI: 10.1093/oso/9780198853985.003.0005

possible to detect the creation of two embryonic, separate medical cultures, one associated with Dissent and the Whigs, the other steeped in Anglican conformism and support for the nascent Tory party. The former owed much to the politics of persecution, and the need for dissenting communities and individual nonconformists to negotiate the radically altered circumstances of life in post-Restoration Britain. Facing a form of social ostracism that left them excluded from the normal avenues of educational and vocational opportunity, many dissenters turned to the practice of medicine and related occupations. The attraction of a medical career was particularly strong for many of those ministers ejected after 1660, large numbers of whom proceeded to establish new ministries that combined pastoral care for the souls of their charges with concern for their physical well-being. This in turn produced what one might describe as a distinctively dissenting approach to specific medico-theological problems, particularly those relating to that traditionally grey area of practice concerned with psychosomatic illness, madness and witchcraft. Contemporaneous with these developments, it is equally possible to detect the emergence in this period of a distinctive Anglican-Tory approach to such issues, one which was diametrically opposed to that of their nonconformist colleagues. However, to understand the origin of these developments, which I discuss more fully in the next chapter, it is first necessary to explore how medicine and its practitioners succumbed to partisanship in the wake of the Restoration.

One of the more notable aspects of the politicization of the medical world in this period, and one shared by both groups, was the extent to which healers of all kinds, including learned practitioners with medical degrees and other qualifications, became increasingly involved in the day-to-day political life of their communities and the wider nation. This was manifest in a variety of ways. In the case of those who hailed from a dissenting or Whig background, there is ample evidence, for example, to demonstrate a willingness to engage in all aspects of religious and political debate, including in many cases a propensity to engage in plotting and other subversive activities against the Stuart regime. As I hope to show, this was no accident or coincidence as physicians and surgeons were inherently well placed to use their medical function to engage in political activism and espionage. In the case of nonconformist medical practitioners, there was the additional stimulus provided by the tendency of many to seek a medical education and qualifications abroad, particularly in the medical schools of Holland, where they freely associated with, and were often supported by, fellow émigrés, political refugees, and co-religionists who had fled persecution in Britain. At the same time, their Anglican and Tory competitors within the medical profession were equally inclined to engage in various aspects of popular politics, either as propagandists for the cause, or, more commonly, as elected officeholders in the towns and cities of England. The second half of the seventeenth century witnessed an influx of medics into the corporate boroughs, both as aldermen and mayors, who used their magisterial powers not simply to purge the miniature body politics of their malignant humours, but also to consolidate their own medical authority and status in what was becoming an increasingly competitive marketplace (discussed more fully in the following chapter). Against this background, then, it is perhaps not too far-fetched to claim that Nedham had a point when he depicted the medical scene in the mid-1670s as riven by religious and political divisions. Indeed, it is the conclusion of this and the following chapter that by the end of the seventeenth and beginning of the eighteenth centuries, and with the onset of party politics and the 'rage of party', it was impossible for those engaged in healing to escape the politicized nature of their calling.

Medical Practitioners on the Margins: Catholics, Baptists and Quakers

Prior to the English civil war, it is probably safe to assume that religious affiliation was largely immaterial for a patient choosing a medical practitioner, particularly among those who subscribed to some version of Protestant belief. The exception may have been the small minority of Catholics who continued to adhere to the old faith, and for whom there were certain advantages in choosing a doctor who shared the same religious beliefs. This was especially true of wealthy Catholic families, who were not only more likely to be able to afford the services of the numerous Catholic physicians who lived in and around London but were also tempted to do so in order to secure medical certificates at politically sensitive moments. Throughout the seventeenth century, for example, prominent Catholic laymen frequently resorted to such measures so as to allow them to travel to the continent for 'health reasons'. Prior to 1640, the government tended to turn a blind eye to these activities, and issued passes for Catholic families to attend continental spas. Occasionally, however, the government did clamp down on popular Catholicism and associated medical rituals, as for example in 1626 when the Privy Council ordered Sergeant Bridgeman, Chief Justice of Chester, to 'prevent the resort of persons ill affected in religion' to St Winifred's well at Holywell in Flintshire. In an attempt to suppress this revered site of healing, local freeholders who lodged Catholic visitors to the wells were bound over by the local justices. The tactic does not appear to have been hugely successful. A decade later, the government was forced to issue further guidelines aimed at preventing such 'pilgrimages'.[2]

These measures were largely half-hearted, however, and evidently were not a great success. More vociferous criticism of Catholic physicians is discernible at grass roots level. In 1624, for example, the Anglican minister John Gee voiced what was probably a common fear among many fellow Protestants when he hinted darkly at the role played by Jesuit priests masquerading as medical doctors.

Having gone to the trouble of compiling a list of Catholic physicians operating in London at this time, he went on to suggest that many were covertly engaged in undercover activity including the oversight of death-bed conversions:

> Whether these, or any of them be allowed by the approbation and authority of the Colledge of Physicians, I know not. But sure it is, that those that take their degrees publiquely in Popish Universities beyond the seas, doe take a solemne oath of obedience to the Pope. And it is vehemently suspected, that some of these have a private facultie and power from the See of Rome, to exercise the authority of Romish Priests in reconciling or absolving their patients, *in articulo mentis*, upon point of death or great danger.[3]

Many of those listed by Gee were able to practise with impunity because they were able to call on the patronage of powerful figures at court. They were also afforded a modicum of protection by their membership of the London College of Physicians, which in the pre–civil war period was a religiously diverse body that paid little attention to individual member's religious predilections. Outside London, of course, Catholic patients, particularly those of low social rank, were often unable to access Catholic doctors. In many instances, moreover, they appeared reluctant or disinclined to make the effort. The casebook of the puritan physician John Hall of Stratford, for example, contains numerous references to Catholic patients, and would appear to substantiate the claim of one of his later editors, the Presbyterian John Bird, that even those who 'hated him for his Religion, often made use of him'.[4] The same was probably true of his puritan colleague John Bastwick (d.1654), who was consulted at Colchester in the 1630s by the local Catholic grandee, Elizabeth Strange, Countess of Rivers.[5] Religious divisions in England prior to the civil war clearly ran deep, but they do not seem to have unduly affected doctor-patient relations. Even in the years immediately prior to the outbreak of hostilities, puritan physicians continued to minister to Anglican clerics, despite wholeheartedly deploring their support for the recent ceremonial innovations and 'superstitions'. The Essex physician, Dr Ady, for example, admonished the Laudian incumbent of Wickham St Paul, Timothy Clay, to leave off his heavy drinking for fear it would send him 'starke mad'.[6]

With the onset of civil war, and the accompanying religious fragmentation that characterized the years after 1640, patients and medical practitioners increasingly gravitated toward co-religionists in seeking or proffering medical advice and assistance. A case in point is suggested by the treatment that the celebrated puritan martyr and physician John Bastwick experienced on his return to London in the early 1640s. Expelled from the London College of Physicians in 1635, he was restored to his fellowship in December 1640 following his triumphal return to the capital from exile on the Channel Islands. His intention was to resume his medical career, but in a work written in 1645 he writes despairingly of the efforts of 'some

Independent doctors and others' to vilify him and undermine his professional reputation.[7] It seems safe to assume that Bastwick's experience was not unique. As we saw in chapter 3, medical success in the 1640s and 1650s largely hinged upon religious and political loyalties. For the emerging sects of this period, whose radicalism largely excluded its members from social and political privileges, there was a tendency to create networks of mutual self-help that increasingly functioned in isolation from mainstream society. This was particularly evident, for example, in the case of the Baptists and Quakers, who often developed their own 'systems' of medical support and advice that were serviced by suitably qualified members of the sect. In the case of the Baptists, the tendency to seek out fellow members for medical relief was probably intensified by the unique approach that many of its early leaders took to conventional medicine and forms of therapeutic intervention. Typical was Hanserd Knollys (1598–1691), who claimed in his autobiography to have dispensed altogether with natural remedies and physic, relying instead on the power of fasting, prayer and anointment by oil.[8] Others, such as the Baptist prophet John Mowlin of Sandwich in Kent, claimed to have received a commission from God to cure the sick and blind. To their opponents, of course, such feats of miraculous healing were deeply suspect. The Presbyterian apologist William Prynne (1660–1669) was convinced that these so-called acts of healing or exorcisms were not only counterfeit but were laid as a trap to make converts to the sectarian cause. Alarmed by the 'dispossessions' carried out by the Baptist preacher, Paul Hobson, Prynne likened such activities to those of the Jesuits, who, as we have already seen, were widely suspected of using medical practice as a cover to make new converts to the old faith.[9]

Once established, the Baptists created their own networks of medical support across the country. The career of apothecary proved particularly helpful in this respect. The example of the London apothecary Jonathan Leigh (d.1717) provides an illuminating example. After serving an apprenticeship in the capital, Leigh was made a freeman of the city in 1671. In the same year, he married Mary Fidsall, the daughter of Samuel Fidsall (d.1668), a Wiltshire clothier, part of whose house was used and subsequently licensed for Baptist worship in 1672. Leigh subsequently took on fourteen apprentices, four of whom were undoubtedly attracted to enrol under Leigh on account of their shared religious and radical backgrounds.[10] Leigh's first apprentice, Thomas Forty, for example, was the son of the Baptist preacher and saddlemaker Henry Forty (d.1693) who ministered to congregations at Totnes in Devon and Abingdon in Berkshire before settling in Southwark. In the year before his son's indentures were signed, Forty was arrested with his wife and children in Exeter where he was accused of being 'a scismaticall person' and was gaoled for refusing to take the Oath of Allegiance. Forty's son Henry, who himself set up as an apothecary in the capital, was one of the principal medical witnesses to attest to the miraculous cures performed by the maid Susanna Arch in 1695.[11] Leigh's other three apprentices—Joseph Batt, Jonathan Gladman and

Samuel Hyde—shared similar radical backgrounds. Batt was the son of Timothy Batt (1613–1692), a leading figure among London Baptists in the early 1640s when he also practised medicine in the capital. He subsequently succumbed to moderation and was ejected from a Somerset living in 1660, though he continued to preach among the dissenters in his native Somerset until his death in 1692.[12] Jonathan Gladman was the son of the radical conspirator John Gladman (d.1688) who narrowly managed to escape with his life in the aftermath of the Rye House Plot.[13] Finally, Samuel Hyde was the son of the Exeter bookseller Michael Hyde (d.1697) who was suspected of selling seditious pamphlets in the city in 1688.[14]

Post-Restoration London, of course, possessed a special allure for wealthy or upwardly mobile dissenters seeking alternative careers for their sons who might otherwise have entered the church or the law. The trade of apothecary was high on that list. As we shall see, large numbers of ejected clergymen also chose this route for their sons after 1660 (see below 190). Provincial practice, however, offered similar advantages, both material and political. In the case of the Baptists, many found the trade of an apothecary congenial to the promotion of their religious and political values. Philip Cary (1637–1705), apothecary, of Dartmouth in Devon, for example, became involved in a heated dispute with fellow nonconformist Richard Burthogge (for whom, see below 212) following a consultation over a gentleman patient. He later published a defence of infant baptism which sparked another debate with the local Presbyterian John Flavell (d.1691) who described Cary as 'the principal Anabaptist in Dartmouth'.[15] Christopher Price (d.1697), who practised as an apothecary in Abergavenny, Monmouthshire, was a leading figure in the Welsh Baptist movement.[16] And elsewhere, Baptists who had briefly enjoyed corporate office during the Interregnum continued to utilize networks of co-religionists to navigate the travails of life in post-Restoration England. Richard Coleman (d.1685), a Leicester apothecary, for example, who was first appointed as a common councilman in the town in 1642 and briefly served as an alderman in 1661, was the earliest known leader of the Particular Baptist movement in the east Midlands town. There, he was able to establish a dynasty of apothecaries that helped to keep alive the flame of Dissent despite the fact that he and his three sons faced constant persecution both in the church courts and at the hands of local magistrates.[17] Evidence of inter-denominational cooperation in Leicester, as suggested by the visit and reception in 1672 of John Bunyan to the town where he was hosted by Richard Coleman,[18] was also evident in the recruitment of new apprentices to the trade. In 1689, for example, Samuel Statham (1672–1732), the son of the ejected London lecturer Samuel Statham Snr (d.1685), was apprenticed to Josiah Coleman (1654–1704), apothecary, of Leicester, the Baptist son of Richard (above). Two years into his apprenticeship, Statham, a Presbyterian by background, and Coleman entered into a business venture whereby the former set up an apothecary shop in his native Loughborough and agreed to split the profits with his master.[19]

Unfortunately, we know little about how medical networks among families like the Colemans of Leicester impacted upon the day-to-day activity of fellow Baptists. Given the fact that so many provincial apothecaries also engaged in general practice, we can safely assume that they travelled widely among neighbouring congregations. Doctors embedded in Baptist communities were well respected, both for their medical expertise and commitment to upholding the values of the sect in the face of persecution. A remarkable example of the close ties that often prevailed between Baptist practitioners and preachers is evident in the forty-year relationship that connected the physician John Roberts (d.1704) and his spiritual mentor and guide Benjamin Keach (1640–1674). Roberts, a member of Keach's congregation at Aylesbury in Buckinghamshire, was reputed to have perfected 'two excellent medicines' the recipes for which he promised to teach Keach's daughter in return for a small allowance for life 'which he performed to the full satisfaction of them both'.[20] Medical self-help was probably the order of the day which in turn encouraged specific families to engage in the cultivation of medical knowledge. The creation of medical dynasties was, of course, a common feature of the world of early modern medicine. Other examples drawn from the annals of the early Baptists, such as the Okeys, also hint at the wide range of opportunities for career progression in medicine in the late seventeenth and early eighteenth centuries. Thomas Okey, the son of the Baptist preacher Thomas Okey Snr (1623–1684), began life as an apothecary in Devizes in Wiltshire but had moved to the parish of St Botolph Aldgate in London by the 1690s where, according to his son, he set up as a 'professor of medicine'.[21] There, two sons John and Thomas (who called himself Thomas Tertius) trained as surgeons. John entered naval service; he was court martialled in 1696 for speaking 'treasonable words' aboard the 'Assistance'. Thomas Tertius fared better. Like his brother John, he began life as a naval surgeon, but following a route common among dissenters, he chose to upgrade from surgeon to physician by travelling overseas to graduate MD at Harderwyck in the United Provinces in 1704.[22] Baptist medical practitioners, like their more moderate brethren among the ranks of the nonconformists, were thus able to establish successful careers in medicine despite the various obstacles posed by hostile lawmakers and defenders of the Anglican Church after 1660. And for the favoured few, a licence from the College of Physicians was not out of the question. John Feake (1676), John Griffith (1670) and Nathaniel Whitehill (1694) were all recipients of the College's largesse.[23]

Despite the tendency then of many early Baptists to shun orthodox medicine and medical practitioners, as congregations became established, so they also became more open to the benefits of natural cures and the usefulness of medical specialists. This is particularly evident from the fact that ministers frequently doubled up as physicians in the service of their congregations. Among those Baptist leaders and preachers who combined pastoral care with a career in medicine were Elias Clarke, John Clarke,[24] Nehemiah Cox (for whom, see below ???), William Crabbe,[25] Charles Maria Duveil,[26] Daniel Fabius,[27] Richard Farmer,[28] Roger Grant,[29] Paul Hobson (below, ???), Philip James,[30] Robert Joney or Jony,[31] Edward Ridgway,[32] John Skinner,[33] Edward Stennett,[34] John Symonds[35] and Joseph Wright.[36] One might speculatively add to this list James Wilmot (1623–1682), pastor of a Baptist congregation at Hook Norton in Oxfordshire. According to the clergyman cum physician John Ward of Stratford-upon-Avon, one Wilmot of Hook Norton claimed to cure the King's evil by blowing a white powder into the eyes of children.[37]

Many of these men were well known to each other and they often cooperated in supporting the education and training of the next generation of Baptist medical practitioners. At the same time, they also, on occasions, collaborated with their dissenter brethren, putting aside doctrinal and other differences to provide medical care to all those suffering persecution. Doctor John Griffin or Griffith (d.1698) of Bristol, a member of the large Baptist congregation that met at Broadmead, thus signed a joint letter with two congregationalist physicians (William Turgis and Ichabod Chauncey) and a Quaker doctor (Thomas Bourne) appealing to local magistrates to improve the unhygienic conditions then prevailing in the city's gaols.[38] The need to work in this way, in a spirit of ecumenicism, became particularly acute after 1660 and the onset of legal persecution and harassment.

Moreover, like their counterparts in more mainstream dissenting circles, Baptist medics were more than willing to utilize the ecclesiastical licensing system to legitimate their practices. Among those who chose this route were Conyers Congrave, William Crabbe, Roger Grant, George Smith and Samuel Taverner.[39] In order to navigate a system that was inherently biased against nonconformists it was essential to have friends in all the right places. The case of Timothy Boyce, who applied for an archiepiscopal licence to practise medicine in several dioceses in central and eastern England in 1679, is illuminating in this respect. His chief sponsor, a Somerset cleric named Thomas Rawbon (d.1692), attested to Boyce's 'loyalty' and appended the signatures of a local minister and two schoolmasters. On the surface at least, there was little reason to suspect the candidate's credentials. Boyce, however, was a Baptist who had initially trained for thirteen years under Dr Elias Clarke at Wantage and had only recently transferred to Daventry, where he seems to have sheltered under the patronage of another Baptist physician Manasseh King (1652–1696). Both Clarke and King provided testimonials and Boyce was duly licensed.[40] Boyce's case is also revealing as it would appear to corroborate the suggestion, made in the previous chapter, of a close link between radical sectarianism and support for iatrochemical forms of cure. According to Rawbon, who was related to Clarke by marriage, the Baptist patriarch of Wantage first employed Boyce as an 'operator in chymistry'. Other Baptists who were attracted to chymical medicine as an alternative to traditional Galenic therapies included the barber surgeon Paul Hobson (along with his radical associates

Ahaseurus Fromanteel and George Kendall), George Jones, William Russell, Thomas Emes and Robert Johnson.

Paul Hobson (1616–1665) was in fact a barber surgeon who advocated the use of natural remedies, becoming a staunch proponent of the benefits of chymically prepared medicines and pills. In the early 1660s, he entered into a partnership with Richard Matthews, whose celebrated pill he sold, and may well have frequented the iatrochemical clubs that proliferated in the capital at this time, many of whose members shared Hobson's heterodox religious opinions.[41] George Jones (d.1676 or 1677), a member of the Baptist congregation that met at Glasshouse Yard, was another who prospered in London through the sale of patent medicines and pills, which were widely advertised in the press. Inevitably, Jones soon fell into dispute with fellow empirics and pillmongers, and a series of broadsides followed in which it is evident that religious tensions (two of his competitors were decried as Quakers) partly underlay the competition for customers and patients.[42] Following his death, Jones' widow Elizabeth married another empiric and chymical physician, John Russell (d.1697) of Holborn, who inherited Jones' London practice.[43] William Russell (d.1702), who was a member of the same Baptist congregation as Jones but seemingly no relation of John Russell, had previously studied medicine at Leiden before acquiring a Cambridge MD by royal mandate in 1688. He too was a passionate advocate of the merits of medicines made by 'Philosophers by Fire' and in 1693 wrote a letter calling for the reform of the medical profession along iatrochemical lines.[44] The surgeon Thomas Emes (d.1707), who later converted to the French Prophets and predicted his own resurrection, was likewise a keen chymist who published two works defending the medicinal virtues of alkaline medicines.[45] Finally Johnson (1640–1706 or 1707) was the author of a medical manual in which he singled out, among others, 'the most famous Helmont' as one of his prime sources of inspiration. He also subscribed to the much-anticipated English edition of Glauber's *Works*. A decade later, he recommended Glauber's *sal miravile* as 'an excellent Lenitive Cathartick'. Johnson was a member of the Baptist congregation of Robert Jemmett (d.1718) which met at Dunning's Alley in Bishopsgate Street. He was also on friendly terms with the celebrated 'empiric' William Salmon; in 1693, he took as apprentice Salmon's stepson, Thomas Herbert, the son of the wealthy Baptist merchant Edward Herbert, with the intention of training him up as a man midwife.[46]

A fondness for the iatrochemical principles of Paracelsus and van Helmont, as I have argued elsewhere,[47] was also a distinguishing feature of the approach of Quaker physicians to the care of the sick. In the case of the early Society of Friends, this was coupled with a growing awareness of the benefits of medical self-help and recourse to medical practitioners who were either fellow Quakers or Quaker sympathizers. By the early years of the Restoration, it seems clear that Friends had forged their own networks of medical practice, often examining potential candidates for their fitness not only as general members but also as potential doctors.[48] The Bristol Quaker Charles Marshall (1637–1698), a prolific author of pamphlets defending the sect, published numerous broadsides aimed at promoting the use of his iatrochemical remedies among his co-religionists. Compared by his wife to the apostle Luke, who 'was both evangelist and physician', he also wrote to fellow Quakers across the country, offering them a combination of spiritual and medical counsel, as, for example, in his advice to the Buckinghamshire meeting in 1689 to avoid 'superfluities in meats or in drink'.[49] Likewise, the German-born iatrochemist Albertus Otto Faber practised mainly among the Quakers, whom he joined in London in the early 1660s. His chymical medicines were sold by a network of Friends in places as distant as Norfolk and Lincolnshire. By 1668 Faber's success among local Quakers precipitated a professional conflict with a rival Quaker physician in Lincolnshire which proved irreconcilable. Shortly after, Faber left the sect, or was 'denied' by them, and began to establish a more broadly based practice in London where his patients included Gilbert Sheldon, the archbishop of Canterbury.[50] Fallings out of this kind were seemingly quite common in the early annals of the Friends. In the same year of Faber's fall from grace, the Quaker physician Dr Gray was attacked in print by the Quaker apostate and fellow practitioner, Nathaniel Smith, in a dispute ostensibly concerned with religion but one that bears all the hallmarks of a medical turf war. Smith initiated the controversy by affirming that Gray had falsely claimed to have discovered the secrets of medicine through divine revelation while in prison. On his release, he subsequently boasted of his ability to cure all diseases 'for which he was much esteem'd of all Friends'. The truth, however, according to Smith was very different, for 'this God of his, was an old Gentle-woman in Islington, Mistriss Slack by name, who... he counted for no better than a devil, when she Su'd him for her bargain... and made him pay for his Revelations, as also for his Doctorship, which he learn'd of her'.[51] The Quakers not unnaturally responded in kind, defending Dr Gray from Smith's aspersions, and asserting instead that it was Smith who was the real charlatan, whose gift of healing, if genuine, was diabolical in origin.[52]

The success of doctors like Faber and Smith among the Quakers, and their subsequent rejection, illustrates one of the dangers faced by medical practitioners in allying too closely with any single religious group or sect. It also led to disputes with medics of other denominations, many of whom were only too happy to undermine their competitor's practices by colluding with the authorities in the persecution of their rivals. Some merely spread rumours about the ineffectiveness of their medicines, as, for example, in 1664, when a Norfolk Friend wrote to Faber recounting how 'several doctors tell the people his medicine will do them more harm than good'.[53] Others, however, were more vindictive. Another supplier of Faber's remedies, Robert Preston, was, according to one of Faber's local supporters and informants in Lincolnshire, imprisoned in 1665 as a 'disaffected person' due to 'the self-endedness of some Phisitians or Apothecaries'.[54] Similar motives almost certainly lay behind the incarceration of the Quaker physician John

Raunce at High Wycombe in 1671. His imprisonment under the terms of the second Conventicle Act of 1670 was instigated by the mayor of the town, Martin Llewellyn (1616–1682), a local physician and Anglican loyalist, who was almost certainly jealous of Raunce's medical standing in the town.[55]

The Emergence of a Dissenting Medical Tradition in Restoration England

The Quakers' tendency to remove themselves from mainstream society and develop their own networks of medical services and personnel represents an extreme position, albeit one that was increasingly fostered by more moderate groups of religious dissenters after 1660 and the imposition of the Clarendon Code. Clergymen of an eirenic spirit, such as Robert Gell (1595–1665), might try to point out the futility of religious divisions by suggesting that no sick man, in his right mind, would reject a sovereign remedy without first enquiring of the healer of 'whose church he were, and what his judgement was concerning predestination, election and reprobation'.[56] But in the land at large, patients were beginning to make such judgements, no doubt encouraged in many cases by a sense of moral outrage and loathing for those Anglican conformists who both upheld, and engaged in, the persecution of 'innocent' nonconformists. In time, such thinking bred a growing sense of injustice and a firm belief that God was on the side of the persecuted. Given that health was widely perceived as God-given, and sickness as the fruit of sin, it is not surprising that many dissenters in the early years of the Restoration began to see the divine hand at work in the various distempers and afflictions that beset their opponents, as well as interpreting their own immunity to disease as evidence of divine approbation. The Quakers were certainly not alone in collecting case histories of persecutors who met fitting ends, many of which involved unpleasant and anti-social diseases such as the pox or plague. Such stories formed part of dissenting culture generally in the years after 1660 and were as likely to be promoted by Presbyterians and Congregationalists as they were by Quakers and Baptists. Equally popular were accounts predicated upon the idea that the true servants of God were afforded divine protection from the worst diseases and afflictions, which were intended as a warning to their persecutors. The Quaker apostate Nathaniel Smith, for example, claimed that the Friends, both in London and Lancaster, boasted of their immunity from the plague, as did the notorious plotter, Colonel Thomas Blood, who argued that his own preservation from the pestilence was a sign of divine approval for his subversive activities against the restored regime.[57]

The firmest evidence, however, for a dissenting medical tradition lies in the extent to which former puritans, and their offspring, were attracted to a career in medicine and related occupations after 1660—a trend that is most manifest among the ranks of those puritan clergymen who were either ejected by the Anglican authorities or were unable, in conscience, to conform to the doctrines and rituals of the restored Church.[58] Citing A. G. Matthews' preface to his revised edition of Edmund Calamy's *Account* of the ministers ousted between 1660 and 1662, Birken suggests that fifty-nine of these men subsequently took up medical practice, many of whom went on to secure some form of medical degree or qualification. Birken also suggests that medicine was a popular career option for the sons of ejected and dissenting ministers, listing thirty-eight examples of this trend. My own survey of these two distinct groups suggests that these figures represent an under-reporting of the actual numbers. A fairer approximation of the numbers in the first category is closer to one hundred, and in the latter seventy-six, though in both cases I suspect that these figures, too, represent under-estimates. One might also wish to include a third category here, the sons of prominent radical or godly families, many of whom had played a prominent role in the political events preceding the Restoration.[59] In what follows, I wish to enquire what we might learn from closer study of these men, and their religious, political and medical careers. In particular, I wish to investigate how nonconformists interacted to create a distinctive dissenting tradition in medicine in the years after 1660, one which was increasingly, if subtly, at odds with the prevailing medical culture of their High Church opponents.

My starting point here is those former ministers who combined preaching with medicine, since such men were regularly on the front line in the conflict with those agencies of the state that were intent on imposing religious uniformity. There can be little doubt that the majority of Calamy's ejected who did practise medicine after 1660 did so while simultaneously ministering to the pastoral needs of their beleaguered and scattered congregations. Over a third of my sample, for example, were to avail themselves of the opportunity to legitimate their ministries by taken out a licence under the terms of the Declaration of Indulgence in 1672. Many others—the vast majority—clearly combined medical and religious functions. Typical, perhaps, was John Bulkley (1619–1690), who, following his ejection from the rectory of Fordham in Essex in 1660, moved to Wapping where, according to Calamy, he administered 'natural and spiritual physick together... And seldom did he visit his Patients, without reading a Lecture of Divinity to them, and praying with them'.[60] Others such as the west-country minister Samuel Stoddon (d.1714) reflected these new arrangements when he described himself in one of his publications as 'medico-theologus'.[61] Given what we have previously observed about pre-civil war puritan misgivings in relation to clergymen who combined the practice of medicine with ministerial duties, the influx of former ministers into the medical profession marked a significant break with tradition. How individuals reconciled their consciences with such practices is not easily determined. To some extent, the argument of necessity, combined with the fact that many of my sample, according to Calamy, practised for free (at least among the poor), may have smoothed the way for such a transition. For the majority, however, one suspects that this radical departure from orthodoxy was justified by the need to be both active and useful in a world that was increasingly hostile to the place of dissenters, especially their leaders, in society. It may also reflect a growing aversion after 1660 toward doctrinal debate as ministers turned instead to focus on the practical, everyday concerns of their beleaguered congregations. The provision of medical services, in this respect, provided one obvious outlet for such men to consolidate their authority among fellow dissenters, as well as an invaluable opportunity to proselytize in their local communities.

Despite Nedham's statement at the beginning of this chapter intimating that the art of healing in Restoration England had succumbed, irrevocably, to the forces of religious partisanship, medicine and acts of healing could also provide a valuable opportunity for men and women of opposing views to bridge the confessional divide.[62] Calamy notes, for example, how on a number of occasions former ministers escaped persecution by ministering to the needs of neighbouring gentry and local justices of the peace. Edward Warren (d.1690), ejected at Colchester in 1662, was said to have 'carry'd himself so affably and courteously to all, that he was generally belov'd... even [among] those who hated him on Account of his Preaching as a Nonconformist, yet lov'd him for the sake of their Bodies'.[63] Likewise Giles Firmin (d.1697), the founder of a dynasty of nonconformist medical practitioners, avoided persecution for illegal preaching because of the 'Favour and Respect [of] the Neighbouring Gentry and Justices of the Peace... on account of their using him as a Physician'.[64] Others cultivated good relations with conformist laymen and clergy, many of whom were themselves ambivalent about the methods used to impose uniformity in church and state. Some of the latter, moreover, clearly colluded with dissenting ministers in promoting their clerical and medical functions. Richard Perrot (d.1671), for example, whom Calamy described as practising physic 'with good Success' after 1660, probably owed much to the support and encouragement that he received from the Yorkshire minister Matthew Robinson (1628–1694), with whom he lived for some time in the 1660s. Robinson, whose sympathy to nonconformists extended to allowing them to preach in his pulpit at Burneston, also practised medicine, his first love, and was prosecuted for the same in 1676 alongside fellow ministers of both the Anglican and dissenting persuasion.[65]

Despite these cross-denominational examples of cooperation and mutual support, it probably remains the case, however, that the principal source of patients for dissenting clergymen-cum-physicians consisted of their fellow co-religionists. In attending to both the physical and spiritual needs of their new congregations, some of these ministers were undoubtedly able to console and affirm waverers in the face of the constant threat of persecution. At the same time, especially where they practised among the poor without seeking payment, many clearly hoped to make further converts to the dissenting cause. Such attempts at proselytizing probably account for the glowing reputations of men like Luke Cranwell (d.1683), the former minister at Derby, who, according to one of his patients, the future astronomer royal John Flamsteed (1646–1719), was 'cried up for cures by the Nonconformist party' in the north Midlands.[66] In certain areas, particularly those where learned physicians were thin on the ground, it is possible that the co-ordinated activities of some energetic dissenting ministers led to their dominating the local medical marketplace. Something akin to this phenomenon seems to have prevailed in and around Newcastle-upon-Tyne, where Richard Gilpin (1625–1700) and his circle of fellow ministers combined an active ministry with the provision of an impressive network of medical services in and around the town. In many respects, Gilpin's life, and his subsequent entry into the medical profession, typified the career profile of those dissenting ministers-cum-physicians who proliferated in England after the Restoration. Eager to promote union among the various 'puritan' factions in the 1650s (he was instrumental in promoting the association movement in his native Cumberland), he might easily have attained a position of prominence in the restored Church, being mooted as a future bishop of Carlisle in some quarters. Unconcerned with the niceties of ecclesiastical governance, he refused to conform and devoted his life instead to pastoral duties and promoting the well-being, both medical and spiritual, of his poor neighbours and fellow dissenters. During the early 1660s, he established leadership over a 'congregation of saints' in Newcastle that met, most appropriately in the context of the present discussion, in the town's barber-surgeons' hall. Here he continued to preach despite the passage of the Five Mile Act, the provisions of which he managed to avoid owing to the intervention of a well-connected friend and fellow nonconformist, Ambrose Barnes, who persuaded local magistrates to turn a blind eye to Gilpin's activities on account of his usefulness as a doctor. By 1668, however, the success of his preaching—on one occasion it was estimated that over 500 people had attended one of his meetings at the barber surgeons' hall—once again led to fears among some members of the town's ruling body that his activities bordered on the subversive. In order, perhaps, to legitimate his career as an established physician, in 1676 he followed the example of many of his fellow ministers by travelling to Leiden in Holland, where he was awarded his MD. On his return, he continued to dominate dissenting politics in the town, and together with neighbouring ministers-turned-physicians, provided one of the chief sources of medical assistance to the people of Newcastle and the surrounding countryside.[67] Among his assistants in the town were John Pringle (d.1692) and William Pell (d.1698), both of whom had been ousted from their livings in the early 1660s and had subsequently taken up the practice of medicine.[68] It was probably no coincidence that another of Gilpin's colleagues, William Durant (d.1683), removed as town lecturer at the Restoration, sent his son John to Leiden in 1669 from whence he graduated MD two years later.[69] Others who fell into this category included Patrick Bromfield, John Lomax

(1635–1693) and Gilbert Rule Snr (d.1701), who all lived close by in the county of Northumberland.[70] Just as importantly, however, Gilpin was careful to ensure that the next generation of dissenting ministers in the town was made in the same mould. His protégé and chosen successor, Timothy Manlove (1663–1699), thus followed in the same footsteps as Gilpin, combining pastoral duties at Durham, Pontefract and Leeds with a burgeoning medical career. In the event, Manlove, who succeeded Pell as Gilpin's assistant at Newcastle in 1699, died after just a few months, closely followed by his mentor the following year, thus bringing to a close almost forty years of devoted ministerial and medical service to the dissenting communities of the north-east.[71]

One of the features of this group of physicians, as Birken has noted, lay in the exceptional extent to which they sought medical qualifications or official approval for their careers as healers. A few, as he remarks, had 'the good sense and fortune to take Cambridge medical degrees in the interregnum'. For the vast majority, however, who wished to legitimate their practice with a university degree the chief destinations were the medical schools of Holland, especially Leiden and Utrecht.[72] For the rest, there were two main sources of official recognition: licences granted by the College of Physicians in London and those issued by the restored ecclesiastical authorities. We have already touched upon the former in relation to what I have perceived as an Anglican distrust of the puritanical leanings of the College and its leadership in the early years of the Restoration (see chapter 4 above). There is little to add here to what Birken has already noted of the role played by the College in this respect. His observation that the peak of support for dissenting ministers coincided with the 1660s, when 'the plight of the ejected was at its worst', seems irrefutable. Equally revealing is the example he quotes of John Hutchinson, who was granted a licence by the College when Dr John Micklethwaite (1612–1683), a former puritan, was censor.[73] Other examples include Ichabod Chauncy and Edward Warren, who were made extra-licentiates in 1666 and 1667, respectively, in both cases following examinations by a committee of members all of whom were known dissenters or sympathetic to dissent (Sir Edward Alston, the President, George Ent, William Staines and John Micklethwaite).[74] On the question of the extent to which ejected ministers and other dissenters managed to obtain episcopal licences, Birken may have underestimated the guile, flexibility and, in some cases, insincerity bordering on duplicity, exhibited by some members of the nonconformist community in gaining such grants. At least thirteen, possibly fourteen, former ministers managed to evade the ecclesiastical authorities in this way, half securing their licences before or shortly after ejection, that is at a time when the licensing bodies may have been least inclined or prepared to impose the new oaths required. Robert Law (d.1685 or 1686), for example, who was licensed in the diocese of Exeter in January 1662, was able to count on the testimonials of two other ministers, both of whom were also ejected later that year.[75] Others employed more crafty subterfuges.

Bartholomew Westley (d.1671), ejected from the curacy of Bridport, Dorset, in November 1662, claimed in his application to have lost his licence in the late wars while fighting for the King. A leading royalist in the neighbourhood, however, described him as 'a rigid, foolish Presbyterian', and there were widespread rumours that Westley had boasted locally of having almost captured the King at Charmouth when he tried to flee the country following the battle of Worcester.[76]

Ejected ministers who turned to the practice of physic after 1660 also played a prominent role, alongside other dissenting physicians, in writing testimonials for those seeking episcopal licences. Ichabod and Isaac Chauncy,[77] Lewis du Moulin,[78] Edward Hulse,[79] Richard Morton,[80] Henry Sampson[81] and Samuel Stoddon[82] all submitted testimonials on behalf of fellow co-religionists and aspiring physicians. There can be little doubt that many of these men, eminent figures in their respective communities, performed a vital role in both encouraging and supporting the medical studies and future careers of a new generation of nonconformist doctors. This is strongly suggested, for example, in the case of those who went abroad to study medicine and frequently expressed thanks to their mentors in the dedications that they attached to their published theses. Henry Sampson (1629–1700) was the subject of at least four such dedications, two of which were penned by students graduating in medicine from his own *alma mater*, Leiden, and all of whom would appear to have been brought up in nonconformist households.[83] Others singled out for similar encomiums included William Floyde,[84] Edward Richardson[85] and Edward Hulse (1638–1711). Hulse in many ways typifies the role played by those doctors who lost their livings or university fellowships at the Restoration in supporting and promoting networks of medical assistance in England thereafter. Forced to quit his fellowship at Emmanuel College, Cambridge, in 1662, Hulse too opted to take a medical degree at Leiden which he dedicated to a number of prominent Suffolk dissenters including Nathaniel Barnardiston and Thomas Bacon. His MD was subsequently incorporated at Oxford in 1670 in honour of the visit of his patron, William, Prince of Orange, and he was made a fellow of the College of Physicians in 1677, acting as censor five years later.[86] He was thus in a strong position to support nonconformist medical practitioners seeking to legitimate their practices through the acquisition of degrees and licences, and the latter reciprocated by, among other things, dedicating their published theses to him. Hulse developed strong bonds with two such medical graduates, Joshua Palmer (*c.*1658–1708) and his nephew William Palmer (*c.*1675–1713), who were awarded their MDs at Leiden in 1682 and 1692, respectively. Both came from impeccable dissenting backgrounds. Joshua was the son of Archdale Palmer (d.1673), one of the leading patrons of nonconformity in Leicestershire in the 1660s and early 1670s. Two months after his graduation, he married Anna Cradock, the daughter of the influential Presbyterian minister Samuel Cradock, who was ejected at North Cadbury in Somerset in 1662 (he was also named as dedicatee in the preface to Palmer's thesis on sudorific medicines). A year later, almost certainly at Hulse's urging, Palmer was made a full licentiate of the College of Physicians.[87] Thereafter, the two men seem to have worked closely together, frequently signing testimonials for candidates seeking licences to practise from the archbishop of Canterbury.[88] Joshua's nephew, William, was educated at the dissenting academy run by John Woodhouse at Sheriff Hales in Staffordshire, before proceeding BA at Cambridge in 1682. He subsequently remembered his old teacher and mentor in 1692 when he dedicated his Leiden MD on wasting diseases to Hulse and Woodhouse, along with his uncle Joshua and his father William. Within a year of graduation, he too received the official sanction of the London College of Physicians, when he was made an extra-licentiate of that body.[89]

The influx of former ministers into the medical profession was impressive, both in terms of numbers and the educational qualifications exhibited by this group of practitioners. Though some had pursued a dual career before 1660, most were new recruits to the profession. For the majority, moreover, the decision to quit the ministry and invade the calling of another highly respected group in society was not taken lightly. Typical, perhaps, was the Somerset clergyman John Oliver, who, in a letter to a colleague, described his intention to take up the study and practice of physic and surgery in 1661. This he would do, he claimed, 'so I may be capable in some country towne or other to get a Livelyhood, as I perceive some as ignorant dunces as I doe, & grow rich too, who have yet only a few english books & receipts'. He was careful to add, however, that 'I do intend to study it seriously, & to lay the best foundation I can in anatomy'.[90] Once ensconced in medical practice, such men usually proceeded to dispense spiritual physic alongside natural medicines. Despite earlier puritanical strictures, later generations of godly ministers found the function of preacher entirely compatible with their medical vocation. Medicine thus offered a profitable and convenient career option for ejected ministers and their sons (see Appendix 2 (b)) which, in the case of the latter, also extended to related fields of medicine such as pharmacy. This is most starkly evident in the case of the recruitment of the sons of ejected ministers to the trade of apothecary in London where once again dissenting ministers were able to exploit denominational networks to place their sons with masters who shared a common religious outlook (see Appendix 2 (c)). Echoing a trend which we have already encountered in the case of the Baptists, 40 sons of ejected clergy were apprenticed to London apothecaries between 1660 and 1700, all but three before 1688. Some, such as William Cornish (d.1733), went on to establish lucrative medical careers.[91] All would appear to have become deeply embedded in dissenting communities that proliferated in London at this time. They and their masters, in turn, often used their wealth to fund the activities of nonconformist ministers in London and beyond as in the case of Matthew Turner (d.1672) who in 1671 left £100 to support one hundred ministers who had suffered ejection.[92] Others, like Edmund Frost, married into the families of dissenting ministers.[93] In this way, the healing arts thus helped to create mutually supportive communities of fellow believers, tied together by bonds of family, kinship and occupation. At the same time and buoyed by a general influx of nonconformists into the medical 'profession' after 1660 (many the sons of godly gentlemen or former servants of the Cromwellian regime), a new generation of medical practitioners, galvanized by their opposition to the constraints of the Restoration settlement, became increasingly engaged in the religious and political debates of the period. As the political crisis enveloping Britain deepened in the aftermath of the Exclusion Crisis, more and more medics from nonconformist backgrounds were thus induced to contemplate and engage in a range of subversive activities many of which were carried out under the cover of their medical function.

Medicine as a Refuge for Plotting and Subversion

One of the untold stories of medicine between the Restoration and the Glorious Revolution concerns the extent to which the art of healing was first politicized, then radicalized, by the turbulent events of this period. We have already seen how these twin processes first took root in England during the years of civil war and Interregnum. After 1649, the competition for medical places, whether in the army, navy, or civil institutions such as hospitals, was increasingly decided by religious and political considerations. At the same time, those practitioners excluded from access to office and the all-important networks of patronage that underlay such appointments, were left with limited choices. Some threw in their lot with the new republican regime, or leastwise temporarily acknowledged the *de facto* authority of successive Interregnum governments. Others chose to lick their wounds and seek support and assistance from among their own kind, either in the exiled royalist communities spread across Europe or among small groups of like-minded dissidents who gathered in places such as the medical schools of Cambridge. At the Restoration, of course, these processes operated in reverse, medicine and medical study now constituting a convenient, and for some attractive and well remunerated, refuge from the winds of change blowing through English society.

Crucially, for those individuals and groups marginalized by the Restoration, medical study and practice also provided an invaluable outlet for a range of activities that might be used to uphold the cause of godly religion as well as promote the 'good old cause' in politics. In the case of religion, we have already noted the extent to which those ejected ministers who took up the practice of medicine after 1660 did so in combination with pastoral and ministerial duties, and in the process helped to console believers while attracting new converts. The government and its local agents were fully aware of such developments. In 1663, for example, James Greenwood, ejected at Kendal in the Lake District a year earlier, was reported to have returned to his old stomping ground where, 'under pretence of phisicke', he was said to be dispersing seditious materials. Three years later, Sir John Birkenhead alerted Sir George Lane, secretary to the duke of

Ormond, to the news that one Isaac Wilson, 'who professes Physick', had travelled to Chester prior to disembarkation to Ireland. He added, ominously, that '[h]e intends to profess Physick there also, [but] only as a Pretense, to go from House to House, with more security'.[94] Others travelled in the reverse direction. In December 1661, Lord Chief Justice Foster recommended that one Timothy Woodroffe, who had come from Dublin a few months earlier and was now practising physic at Gilgarra in Cumberland, should be imprisoned immediately until he had provided a satisfactory explanation for some 'mystical words' that he had spoken in relation to a prediction that 'a storm is coming'.[95]

As these examples suggest, one of the great advantages that medical practitioners, surgeons as well as physicians, possessed was the relative freedom which they enjoyed to move around the country, as well as cross seas and national boundaries. This, in turn, almost certainly fed the paranoia of local magistrates, government agents and local informers who were constantly on the lookout for such unusual comings-and-goings. Such fears almost certainly explain the interrogation of one Captain John Davis, a surgeon of Portbury, Somerset, in November 1663, when various neighbours informed local magistrates that they had heard much suspicious riding at night between Davis's house and the village of Portbury about the time of the late plot. Other witnesses intimated that Davis had become disaffected because he had been overlooked for a post at court (presumably as a surgeon to the King or royal household), but Davis, on examination, denied the inference, pledged his loyalty to the King, and claimed only that his nocturnal visitor was a local physician, one Parsons, who came 'to prescribe unto some of his family that then lay sicke of the small pox'.[96] Similar anxieties on the part of the authorities would appear to have prompted the arrest and examination of Samuel Ker or Carr, a Scottish surgeon, who was suspected of acting as a general go-between and passing letters from Holland to prisoners in England in 1666.[97] Evidence gleaned from the state papers and other sources confirms that surgeons were very prominent in plotting against the government of Charles II. From the early years of the Restoration, they were frequently arrested on suspicion of engaging in treasonous activity. Robert Wills and Giles Horsington of London, and Thomas Fox of Canterbury, all surgeons, were accused in 1660 of uttering seditious words.[98] In all three cases, the object of the men's ire was George Monck, the architect of the Restoration, and it may well be that their antagonism toward the new political settlement, and Monck's role in it, was partly motivated by concern for the loss of lucrative posts as surgeons in the Commonwealth armies. This would certainly make sense in the case of Horsington, who had served as surgeon to the parliamentary armies in Ireland, as well as profiteering from the sale of appropriated royalist lands in 1653.[99]

Surgeons continued to be arrested on suspicion of uttering seditious words and plotting throughout the 1660s. Many were devoted supporters of republicanism and the good old cause. Thomas Hill of Taunton, for example, was arrested and questioned in 1664 in relation to his knowledge of the whereabouts of the radical republican and conspirator, Richard Bovet.[100] Two years later, his Somerset colleague, Roger Toose, variously described as a surgeon and 'practiser of physic', was imprisoned in Wiltshire for speaking subversive words and disparaging the government. He was subsequently transferred to the Gatehouse at Westminster, from where he appealed to Lord Arlington for release on the grounds that he was drunk when he spoke the alleged words.[101] In the same month that Toose was languishing in Westbury gaol, Edward Page, a surgeon of St Katherine's, London, was facing equally serious charges. According to notes prepared by that hammer of dissent, Lord Chief Justice Keeling, Page was accused of saying that 'Cromwell's government was far better than the present, and that all the lords spiritual were rogues'. He also spoke ill of the King. Like Toose, Page denied the charge, arguing in predictable fashion that his prosecutors were acting out of malice due to an outstanding lawsuit pending between himself and his detractors. It is tempting to speculate that Page might be the same as the Mr Page, a London surgeon and close associate of the Whig exclusionist, Roger Whitley of Chester, upon whom he regularly attended during the latter's frequent visits to the capital between 1685 and 1687. In his diary, Whitley frequently refers to using Page's services as a surgeon, as well as socializing with him at various political clubs in the city.[102]

During the early years of the Restoration, physicians, surgeons, and others masquerading as medical practitioners were frequently accused of fomenting political discord and engaging in rebellion. Others were placed under close supervision and their movements carefully monitored.[103] Surveillance of individuals went hand in hand with a general preoccupation on the part of the government to police specific geographical locations, some of which, such as spas, provided a particularly conducive space for medical practitioners and others to engage in plotting and other acts of subversion. Loyal agents of the restored Stuart regime were only too aware of the threat posed by large numbers of visitors to the countries' many spas, and their potential use as a convenient rendezvous for the disaffected, since many former royalists had utilized them for the same purpose during the Interregnum.[104] It is therefore probably no coincidence that the radical Baptist and physician John Vernon (d.1667), who was gaoled and subsequently banished for life for acts of subversion in 1661, ended up practising medicine at Epsom in Surrey, a popular resort for Londoners wishing to take the waters and commune away from the glare of government spies.[105] As such places grew in popularity, partly in response to new ideas about sociability and genteel leisure, but also because they provided a degree of anonymity, they also became the object of increased official scrutiny and not without reason.[106] Gatherings of suspected plotters were reported at Tunbridge Wells in 1682 and at Scarborough and Epsom in 1683. In the latter case, a local magistrate specifically warned the government that, in the aftermath of the abortive Rye House Plot, the spa at Epsom was being frequented by rebels and subversives 'on pretence of drinking the waters'.[107] In the same year, Edward Mathews was arrested at the Surrey spa, charged with calculating the King's nativity and predicting his imminent death.[108]

The one place, however, that the governments of Charles II and James II would most like to have policed and controlled lay beyond their jurisdiction, a situation that was widely exploited by the growing chorus of critics of the Stuart regime and its perceived absolutist tendencies. Throughout the first half of the seventeenth century, Holland had provided a safe sanctuary for religious and political refugees from England. Now, in the aftermath of the Restoration and the onset of religious and political persecution, it once more became a popular destination for a range of dissidents, some of whom opted to study medicine in what were widely perceived at the time as the most advanced medical schools in Europe. Leiden and Utrecht thus became a magnet for English and Scottish medical students in the period from 1660 to 1700. Typically, they hailed from nonconformist (or in the case of the Scots, covenanting) backgrounds. Some stayed for three years or more and completed a full course of study. Others either curtailed their studies and moved on, or, as in the case of the majority, submitted their medical theses for examination and returned to Britain after the briefest of sojourns. Regardless, however, of the method undertaken, there can be little doubt that the experience for many of these students was a formative one that helped, among other things, to raise the profile of physicians within the embryonic dissenting communities that were taking shape after 1660. Moreover, and critically for this study, study overseas in Holland also assisted that process of politicization and radicalization which I have identified as a key feature of the medical history of Britain in this period.

Between 1660 and 1699, 152 English-born students proceeded to the degree of MD from one of the three main Dutch medical schools at Leiden, Utrecht, and Harderwyck. Of that number, fourteen were former ministers or fellows, expelled after 1660, fifteen were the sons of the same, and another thirty-one have been identified as possessing strong connections with the families of well-known religious and political dissidents in England. In addition, large numbers of English (and Scots) enrolled briefly as medical students without, for whatever reason, completing their studies. Many of these too came from radical religious and political backgrounds. Closer study of British visitors to Holland in this period can tell us a great deal about the relationship between medicine and politics in the Restoration. Though we know surprisingly little about the way in which British residents and travellers in Holland interacted with their Dutch hosts, we do know that from an early date the Dutch influence on the religious and political sensibilities of English visitors was far-reaching.[109] Its republican and 'democratic' political traditions, allied to Holland's famed (or in many circles, infamous) reputation as one of the most religiously tolerant societies in Europe, made it a natural refuge for English and Scottish dissidents seeking asylum and almost certainly reinforced the radical aspirations of those that fled there after 1660. As we shall see, our sample of medical students was not immune from this process, the universities of Leiden and Utrecht, along with the larger cities of Rotterdam and Amsterdam, offering a thoroughly congenial atmosphere in which to live and study, as well as to encounter, and in some cases imbibe, the latest ideas on a broad range of medical, philosophical, religious, political and social issues. Holland, in short, provided a home from home for the radical British émigré community in which our group of medical students, a small minority of the whole, were destined to play a disproportionately significant role in promoting the twin causes of religious dissent and political opposition to the 'absolutist' aspirations of the restored Stuarts.

In broad terms, the medical students I have identified here as drawn from the ranks of the dissenting-republican-Whig wing of English politics fall into two main categories. In the first instance, we have those (probably the majority) who emanated from such a background and were probably sponsored by supportive networks from within their respective communities, but who remained politically inactive, i.e. they declined to engage in open dissent or plotting. In contrast to this group, there existed a significant minority of students who combined medical study with active resistance to the restored regime of the Stuarts. In some cases, as we shall see, these men came to Holland with the explicit intention of using their studies as a cover for insurrectionary plotting. Others were drawn from the ranks of the first group and were recruited to the 'good old cause' and later radical Whiggism while studying at places like Leiden and Utrecht. Interaction between the two groups almost certainly occurred, though this is not always readily apparent from the sources that have survived.

We know precious little about the majority of those English medical practitioners who chose to study in Holland between 1660 and 1700. Apart from the seminal research of the Scottish physician and medical historian, Robert William Innes Smith (1872–1933), little else is known about this distinctive group of medical men or the nature of their experiences as students in the Dutch medical schools. In most cases, such as Leiden, it is possible to locate where such individuals lived and lodged. While some resided with their professors, the majority were to be found lodging in a small enclave close to the English church in the town.[110] Given the fact that so many of these students shared similar religious and political backgrounds, it seems likely that they also forged close bonds of friendship and collegiality. The Leiden graduate Christopher Love Morley (d.*c.*1707), for example, alluded frequently to his friendship with fellow English student, James Oviatt, in a work published shortly after his return to England in 1680.[111] A particularly rich but under-explored source for discovering more about the backgrounds of these students, particularly their religious and political affiliations, can be found in the dedications that most appended to the medical theses which they published on completing their studies. In the case of Oviatt, for example, it seems fair to conclude that he came from a nonconformist background as two of his listed dedicatees, the clergymen Henry Hickman (d.1692) and John Goldwire (d.1690), had been ejected in 1662. Hickman's appearance is not surprising as he served as pastor of the English church at Leiden during the period of Oviatt's residence in the town (see further below). Goldwire, who taught school at Broadlands, near Romsey, may have been Oviatt's schoolmaster since the latter's family home was in nearby Southampton.[112] The names of ministers deprived of their livings in the early 1660s not surprisingly recur in countless other dedications penned by the grateful beneficiaries of their support and largesse. Some were clearly named for the role which they had played as schoolmasters and mentors to future medical graduates. Samuel Jordan and William Higginbotham, for example, who obtained MDs at Leiden in 1678 and 1693, respectively, both appended dedications to their former headmasters and tutors.[113] Another subset of dissenting clergymen who appear regularly in these dedications are the various ministers, all deprived at the Restoration, who acted as pastors to the various English churches established in the United Provinces. Edward Richardson, Matthew Newcomen, John Spademan and Henry Hickman were all honoured in this way.[114] Hickman, for example, who ministered to the English community at Leiden between 1675 and 1692, was the subject of five such dedications.[115] He may even have entered Leiden as a medical student himself in 1675; his son, William (b.1668) was studying medicine there in the 1680s.[116] Little firm evidence survives detailing precisely what role men like Hickman played in the careers of these nonconformist medical students who flocked to places like Leiden in the 1670s and 1680s. It seems likely, however, that spiritual guidance and financial support were high on the agenda. Hickman's predecessor as pastor at Leiden, Edward Richardson (1670–1675), who was himself a Leiden medical graduate, offered these and much more. Fluent in the native language, in 1677 he published a Dutch primer for English students as well as offering his services as a translator.[117] Such activities, as we shall see, also carried sinister overtones, and were linked in the minds of English government spies with what they saw as a general plot, masterminded by dissenters and former radicals in Holland, to subvert the government of Charles II.

Given the extent to which religious and medical functions had become entwined in the world of post-Restoration dissent, we should not be overly surprised by the large numbers of dedications in medical theses to former clergymen. More significant, perhaps, were those dedications to leading lay figures and patrons in England, many of whom played a critical role in fanning the flames of opposition to the governments of Charles II and James II. These not only reveal much about the close relationships forged by physicians and politicians who shared a common religious and political agenda, but they also have much to tell us about the important networks of support that stretched across the North Sea and linked those in exile with dissenting, and after 1679 Whig, communities at home. Among those, for example, so honoured were well-known dissidents such as the former army officers John Braman (*c.*1625–1703) and Robert Venables (d.1687), the exclusionist MPs Sir Edward Harley (1624–1700), Sir William Ayscough (1614–1695) and Hugh Boscawen (1625–1701), and the prominent patron of London dissent, Henry Ashurst (d.1680)[118]. Associations of this kind suggest close links to the radical underground, and in some cases to the murky world of Restoration subversion peopled by former Cromwellians and other inveterate opponents of restored monarchy. In some cases, the relationship was based on close family ties. Samuel Desborough or Disbrowe, who graduated from Leiden as MD in 1668, was in all probability the son of Cromwell's major-general and brother-in-law, John Disbrowe.[119] The Presbyterian, Thomas Gibson (d.1722), who proceeded to his medical degree at Leiden in 1675, later married Anne, the youngest daughter of Richard Cromwell.[120] Former servants of the Cromwellian state also sent their sons abroad to study medicine in Holland. Bulstrode Whitelocke, son of the administrator and diplomat of the same name, was enrolled as a medical student at Leiden for three years, between 1668 and 1671, though he failed to graduate. Likewise, Andrew Birch (MD Leiden, 1674) dedicated his thesis on scurvy to his father, Thomas, a former army officer and loyal MP in the 1640s and 1650s who, after the Restoration, continued to ensure that Birch chapel remained 'a haven for nonconformist ministers'.[121] Close study of the remodelled corporations of England after 1660 provides further examples of strong links between religious and political dissent and support for those from nonconformist backgrounds who wished to study medicine abroad. Charles Glyde (d.1690), Andrew Jeffery and Nathaniel Slade, students at Leiden after the Restoration, were the sons of prominent citizens in Exeter who were all active opponents of the religious policies of the crown.[122] Similarly, Arthur Parsons (d.1698), the father of the medical student of the same name who graduated from Harderwyck in 1678, was a wealthy clothier from nearby Taunton who left an endowment for the education of young men designed for either the Presbyterian or Congregational ministry.[123] Another incentive for prominent citizens to send their sons to study medicine at places like Leiden may well relate to the fact that many of the towns and cities concerned retained strong trading links with Holland. This was certainly true of our Exonians, and may also account for the decision of George Spelman (d.1669), a merchant and prominent figure in oppositionist circles in disaffected Yarmouth, to direct his son Samuel to Leiden in 1664.[124] Twenty years later, the Baptist minister and physician, Nehemiah Cox (d.1689), dedicated his Utrecht MD to the prosperous London merchant and fellow Baptist, William Kiffin (1616–1701), much of whose wealth was based on trade with Holland.[125]

The subjects of these dedications undoubtedly reveal much about the elaborate networks that religious and political dissidents (usually one and the same) established after 1660, and which helped to forge communal solidarity in the face of intermittent persecution and exclusion from so many areas of life in Restoration England. And while it would be a mistake to over-exaggerate the extent to which many dissenters and dissidents accepted their fate, including permanent exclusion from the body politic, the tide of events was moving inexorably toward political stalemate. By the end of Charles II's reign and amid growing political divisions in the wake of the Exclusion Crisis, ever growing numbers of the King's subjects were becoming convinced of the hopelessness of their situation and were thus moved to contemplate a range of radical measures, including revolutionary violence, in order to effect political change. The failure of the exclusionist movement, followed by the years of Tory reaction, hardened these divisions and encouraged desperate men to seek desperate remedies. Throughout this period, but especially after 1682, the United Provinces provided a safe sanctuary for English dissidents eager to plot the downfall of what many saw as a vindictive and degenerate regime. At the same time, its medical schools attracted more English and Scottish students than at any other time either before or since. In the following section, I should like to explore the possibility that these two phenomena were not in fact coincidental, but were rather inter-related, providing further evidence of the disproportionate influence exerted by medical men in the political arena in the second half of the seventeenth century.

'A Fruitful Mother of Such English Brats': Holland, the Dutch Medical Schools and Political Opposition to the Stuarts

By the early 1680s, the subversive potential of medical practice and study was firmly established in England. The ability of surgeons and doctors to move around the country, often at night or on Sundays, and to travel long distances to minister to sick patients provided a convenient cover for all manner of extra-mural activities, including the conveyance of sensitive religious and political documents and other forms of communication. Messages might themselves be encoded in medical language in what contemporaries saw or suspected as a specific form of cant or insurrectionary code. These developments almost certainly date from 1640s and 1650s, when, as we have seen in chapter 3, numerous medical practitioners were rewarded for their service to first Parliament and then the Cromwellian state through a variety of means, including access to political power and the profits of office. The growing status of medical men in the 1640s and 1650s clearly reflected the expanding contribution that many of their number made in these years as agents of the state. In addition to serving the various governments of the day as officeholders, medics loyal to the cause often served the interests of the state in various ways. In May 1649, for example, it was reported from Northampton that news of the Leveller seizure of the town was immediately brought to the attention of Cromwell by one of the town's aldermen, a physician, who hid a letter addressed to the army-general 'in the bottom of a box of pills'. On another occasion in 1658, a Suffolk doctor named Nicholas Murton was able to extract information about a royalist plot from one of his patients during a medical consultation.[126] These subterfuges were not confined, of course, to supporters of the new regime. Royalist medics had long engaged in such surreptitious activity. In 1646, for example, the loyalist go-between and cleric, Michael Hudson, sought to avoid the parliamentarian authorities and travel to France 'for the Improvement of his profession' by using a false passport in the name of his brother-in-law, the physician Francis Cross.[127] During the 1650s, royalist doctors and surgeons engaged in a range of espionage, frequently moving to and fro between England and the continent as agents in various conspiracies. Not surprisingly, when the tables were turned after 1660 vanquished Cromwellians and others who sought to overthrow the restored regime soon resorted to similar tactics.

One of the first of the new breed of plotters to appreciate the advantages to be gained by combining the practice of medicine with subversion was the former Yorkshire preacher, Edward Richardson (1617–*c.*1678). Richardson was well placed to exploit the potential of a base in Holland, as he had resided and ministered to English congregations there in the 1640s and was a fluent native speaker. In April 1664, he submitted a thesis on diseases of the kidney and was immediately awarded his MD by the university of Leiden, assisted no doubt by the fact that he was able to show a licence from the London College of Physicians (granted by 'friends' within that body in November 1662).[128] Thereafter, he resided primarily in Holland, keeping some distance between himself and the English authorities, which suspected him of constantly plotting against the restored regime. All the while, he continued to combine medical practice with pastoral duties, acting as minister to the English congregations at Haarlem (1665–1670) and Leiden (1670–1675). He also encouraged and supported young English medical students seeking qualifications from his *alma mater* and was rewarded in typical fashion with dedicatory epistles appended to completed theses.[129] He was also instrumental, according to the Quaker historian Gerard Croese (1642–1710), in persuading the young Anglo-Dutch Quaker, Jan Coughen, to study medicine at Leiden. Coughen was the son of the merchant Laurence Coughen and was born in Amsterdam about 1638. Educated at Cambridge, he was destined for the priesthood before converting to Quakerism in about 1663. He probably met Richardson the following year, when he was laid up sick in Amsterdam, and subsequently enrolled for medical study at Leiden in early 1665, when the Quaker William Caton reported that Coughen had 'gone againe to the filthy fountains of the universitie to drink yet deeper of the foul streams thereof, that thereby hee may become a doctor'. On his return to England, he took up the practice of medicine, receiving a licence from the College of Physicians in London in July 1672. He was subsequently to play a leading role in the foundation of the Philadelphian Society, a move hinted at by Croese who claimed that he later sought to 'introduce a new Model of Doctrine and Discipline [and] of obliging all

Christians to concentrate in one common faith, and interpose their interest and power, for reconciling the differences of religion amongst all who profess'd the Name of Christ'.[130]

As for Richardson's conspiratorial activities, these are charted in the state papers, where he is frequently mentioned in the early 1660s as one of the leading lights advocating insurrection in the north of England. Accused of complicity in the Farnley Wood Plot of 1663, he may well have used his medical connections to instigate a rebellion in the north. One of those who informed against him in 1663 subsequently intimated that much of the planning for this conspiracy took place 'at the Spaw' (presumably Scarborough), where Richardson and fellow medical practitioners were able to associate freely with their 'patients'.[131] Among those who participated in these meetings was the radical Baptist and surgeon, Paul Hobson, who travelled the countryside under various aliases, including Dr Smith and, according to Richardson, Dr Love.[132] Imprisoned at York, Richardson managed to escape and make his way to Holland, where his activities were closely monitored and his post intercepted. Despite his protestations to the contrary, there seems little doubt that he continued to play an important role in coordinating opposition to the restored Stuarts from his base in Holland. He was particularly energetic in printing and translating subversive literature intended for export to England.[133] Richardson may also have been the brains behind a plot, uncovered in December 1665, to re-fan the flames of rebellion in his native Yorkshire. Among the conspirators on this occasion were said to be Joseph Flather, father-in-law of Henry Bradshaw, the brother of the regicide, and Captain John Hodgson, both of whom practised medicine in Yorkshire. According to the chief informant, Flather had recently been released from incarceration at York on the intervention of the duke of Buckingham after promising that he would focus solely on his medical practice and forswear further involvement in insurrectionary activity.[134] Hodgson, on the other hand, was still in prison, having been arrested along with Richardson in 1663, but the fact that it was rumoured that the plot was to be initiated by 'some people come out of Holland lately' suggests that the latter may have played some hand in the proceedings.[135] In later years, Richardson was again rumoured to be heavily involved in translating subversive literature. In 1681, William Carr, the English consul in the Netherlands, accused the Whig plotter Lord Howard of Escrick of seeking to persuade Dr Richardson, the 'architect of the northern rebellion', to put to good use his linguistic abilities by translating seditious documents for the insurgents.[136] Others alleged that while he was resident at Haarlem in the early 1670s, Richardson kept close company with the infamous plotter, Colonel Scott, and had frequent access to him both at Amsterdam and Leiden. Given Scott's own medical interests, especially in alchemical and iatrochemical secrets, it seems clear that the two shared more than just a common purpose in plotting the overthrow of Charles II.[137]

In the light of what we know about the activities of men like Richardson, it seems highly likely that many more English students who enrolled in the medical schools of Holland did so in the knowledge that they were likely to encounter a well-established network of English expatriates and émigrés, some of whom were engaged in the serious business of plotting regime change in their native land. By the early 1680s, following the defeat of the exclusionist cause and the onset of Tory reaction, the steady flow of disgruntled and alienated opponents of Stuart absolutism to Holland gave way to a major diaspora of both moderate and radical elements within the Whig movement. At the same time, the Dutch universities were reaching the peak of their popularity with British medical students. Given the religious and political backgrounds of these students, it should come as little surprise to discover then that the medical schools frequently acted as important recruiting grounds for those plotting serious acts of subversion, and even rebellion, in their homeland. The Whig background of many of these potential recruits has rarely been noted. Strange Southby, for example, who enrolled as a medical student at Leiden in November 1682, was expelled from Oxford as a 'green ribband man' for attempting to justify the regicide. He was also well connected to leading figures within the radical Whig movement. His father Richard (*c.*1624–1704) was a fellow member of the Green Ribbon Club, while his brother John was married to Mary Trenchard, the sister of the Whig politician and plotter, Sir John Trenchard (1649–1695). The family were placed under close surveillance by the government in the aftermath of the Rye House Plot. Under the circumstances, it is highly likely that Trenchard availed himself of his brother-in-law's Dutch connections following his flight to Holland after the defeat of Monmouth's rebellion in 1685.[138] Another medical student at Leiden who had engaged in radical politics before travelling to Holland was Richard Gilpin's future son-in-law, Jabez Cay (d.1702), of Newcastle-upon-Tyne. While a student at Edinburgh in 1682, he had engaged in the university's traditional pope-burning ceremony, an inflammatory act in more ways than one as the Catholic duke of York was serving at the time as high commissioner to Scotland. Cay was subsequently banished, and seems to have spent much of the 1680s travelling around Europe as a medical student before graduating at Padua in 1688.[139] Such men made ideal recruits to the radical cause, particularly after 1683 and the failure of the Rye House Plot when a desperate opposition, primarily based in Holland, began to lay plans for a full-scale insurrection in England led by the King's bastard son, the duke of Monmouth. In the event of armed conflict, surgeons and physicians were expected to play more than just a medical role. This was particularly true in the case of Hugh Chamberlen the younger (1664–1728), grandson of the famous man-midwife, Peter Chamberlen, who seems to have shared his illustrious forbear's attachment to radical causes. Admitted to the medical school at Leiden in October 1684, he was soon recruited by Monmouth's agents and was one of the first to land at Lyme Regis in June 1685, from where he travelled the country drumming up support for the invasion. Following the duke's defeat at Sedgemoor, Chamberlen managed to make his way back to Holland, where, with other fugitives, he allegedly spent his time spreading reports that Monmouth was still alive.[140] Chamberlen was later reprieved, as was the duke's own surgeon, Joseph Gaylard, the son of the Devon nonconformist minister, Robert Gaylard. Arrested in the aftermath of the rebellion, Gaylard returned to Holland, where, in 1688, he obtained a medical degree from Leiden.[141] Likewise William Oliver (1659–1716), son of an ejected minister, combined medical study with plotting. He enrolled at Leiden in December 1683 as part of the general diaspora of English radicals in the wake of the Rye House Plot, and later fought alongside Monmouth at Sedgemoor. Unlike his master, who refused to escape with him via the coast and Wales, Oliver avoided detection and returned to the continent and Holland, where in 1687 he was allegedly associating with 'several of Monmouth's friends'.[142] Whereas most of the men cited here went on to practise medicine, many establishing lucrative practices and obtaining important posts in England after the Revolution, others simply used enrolment at the Dutch medical schools as a convenient bolt hole to escape persecution in England. Joseph Hallett, for example, yet another son of an ejected west county minister, almost certainly entered Leiden as a medical student in July 1685 with no intention of graduating. His greater concern was to avoid the attention of the authorities in the wake of the rebellion, his father having been placed under arrest in Exeter.[143]

Other medics attached to Monmouth were less fortunate. Benjamin Temple, who travelled to Holland to obtain a medical degree in the early 1680s, was likewise recruited by agents of the duke of Monmouth. Captured after the abortive rebellion, he fell victim to Judge Jeffreys and was executed along with hundreds of other rebels at the ensuing bloody assizes.[144] The physician Richard Evans and surgeon Robert Thatcher almost certainly joined Temple on the gallows.[145] The surgeon Henry Pitman was more fortunate. Condemned to death, his sentence was commuted at the eleventh hour to deportation and transportation into slavery in Barbados. His subsequent adventures, including a brief period shipwrecked on a Caribbean island where he became engrossed in the study of the local marine and vegetable life, formed the core of a fascinating autobiography published on his return to England in 1689. Ever the opportunist, Pitman used this work as a platform to sell patent medicines, some of which he advertised in an appendix to the main pamphlet.[146]

In many respects, men like Pitman probably represented small fry in the eyes of a government determined to crush dissent, particularly from within the ranks of the governing classes, so many of whom sent their sons abroad during the years of Tory reaction and in the aftermath of the defeat of the rebels at Sedgemoor. Holland thus became the focus of a concerted campaign of government-funded espionage aimed at infiltrating the ranks of the rebels, a strategy that bore considerable fruit as evidenced by the mass of surviving reports compiled by government spies based in Holland in these years. At least one English agent operating in Utrecht in the mid-1680s managed to gain access to the rebels by posing as a physician.[147] There was nothing particularly novel about this tactic. Edward Riggs, ejected from a living on the Isle of Thanet and subsequently arrested in the wake of Tonge's Plot in 1662, became a government spy and, masquerading as a physician at Amsterdam, kept the authorities informed as to the whereabouts and proceedings of his former colleagues.[148] Likewise, in England, Nicholas Butler and the Scots-born physician, Thomas Burnett, were used by the government to infiltrate the ranks of various enemies of the state. Butler (d.1700) was rewarded for his efforts in spying on the nonconformist community with the grant of a mandated MD from the King in 1670.[149] Burnett, on the other hand, who had strong connections with the Scottish covenanters, was said by fellow agent, Colonel Scott, to have wormed his way into the inner sanctum of 'those Gentlemen from ye North' on the pretence of being an enemy to Lauderdale despite the fact that he was secretly receiving a state pension.[150] Back in Holland, the English government tried other measures to exert pressure on the Dutch government to clamp down on the 'illegal' activities of the exiles, though this effort was mostly in vain. Aware of the fact that English and Scottish radicals were enrolling at the Dutch universities as a pretext for plotting,[151] the government even attempted on occasion to halt the award of degrees on the grounds that the recipient was wanted for outlawry in Britain. In 1684, for instance, an attempt was made to bring pressure to bear on the university of Leiden to halt the promotion of the Scottish medical student Duncan Cummings (d.1724) to his MD, but the Dutch authorities refused to accede on the grounds that they had no jurisdiction over such matters.[152] Even more indicative of the helplessness of the government was the case of fellow Scot William Blackadder (1647–1696), who, following the award of his MD at Leiden in 1680, became involved in the earl of Argyll's expedition to Scotland in 1685 and lingered in prison for over a year. He was finally freed, however, in 1686, through the intervention of one of his former Dutch patients, Pensionary Fagel, who secured his release on the grounds that he was a naturalized Dutchman.[153]

Holland undoubtedly provided a safe and convenient refuge for British radicals in the period after 1660, medicine and medical study providing a useful alibi for subversion and conspiracy. Those who crossed the North Sea to acquire medical degrees from Leiden and Utrecht naturally gravitated to the expatriate communities in these and neighbouring towns and cities and were frequently drawn into the various plots that were hatched there, especially in the years following the collapse of the exclusionist cause, the Rye House Plot and defeat of Monmouth's Rebellion. In some cases, the link between medical study and plotting was all too evident in the political associations revealed by the dedications prefixed to published medical theses. In 1684, for example, the Bristol physician-cum-minister, Ichabod Chauncy (1635–1691), who fled England in that year after being implicated in the Rye House Plot, provided unwitting testimony to his radical associations when he included among the dedicatees to his Leiden thesis the woman he referred to as his 'foster mother', Mrs Smith.[154] Smith, the widow of a wealthy London sugar-baker, was a major political and financial supporter of what Ashcraft has termed 'the revolutionary movement' in Holland in these years. Prior to removing from England in the wake of the Plot, she and her husband had provided a safe house for many of the most important figures in the opposition to Charles II. Later in Holland, she (her husband died shortly after arrival) made her home at Utrecht, and from there provided vital financial assistance to both the Earl of Argyll and the Duke of Monmouth in their plans to equip forces for imminent insurrections in Scotland and England.[155] Just as important as women like Mrs Smith, however, were the pre-existing networks of radical associations and clubs in England that medical men like Chauncy inhabited prior to their arrival in Holland, which often provided newcomers with an entrée into the world of international sedition. Chauncy, for example, who ministered to an Independent congregation in Bristol, was instrumental in establishing exclusionist political clubs in the city, whose members included the radical lawyer and Dutch émigré, Nathaniel Wade (d.1718).[156] Through intermediaries such as Wade, Chauncy rapidly entered the innermost circle of the English and Scottish insurgents in Holland. In 1685, he was reported by a government spy to be living with the Whig rebel and activist Thomas Dare (d.1685), an intimate acquaintance of John Locke, Argyll and Monmouth.[157] Later that year, Chauncy was observed with other radical leaders discussing the disastrous aftermath of Monmouth's rebellion in an Amsterdam coffee house. He was finally pardoned in the spring of 1686, but on his return later that year he was again arrested and interrogated. His admission that he was merely delivering personal letters for the Whig lawyer and propagandist Thomas (alias 'Postscript') Hunt (d.1688) was unlikely to have endeared him to the authorities.[158]

For most Englishmen (and Scots) who chose to study medicine or receive a medical qualification from a Dutch university after 1660, the experience almost certainly fostered a hardening of attitudes toward their High Church Anglican and Tory rivals back home. In addition to exposing this group of scholars to what was arguably the most advanced medical training in late seventeenth-century Europe, it also enabled the same men to mix freely with Dutch and English radicals, many of whom shared the same religious and political principles. On returning to England, many of these newly qualified medical practitioners were destined to play a pivotal role in the medical and political lives of their communities. This was particularly evident, as we have seen, in the case of those who combined pastoral duties with a medical practice. Men like Richard Gilpin at Newcastle-upon-Tyne were enormously influential in ministering to the spiritual and physical needs of their congregations and providing leadership in times of hardship and persecution. Others such as Samuel Spelman, who set up in medical practice at Yarmouth after receiving his degree at Leiden in 1664, actively engaged on the political stage by dispersing what opponents described as seditious and scandalous libels, many of which were probably imported from nearby Holland.[159] Spelman, in all probability, was radicalized by his experiences abroad as a medical student. But it is equally important to acknowledge, as in numerous of the cases cited above, that many of those who travelled to Holland after 1660 in search of a medical education emanated from towns and cities in which dissenting communities had already begun to establish important networks of medical self-help. In Bristol, for example, Ichabod Chauncy and other nonconformist physicians combined to petition the authorities to act to alleviate the chronic plight of those Quakers imprisoned in the city's gaol.[160] Throughout England, nonconformist medical practitioners, or those sympathetic to the dissenters' plight, assisted their co-religionist colleagues in a myriad of ways. We have already noted, for example, the frequency with which many dissenters circumvented the ecclesiastical licensing system, typically through the intercession of supportive friends and colleagues from within the medical profession who signed licence applications and provided glowing testimonials. Many no doubt adopted the same stratagem of those fellow dissenters who sought local political office after the Restoration, temporizing with the powers-that-be under the guise of partial conformity. Others found a congenial host in the London College of Physicians, the leadership of which by the early 1680s had turned this august body into a stronghold of Whiggism and dissent. Throughout the 1660s and 1670s the puritanical governing clique had done all in its power to extend its support to deprived ministers and other dissenters seeking alternative careers in medicine. Licences were freely offered and granted, and the creation of new titles afforded an important source of medical patronage that nonconformist physicians, ultra-conscious perhaps of the need to secure legitimation, were only too eager to accept. On 30 September 1680, amid a growing crisis in church and state, the College took the provocative step of creating yet more honorary fellows, the vast majority of whom on this occasion were clearly antipathetic to the religious and political policies of the crown.[161] The medical advantages that accrued from an affiliation of this kind were obvious. The new fellows gained status and authority, an important acquisition given that many either possessed no formal medical qualifications or had secured degrees from foreign universities, which were suspect in the eyes of their political opponents and rivals. But just as important were the channels of communication that were created by such networking that could easily be exploited for religious and political ends as much as medical ones. Indeed, by the late 1670s and early 1680s there is growing evidence to suggest that these networks were increasingly being used for precisely such ends.

Medicinal Networks, Plots and the Whig Cause

The political crisis engendered by the Popish Plot and the ensuing demand of a Whig opposition to exclude the King's brother from the succession to the throne has an interesting medical dimension that has previously evaded the notice of historians. The Plot itself was first brought to the King's attention through the offices of some of his own chymical acquaintances and medical servants at court. The central figures here were the chymist and royal physician Sir Richard Barker and Christopher Kirkby, a shadowy figure who seems to have acted as some form of chymical operator or laboratory assistant at Whitehall. Using their connections at court, these two men were able to facilitate the access of a third man, Israel Tonge (1621–1680), one of the chief actors in the plot, to the Lord Treasurer, and through him to the King, who was thus informed of the threat to his life reputedly posed by a group of Catholic desperadoes.[162] Barker we have previously encountered as a signatory to the abortive Society of Chymical Physicians in 1665. Despite the failure of the chymists, Barker's career subsequently flourished. In December 1673, he joined the ever-growing ranks of royal physicians, the majority of whom as we have seen were chymically inclined, and was knighted by a grateful monarch. He also grew exceedingly wealthy. His staunch anti-Catholicism, combined with his support for ecumenical Protestantism, brought him into contact with Tonge, who shared Barker's passion for chymistry.[163] Among other forms of support, Barker, as patron, bestowed upon Tonge the living of Avon Dassett in Warwickshire. He was also responsible for introducing him to Titus Oates, whose son, Samuel, was a beneficiary of Barker's largesse.[164] Less is known about the third figure, Christopher Kirkby, who was clearly instrumental in smoothing the way for Tonge's meeting with the King. Kirkby was in fact a merchant, who was clearly well respected for his chymical abilities, both within and outside the court. He was well known, for example, to Robert Boyle, with whom he corresponded for over twenty years, and also supplied material of scientific interest to Henry Oldenburg, some of which was published in the *Philosophical Transactions.*[165] The shared interest of all three men in chymistry was probably no coincidence. Not only did it provide a convenient entrée into the inner recesses of the court, but it also, in certain respects, provided a form of intellectual legitimation for moral and political practices and beliefs consonant with an eirenic and conciliatory strain of Protestant belief.[166]

In the panic that followed the publication of the Plot, medical men continued to play a prominent role. Some, such as Hugh Chamberlen the elder, were active as magistrates and used their judicial powers to round up, search and question Catholics in London who were suspected of involvement in the plot. He may also have used this as an opportunity to settle old scores with rival Catholic physicians; among those he examined was John Butler (d.1681), physician to the duke of Norfolk.[167] Butler was not the only physician of his confession to suffer.

William Fogarty, physician to the duke of Ormond, died in custody in 1678.[168] In the meantime, Sir George Wakeman,, physician to the Queen, was tried but ultimately acquitted of attempting to poison the King.[169] Other Catholic physicians arrested and interrogated in the wake of the discovery of the plot included the Derbyshire practitioner Richard Needham.[170] There can be little doubt that news of the plot and subsequent arrests spread panic in the ranks of the Catholic community. As physicians would appear to have been particularly vulnerable to accusations of complicity in the plot, many reacted by fleeing the country.[171] Others like John Betts (*c*.1623–1695) either lost office (his membership of the London College was suspended from 1679 to 1684) or, as in the case of Walter Harris (d.1732), publicly recanted and espoused the Protestant faith.[172] Briefly, Whig physicians prospered at the expense of their Catholic colleagues and sympathizers, but the victory was short-lived. Chamberlen, a prominent Whig, ultimately paid the price for his political allegiance. In November 1682 he was dismissed from office as a royal physician and replaced by the Tory loyalist Robert Brady. A year later, he was said to be part of the coterie waiting on the duke of Monmouth whom he defended from the accusation that he had taken part in the Rye House Plot.[173]

Chamberlen was not alone among the Whig medical fraternity in suffering for his political beliefs. The medical practice of the eminent physiologist and royal physician Richard Lower (1631–1691)[174] suffered greatly in the wake of the Tory reaction as many of his court-based patients deserted him and opted instead to seek the medical advice of rival loyalists such as Thomas Short.[175] Likewise, it was widely rumoured that the Whig President of the London College of Physicians, Thomas Coxe (1615–1685), was forced out of office in 1683 for his political sympathies.[176] Similar purges were conducted in the London hospitals, where medical practitioners suspected of holding Whig views, or allying with Whigs and dissenters, found themselves the victims of political partisanship.[177] Some even paid for their convictions with their lives. The radical Baptist, Charles Bateman (d.1685), formerly surgeon to the earl of Shaftesbury and a long-time advocate of insurrection (he was a member of the Green Ribbon Club), was ultimately tried and executed for his role in promoting the Whig cause.[178] Bateman would appear to have served the 'faction' in various ways. In addition to sheltering fugitive Whigs such as Sir Patience Ward (1629–1696), he provided a conduit for rebel funds. On another occasion in December 1682, at the height of the political furore over the shrieval elections in London, he was said to have supplied bottles of sack to three men pilloried in Gracechurch Street, who then proceeded to drink healths to the King, Monmouth and Shaftesbury.[179]

Networks of like-minded physicians and surgeons can also be found operating outside London in this period, some of whom clearly used their medical practice to further their political aims. In some cases, well-connected medical practitioners facilitated communication between radical groups in the capital and the provinces. The nonconformist surgeon John Friend (d.1706), for example, seems to have taken on this role in the Somerset town of Taunton, one of the major provincial strongholds of Whiggism and dissent. In 1683, he was acting as a recruiting sergeant in the town and surrounding countryside for the duke of Monmouth, no doubt trading on his close connections with the radical lawyer and member of the Green Ribbon Club, John Trenchard (1649–1695).[180] Taunton had a track record of producing radical medics. The town's MP in the 1650s was the staunch commonwealth man John Palmer (for whom, see above ???–???). Taunton's coffee houses, like those at London, also provided good opportunities for local dissidents to discuss the latest political news and speculate on future developments. Again, medics feature prominently in the confessions of reluctant informants and witnesses to such discussions. In September 1683, for example, one Hoit, described by an informer as an MD of Tiverton in Devon, was overheard discussing insurrection in a Taunton coffee house with a nonconformist minister Robert Carel.[181] More often than not, however, as many of the examples cited above suggest, it was surgeons who seemed to have been most prominent in proffering their services to the radical cause. Many travelled incognito or under a string of aliases, all sheltering under the pretence of pursuing their chosen profession. Typical was the case of John Stone, alias Jones, alias Whitacre, who was arrested and examined at Gloucester in June 1685. Accused of fomenting rebellion and travelling the country in search of supporters for the duke of Monmouth, he claimed to have lived and practised surgery in London for almost twenty years before uprooting to the west country and wandering through various towns and cities (Chepstow, Bristol, Monmouth, Hereford, and Gloucester) in pursuit of patients and, in his own words, 'to seeke for Cures'. The examining magistrate, however, clearly thought otherwise, concluding that Stone was 'a Rogue', who wandered the country propagating his 'Mischeivous Designs'. He was also a determined character; despite 'all the Arts and Methods' at his disposal, the loyal JP was unable to 'bring him to any Confession of his accomplices or Adherents'.[182]

Surgeons like Friend and Stone were clearly part of a much wider network of organized political dissidence, the focal point of which is often difficult to trace. Such networks, however, were clearly highly developed in England by the late 1680s and are perhaps best observed in the corporate towns and boroughs, where social elites gathered in this period to discuss the latest political news and gossip as well as consult with their surgeons and physicians. The latter, in particular, were chosen not simply on the grounds of professional competence, but also with respect to their religious and political allegiances. A good example of this process in action is provided by the city of Chichester in Sussex, which, in common with many other corporate towns in this period, was riven by political conflict. At the heart of the Whig cause here were two powerful townsmen, John Braman and John Farrington, along with an important ally in the cathedral close, canon

Henry Eedes (d.1703). Braman was the guardian of Thomas Aylwin, who graduated MD at Leiden in 1682. A former Cromwellian army officer, he served as MP for the city throughout the Exclusion Crisis and was consistently suspected thereafter of plotting against the crown and providing support for the cause of the duke of Monmouth, whom he warmly welcomed to Chichester in 1683.[183] Farrington, like Braman, was a patron of the city's nonconformists, who, with other members of his family, was active throughout the 1680s in support of the Whig cause.[184] Both men found support from an unusual source in the shape of Henry Eedes, who was described in 1677 by his bishop as 'the great patron & friend of Corbet the great conventicle preacher of this towne'. He, too, was widely suspected of supporting the duke of Monmouth on his first visit to the city in 1679, and was subsequently accused, along with Braman, of involvement in the Rye House Plot.[185] In cultivating the cause of the Whigs and dissenters, this triumvirate relied heavily on the support of fellow citizens and clients among whom the city's medical practitioners were notably conspicuous. In 1685, for example, a government spy (in all probability, Ezekiel Everest, a native of Chichester, who had recently returned from Holland) reported to his superiors that Robert Haslen, an 'apothecary', along with one 'Barnham Dr in phisick', had endeavoured to ride out of the city after curfew in order to alert Major Braman to an attempt by government messengers to arrest him and thus facilitate his escape from the clutches of the law. Everest was well informed, for he added that about five years earlier, Haslen had been indicted for speaking treasonable words against the late King, Charles II, and his brother, the duke of York, 'saying that the King had no title to the crown & that both his Majestie & the Duke of Yorke were illegitimate'. Owing to the temper of the times, however, 'the faction prevailed to have him acquitted by a ignoramus jury'. Haselin, who held an ecclesiastical licence to practise medicine and was probably a nonconformist, possessed influential connections and later served as mayor of Chichester.[186] So did his associate on this occasion, Dr Barnham Dobell (d.1694). Dobell was a graduate of Padua, who settled in the city in the 1660s and was closely connected to the circle of John Farrington Snr, whose daughter he married in 1669.[187] As these examples suggest, medical men were often usefully employed in the service of the 'faction'. In another incident in the city at the height of the political crisis engendered by Charles' decision to dissolve the third Exclusion Parliament, allegations were made that William Peachey (d.1702) had been negligent in his duties as a surgeon and medical practitioner in failing to assist one Richard Habin, a Tory informer, who had been attacked and beaten by a servant of the Whig grandee, John Farrington. According to one witness, cited in a contemporary pamphlet account, Peachey was well known as 'a Friend to Mr. Farington and the Party', a state of affairs that left the 'impartial' reader in little doubt as to who should be held responsible for the subsequent death of the unfortunate Habin.[188]

By the early 1680s, many medical practitioners were closely bound together by ties of marriage, education, religion, patronage, and occupation, all of which helped to reinforce their commitment to the Whig cause. These ties, moreover, often extended beyond local horizons and narrow urban constraints. A particularly good example of this process of medical networking, where professional interests would appear to have intersected with a commitment to radical religious and political change, is evident in the case of the Essex doctor and eminent amateur botanist, Samuel Dale (1659–1739). In an incident unnoticed by his biographer, Dale was accused in September 1683 of engaging in insurrectionary activity in the aftermath of the Rye House Plot. More specifically, he is alleged to have shown an associate a pair of pistols and to have told him 'he knew not but he might shortly discharge them in the [Duke of] York's bowels'. What makes this seemingly isolated incident so intriguing is that just over a year earlier Dale, an apothecary in his native Braintree, had obtained an archiepiscopal licence that allowed him to augment his living by practising medicine. In addition to the customary signatures of grateful patients, Dale was able to call on the support of two fellow licentiates, Blaise or Blaze Allen and Christopher Packe, both of whom would appear to have shared his predilection for radical politics.[189] Allen (d.1703), who practised physic in Somerset and later in London, was long suspected of involvement in subversive activity and plotting. In 1661, for example, he was allegedly present at a gathering of almost one thousand dissidents in Somerset, where he is said to have told one of the local justices that 'he need not be so harsh, [for] it would be their turn soon'. He was subsequently arrested and imprisoned in neighbouring Wiltshire, where he was described as one 'eminent to promote faction & sedition'. Within two years, he was nonetheless licensed for medical practice by the archbishop of Canterbury and, in addition to supplying testimonials for both Dale and Packe (in 1674), signed numerous others on behalf of local practitioners.[190] Allen was, in all probability, connected to Dale through ties of kinship, as he was the father of Dale's close associate, fellow dissenter and brother-in-law, Benjamin Allen (1663–1738), who, like Dale, practised medicine at Braintree after the Glorious Revolution.[191] Benjamin, too, was a committed Whig, who probably fell out with his brother-in-law in the 1690s over political differences.[192] Christopher Packe (d.1714) was a leading proponent of Helmontian medicine in London, and was closely related to the Cromwellian mayor of the city, Sir Christopher Packe (d.1682), who was instrumental in promoting the early medical career of his young relation. Packe's Whig sympathies are evident in the comments that he made in his published writings regarding his patients. In 1688, for example, he alluded to curing a niece of the Whig martyr Elizabeth Gaunt, 'who was unhappily executed the same day that the Worthy Alderman [Henry] Cornish also fell a Sacrifice to the Iniquities of those Times'.[193] Like many other Whigs, Packe was also a practising nonconformist. At his death in 1714, he was a member of the congregational church that met at

Ropemakers Alley in Little Moorfields under the leadership of John Asty (1675–1730), whom he asked to preach his funeral sermon.[194]

What is particularly noteworthy about this and other examples is the extent to which the relationship between these three men transcended geography. Medical friendships and shared professional interests, often affirmed by familial ties, helped to reinforce political solidarity and create the sense of a nationwide movement of opposition to what they and others increasingly perceived as the tyranny of the Stuarts. This is evident in the career of the most famous proponent of reform, the political theorist and philosopher John Locke (1632–1704), who was forced to endure a six-year exile in Holland on account of his connections and activities in the upper echelons of the Whig movement. It is easy to overlook the fact that Locke was first and foremost a practising physician, who spent much of his time in Holland discoursing with Dutch physicians. While abroad, he maintained contact with medical friends and colleagues in England, the majority of whom would appear to have shared his political opinions as well as his passion for iatrochemistry. David Thomas and Charles Goodall, for example, were, like Locke, keen devotees of chymical medicine who assisted him in various ways before, during, and after his exile in Holland. Thomas (*c.*1634–1694) was a provincial physician, based in Salisbury, who first encountered Locke at Oxford in the mid-1660s when the two men became engaged in chymical research. Like Locke, Thomas was an admirer of van Helmont and in later letters to his friend expressed great excitement at the prospect of a visit when the two men might indulge their shared passion for labouring in the laboratory. He also moved in the same political circles as Locke, standing on friendly terms with James Tyrell, as well as acting as physician to the household of the earl of Shaftesbury, whose family seat, Wimbourne St Giles, was within an easy ride of Thomas's home at Salisbury.[195] Goodall (*c.*1642–1712), a graduate of Leiden (MD 1670), was a later acquaintance of Locke, the two men probably meeting for the first time in about 1680 when the former, an outspoken supporter of the rights of the London College of Physicians, was living on the College's premises at Warwick Lane. Shortly thereafter, Locke recommended that his friend and fellow Whig activist Edward Clarke (d.1710) should seek Goodall's advice with regard to taking the waters (he subsequently became his patient). In May 1683, Locke briefly lodged with Goodall, before departing in haste for Holland, when he was forced to ask his friend and fellow Whig to look after some of his possessions. Five years later, it was Goodall who was the first to regale Locke with the news of the flight of James II, and the arrival of William of Orange, whom, he claimed, had saved the country from 'popery and slavery'.[196] Like Thomas, the close friendship of the two men may have been sealed by their mutual interest in chymistry. Goodall had in fact been appointed physician and chymist in ordinary to Charles II in February 1671. Three years earlier, he had written to Robert Boyle recommending the use of Delaune's pill and discussing the usefulness of various chymical recipes, including a 'grand

Arcanum' that cured epileptic, hysteric and convulsion fits. At the same time, he asked Boyle to respond by sending chymical preparations recently recommended by Daniel Coxe in his book against the apothecaries.[197]

Locke's network of connections extended to two other men whose politico-medical profiles were remarkably similar to those of Thomas and Goodall. Locke's friendship with fellow Whig apologist, Richard Burthogge (1638–1705), did not begin until about 1694 but the two men shared much in common. Burthogge, who was awarded his MD from Leiden in 1662, came from a family of Devon nonconformists and practised medicine in that county for over forty years. Like Locke, he seems to have been attracted to iatrochemistry, his thesis (on the stone) containing copious references to Helmontian concepts such as the archeus as well as referring to the works of other chymists including Quercetanus, Poppius and Faber.[198] Burthogge was also active in politics, both as a writer and, briefly, in 1687–8 as a burgess and JP in the remodelled borough of Totnes.[199] It is his philosophical writings, however, that have elicited most historical attention and have led modern-day commentators to 'place him squarely within the anti-dogmatic, broad-church, tolerationist tradition' of writers like Locke. Burthogge himself hailed Locke as 'one of the greatest masters of reason' and dedicated his *Essay Upon Reason* (1694) to him, in return for which Locke sent him copies of his book opposing bishop Stillingfleet. In 1699, Burthogge dedicated another of his works, *Of the Soul of the World*, to his friend and they continued to correspond on philosophical and theological matters until 1703.[200] In this last work, Burthogge cited an article from the Royal Society's *Philosophical Transactions* written by yet another medical colleague, friend and political ally of Locke, Daniel Coxe (1640–1730).[201] Coxe was an early convert to Helmontian chymistry and, like Thomas, Goodall, and Locke, corresponded with Robert Boyle on chymistry and related issues. He was also a dissenter and active Whig (for which he was arrested in 1685) and was on close terms with Locke, who lent him books and consulted with him over the cure of venereal disease.[202] Coxe's radical credentials were impeccable. From the 1650s, he and his father, Daniel, a former servant of the early Cromwellian state, were on close personal terms with Major-General John Lambert (1619–1684), one of whose daughters Coxe Jnr later married.[203] By the early 1680s, Dr Coxe was actively supporting the Whig petitioning campaign in London as well as using the law courts to undermine his political opponents. In October 1681, for example, he laid informations against the Tory Lord Mayor of London, Sir John Moore, whom he claimed to have overheard say that the Popish plotters had been justly punished and no longer offered a threat to the safety of the kingdom. He was also alleged to have said that '[t]here was a Restlesse active sort of people of Common wealth principles that were Endeavouring to bring us into Confusion and that the Government had cause to have as watchfull an Ey over them as over the Papists'—a comment aimed at men like Coxe and Locke who stood in the vanguard of the Whig movement.[204]

What common threads, then, can we detect here, and how might they inform our greater understanding of the relationship between medicine and politics in later Stuart England? One striking feature is the extent to which all five men shared an interest in medical and scientific innovation. More specifically, their profound interest in the new iatrochemical ideas and beliefs of physicians like van Helmont, allied to a general openness to empirical methods and techniques in medicine, is indicative of what one might loosely term a 'progressive' approach to healing in Restoration England. In addition, two figures stand out as significant influences on their scientific and medical careers: Robert Boyle and Thomas Sydenham. Four of the five (Burthogge was the exception) were on friendly terms with Boyle and communicated regularly with him in the 1660s, often supplying or requesting information relating to their mutual interests in medicine and chymistry. Sydenham, however, was probably the greater influence. He was intimately acquainted with Coxe, Goodall and Locke, and worked closely with all three in researching areas of mutual medical concern. Coxe, for example, who claimed to have converted Sydenham to the merits of chymistry in 1666, was engaged at the same time in assisting him in his pioneering work on the nature of fevers.[205] Likewise, Goodall worked closely with Sydenham on various projects related to the latter's research into the natural history of disease, the two men forming something of a mutual admiration society judging from the frequency with which they extolled each other's work and good character in the prefaces to their various publications. It has also been suggested that Goodall was responsible for introducing Locke to Sydenham.[206] Sydenham's impact on this closely connected group of physicians was probably most evident in the extent to which they shared and developed his emphasis on the need to pursue an empirical approach to medical practice based on improved clinical awareness of the needs of patients. Coxe's anonymously published assault on the apothecaries in 1669 was thus predicated on the grounds that physicians should prepare their own medicines because they were the fittest judges of what may or may not cure their patients.[207] Goodall's empirical credentials, which may appear ironic given his later assault on uneducated and illicit practitioners on behalf of the College of Physicians, are evident in his correspondence with Boyle, cited above, in which he advertised the merits of various nostrums, some of which he derived from a Suffolk neighbour, Madam Saxford. Locke, too, shared and encouraged Sydenham's empirical approach to healing. Shortly after their first meeting, he wrote two medical treatises, both unpublished, which 'expressed a profound scepticism about our capacity to discover the nature of disease, and advocated a purely empirical approach to medical practice'.[208]

Sydenham, of course, shared much else in common with these fellow physicians, including an instinctual aversion to the religious and political agenda pursued by Charles II in the last years of his reign.[209] In all but one case, they shared remarkably similar backgrounds, their fathers having served and supported the parliamentarian-puritan cause in the years before 1660. They also acquiesced in the return of the Stuarts in the hope that it offered the best opportunity to restore harmony and order to the body politic. Some, such as Burthogge, opted out, unable to accept the new strictures imposed on tender consciences in the 1660s. Others, such as Locke, were more gradually persuaded of the need to strive for greater religious freedom and the establishment of a broad-based, national church able to accommodate moderate dissent. By the 1680s, all were active in Whig politics in some form or another. Whether or not they would have agreed with the drift of Marchamont Nedham's comment, with which we began this chapter, that medicine in Restoration Britain had witnessed the emergence of a distinctive new voice, one shaped by the experience of dissent and persecution, is impossible to say. There is little doubt that Nedham's depiction of events on the ground was to some extent exaggerated. Medical practitioners from dissenting and Whig backgrounds never entirely turned their backs on professional colleagues and friends who opted to support the status quo. Sydenham, for example, dedicated his work on gout and dropsy to his friend Thomas Short, a convert to Roman Catholicism who retained his fellowship at the London College after the Popish Plot revelations (below 277). Others such as Charles Goodall probably survived the Tory backlash after 1682 in part through the intercession of well-placed acquaintances such as the Anglican clergyman and apologist William Clagett (1646–1688), who described Goodall in 1686 as his 'honoured friend'.[210] The events of the last years of Charles II's reign, however, clearly polarized religious and political opinions in the country to an unprecedented extent, and the world of medicine was not immune to these developments. Utilizing a range of networks both familial and collegiate, dissenting medical practitioners often acted as one to validate and promote their careers as healers. At the same time, they almost certainly used their medical connections in order to bolster opposition throughout England to what they perceived as the growing threat of an absolutist, Catholic state.

The extent to which such connections permeated the provincial medical scene is particularly well illustrated by the example of Dr William Jacob (*c.*1623–1692), whose professional and political interests intersected on numerous levels with those of Sydenham and Locke. Jacob, who graduated MD at Oxford in 1660, practised physic at Canterbury in Kent where he later served as the city's MP (first elected in March 1679).[211] Shortly after his election, Sydenham wrote to Locke requesting that he present his services to Jacob, 'of whom I have received so good a character of his integrity that I should be very glad if you could settle an acquaintance between us'. Locke was staying at the time with Dr Jacob, the two men exchanging medical recipes and other gossip (including Jacob's account of a haunting at his house which Locke copied down verbatim in his journal). Clearly the two men shared much in common, both in terms of their approach to medicine and contemporary politics. A year later, for example, Jacob penned a letter to Locke in which he claimed to:

> have often thought how desirable a paper commerce might be betweene Physitians living at some convenient distance, especially in empiricall medicine. For usually the presse gives us notice of what hypotheses rise and fall in the world, but for the Arcana's, men usually suppresse them, or doe not deliver them faithfully and fully provd by many successes.[212]

Jacob's interest in exchanging medical gossip and remedies may well have been genuine rather than an example of medical 'cant', but it is equally plain that the two men were cut from the same political cloth. Jacob, as MP for the city, voted for exclusion in 1680 but was not re-elected in the fresh elections later the same year. Back in Canterbury, he became increasingly active in exclusionist and dissenting circles. In June 1682, for example, he tried, with other Whigs in the city, to present a petition to the King requesting that the succession pass to the duke of Monmouth. A month later, he wrote to one of his patients in Rye in Sussex, lamenting the fact that he had just spent the better part of a week at Maidstone 'in order to testify in a good cause & for a worthy Justice, unworthily Treated by a sort of vermin called Informers'. Typically, he concluded by recommending one of his own medicines for the recipient's gout.[213] The patient in question, Thomas Markwick, was a prominent nonconformist, and it was among the dissenters that Jacob would appear to have primarily moved. Like so many medical practitioners who shared his religious sympathies, he may also have acted as a patron to co-religionists seeking medical qualifications abroad. In 1680, for example, John Bemister of Canterbury, the son of a local surgeon and prominent dissenter, dedicated his Leiden MD on dysorexia, an eating disorder akin to anorexia nervosa, to Jacob and other city radicals.[214] A year earlier he was the recipient of a similar dedication at the hands of the Leiden MD, Peter Peters (1656–1697) of Canterbury, an honour he shared with the latitudinarian and fiercely anti-Catholic dean of Canterbury, John Tillotson (1630–1694).[215]

A Dissenting Medical Tradition?

What then, we might ask, was distinctive about the medical culture of Britain's dissenters after 1660? While it is not possible to provide definitive answers here, some preliminary conclusions are possible. In the first place, the growing interest in dissenting medical circles after 1660 in iatrochemical methods and principles strongly suggests that by the end of the seventeenth century no single religious group or denomination was responsible for promoting the therapeutic benefits of chymical medicines. Whereas, it has been argued, the generality of mainstream puritan physicians and theologians before the Restoration had expressed concerns, both medicinal and moral, about the virtues of medicines made according to the principles of men like Paracelsus and van Helmont, after 1660 there was a sea-change in attitudes among those who stayed loyal to their Presbyterian and Congregational roots. One explanation for the growing faith of physicians from dissenting backgrounds in chymistry may be found in the fact that so many were now receiving their training in Dutch universities, where chymistry formed such an important part of the medical curriculum. At Leiden in particular, under the aegis of men like Franciscus de la Boë Sylvius (1614–1672), who held the chair of medicine from 1658 until his death in 1672, chymistry became not only fashionable but, shorn of its earlier mystical associations, part of mainstream medical culture and education. Sylvius's influence upon his English students is evident both in the dedications which they wrote in the preface to their medical theses, but also in their own writings and research.[216] The Dutchman had partly 'tamed' the excesses of earlier chymists like van Helmont by adopting the mechanistic principles of Descartes and applying them to his own chymical research. In many respects Sylvius's programme paralleled the work of influential figures such as Robert Boyle in England, whose corpuscularian ideas were readily assimilated by a new generation of English physicians, eager to exploit the therapeutic potential of chymistry. Boyle's influence in this respect, as well as his marked ambivalence toward conventional medicine and medical practice, was especially well received in dissenting medical circles. His writings, for example, were frequently cited and praised by nonconformist practitioners such as John Reynolds,[217] Anthony Smith[218] and John Peachey,[219] while a large number of medics from dissenting backgrounds eagerly corresponded and often met with Boyle in order to discuss areas of mutual concern.[220] Some of these men, such as Samuel Haworth (below), have been rather too readily dismissed by modern commentators as 'empirics' and 'quacks', though it is highly unlikely that Boyle himself would have concurred. Indeed, one aspect of Boyle's medical outlook that so appealed to men like Sydenham and Locke, as well as a broad spectrum of medical practitioners in the late seventeenth century, was his apparent openness to new cures irrespective of their origins. When Sydenham wrote to Boyle in 1668, commenting on the manner in which he had been marginalized and sneered at by established (i.e. collegiate and university-educated) physicians, and deriding their excessive 'bookishness', he must have been aware that his complaints were likely to meet with a sympathetic ear.[221] Other admirers of Boyle echoed Sydenham's lament for the state of medicine. The nonconformist William Westmacott, for example, whose medical education largely consisted of a series of apprenticeships, probably spoke for many others of his background when he commented in 1694 that '[n]o letter'd hypothesis in the theory, nor a diploma of MD, painted as a reward, can make a man the true servant of nature'.[222] In a similar vein, the celebrated 'empiric' John Colbatch (d.1729) elevated 'ocular demonstrations' over university learning, while simultaneously praising 'that Admirable and never sufficiently to be valued Mr. Boyle' above all others as the chief exponent of the new experimental philosophy, which, he believed would provide a suitable foundation for the perfection of medicine.[223]

One element of Boyle's approach to medicine that struck a particularly responsive chord among contemporary medical practitioners was his conviction that physicians should make and compound their own medicines. Echoing the complaints of his friend Thomas Sydenham (above), Daniel Coxe wrote to Boyle in 1666 recounting how he had been scorned and rebuked by his more senior colleagues for refusing to accept fees and making his own medicines. Just over twenty years later, when five enterprising medics attempted to establish a profit-sharing group practice in London that, if successful, would have undermined the traditional tripartite division of medicine in the capital, they did so by citing the example of Robert Boyle, he being 'a Master of many noble Preparations in Medicine'.[224] In the intervening years, it is probably fair to say that some strides had been made toward achieving this goal. Coxe himself, as we have seen, had been one of the first to set the ball rolling in 1669, when he published an anonymous pamphlet arguing that physicians, rather than apothecaries, should compound their own medicines. A year later, one of the College's own members, the librarian Christopher Merret (1614–1695), issued a further defence of this approach, citing, among others, the example of the celebrated nonconformist Richard Baxter with whom he had recently conversed on the subject.[225] Intriguingly, in a letter written by the College's apologist Henry Stubbe to Boyle in 1670, the former effectively laid the blame for the various attacks on the College's integrity emanating from the chymists and Royal Society on Boyle, citing the section in his *Usefulness of Natural Philosophy* (1663) as the source of their discontent.[226] The tensions exposed by these debates no doubt proved unwelcome to Boyle, who consistently sought to avoid the limelight on these occasions. It did not, however, lead to a cessation of interest in his writings and work which continued to evoke the admiration of a wide cross-section of the medical community both during his lifetime and after his death in 1691. Throughout his life Boyle was appealed to as an umpire in medical disputes,[227] became the subject of numerous dedications by physicians,[228] and was sought after as a patron by medical students.[229] His theories, moreover, were widely adopted and adapted by medical men in order to promote medical and natural philosophical innovation.[230] Boyle then clearly attracted a wide following in medical circles, and not just from those inclined toward or sympathetic to dissent. By the end of the century, support for Boyle's corpuscularian programme allied to his aversion for conventional physic and its prescribed organizational forms possessed, by and large, broad appeal and was not restricted to partisan lines. The single exception relates to an aspect of Boyle's natural philosophy that was to prove inordinately attractive to nonconformist medics, namely Boyle's overwhelming desire to conserve a role for the operation of spirit or immaterial substances in the sublunary world. The appeal of such thinking is neatly captured in the work of the 'empiric' Samuel Haworth, who specifically invoked Boyle's views on spirit and his corpuscularian approach to nature in order to establish a new etiology of disease and a reformed medical practice. Haworth, the son of an ejected minister, was conversant with most of the major scientific and medical developments of his day and argued in favour of revealed religion as a bulwark against Hobbesian atheism.[231] Other admirers of Boyle drawn from the ranks of the dissenting medical community regularly regaled him with instances of preternatural events in the knowledge that they would receive a warm reception. Concerns of this nature, especially those that helped to illuminate the bewilderingly fuzzy boundary between the natural and supernatural, or material and spiritual worlds, were to prove inordinately attractive to medical practitioners operating in and among Britain's dissenting communities. In practical terms, the exploration of this contested intellectual borderland found particular expression in the desire of dissenting physicians to defend the existence of witches and witchcraft, and to maintain the reality of a range of 'supernatural', or more properly preternatural, afflictions.[232] At the same time, the stance taken by this group of practitioners stands in stark contrast to the approach adopted by others within the medical profession, especially those of a strong Anglican or Tory bent, who consistently rejected the reality of such phenomena. Before looking at these developments in more detail, however, it is first necessary to turn our attention to this latter group, and to chart the various ways in which they too were becoming politicized and engaged in matters of state after the Restoration.

Notes

1. F. de la Boë Sylvius, *A New Idea of the Practice of Physic… Whereunto is Prefixed a Preface… by Dr. Mar[chamont] Nedham. Translated… by Richard Gower* (London, 1675), preface dated 13 October 1674.
2. *Acts of the Privy Council of England 1625–1626* (London, 1934), 452; *CSPD, 1636–1637*, 419–20. The pre-civil war state papers are replete with examples of London-based Catholic physicians, many protected by powerful patrons at court, supplying medical certificates for co-religionists. Typical was Dr William Gibbes, physician to Queen Henrietta Maria, who was repeatedly presented for recusancy in the early 1630s but continued nonetheless to practise at court as well as intervene in cases of imprisoned priests suspected of promoting the old religion; J. C. Jeaffreson (ed.), *Middlesex County Records*, 4 vols (London, Middlesex County Rec. Soc., 1886–92), iii,19, 25, 35, 38, 130, 131, 135, 136. Equally active in this respect was the royal physician Sir Thomas Cademan or Cadyman (*c.*1590–1651), who was elected a fellow of the London College of Physicians in 1630, and his colleague John Gifford (d.1647). For Cademan, see *ODNB*. For Gifford, see Munk, i, 114; *CSPD, 1628–1629*, 174, 409; *CSPD, 1631–1633*, 224, 268.

3. J. Gee, *The Foot out of the Snare* (London, 1624), X2r. Gee, who had flirted with Catholicism in Lancashire, was forced to recant the error of his ways following the revelation that he had been present in London in October 1623 at the incident known as the 'fatal vespers' when, following the collapse of a building in Blackfriars, almost one hundred Catholic worshippers died. *The Foot out of the Snare* was partly published as a form of penance, and went through four editions in a single year, 1624. All but the first edition contained the list of Catholic physicians. Three years after the publication of Gee's work, Peter Hambleton, a Roman Catholic priest masquerading as a physician, was arrested at Rochester; *CSPD, 1627–1628*, 367, 368. For Gee's identification in 1624 of, among others, the Scottish-born Catholic physician John Eglisham who was to play such a pivotal role in popularizing the idea that James I was murdered by his Protestant physicians, see A. Bellany and T. Cogswell, *The Murder of James I* (New Haven & London, 2015), 125–8.
4. J. Hall, *Select Observations on English Bodies* (London, 1657), A5v. Hall's patients, including their religious affiliations, are discussed in a modern edition of the physician's casebook; see J. Lane, *John Hall and His Patients: The Medical Practice of Shakespeare's Son-in-law* (Stroud, 1996).
5. [J. Bastwick], *Flagellum Pontificiis et Episcoporum Latialium* (Amsterdam?, 1635), 72. For Bastwick's authorship of this inflammatory work, copies of which had been sent to members of his *alma mater*, Emmanuel College, see the letter of Henry Smith to Dr Sancroft, Master of Emmanuel, asking him to investigate; CUL, MS Mm.I.45, 126.
6. BL, Add. MS 5829, fo. 17. There were two physicians of this name, probably brothers and both seemingly inclined to puritanism, operating in Essex at this time. Edward Ady, a former student of puritan Emmanuel College, Cambridge, was made an extra licentiate of the London College of Physicians in September 1631. He would appear to have been on friendly terms with the eminent puritan Daniel Rogers (1573–1652), who was minister of Ady's home parish of Wethersfield; T. Webster and K. Shipps (ed.), *The Diary of Samuel Rogers, 1634–1638* (Woodbridge and Rochester, NY, 2004), 13; Venn, i, 8; Munk, i, 204–5. For the puritan credentials of the witchcraft sceptic Thomas Ady, see my *Witchcraft, Witch-Hunting, and Politics in Early Modern England* (Oxford, 2016), 164–71.
7. RCPL, Annals, iii, 281, 350, 438; J. Bastwick, *The Second Part of the Book Called Independency Not Gods Ordinance* (London, 1645), 48–50.
8. H. Knollys, *The Life and Death of... Mr Hanserd Knollys* (London, 1692), 35–6. Knollys was following the biblical injunction laid down in James 5: 14–15. Further examples of this form of faith healing among the Baptists and other sects are discussed in K. V. Thomas, *Religion and the Decline of Magic: Studies in Popular Beliefs in Sixteenth- and Seventeenth Century England* (London, 1971), 126–7.
9. [J. Mowlin], *The Divell in Kent, or His Strange Delusion at Sandwitch* (London, 1647); W. Prynne, *A Fresh Discovery of Some Prodigious New Wandring-Blasing-Stars, & Firebrands Stiling Themselves New-Lights* (London, 1645), 13–14 [mispaginated in original].
10. SAL, MS 8200/2 [court minutes, 1651–1680]; WSA, D1/62 [marriage licence bonds and allegations, diocese of Salisbury, 1671–80]; F. Bate, *The Declaration of Indulgence 1672: A Study in the Rise of Organised Dissent* (London, 1908), Appendix 7, liii, liv; TNA,

PROB 11/327, fos 174v–175r [will of Samuel Fidsall, clothier, of Devizes, Wiltshire, 28 April 1668, pr. 9 June 1668]. Leigh's daughter Hannah married Francis Merewether (*c.*1674–1718), sheriff of Wiltshire in 1699–1700 and Whig MP for the county in 1701 and 1703–5. Leigh grew rich as one of four apothecaries, all supportive of the government, supplying medicines to the army and navy from a laboratory at the Savoy; WSA, 2106/90; 1656/2 [parish registers of St Mary's, Devizes, Wiltshire, 1659–1713, sub marriages, 19 October 1697]; S. Baston, *Baston's Case Vindicated, or a Brief Account of Some Evil Practices of the Present Commissioners for Sick and Wounded* (London, 1695), 47–50.

11. SAL, MSS 8200/2 and 3 [court minutes, 1651–1680; 1680–1694]; DRO, C/1/65 [Exeter City Archives, Quarter Sessions Order Book, 1660–72], fos 348v–349r; SHC, SW 23/423 [will of Henry Forty, gospel minister, of St Olave, Southwark, Surrey, 14 May 1692, pr. 13 January 1692/3]; *A Relation of the Miraculous Cure of Susannah Arch, of a Leprosy and Ptysick* (London, 1695); For Henry Forty, see especially https://www.abingdon.gov.uk/abingdon_people [accessed 15 June 2022]. For Susanna Arch, see note 88.
12. SAL, MS 8200/3 [court minutes, 1680–1694]; *Cal. Rev.*, 37; S. Wright, *The Early English Baptists, 1603–1649* (Woodbridge, 2006), 87–9.
13. SAL, MS 8200/3 [court minutes, 1680–1694]; For Gladman, see *ODNB*. Gladman is described as a sadler in the record of his son's apprenticeship. He was buried at St Botolph Bishopsgate, London, on 19 December 1688. In his will, made the same year, he mentions his son Jonathan, then apprenticed to Leigh, who did not subsequently pursue a career as an apothecary. Instead, he joined his brother as a trader with the East Indies and died as the commander of a ship bound for Guinea, where he became involved in a slave rebellion led by John Kabes; LMA, P69/BOT4/A/002/MS04516/001 [parish registers of St Botolph Bishopsgate, London, 1677–1701]; TNA, PROB 11/395, fos 29v–30r [will of John Gladman, gentleman, of St Botolph Bishopsgate, London, 21 April 1688, pr. 18 April 1689]; *A Collection of Voyages and Travels... in Six Volumes. Volume V* (3rd ed., London, 1746), 439.
14. SAL, MS 8200/3 [court minutes, 1680–1694]; M. Scott (ed.), *Apprenticeship Disputes in the Lord Mayor's Court of London 1573–1723* (London, BRS, Apprenticeship Series, vol.1, Part 2, 2016), 1177; *CSPD, 1697–1689*, 153. Hyde's Exeter premises were also an outlet for Bromfield's cure-all pill; M. Bromfield, *A Brief Discovery of the True Causes, Symptoms, and Effects of the... Scurvy* (London, 1678), 15.
15. P. Cary, *A Disputation between a Doctor and an Apothecary, or, a Reply to the New Argument of Dr R. Burthogge, MD. for Infant's Baptism* (London, 1684); *idem*, *A Solemn Call unto All That Would Be Owned as Christ's Faithful Witnesses... Or, A Discourse Concerning Baptism* (London, 1690); *idem*, *A Just Reply to Mr John Flavell's Arguments By Way of Answer to a Discourse Lately Published, Entituled, A Solemn Call* (London, 1690); J. Flavell, *The Whole Works of the Reverend Mr. John Flavel* (London, 1701), vol.1, 'The Life of Mr John Flavel', unpaginated. Cary was the brother-in-law of the radical physician Benjamin Worsley (d.1677) who may have inclined towards Socinianism. It has also been suggested that he may have been the brother of the mystical fifth monarchist cum alchemist, Mary Rand, née Cary (a sister Mary was baptized at Dartmouth in 1622); T. Leng, *Benjamin Worsley (1618–1677): Trade, Interest and the Spirit in Revolutionary England* (Woodbridge, 2008), 176–83.

16. For Price, see *Dictionary of Welsh Biography.*
17. G. Lyon Turner, 'Bunyan's Licence under the Indulgence', *Transactions of the Baptist Historical Society*, 6 (1919), 129–37.
18. Bunyan's meeting took place at the house of the ejected minister Nicholas Kestian or Kestin (d.1686). Richard Coleman's house was not licensed for worship until a few months after Bunyan's visit; Bate, *Declaration of Indulgence*, Appendix 7, lxxii.
19. D. L. Wykes, 'The Autobiographical Account of a Leicestershire Apothecary: Samuel Statham, *c.*1673–1732', *The Leicestershire Historian*, 3 (1990), 6–16. Josiah's brothers Jonathan (1646–1689) and David (1647–1715), who also traded as apothecaries, were prosecuted by the authorities for not attending their parish church in 1687; LRRO, ID 41/13/82.
20. T. Crosby, *The History of the English Baptists*, 4 vols (London, 1738–40), iii, 146–7. The aged Dr Roberts and his wife Prudence followed Keach to London and were buried in 1704 in Southwark where Keach had established his final ministry; LMA, P92/GEO/143 [parish registers of St George the Martyr, Southwark, Surrey, 1695–1732].
21. Interestingly, Thomas Okey was licensed to preach as an 'anabaptist' in the Devizes home of widow Fidsall, the mother-in-law of the London apothecary, Jonathan Leigh (above). It is tempting to speculate that Leigh may have played some part in assisting the relocation of Okey the apothecary to London sometime in the 1680s or early 1690s; Bate, *Declaration of Indulgence 1672*, Appendix VII, liv; WSA, 1597/2 [parish registers of St John the Baptist, Devizes, Wiltshire, 1653–1705].
22. For John Okey (b.1678), see TNA, ADM 1/5257/5, fos 5, 7; TNA, PROB 11/489, fos 1v–2r [will of John Okey, surgeon, of St Botolph without Aldgate, Middlesex, 16 March 1703/4, pr. 5 June 1706]. For Thomas Tertius Okey (b.1674), see Innes Smith, 173; D. Pearson, bookowners.online, sub Okey, Thomas Tertius; TNA, PROB 11/519, fo. 258v [will of Thomas Okey, surgeon to HM regiment of foot under Colonel William Evans, 27 June 1704, pr. 13 February 1710/11]. In the preface to his published thesis, Okey described himself as 'for many years engaged in various conflicts in the English navy'. The main work also contains a flattering reference to Dr William Salmon, the celebrated 'empiric' and nonconformist sympathizer, whom he lauded as a modern Hippocrates; T. T. Okey, *Disputatio Medica Inauguralis de Febre Quartana* (Harderwyck, 1704), B3r–v.
23. John Feake (d.1700) was the son of the fifth monarchist Christopher Feake (d.1683). He graduated MD from Leiden in 1670 and practised medicine at Salisbury in Wiltshire; Innes Smith, 83, Munk, i, 389; WSA, 1901/2 and 3 [parish registers of St Edmund's, Salisbury, Wiltshire, 1653–1699; 1699–1767]; P4/1700/8 [will of John Feak or Feake of Salisbury, Wiltshire, 29 September 1699, pr. 16 July 1700]. Nathaniel Whitehill (1670–1725 or 1726) was a member of the thriving Baptist community at Wantage which produced numerous preacher physicians (for which see below note 39); Munk, i, 510; TNA, PROB 11/607, fos 314r–v [will of Nathaniel Whithill, physician, of Wantage, Berkshire, 25 November 1725, pr. 16 February 1725/6]. For Griffiths, see below note 38.
24. John Clarke (1609–1676) may have attended Leiden before emigrating to Boston in Massachusetts in 1637. On returning to England in 1651, he established a Baptist congregation at Worcester House in London and was active as a proponent of fifth monarchist beliefs. He returned to Newport, Rhode Island, in 1661, having been

released from imprisonment in the wake of Venner's rising; B. S. Capp, *The Fifth Monarchy Men: A Study in Seventeenth-Century English Millenarianism* (London, 1972), 246. Clarke described himself as a physician in the frontispiece to his *Ill Newes from New England: Or, A Narrative of New-Englands Persecution* (London, 1652).

25. William Crabbe was instituted as a Baptist preacher at North Bradley in Wiltshire in 1654. The village was a centre of local Baptist activity and was infamous in the early years of the Restoration for its nonconformity. Crabbe and his co-religionists almost certainly owed a debt of gratitude to the local lord of the manor, William Trenchard, who was also a JP. Despite his radical background, Crabbe, a surgeon, acquired a licence to practise his faculty from the diocesan authorities in Salisbury in 1664. Ten years later, he, or his son of the same name, was forced to swear the oath of allegiance and supremacy following his arrest for attending a meeting of 'Anabaptists'; *CSPD, 1654*, 32, 54; E. Crittall (ed.), *VCH, Wiltshire. Vol. 8* (London, 1965), 228; WSA, D1/22/2, fo. 15v; D1/14/2/1/25.
26. Jewish by birth, Duveil became a Baptist preacher to a congregation in Gracechurch Street after multiple conversions. He took up medicine for his maintenance and 'was very skilful therein'; Crosby, *History of the English Baptists*, iii, 108–9.
27. Fabius, variously described as a practiser of physic, apothecary and chymist, was host to a Baptist meeting in his house in Everton, near Liverpool, Lancashire; O. Knott, 'The Baptists of Liverpool in the Seventeenth Century', *Baptist Quarterly*, 4 (1928–9), 219–22; D. Harley, '"Bred Up in the Study of That Faculty": Licensed Physicians in North-West England, 1660–1760', *Medical History*, 38 (1994), 408n. The Baptist minister-cum-physician Philip James (1668–1748) studied under Fabius while Fabius' son Daniel followed in his father's footsteps.
28. Richard Farmer (d.1688), variously described as a yeoman, gentleman, and trader in silk, was the head of a Baptist congregation at Arnesby in Leicestershire. He was imprisoned during Monmouth's Rebellion and faced constant persecution for his Baptist faith. Farmer, of nearby Kilby, left all his physic and surgery books to his daughter Anne; A. Betteridge, 'Early Baptists in Leicestershire and Rutland', *Baptist Quarterly*, 26 (1976), 211; LRRO, archdeaconry court of Leicester wills, will of Richard Farmer, gent, of Kilby, Leicestershire, 10 September 1687, pr. 1688.
29. For a short account of the medical career of the royal oculist Roger Grant (d.1724), see *ODNB*. According to the archiepiscopal licence awarded to Grant, of Westport in Wiltshire (where he was described in 1702 as a Baptist preacher) in 1704, he had long practised as an eye specialist. Among his detractors, Timothy Childe claimed in an anonymous publication in 1709 that Grant's medical practice was partly motivated by a desire to proselytize for the Baptist cause; *ODNB*, sub Grant, Roger; WSA, 1589/47 [parish registers of Westport St Mary, Wiltshire, 1678–1795]; LPL, VX 1A/10/377; VG 1/6, fo. 196v; Tenison 1, fo. 153; *Account of a Miraculous Cure of a Young Man in Newington* (London, 1709); LMA, MS 9172/122/103 [will of Roger Grant, esquire, of St Dunstan's, Stepney, Middlesex, 2 April 1724, pr. 9 April 1724]. Another Baptist who saw profit in medical specialization was William Atkins, a member of White's Alley congregation in London, who claimed a special gift, bordering on the miraculous, in the cure and treatment of gout; W. Atkins, *A Discourse Showing the Nature of Gout*

(London, 1694); Angus Library, Regent's Park College, Oxford, minutes of the church book of the White's Alley Baptist meeting, 1680–1700, fos 111r, 122r, 124r, 125r, 126r [which confirms that Atkins was living in Old Jewry, London, at the same time that he was accused of acting like a schismatic].

30. Philip James (1668–1748), who trained under Daniel Fabius (note 27), was a Baptist preacher and physician at Lichfield, Warwick, and Hemel Hempstead; W. Urwick, *Nonconformity in Hertfordshire* (London, 1884), 441–2.
31. Robert Joney or Joney (d.*c.*1703), a barber surgeon of Princes Risborough, Buckinghamshire, was 'a somewhat unstable pillar in the church of Cuddington or Ford' where he preached among local Baptists; A. H. J. Baines, 'The Signatories of the Orthodox Confession of 1679', *Baptist Quarterly*, 18 (1957–8), 80–1; W. Le Hardy (ed.), *Buckinghamshire Sessions Records. Vol.1 1678 to 1694* (Aylesbury, 1933), 294, 297.
32. Edward Ridgway, variously described as a 'chymist' and barber in contemporary sources, was minister to a Baptist congregation at Angel Alley in London from 1715 until his death in about 1749. He had been a resident of the parish of St Giles Cripplegate in London since at least 1696 when he married his first wife Jane Adderley; Joseph Ivimey, *A History of the English Baptists*, 4 vols (London, 1811–20), vol.3 (1823), 541; TNA, PROB 11/789, ff.355v–356r [undated will of Edward Ridgway, citizen and barber, of Hoxton in St Leonard's, Shoreditch, Middlesex, pr. 26 August 1751]; LMA, P69/TRI2/A/010/MS 09245 [parish registers of Holy Trinity, Minories, London, 1694–1713].
33. For Skinner, see Appendix 2 (a).
34. Edward Stennett (d.1705) was a former parliamentary army chaplain who led a Seventh Day Baptist congregation at Wallingford in Berkshire after the Restoration. According to his son Joseph, Edward took up medicine 'by the practice of which he was enabled to breed up his children, and to give them a liberal education'. This was achieved despite frequent persecution. On one occasion, a local clergyman, with whom Stennett had previously been on good terms, supplying medicine *gratis* to his family, was complicit in bringing him to trial at the Newbury assizes under the Conventicle Act. Edward's son Jehudah (d.1718) followed his father into medical practice, establishing himself as 'an eminent physician' at Henley upon Thames in Oxfordshire; Capp, *Fifth Monarchy Men*, 263; J. Stennett, *Works*, 4 vols (London, 1731–2), i, 4–5, 7.
35. According to a diocesan survey of medical practitioners conducted in 1665–6, Symonds, of Farringdon, Devon, was 'a person of no note or Learning, an Anabaptist, and one that keeps Conventicles, he is neither Licenced nor conformable'. He was reputed to hold Baptist meetings at Ottery St Mary. He may be the same as the John Simmins who was buried at Farringdon on 13 February 1672/3; LPL, MS 639, fos 306v, 398v; DRO, PR 362–364/33/1; E. A. O. Whiteman, 'The Episcopate of Dr Seth Ward, Bishop of Exeter (1662 to 1667) and Salisbury (1667 to 1688/9)', Ph. D. (Oxford, 1951), 142–143; DRO, 3167A/PR/1/1 [parish registers of Farringdon, Devon].
36. Wright (1623–1703) practised medicine at Maidstone in Kent and suffered frequent bouts of imprisonment for his beliefs. On one occasion in 1684 he appealed to the Privy Council to allow him his liberty in order to 'exercise his faculty of Midwifury'. Wright was a close friend and business associate of the Jeakes of Rye in Sussex. He or his son,

described only as Dr Wright, may have been practising in Rye in 1696; Crosby, *History*, iii, 116; J. S. Cockburn (ed.), *Calendar of Assize Records, Kent Indictments, Charles II 1676–1688* (London, 1997), 143; TNA, PC 2/70, 200–1; M. Hunter and A. Gregory (eds), *An Astrological Diary of the Seventeenth Century: Samuel Jeake of Rye 1652–1699* (Oxford, 1988), 238–40, 257; ESxRO, FRE 5301 [Samuel Jeake the younger to his wife, Elizabeth, 26 March 1696]; 5302 [same to same, 4 April 1696].

37. Crosby, *History*, iii, 124–5; FSL, V.a.293, fo. 82r. More probably Wilmot the healer was Samuel Wilmot, brother of the preacher, whose shop in Hook Norton was an outlet for the remedies of fellow Baptist and London pillmonger George Jones (for whom, see below note 43). Jones claimed to have cured Wilmot's daughter Mary of the evil and scurvy with his pills; *George Jones of London, Student in the Art of Physick and Chyrurgery* (London?, 1675?), 4; *George Jones of Hatton Garden, Holborn... His Book of Mighty Cures* (London?, 1675?), 20. Given the chymical interests of so many early Baptists, the Wilmots of Oxfordshire may have been related to the chymist Wilmot of Wood Street in London who was employed as a 'refiner' by the earl of Pembroke in 1662; FSL, V.a.292, fos 69r, 75v, 84v.
38. Griffiths briefly attended Oxford in 1658 but did not graduate. He was made an extra licentiate of the London College of Physicians in 1670. Griffiths, who died and was buried in London in 1696, left three boxes of Peruvian Bark, a fever cure, to his wife and daughter which he would appear to have accessed via a Bristol apothecary (James Freeman) trading at Cadiz; Foster, ii, 610; Munk, i, 359; LMA, P69/MGT1/A/001/MS04346/001 [parish registers of St Margaret, Lothbury, London, 1558–1736]; TNA, PROB 11/430, fos 236v–237v [will of John Griffith, physician, of Bristol, 25 January 1695/6, pr. 5 March 1695/6]. A radical Whig, Griffith also worked alongside Congregational colleagues in securing ecclesiastical medical licences; see below ???.
39. Conyers Congrave, like Richard Coleman, was an early convert to the Baptists in Leicester in the 1650s and a leader of the sect thereafter. He was licensed to practise surgery in the diocese of Lincoln in 1662; R. A. McKinley (ed.), *VCH. Leicestershire. Vol. 4* (London, 1858), 391; LAO, Dioc/Sub/I, fo. 253v. George Smith was a leading member of the congregation of the London Baptist Robert Jemmett (d.1718) and was licensed to practise surgery in the diocese of London in 1700. Both men were close friends of the Helmontian physician Robert Johnson (above 182); TNA, PROB 11/521, fos 140v–141r [will of George Smith, surgeon, of London, 28 November 1705, pr. 28 May 1711]; Bloom and James, 69. Samuel Taverner, the son of Captain Samuel Taverner (1621–1692), the radical Baptist preacher and captain of Deal Castle in the 1650s, was licensed to practise surgery in the diocese of Canterbury in 1680; CCAL, DCb/L/R/23, fo 52a. For Crabbe and Grant see notes 25 and 29 above.
40. LPL, FII/20/15a-d; F1/D, fo. 217. Clarke served as a deacon in the Wantage Baptist church and was an associate of the pastor Robert Keate and London businessman William Kiffin, who had links with the town. Clarke himself had attempted to secure a licence to practise medicine from the bishop of Salisbury in 1664 and 1667. Despite securing numerous testimonials, including that of the rector of All Cannings in Wiltshire, no licence would appear to have been issued; TNA, C 111/190/31; WSA, D1/14/1/1b, nos 14, 15, 98. Manasseh King was the son of the Baptist preacher of the same name who operated from a base at Coventry where he died in 1696. Manasseh

King Jnr later set up in practice at Newbury in Berkshire where he was admitted to the common council in January 1688 following the purge of the corporation; Crosby, *History*, iii, 115; F. Bate, *The Declaration of Indulgence 1672: A Study in the Rise of Organised Dissent* (London, 1908), Appendix 7, lii; W. Money, *The History of the Ancient Town and Borough of Newbury in the County of Berks* (Oxford, 1887), 309–10, 317; Berkshire RO, D/A1/201/35 [administration of the will of Manasses King, physician, of Newbury, Berkshire, 1696]. As for Boyce, he later returned to Wantage, where he succeeded to Clarke's practice; WSA, P23/406 [will of Timothy Boyce, physician, of Wantage, Berkshire, pr. 1721].

41. A. Matthews, 'A Precious Pearl', appended to R. Matthews, *The Unlearned Alchymist* (London, 1663), 1–2; G. Starkey, *The Admirable Efficacy, and Almost Incredible Virtue of True Oyl, which is made of Sulphur-vive*, in W. Cooper (ed.), Collectanea Chymica: A Collection of Ten Several Treatises in Chymistry (London, 1684), 150. The latter has a separate titlepage, dated 1683, and is a reprint of the original pamphlet first published in 1660, the sole surviving copy of which is in the Library of Congress, Washington DC. For Matthews' links to the Baptists and other radical sects, see above 138, 182. Hobson suffered long periods of imprisonment after the Restoration on suspicion of plotting against the restored Stuarts.
42. Jones, originally from Gloucestershire, had settled in London in about 1669. In his will, made in 1676, he left the profits of the residue of his estate to be used 'for the preserving upholding and incouraging the service and worship of God and the ministry thereof in and amongst the Church congregation or People of Christ though ignorantly called Anabaptists meeting now in Glassehouse Yard in Goswell Street in the parish of St Buttolph without Aldersgate'; TNA, PROB 11/353, fos 47r–48r [will of George Jones, gent, of Hatton Garden, St Andrew Holborn, Middlesex, 20 November 1676; pr. 22 January 1676/7]. Some time around 1674, Jones published *Hell's Cabal, or the Devilish Plots of Envy and Malice, against Dr Jones, and His Friendly Pills Discovered*, in which he attacked his four main rivals whose names are thinly disguised. The two Quakers were identified as William Salmon and Richard Fletcher who with Matthew Bromfield and Humphrey Nendick were viciously traduced as servants of the Devil. Salmon (1644–1713) was probably a Quaker sympathizer rather than a member. Fletcher, on the other hand, was a Quaker and a Helmontian, who compared the pretensions of the College of Physicians to the infallibility of the Pope for compelling men to obey their dictates; TNA, RG6/499 [register of Quaker burials, London and environs, 1660–1700], 22 December 1672 and 23 October 1680]; R. Fletcher, *The Character of a True Physician* (London, 1676), 20–1; *idem*, *Starkey Revived, or, Collections out of Nature's Explication, and Helmont's Vindication, Being a Short Examination of the State of Physick as Now Practised* (London, 1676).
43. There is no definitive proof that John Russell was a Baptist. An astrological physician and author of almanacs (he was on friendly terms with John Partridge), Russell's marriage to Jones' widow, whom he accused of living beyond her means, led to a bitter dispute with the trustees of the Glasshouse Yard meeting who contested Jones' will. Russell was also an associate of the prominent iatrochemist Christopher Packe whom he mentions in his will and who in turn mentioned Russell's son-in-law Samuel Warburton (d.1709) in his own will of 1714; B. S. Capp, *Astrology and the Popular*

Press: English Almanacs 1500–1800 (London & Boston, 1979), 328; J. Partridge, *Merlinus Liberatus. An Almanack... 1697* (London, 1697), C7; TNA, PROB 11/441, fos 260r–261v [will of John Russell, physician, of St Andrew Holborn, Middlesex, 18 March 1696/7, pr. 13 November 1697]; Angus Library, Regent's Park College, Oxford, Church Book of the Glasshouse Yard Baptist meeting, 1680–1740, 195, 199, 201, 210, 229; TNA, C6/305/28; TNA, PROB 11/541, fos 267v–272r [will of Christopher Packe, licentiate physician, of St Giles without Cripplegate, London, 1 April 1714; pr. 9 August 1714].

44. For Russell's activities as a leading London Baptist, see the article by Michael Davies in the *ODNB*, which makes no mention of his passion for chymistry. In addition to subscribing to Christopher Packe's edition of the *Works* (1687) of the Dutch iatrochemist Johann Rudolph Glauber (1604–1670), Russell signed letters testimonial on behalf of the chymical physician George Deane of Wokingham in 1695. In 1693, both he and Deane wrote to the Helmontian Packe (for whom, see above 210), commending the virtues of his various preparations. He was living in the Barbican at the time, from where in 1695 he advertised the merits of his pills in the cure of venereal disease; LPL, VX 1A/10/286/1–2; C. Packe, *Mineralogia, or, An Account of the Preparation, Manifold Vertues, and Uses of a Mineral Salt, Both in Physick and Chyrurgery* (London, 1693), 40–3, 44–5; J. Jackson, *Enchiridion Medicum Theoretico-Practicum; sive Tractatus de Morborum Theoria & Praxi* (London, 1695), 246.
45. For Emes, see *ODNB*. He was described as a 'chymist' in the record of his burial at Bunhill Fields; LMA, P69/GIS/A/002/MS06419/013 [parish registers of St Giles Cripplegate, London, 1703–1711].
46. R. Johnson, *Enchiridion Medicum; or a Manual of Physick* (London, 1684), A2r; *idem*, *Praxis Medicinae Reformata: Or, The Practice of Physick Reformed* (London, 1700), x; TNA, PROB 11/492, fos 284r–285v [will of Robert Johnson, gent, of St Clement Danes, Middlesex, 27 July 1706, pr. 7 February 1706/7]; R[obert] Johnson, *An Almanack for the Year 1683* (London, 1683), preface by William Salmon; Scott (ed.), *Apprenticeship Disputes in the Lord Mayor's Court of London 1573–1723*, 512. The tangled web of intellectual and religious networks inhabited by Salmon, including those of his Bristol wife Anne, are fully explored in a forthcoming study of Salmon by Jonathan Barry. Johnson was the son of a Somerset clergyman whose fitness to hold the cure was questioned by the diocesan authorities in 1636; Somerset Heritage Centre, D\P\PET.S/2/1/1 [parish registers of South Petherton, Somerset, 1574–1674]; D\D\Ca 310 [10 November 1636].
47. P. Elmer, 'Medicine, Science and the Quakers: the "Puritanism-Science" Debate Reconsidered', *Journal of the Friends Historical Society*, 54 (1981), 265–86. Space here prevents a full discussion of the wealth of new evidence that I have since found relating to the Quakers and medical practice. Much of it confirms the situation depicted in my early article, particularly in relation to the almost total obsession on the part of early Friends with chymical physic. I hope to publish on this subject in due course.
48. See, for example, the case of John van Rabat, who was examined and rejected, both as member and doctor, in Somerset in 1692; C. Morland (ed.), *The Somersetshire Quarterly Meeting of the Society of Friends, 1668–1699* (Woking, Somerset Rec. Soc., vol. 75, 1978), 218–21, 226.

49. C. Marshall, *A Plain and Candid Relation of the Nature, Use, and Dose of Several Approved Medicines* (London, 1670; 2nd ed., 1681), 8 [list of outlets]; T. Chalk (ed.), *The Journal, Together with Sundry Epistles and Other Writings of Charles Marshall* (London, 1844), xxvi; B. S. Snell (ed.), *The Minute Book of the Monthly Meeting of the Society of Friends for the Upperside of Buckinghamshire, 1669–1690* (High Wycombe, Buckinghamshire Rec. Soc., vol. 1, 1937), 221 and n.
50. H. Sampson, 'Dr Faber and His Celebrated Cordial', *Isis*, 34 (1942–3), 472–96. In this dispute, Faber's opponent insinuated that he had joined the sect for mercenary ends and to further his practice. A similar accusation was made against the astrological physician and Quaker sympathizer, William Salmon; see W. Salmon, *An Apology for the Innocency and Justice of the Quakers Cause* (London, 1674), 45.
51. N. Smith, *The Quakers Spiritual Court Proclaim'd* (London, 1668), 39–40.
52. In this pamphlet, the Quaker apologist characterized Smith as one who frequently spoke of 'the power of conjurations, and how the devil might be raised, and what he could do, as if he had great knowledge in such Diabolical Acts'. He was also reputed to possess great skill in palmistry and other magic arts, which he had briefly practised in Ireland in the 1650s; J. R., *The Innocent Assemblies, and Good Order of the People of God (called Quakers) Vindicated* (London?, 1669), A2v; 23. The author, J. R., was probably the Quaker physician John Raunce who practised at High Wycombe in Buckinghamshire (see below). In 1650, he had published a scathing attack on judicial astrology which he condemned as a form of witchcraft; J. Raunce, *Astrologia Accusata Pariter & Condemnata. Or the Diabolical Art of Judicial Astrologie, Receiving the Definitive Sentence of Final Condemnation* (London, 1650). The Quaker, Dr Gray, was in all probability Isaac Gray or Grey, physician and gentleman, who was tried at the Old Bailey for refusing to swear the oath of allegiance in June 1662. One of his fellow prisoners on this occasion was the Quaker John Bolton, a London goldsmith, who published a second rebuttal of Nathaniel Smith in 1669; Besse, *Sufferings*, i, 369–73; J. Bolton, *A Justification of the Righteous Judgement of God on Nathaniel Smith* (London?, 1669).
53. TNA, SP 29/100/110 [John Laurence of Wramplingham to Faber, 24 July 1664].
54. FHL, Martin Mason MSS, fos 63, 80. Similar intentions would appear to have underpinned the efforts of two apothecaries, in combination with local surgeons, barbers and others, to drive the Quaker apothecary Richard Pearce out of the city of Limerick in Ireland; Besse, *Sufferings*, ii, 463.
55. LPL, MS 639, fos 211r, 212v, 213v; TNA, PC 2/63, fos 64v, 67r, 72r; Besse, *Sufferings*, i, 80. Llewellyn (1616–1682), one of the leaders of the 'loyal' party in Wycombe, was responsible for waging a long and bitter campaign against dissenters and their sympathizers in the town, provoking, in the process, deep divisions within the ranks of the corporation; P. D. Halliday, *Dismembering the Body Politic: Partisan Politics in England's Towns 1650–1730* (Cambridge, 1998), 119–20; R. W. Greaves (ed.), *The First Ledger Book of High Wycombe* (London, Buckinghamshire Rec. Soc., vol. 11, 1947), 184–205. In 1672, following the release of Raunce, Llewellyn, who had a reputation as a poet, published *Wickham Wakened: or, the Quaker's Madrigal* (1672). In a note on a copy of this work in the Bodleian Library, the Oxford antiquarian Anthony Wood has written that the subject of Llewellyn's ribald verse was one 'Hirze',

a Quaker, who 'takes much from Lluellin's practice'; Bodl., Wood 645 (21). I have not been able to trace Hirze, who must have been either a colleague of Raunce's, or perhaps an error in transcription for Raunce himself.

56. R. Gell, *EIPHNIKON: or, a Treatise of Peace Between the Two Visible Divided Parties* (London, 1660), a3r. Gell, of course, had earlier been an advocate of the 'miraculous' stroker Matthew Coker, part of whose mission to heal the sick, like that of the Irishman Greatrakes, was tinged with a desire to promote religious reconciliation among Protestants; P. Elmer, *The Miraculous Conformist: Valentine Greatrakes, the Body Politic, and the Politics of Healing in Restoration Britain* (Oxford, 2013), 75–6.
57. Smith, *Quakers Spiritual Court Proclaim'd*, 10; A. Marshall, 'Colonel Thomas Blood and the Restoration Political Scene', *The Historical Journal*, 32 (1989), 563. Charles II was sufficiently alarmed by these claims to enquire whether any Quakers had died of the plague in 1665. On being told that they had suffered as others, the king was reassured that the punitive policies adopted toward the sect could not be used by his opponents as a stick to beat his government; W. G. Bell, *The Great Plague of London in 1665* (London, 1951), 181.
58. The case for a dissenting medical tradition was first made by William Birken in his 'The Dissenting Tradition in English Medicine of the Seventeenth and Eighteenth Centuries', *Medical History*, 39 (1995), 197–218. What follows is an attempt to build on Birken's work and to demonstrate more fully just how the dissenters developed networks of support and in the process created a separate medical identity.
59. My revised figures for the first two categories, with lists, are included in Appendix 2 (a) and (b). I cite numerous examples of the third type—the sons of godly laymen and politicians—elsewhere throughout this chapter.
60. *Cal. Rev.*, 85; E. Calamy, *An Abridgment of Mr Baxter's History of His Life and Times. With an Account of the Ministers, &c who were Ejected after the Restauration of King Charles II*, 2 vols (2nd ed., London, 1713), ii, 311–12.
61. Stoddon described himself thus on the titlepage of a manuscript collection of sermons entitled *Gemitus Sanctorum* (1702), the original of which is in the Congregational Library, London. For Stoddon's reputation as a specialist in treating the distracted, see P. Elmer, *Witchcraft, Witch-Hunting, and Politics in Early Modern England* (Oxford, 2016), 209 and n.
62. This is the essential thrust of my account of the Greatrakes affair in 1665–6.
63. *Cal. Rev.*, 511; Calamy, *Abridgment*, ii, 293. For Warren, and his cordial relations with puritanically inclined members of the London College of Physicians, see above 188 and n.
64. *Cal. Rev.*, 197; Calamy, *Abridgment*, ii, 296. It may also have helped Firmin's case that he was reluctant to accept deprivation in 1662 and continued to attend his local church for monthly sermons thereafter. He, too, dispensed medicines to the poor *gratis*, and charged very moderate fees to the better off. His son, Nathaniel, and grandson, John, both practised medicine; for the former, see Appendix 2(a).
65. *Cal. Rev.*, 387; J. E. B. Mayor (ed.), *The Life of Matthew Robinson* (Cambridge, 1856); *ODNB*, sub Robinson, Matthew; J. Raine (ed.), *Depositions from the Castle of York Relating to Offences Committed in the Northern Counties in the Seventeenth Century* (Durham, Surtees Soc., vol. 40, 1861), 224–5. Among those prosecuted with Robinson for practising medicine without a licence was the former curate of Tong in Yorkshire,

Richard Coore. This prosecution was almost certainly part of a wider campaign, initiated by a group of qualified physicians in Yorkshire, the majority ardent Anglicans, to root out illicit practice and what they saw as the encroachments of empirics; see below 306 n.93.

66. *Cal. Rev.*, 142; F. Baily (ed.), *An Account of the Revd John Flamsteed, the First Astronomer Royal* (London, 1835), 11. Flamsteed, who found no relief from Cranwell's ministrations, was eventually sent by his father to Greatrakes in Ireland for cure. Among Cranwell's other patients was the godly minister John Hieron (1608–1682), whose death he attributed to 'a decay of Nature, whereby his Blood was stagnated'; R. Porter, *The Life of Mr John Hieron* (London, 1691), 53. It is possible that Cranwell's impulse to take up medicine after the Restoration was partly motivated by his deep-seated desire for a moderate settlement in church and state. In 1661, for example, he made a plea for moderation along the lines laid down at Breda by Charles II, whom he described as one 'who seeketh to heal by a gentle hand'; L. Cranwell, *The Holding the Bishop and Presbyter Equall, Vindicated from Heresie* (London, 1661), A2v.

67. *ODNB*; *Cal. Rev.*, 223–4; Innes Smith, 94; *CSPD, 1668–1669*, 73, 78, 91, 269, 342; H. Bourne, *The History of Newcastle upon Tyne. Or, the Ancient and Present State of the Town* (Newcastle, 1736), 240–1. Gilpin and his co-religionists were undoubtedly encouraged in the use of the barber surgeons' hall by the fact that it lay outside the immediate jurisdiction of the town's magistrates; ibid., 137. The dissenters' virtual monopoly of medical services in Newcastle at this time, spearheaded as it was by Gilpin, is further illustrated by the marriage of the latter's daughter, Dorothy (1668–1708), to the physician and nonconformist Jabez Cay (d.1702). For Cay, see above 201.

68. For Pringle, who was reported preaching with Gilpin at the barber surgeons' hall in Newcastle in November 1668, see *Cal. Rev.*, 400; *CSPD, 1668–1669*, 73. In common with many of his ilk (see above 129–31), Pringle, shortly after being deprived of his living, took the precaution of obtaining a licence to practise medicine from the College of Physicians in London. For Pell, see *Cal. Rev.*, 385; *ODNB*; Calamy, *Abridgment*, ii, 288–90.

69. Innes Smith, 76; *Cal. Rev.*, 174. Durant's father, William, assisted Gilpin in conducting conventicles at the barber surgeons' hall in Newcastle. In addition to his father, John dedicated his Leiden thesis on erysipelas to the renowned Dutch physician and professor Franciscus de la Boë Sylvius, and his uncle, John Durant (1620–1689), a congregational minister at Canterbury. Interestingly, the nonconformists in Canterbury seem to have been equally active in promoting medical talent from amongst their ranks; see above 214–15. Shortly after his return to England, and following a recent visit to Robert Boyle in London, Durant wrote to the natural philosopher with detailed observations on the mining of local coal and ores and a recent coalfire in the vicinity of Newcastle. These were later published in the *Philosophical Transactions*; Boyle, *Correspondence*, iv, 379–81 [Durant to Boyle, 9 February 1674].

70. For Bromfield, see *Cal. Rev.*, 77. Lomax set up as a physician, surgeon, and apothecary at nearby North Shields; *Cal. Rev.*, 327. Rule acquired a Leiden MD in 1665 and, like other puritan physicians, demonstrated a keen interest in rickets which was the subject

of his thesis. The work was dedicated, among others, to the nonconformist physician John Micklethwaite, a prominent figure in the affairs of the London College of Physicians after 1660; *Cal. Rev.*, 420; *Innes Smith*, 200; *ODNB*, sub Rule, Gilbert.

71. For Manlove, see *ODNB*. Gilpin preached Manlove's funeral sermon, in the preface to the published version of which one J. T. praised Manlove for his precocious talents as both a preacher and a doctor; R. Gilpin, *The Comforts of Divine Love Preach'd upon the Occasion of the Much Lamented Death of the Reverend Mr Timothy Manlove* (London, 1700). Manlove was admitted as an extra licentiate of the Royal College of Physicians at London on 1 June 1694; Munk, i, 509.
72. Between 1660 and 1699, 97 Englishmen graduated MD from Leiden and a further 49 from Utrecht. Six more Englishmen graduated MD from the Dutch medical school at Harderwyck between 1674 and 1697.
73. Birken, 'Dissenting Tradition in English Medicine', 200–3.
74. RCPL, Annals, iv, fo. 90a. Warren was examined on 25 June 1667 and admitted to practise as an extra-licentiate on 31 July 1667; Munk, i, 355. He was also on good terms with Charles Goodall, who later played a key role in defending the integrity of the College against interlopers and probably shared Warren's religious disposition. In an undated letter, Warren wrote to Goodall enclosing a receipt for a medicine that the latter presumably intended to forward to Robert Boyle; Royal Society Library, Boyle Letters, vol. 5, fos 117–18.
75. *Cal. Rev.*, 317; DRO, PR 518, sub Hennock; I. Mortimer, 'Index of Medical Licentiates, Applicants, Referees and Examiners in the Diocese of Exeter, 1586–1783', *Transactions of the Devonshire Association*, 136 (2004), 119. Law's application, dated 6 October 1661, refers to his 'having for divers years last past addicted himself to the study and practice of physicke' and was supported by Joshua Bowden, vicar of Ashburton (ejected 1662, though he subsequently conformed) and Robert Wolcombe, rector of Moreton Hampstead (ejected 1662).
76. *Cal. Rev.*, 251; LPL, FII/3/277; F1/C, fo. 107v; Bodl., Tanner MS 54, fo. 2r. Westley had in fact established a long-standing reputation as a physician some time before the Restoration; see J. H. Bettey, 'Contrasts among the Dorset Clergy during the Seventeenth Century', *Notes and Queries for Somerset and Dorset*, 32 (1986–1990), 849.
77. Ichabod acted as a referee for Nathaniel Blinman, the son of an ejected Somerset minister; see below note 160. Isaac signed letters for William Gostwick of Reading in 1681; LPL, VX 1A/10/165/1–2.
78. Du Moulin provided testimonials for Maturin Montallier (London, 1669), Daniel Monke (Nuneaton, Warwickshire, 1675) and Thomas Broomhall (Middlewich, Cheshire, 1677); Bloom and James, 61; LPL, VX 1A/10/77; W. F. Irvine (ed.), *Marriages Licences Granted Within the Archdeaconry of Chester in the Diocese of Chester* (Lancashire and Cheshire Rec. Soc., vol. 69, 1914), 186. As an Oxford don, he was also responsible for providing a testimonial on behalf of the well-travelled mountebank John Ponteus or Puntaeus (d.1674), who was seeking a surgeon's licence from the University in 1649; Bodl., UOA, NEP/supra/Reg Qa [Register of Congregation], fo. 170v.
79. Letters testimonial on behalf of: Francis Bogas (Dickleburgh, Norfolk, 1679); Thomas Fairfax (Needham Market, Suffolk, 1687); Stephen Everard (Faversham, Kent, 1687);

LPL, VX 1A/10/121; VX 1A/10/239/1–2; FII/28/28a-e. For the nonconformist associations of Fairfax and Everard, and those of Hulse's colleague Joshua Palmer, who also supported the applications of the same two men, see below, note 88.

80. Letters testimonial on behalf of: John Allen (Kidderminster, Worcestershire, 1673–4) and John Chester (Ewell, Surrey, 1683); LPL, VX 1A/10/47/3; FII/24/15. Allen may have carried the taint of nonconformity. In 1665, the curate provided a certificate confirming that Allen's wife had given thanks after birth in the prescribed fashion in the parish church of Kidderminster; WRO, 795.02/2302/11/2491. For Chester, father and son, see Appendix 2 (a) and (b). For Morton, a senior figure in the London College of Physicians after 1679 who was widely respected in dissenting circles, see *ODNB*; Munk, i, 398–400; R. R. Trail, 'Richard Morton (1637–1698)', *Medical History*, 14 (1970), 166–74.
81. Letters testimonial on behalf of: John Allen (above) and Jonathan Kestin (Fleckney, Leicestershire, 1691); LPL, 1A 10/47/2; 1A 10/272. For Sampson, who developed an extensive practice among fellow nonconformists and harboured ambitions of publishing a history of dissent in which he hoped to portray his co-religionists as 'a Considerable... injured & misjudged people', see *ODNB* and Appendix 2 (a).
82. Stoddon signed letters testimonial on behalf of John Skinner of Brompton Ralph, Somerset, in 1686; LPL, VX 1A/10/232/1–3. For Stoddon, see Appendix 2 (a) and above 185.
83. Innes Smith, 30, 58, 66, 102. The most prominent of the four was his half-brother Nehemiah Grew (1641–1712), who graduated MD from Leiden in 1671. In addition to Sampson, Grew dedicated his thesis on nervous fluids to his father Obadiah and the physician Abraham Clifford, both of whom had suffered the loss of their livings in 1662. Of Sampson's other protégés, Samuel Cromwell (MD Leiden, 1692) was almost certainly related to the ejected Nottinghamshire minister, John Cromwell. Likewise, Edmund Devis (MD Utrecht, 1692) was well connected in dissenting circles in his native Warwick. Joseph Bridges' dissenting credentials are suggested by the fact that he was responsible, in the year of his graduation at Utrecht (MD 1697), for publishing an English translation of Nehemiah Grew's *A Treatise of the Nature and Use of the Bitter Purging Salt* (London, 1697), which carried the imprimatur of the President and censors of the College of Physicians in London.
84. Floyde, who graduated MD at Cambridge in 1661, practised medicine at Ipswich in Suffolk, where he acted as mentor to the sons of two former ministers (both ejected) and local residents, Robert Brinsley (d.1684) and Thomas Fones (1642–1679); Innes Smith, 30, 86. See also below Appendix 2 (b).
85. Richardson, who served as the minister to the English church at Leiden between 1670 and 1675, was the subject of dedications by William Lovell (MD 1673) and John Hodgson of Yorkshire (MD 1677); Innes Smith, 144. I suspect that the latter was either the son of, or closely related to, the Yorkshire radical and medical practitioner, Captain John Hodgson, who was almost certainly known to Richardson because of their joint engagement in plots against the government of Charles II in the 1660s and 1670s. I discuss Richardson's involvement in these activities, and the more general issues arising from the close connections between medicine and subversion after 1660 more fully above 199–201.

86. *ODNB*; *Cal. Rev.*, 283; Innes Smith, 123; Munk, i, 397–8.
87. Innes Smith, 176; Munk, i, 429; *Cal. Rev.*, 141; In his will of 1672, Archdale Palmer made bequests to five dissenting ministers who were all active in Leicestershire and had formerly been ejected at the Restoration; TNA, PROB 11/342, fos 499v–500v [will of Archdale Palmer, esquire, of Wanlip, Leicestershire, 3 April 1672; pr. 20 September 1673].
88. In 1687, Hulse and Palmer were joint signatories to the applications of Thomas Fairfax, of Needham Market, Suffolk, and Stephen Everard of Faversham, Kent; LPL, VX 1A/10/239/1–2; Sancroft, fo. 268v [Fairfax]; LPL, FII/28/2/28a-e [Everard]. Fairfax (b.1654) was the son of the nonconformist preacher, John Fairfax (d.1700), who was ejected from the living of Barking, adjacent to Needham Market, in 1662 and was ten years later issued with a licence to preach there under the terms of the Declaration of Indulgence; *Cal. Rev.*, 189; *ODNB*, sub Fairfax, John. Everard, too, may have been a nonconformist. In addition to Hulse and Palmer, his application was signed by a third physician, Charles Nichols (d.1718), son of the celebrated dissenting minister of the same name. Nichols, who held an MD from Caen (1679) and a licence from the College of Physicians, almost certainly shared his father's religious affiliations. In 1695, he attested to the miraculous cure of one of his former patients, Susanna Arch, a member of the nonconformist congregation of Thomas Beverley in London. The incident is recounted by Jane Shaw, who mistakenly refers to Nichols as an apothecary; *Cal. Rev.*, 365–6; Munk, i, 476; Venn, iii, 254 [who confuses the father with the son]; *A Relation of the Miraculous Cure of Susannah Arch*, 13, 19; J. Shaw, *Miracles in Enlightenment England* (New Haven & London, 2006), 132–3.
89. Innes Smith, 177; Munk, i, 497; Venn, iii, 302. For Woodhouse and his Staffordshire academy, which he oversaw from 1676 to 1697, see *Cal. Rev.*, 544. William Palmer Snr (d.1692 or 1693) carried on the family tradition of providing financial and other support to local dissenting ministers. In his will of 1692, he made provision for four nonconformist preachers, all of whom had lost their livings at the Restoration; TNA, PROB 11/415, fos 197v–199r [will of William Palmer, esquire, of Wanlip, Leicestershire, 12 April 1692; pr. 14 July 1693].
90. Bodl., Rawlinson Letters 109, fo. 83r [J[ohn] O[liver] to John Thornton, chaplain to William Russell, earl of Bedford, 19 July 1661]. I identify John Oliver as the author on the grounds that his letter is signed and dated from 'Mont', i.e. Montacute in Somerset, where Oliver resigned as vicar in 1661; *Cal. Rev.*, 373. I have not discovered any evidence to suggest that he did in fact take up the study and practice of medicine. For Oliver's friendship with John Beale, whom he was unable to forgive for opting to conform in 1662, see Elmer, *Miraculous Conformist*, 146.
91. See Appendix 2 (c).
92. TNA, PROB 11/340, fos 51r–55r [will of Matthew Turner, apothecary, of St Benet Gracechurch, London, dated 1 June 1671, 5 June 1671 and 15 February 1671/2, pr. 23 September 1672].
93. For Frost's extensive dissenting connections, see Appendix 2 (c), under Thomas Wilson. Frost, of Suffolk, like Cornish, set up as a physician. Both men legitimated their practice through the acquisition of a licence from the College of Physicians.

94. *Cal. Rev.*, 234; TNA, SP 29/88/59; Bodl., Carte MS 35, fo. 28; MS 219, fo. 61. Given the importance of Holland as a refuge for English medical practitioners (discussed more fully below), it is worth noting that Wilson (probably not his real name) was reported by Birkenhead to have recently spent time in Holland from whence he had returned 'so hotter'.
95. *CSPD, 1661–1662*, 186. Woodroffe's brother-in-law, John Fletcher of Dublin, was also examined and confessed that Woodruffe, the youngest son of Timothy Woodroffe, minister of Kingsland, Herefordshire, was an evil liver and 'a great grief to his family'; ibid. Woodroffe (b.1632), who briefly spent time at Oxford without graduating, was granted a licence to practise medicine by the College of Physicians in 1653. He subsequently practised medicine in St Albans, Hertfordshire, and Berkshire where he was licensed by the dean of Salisbury in 1674; Foster, iv, 1676; Munk, i, 268; WSA, D5/9/2, fo. 1r.
96. Somerset Heritage Centre, Q/SR/104/30–31. Interestingly, just a month before the incident described here, John Davis of Portbury was licensed to practise physic and surgery in the diocese of Bath and Wells, possibly as a convenient cover for acts of subversion; Somerset Heritage Centre, DD\Bs/39, 1 October 1663.
97. *CSPD, 1665–1666*, 267–8. A year later, Ker or Carr was mentioned in a letter written by one John Thomson, of Rotterdam, to John Drysdale, a prisoner in England, where Thomson informed his son-in-law that Ker, the surgeon, 'will give such money as he needs to release and carry him to [his native] Scotland'; *CSPD, 1666–1667*, 517. Ker was probably a fellow Scot, referred to in another letter as Mr Carr, now living at Colchester; ibid.
98. Wills was bailed to appear at the next assizes at Wiltshire to answer for words spoken against Monck; TNA, ASSI 24/1, 19 April 1660. Horsington and Fox both accused Monck of fomenting the White Plot (December 1660) in order to precipitate another conflict (and presumably destroy the 'good old cause' once and for all); *CSPD, 1660–1661*, 418, 423. For discussion of the plot, see R. L. Greaves, *Deliver us From Evil: The Radical Underground in Britain, 1660–1663* (Oxford, 1986), 35–40.
99. For Horsington, see the entry for his brother, Thomas, in Appendix 1 (a). Disaffection among the ranks of surgeons in the armed forces is also suggested by the case of one Jennings, a former naval surgeon, who was accused in 1670 of being a 'great crony' of Colonel Thomas Blood and suspected of complicity in the plot to assassinate the duke of Ormond; *CSPD, 1670, with Addenda 1660–1670*, 594. For Blood, who briefly professed the practice of medicine in this period while plotting against the government, see below ???–???. He later apprenticed his son, under the alias Thomas Hunt, to one Samuel Holmes, variously described as an apothecary and surgeon, who served in Colonel Goffe's regiment and was suspected of involvement in an earlier attack on the duke of Ormond in 1663; Marshall, 'Colonel Thomas Blood and the Restoration Political Scene', 564 and n.
100. Hill, described by another deponent as a surgeon, claimed to practise physic at Taunton 'being allowed by the Hall in London'; *CSPD, 1663–1664*, 590, 598. He may be the same as the Mr Hill, described as 'Cromwell's surgeon', who was allegedly involved in a plot to assassinate the King in 1662; Greaves, *Deliver us From Evil*, 102. I have not been able to trace any surgeon of this name attending on Oliver Cromwell.

101. *CSPD, 1665–1666*, 443, 451; *CSPD, 1666–1667*, 69, 76, 112, 205, 242. Evidently, Toose was widely seen as a man of loose morals. In June 1664, he was accused of being the reputed father of a bastard child, as well as trying to seduce two women; Somerset Heritage Centre, Q/SR/106/14.
102. *CSPD, 1665–1666*, 442–3; Bodl., MS Eng. Hist. c.711, fos 27r and *passim*. For Whitley (1618–1697), see the entry in the *ODNB* by Paul Halliday. For other examples of surgeons accused of disaffection to the government in this period, see *CSPD, 1665–1666*, 102 [one Jones, described as such by Monck, now duke of Albemarle, in December 1665] and above 192–3.
103. Dr Gabriel Barber, for example, gave security to live peaceably in 1666. Seven years earlier, he had presented a petition to Parliament on behalf of the town and county of Hertford calling for a restoration of all army officers previously displaced and proposing that 'the Militia may be settled in the hands of those that have faithfully adhered to the Good Old Cause, in opposition to Monarchy, Name and Thing'; *The Humble Petition of Divers Inhabitants of the County of Hertford... Presented to Parliament by Dr Barber... May 13. 1659* (London, 1659); *CSPD, 1665–1666*, 183. Barber (d.1691) was a Cambridge MD, who practised medicine in the town of Hertford; Venn, i, 81.
104. In July 1659, for example, royalist plotters were said to be congregating at the wells at Tunbridge and Bath; *CSPD, 1659–1660*, 50, 61. During the 1650s, the state papers contain numerous references to prisoners of the state and other suspects gaining medical affidavits requiring them to take the waters on health grounds. Many are signed by physicians who were clearly acting on political as much as health grounds. For examples, see *CSPD, 1650*, 216, 253; *CSPD, 1655–1656*, 5, 36, 63, 131. In puritan eyes, the baths were often associated with vice and immorality; see John Bond, *Occasus Occidentalis: or Job in the West* (London, 1645), 31.
105. Capp, *Fifth Monarchy Men*, 204, 267. I strongly suspect that Vernon, a fifth monarchist and author of several millenarian tracts, was responsible for the plague tract entitled *Golgotha, or a Looking-Glass for London, and the Suburbs Thereof* (London, 1665), which appeared under the initials J. V. Not only does this work describe the plague as a sign of 'the near approaching Kingdom of Christ Monarchicall in the Earth' (6), but the author also demonstrates some knowledge of medicine, commending the work of the chymical physician Roger Dixon, as well as a medicine called 'Spirit of Sulphur, which I advise all to have by them' (16). Nonetheless, the author was generally disparaging of physical remedies for the plague, and he specifically condemned the practice of shutting up the infected on the grounds that it was not warranted by scripture. Dixon was the author of numerous self-help manuals, as well as a tract on the plague. A surgeon in the parliamentary armies, he was granted a licence by the bishop of London in May 1661. Dixon would appear to have favoured Helmontian medicines. In 1663, he commended the recent publication of van Helmont's works; Bloom and James, 29; TNA, SP 28/3B/I, fo. 397; 28/3/B/II, fo. 411; 28/10, fo. 282; 28/121B/I and II, *passim*; 28/143, fo. 38; R. Dixon, *Consultum Sanitatis, A Directory to Health* (London, 1663), 13 and *passim*.
106. Even the government's opponents tacitly agreed with this analysis. In April 1670, one John Lerie wrote to the King protesting at the recent passing of the Conventicle Act

and the foundations upon which it rested, namely the notion that conventicles were being used as a pretext for plotting. In response, Lerie argued that it was 'a thing utterly impossible, and beyond all precedent, that such open and public assemblies should be a place for setting such wickedness on foot, whereas taverns, coffee houses, bowling greens, Tunbridge waters, horse races, fairs, markets, or private chambers, are the places where men may more conveniently resort to transact such matters'; *CSPD, 1670, with Addenda 1660–1670*, 151.

107. *CSPD, 1682*, 303; *CSPD, 1683–1684*, 39, 46–7; *CSPD, July–September 1683*, 172.

108. *CSPD, July–September 1683*, 81; *CSPD, 1683–1684*, 37. The nonconformist minister Matthew Meade (d.1699), whose son Richard was to become one of the most celebrated physicians of his age, successfully petitioned (he suffered from the stone) to be allowed to attend the spa and take the waters on health grounds. He was suspected at the time of having participated in the Rye House Plot; *CSPD, July–September 1683*, 113, 195, 211, 214.

109. To take just one example, the English minister and republican apologist Hugh Peters (1598–1660), who acted as preacher to the English church at Rotterdam in the 1630s, cited the example of Holland and the city of Amsterdam as a model for social, political and medical reform in the early years of the commonwealth; see H. P[eters], *Good Work for a Good Magistrate* (London, 1651), 12, 18–19, 33 and unpaginated post-script.

110. The English church was situated underneath the town library and adjacent to the celebrated anatomy theatre; P. Skippon, 'An Account of a Journey Made Thru' Part of the Low Countries, Germany, Italy, and France [1663–1665]', in *A Collection of Voyages and Travels... in Six Volumes* (London, 1732), vi, 400.

111. C. L. Morley, *De Morbo Epidemico* (London, 1680), 139, 157, 173. For Morley and Oviatt, see Innes Smith, 164, 175. Morley's lecture notes and case histories, extending to 36 volumes of manuscript notes, mainly in Latin, provide one of the best sources for an understanding of the experience of English medical students at Leiden in this period; BL, Sloane MSS 1256–1280, 1282–1294, 1297–1299.

112. Innes Smith, 175; *Cal. Rev.*, 226. In the same year that Goldwire (d.1690) was licensed as a Presbyterian to preach at Romsey, Esther Oviatt, James' grandmother, was likewise issued with a licence for her house at Eling, just outside Southampton. She was later prosecuted in 1676 for allowing her home to be used for a conventicle; Bate, *Declaration of Indulgence 1672*, Appendix 7, xxix, lxviii; Hampshire Record Office, Q1/5, 138 [Winchester Quarter Sessions, 3 October 1676]. The medical student James Oviatt was the son of a Southampton merchant by the same name. His father does not appear to have been active in the government of the town and rarely appears in the municipal records. In 1661, however, he did ask to be discharged from holding the office of bedel in the ward of Holy Rood to which he had been elected; Southampton City Archives, SC2/1/8, fo. 159r. James Oviatt Jnr clearly shared his family's Presbyterianism. In his will of 1702 (where he is described as a gentleman, living at Romsey), he granted an annuity of £10 and a six-volume edition of Ogilby's *Atlas* to Goldwire's son, also John (d.1713), who continued to run the dissenting academy at Romsey begun by his father; TNA, PROB 11/472, fos 79v–80r [will of Jamess Oviatt, gent, of Romsey, Hampshire, 27 July 1702; pr. 25 October 1703].

113. Innes Smith, 130, 112. Jordan dedicated his thesis on hysteria to the eminent nonconformist clergyman Samuel Cradock (d.1706), who had probably been responsible for the education of the young Jordan at the dissenting academy that he ran at Geesings, near Wickhambrook, in Suffolk. Samuel Jordan was probably the same as the 'Nephew Jorden', whom Cradock described in 1674 as among 'those young men I have with me in their Greek and Latin'; *Cal. Rev.*, 140–1; Bodl., Rawlinson Letters 51, fo. 34 [Cradock to Edward Terry, 5 May 1674]. Jordan later practised medicine at Sudbury in Suffolk, and was still alive in 1695; LPL, VX 1A/10/144/1–3; VX 1A/10/255/2; WSkRO, EE/501/17/26. Higginbotham's thesis was explicitly dedicated to his tutor Richard Frankland and Robert and Samuel Eaton of Manchester, father and son. For Frankland and the Eatons, see *Cal. Rev.*, 177, 211–12.
114. For Spademan and Newcomen, see Innes Smith, 51, 59. The latter was thanked by the former minister Francis Cross (d.1675), who graduated MD at Leiden in 1664; Appendix 2 (a). Spademan, pastor at Rotterdam, was the subject of a dedication by Thomas Colton (MD Leiden, 1691; d.1731), who later combined the practice of medicine with that of preaching to a dissenting congregation at York. Colton also thanked his patron, Sir William Ayscough (below note 118), and the Reverend John Shower (1657–1715), who was resident at Rotterdam between 1687 and 1691 and served as evening lecturer to the English church there. In July 1685, Shower was alleged to have preached before the duke of Monmouth at Amsterdam prior to his embarkation for England. He was also responsible for preaching the funeral sermon of the physician-cum-minister, Nehemiah Grew; *ODNB*, sub Shower, John; BL, Add.MS 41,817, fo. 237r.
115. James Oviatt (1679), Ichabod Chauncy (1684), Charles Morton (1683), Nicholas Paunceforte (1690) and William Smith (1684); Innes Smith, 44, 165, 175, 179, 217.
116. I have not been able to corroborate Stephen Wright's statement that Henry Hickman was admitted to study medicine at Leiden, as pastor of the English church there, on 18 April 1675. His admission is not cited by Innes Smith; *ODNB*, sub Hickman, Henry. Henry's son William did dedicate a series of exercises undertaken as part of his studies at Leiden to his father in 1688; Innes Smith, 117.
117. Innes Smith, 194. For Richardson, see above 199–201.
118. Innes Smith, 10 [Braman], 11 [Harley], 51 [Ayscough], 77 [Venables], 105 [Boscawen], 239 [Ashurst]. Ayscough, MP for Thirsk in 1645 and 1681, was a Presbyterian who was suspected of plotting in the immediate aftermath of the Restoration and again after the Rye House Plot; Henning, i, 576 and above note 114. Boscawen and Harley were likewise Presbyterians whose patronage of Joseph Halsey and John Bagley, respectively, stemmed from a desire to assist the sons of two ejected ministers. In Halsey's case, the link was very close as his father, also Joseph, had acted as Boscawen's long-time personal chaplain; *Cal. Rev.*, 21, 244; Henning, i, 686–90; ii, 494–7. For Braman, see above 208–9. For Ashurst, see *ODNB*.
119. Desborough's Leiden thesis of 1668 was dedicated to his father John, uncle Samuel, his teacher Professor Johannes van Horne (1621–1670), a pioneer researcher into the lymphatic circulation, and, most tellingly perhaps, the Anglo-Dutch merchant, George Gosfright (d.1694); Innes Smith, 68. In 1671, a correspondent of the Irish stroker Valentine Greatrakes noted that the plotter Major-General John Disbrowe

(1606–1680), prior to making his peace with the English authorities, had been living in the house of the Amsterdam merchant George Gosfright, who subsequently accompanied him back to England. Gosfright himself was a committed republican who had lived in England before the Restoration. Among his closest associates was the Baptist William Kiffin, whom he probably helped to export factious books to England in 1668; for further details see Elmer, *Miraculous Conformist*, 237 and n.

120. Innes Smith, 93. The recent biography of Gibson in the *ODNB* clearly errs in a number of significant respects. He could not have been granted a Lambeth MD in 1663, as he was only about fifteen years old at the time. Moreover, he could not have been removed from the list of fellows of the London College of Physicians in 1687 on account of his marriage to Anne Cromwell as this did not take place until 1698; *ODNB*, sub Gibson, Thomas.

121. Innes Smith, 249. Birch, who was related to the physician-cum-minister Robert Birch, former incumbent of the family living at Birch in Lancashire, later practised medicine at Manchester; Innes Smith, 22; *ODNB*, sub Birch, Peter. Andrew is not mentioned, however, in the entry for his father in the *ODNB*.

122. Innes Smith, 96, 127, 215. Glyde and Jeffery were clearly close acquaintances, entering Leiden on the same day (19 April 1686). The former spent four years as a medical student at the Dutch university and probably died there in 1690. The latter, who enrolled as a philosophy student, certainly moved in medical circles, writing a published 'exercise' on the air and lungs. He also befriended the young Dutch medical student Hermann Boerhaave. Nathaniel Slade graduated MD in 1667. He is probably the physician of the same name who was appointed physician in ordinary to Charles II in 1681, and who later subscribed to Christopher Packe's translation of the *Works* (1689) of Glauber. Slade's father, Samuel, who served as a loyal alderman in the 1650s, resigned from the corporation at the Restoration and retired to his family home at Otterton outside the city; DRO, ECA 10, fos 44r, 79v, 138r. Jeffery's father, also Andrew, was jailed in 1670 for holding a conventicle in his house and contemptuously refusing to give surety. He was later appointed to the aldermanic bench under the new charter of James II in March 1688, as well as serving as deputy lieutenant of the city in the same year; DRO, ECA, C/1/65, fos 356r, 362r; *CSPD, 1687–1689*, 160, 228. Jeffery was almost certainly an ally of Charles Glyde's father, William, who, despite a royalist upbringing, sat as Whig MP for Exeter in the first two exclusion parliaments and was a staunch supporter of Dissent and dissenting ministers in the city; Henning, ii, 398–9; *CSPD, 1668–1669*, 350; TNA, PC 2/67, 123; *CSPD, 1679–1680*, 566–7; DRO, ECA C/1/66, fo. 19v; *CSPD, 1 January–30 June 1683*, 210, 224; *CSPD, 1687–1689*, 160.

123. Innes Smith, 178 [who corrects Foster in ascribing Parsons MD to Harderwyck rather than Groningen]; Somerset Heritage Centre, DD\SP/319/6. In addition to his parents, Parsons dedicated his thesis on kidney and bladder stones to his professor at Harderwyck, Charles Drelincourt, the Exeter physician Thomas Waterhouse and three local clergymen, all ejected at the Restoration, George Newton (d.1681), John Gardiner and Francis Fuller (d.1701). The latter's son, also Francis, wrote on medical matters; see *Cal. Rev.*, 215, 217, 364–5; *ODNB*, sub Fuller, Francis and Appendix 2 (b).

124. Spelman, who entered puritan Emmanuel College, Cambridge, in 1659, but promptly left at the Restoration, was admitted to Leiden as a medical student in September 1662 and graduated MD eighteen months later in May 1664; Innes Smith, 219; Venn, iv, 131. In addition to his father, Spelman dedicated his thesis on hemorrhoids to a number of leading figures among Yarmouth's large dissenting population including the deprived town lecturer William Bridge (d.1671), and Francis Brewster, a prominent patron of the godly cause in Suffolk after the Restoration. In 1674, for example, his house at Wrentham was the site of an alleged conventicle, and he played a central role in establishing a Congregational church in the village under the leadership of William Ames (d.1689) which townsmen from nearby Yarmouth (in Norfolk) frequently utilised in order to avoid prosecution; *CSPD, 1673–1675*, 396; DWL, Harmer MS 76.7 [Records of the Congregational Church at Wrentham], fo. 21 and *passim*. There was a long history of Yarmouth puritans and dissenters using the Low Countries as a bolthole to avoid persecution. William Bridge himself had taken this route in 1636, following his deprivation by bishop Wren. He subsequently served as minister to the congregational church at Rotterdam and was granted honorary admission to Leiden University in 1639, links that no doubt proved extremely useful to the next generation of dissenting émigrés who sought refuge in Holland after the Restoration; *Cal. Rev.*, 74.
125. Innes Smith, 55. Cox was the son of an early convert to the Baptists, Benjamin Cox (d.*c.*1663), and a member of John Bunyan's congregation at Bedford. He suffered frequent periods of imprisonment before removing to London, where he acted as pastor to a Baptist congregation in Petty France. Cox would appear to have turned to the practice of medicine sometime in the early 1680s at roughly the same time that he was forced to flee to Holland to avoid prosecution in the wake of the Tory reaction. In 1687, he received a royal grant of immunity from prosecution as a nonconformist, and in the same year was elected a fellow of the Royal College of Physicians; *ODNB*, sub Cox, Benjamin; BLARS, HSA/1671 W/15 and S22; *CSPD, 1686–1687*, 335; Munk, i, 475–6. Kiffin was a colleague of Cox's father. In 1677, he signed, with five others, a preface to Cox's *Vindiciae Veritatis, or a Confutation of the Heresies and Gross Errours Attested by Thomas Collier* (London, 1677). Kiffin was also a former associate of the radical Anglo-Dutch merchant George Gosfright (above note 119).
126. *A Perfect Diurnall of Some Passages in Parliament*, no.303 [21–28 May 1649], 1534 [error in original pagination]; Thurloe, *State Papers*, vii, 41.
127. CUL, MS Mm.I.45, 408–9, 415, 416; *HMC. Thirteenth Report, Appendix, Part 1. The Manuscripts of the Duke of Portland. Vol.1* (London, 1891), 368–70, 371, 372, 381.
128. Innes Smith, 194; Munk, i, 307; *Cal. Rev.*, 410–11. Richardson's first wife Dorcas, the daughter of Julius Herring, minister of the English church at Amsterdam (1637–1645), died in 1651. By his second wife, otherwise unknown, Richardson had a son, Daniel, who entered Leiden as a medical student, aged 20, in 1678. He enrolled on the same day as another English medical student, Thomas Bowles, and lodged with him in the house of Nicholas Bert on the Nonnesteegh. It is probably safe to assume that Bowles was the son of Edward Richardson's former colleague, Edward Bowles (d.1662), who lost his place as preacher at York Cathedral at the Restoration; Innes Smith, 193; Leiden University Archives, ASF 12, 60; *Cal. Rev.*, 67.

129. Innes Smith, 119, 144 [dedications of John Hodgson, MD Leiden, 1677, and William Lovell, MD Leiden, 1673]. I discuss the possible significance of the Hodgson dedication above, note 85.
130. G. Croese, *The General History of the Quakers*, 2 vols (London, 1696), ii, 27–8; Venn, i, 405; *Album Studiosorum Academiae Lugduno Bataviae MDLXXV–MDCCCLXXV* (The Hague, 1875), 520; W. I. Hull, *Benjamin Furly and Quakerism in Rotterdam* (Swarthmore, PA, 1941), 21n–22n, 24–5; Munk, i, 366; A. Hessayon, 'Lead's Life and Times (Part Two): The Woman in the Wilderness', in A. Hessayon (ed.), *Jane Lead and Her Transnational Legacy* (London, 2016), 51. I'd like to thank Dr Hessayon for kindly alerting me to his work on Jane Lead and the Philadelphians. I discuss the disproportionate role played by medical men in the early Philadelphian Society in my '"Under the Operation of a Higher and Exalted Mind": Medicine, Mysticism and Social Reform in Restoration England', in H. C. Powell and C. J. Saunders (eds), *Visions and Voice-Hearing in Medieval and Early Modern Contexts* (Palgrave Studies in Literature, Science and Medicine, Palgrave Macmillan, 2021), 281–304.
131. TNA, SP 29/302/136.
132. *CSPD, 1663–1664*, 263, 324, 521. Hobson, too, had links with Holland. In 1661, the Dutch-based Quaker William Caton reported that Hobson was present at a meeting of religious radicals in Rotterdam; FHL, Swarthmore MSS, vol. 1, no. 322. Later that year, it was reported that one Love and various disaffected émigrés had landed at Lowestoft in Suffolk. Of Love, the government's informer reported that he 'gave himself out at Rotterdam for a doctor of physic, but was a holder forth at a private assembly of Independents there, where the regicides and such like men meet'; *CSPD, 1661–1662*, 79. In all probability, this was Hobson, and not Nicholas Love, an associate of various regicides, as suggested by Richard Greaves; Greaves, *Deliver Us From Evil*, 94–5. Back in England, Hobson suffered frequent and sustained periods of imprisonment, dying in London in 1665. In his will, he was described as a citizen and barber surgeon of London, but elsewhere he gave his profession as that of doctor of medicine; *ODNB*; *CSPD, 1661–1662*, 62, 549, 559, 564; LMA, S[essions] F[ile] 163, recognizance no. 27 [26 June 1662]; *CSPD, 1663–1664*, 245, 247, 537, 574, 670; *CSPD, 1664–1665*, 22, 168, 186; TNA, PC 2/58, fo. 65v; TNA, PROB 11/321, fos 58r–59v [will of Paul Hobson, citizen and barber chirurgeon, of London, 12 March 1663/4; pr. 13 June 1666]. Hobson was in fact the son of a London barber surgeon, and was a freeman of the Barber Surgeons' Company in 1646 by virtue of his father's standing; Guildhall Library, London, MS 5265/1 [Barber Surgeons' Company, Freedom and Admissions, 1522–1664], fos 66, 102.
133. *CSPD, 1663–1664*, 324, 505, 521. In November 1663, one Robert Stent, a leather seller, admitted during interrogation that he had consulted Dr Richardson while in Rotterdam. He was discovered with a letter addressed by Richardson to Peter Jennings, a London apothecary, in which the former claimed to live in Holland 'for freedom of conscience' and asked that the latter might furnish Stent with 'Galenical extracts for obstructions of the liver'. Given the authorities interest in the details of this letter, it seems likely that some at least suspected here an example of medical cant, i.e. the use of medical language to disguise the true, subversive intent of Richardson's instructions; ibid., 352. In another intercepted letter, written during the Second

Anglo-Dutch War, Richardson wrote to Edmund Custis, an English merchant resident in Bruges, protesting that he 'is of no party but that of Jesus against wickedness', and that he desired the ruin of no man, 'especially not of his native country nor King, and concerns himself not in the war, but prays for the safety of the place and people where he enjoys the freedom which few kings on earth are willing to give'. He added somewhat cryptically that 'greater things are on the wheel', and hoped soon to be found in Mount Zion; *CSPD, 1666–1667*, 44. For Custis, who later provided Samuel Pepys with information relating to the activities of Richardson's friend and fellow plotter Colonel Scott, see Bodl., Rawlinson MS A 176, fos 62–70.

134. *CSPD, 1665–1666*, 115.
135. R. L. Greaves, *Enemies Under His Feet: Radicals and Nonconformists in Britain, 1664–1677* (Stanford, 1990), 36–7; Greaves, *Deliver us From Evil*, 31, 199. For Hodgson and Richardson, and possible links between the two suggested by the dedication of John Hodgson's medical thesis on chlorosis (a form of green sickness that particularly effected anaemic women) to Richardson in 1677, see above note 85. Captain John Hodgson, who lacked formal medical qualifications, was later indicted for practising medicine without a licence; *ODNB*, sub Hodgson, John.
136. R. L. Greaves, *Secrets of the Kingdom: British Radicals from the Popish Plot to the Revolution of 1688–1689* (Stanford, 1992), 26. It is hard to reconcile these accounts of Richardson with Greaves' view, expressed elsewhere in his trilogy of Restoration radicalism, that he 'shunned radical schemes after fleeing to the Netherlands'; cf. *idem*, *Enemies Under His Feet*, 199.
137. Bodl., Rawlinson MS A 176, fos 21, 32v. It would be good to know more about this elusive and enigmatic character, Colonel John Scott. A close associate of both the duke of Buckingham and the earl of Shaftesbury, Scott was very active in Whig circles in the 1670s and early 1680s. George Starkey described him in 1662 as a 'German... chymist who hath done wonders'; R. Ashcraft, *Revolutionary Politics and Locke's* Two Treatises of Government (Princeton, NJ, 1986), 130–4; FSL, V.a.292, fo. 73r. The only full-length study of Scott is that by L. T. Mowrer, *The Indomitable John Scott* (New York, 1960).
138. Innes Smith, 218; *CSPD, July–September 1683*, 227; R. A. Beddard, 'Tory Oxford', in N. Tyacke (ed.), *The History of the University of Oxford: Seventeenth-Century Oxford* (Oxford, 1997), 898–9; *ODNB*, sub Trenchard, Sir John; Henning, iii, 548. Southby was still at Leiden as late as August 1684, when he supplied a carmen in praise of his fellow student, Edward Wetenhall (d.1733), the son of the 'moderately ecumenical' bishop of Cork and Ross, Edward Wetenhall (1636–1711), who opposed the government's campaign of repression against conventicles in 1683. There is no record of Southby's graduation as a doctor at Leiden or anywhere else in Holland; Innes Smith, 246; *ODNB*, sub Wetenhall, Edward.
139. Innes Smith, 43. For Cay's father-in-law, Richard Gilpin, see above 187–8.
140. Innes Smith, 44; BL, Add. MS 4460, fo. 63v; BL, Add. MS 6845, fo. 286r; Venn, i, 317. The government continued to track Chamberlen's movements after his return to Holland, aware of the central role he had played in promoting Monmouth's cause. In the spring of 1686, for example, a government spy stationed at Utrecht noted that Chamberlen, 'son of Dr Chamberlain the man midwife aged about 17 [*sic*], who is said

to have been concern'd with the late Duke of Monmouth', was shortly expected in the city. A few months later, in June 1686, he was granted an official pardon; BL, Add. MS 41,812, fos 212v, 236r; Add. MS 41,818, fo. 257; *CSPD, 1686–1687*, 163. Helen King's entry for Chamberlen in the *ODNB* seriously confuses the father and son, both called Hugh, as well as erroneously suggesting that Hugh Chamberlen the younger 'held political and religious affiliations very different from those of his father, who was a whig and a baptist'. Both father and son were committed Whigs, and, *pace* King, the former's career at court was most certainly affected for the worse by his political beliefs. In November 1682, Hugh Chamberlen Snr was discharged as personal physician to Charles II and replaced by the ultra-loyalist, Robert Brady; TNA, LC 3/26, fos 141, 143; 3/24, fos 16, 17; LS 13/197, fo. 84. For Hugh Chamberlen the elder's political activism, see above 206–7.

141. Innes Smith, 92; *Cal. Rev.*, 219; W. M. Wigfield, *The Monmouth Rebels 1685* (Gloucester, 1985), 67. Like Chamberlen, Gaylard achieved respectability in his chosen profession after the Glorious Revolution, no doubt assisted by the fact that he had backed the right horse. Both were admitted to the Royal College of Physicians in London in 1694 (Chamberlen as a full member, and Gaylard as a candidate), and both were honoured by the University of Cambridge with MDs (Chamberlen, by royal mandate, in 1690, while Gaylard's Leiden MD was incorporated there in 1693). Gaylard, moreover, was appointed physician to the armed forces in the West Indies in 1702; Munk, i, 504.
142. For Oliver see *ODNB*; *Cal. Rev.*, 373–4; Innes Smith, 173; J. Oldmixon, *The History of England, During the Reigns of the Royal House of Stuart* (London, 1730), 704; J. Dunton, *The Life and Errors of John Dunton Late Citizen of London* (London, 1705), 211. The bookseller and Whig sympathizer John Dunton (1659–1732), who encountered Dr Oliver and his political associates at Amsterdam in 1687, claimed to have been introduced to Leiden by one 'Dr Rolf'. It is tempting to speculate that Dunton's contact was Thomas Rolfe (d.1713), who had entered Leiden as a medical student just a few months before Oliver in October 1683. Rolfe almost certainly knew Oliver. In 1704 the two men signed a testimonial on behalf of Nathaniel Firmin of Essex, a candidate for an archiepiscopal medical licence; Dunton, *Life*, 208; Innes Smith, 198; LPL, VX 1A/10/376. If Rolfe, too, combined medical study with conspiratorial politics during his stay in Holland, then it is possible that he may have been related to the former army officer and plotter, Major Edmund Rolfe, who died at London in 1668. Details of his background are scant, but he was probably the second son of the nonconformist apothecary Thomas Rolfe who left £20 in his will for the relief of those ministers or 'Preachers of God's word now silenced and deprived of their livings'. Thomas named his 'loving friend' Edmund Rolfe, scrivener, as one of the overseers of his will; TNA, PROB 11/379, fos 71r–72r [will of Thomas Rolfe, apothecary, of London, 13 October 1683; pr. 7 January 1684/5].
143. Innes Smith, 105; *Cal. Rev.*, 243; *ODNB*, sub Hallett II, Joseph; Leiden University Archives, ASF 12, 275 [Hallett was lodging at the house of Hester Tebow in Leiden].
144. Harley, '"Bred Up in the Study of That Faculty"', 403. Temple was probably the same person as the Dr Temple, who was made a freeman and burgher of the city of Amsterdam in December 1683 through the intervention of Abraham Keck, a Dutch

merchant responsible for assisting and befriending numerous exiled English radicals in this period. In a list of recently appointed burghers, drawn up two months later, Temple was described as wanted for 'speaking treason'; BL, Add. MS 41,809, fo. 206; 41,811, fo. 121; Ashcraft, *Revolutionary Politics*, 419. Prior to studying in Holland, Temple had been granted a licence by the London College of Physicians with the proviso that he should consult with more experienced colleagues in the future; Munk, i, 393.

145. The forfeited lands of Richard Evans, doctor in physic, of Cotleigh in Devon, were granted to Colonel John Hope of Westminster and others, in 1688; *Calendar of Treasury Books*, viii, iv, 2002–6. Thatcher, of Wedmore in Somerset, was tried and listed for execution at Wells, and his lands declared forfeit, though no official record of his execution survives. He was licensed to practise surgery in the deanery of Wells in 1675; Wigfield, *Monmouth Rebels*, 169; Somerset Heritage Centre, D\D/Bs/42, sub 4 September 1675.

146. [H. Pitman], *A Relation of the Great Sufferings and Strange Adventures of Henry Pitman, Chyrurgion to the Late Duke of Monmouth* (London, 1689). Pitman excused his role in the Monmouth rebellion by claiming that he had been importuned by family and friends to fight for the duke. In mitigation of his offences, he also professed to have cared for the sick and wounded on both sides.

147. BL, Add. MS 41,812, fo. 34v.

148. *Cal. Rev.*, 412; A. Marshall, *Intelligence and Espionage in the Reign of Charles II, 1660–1685* (Cambridge, 1994), 145–6. Marshall is one of few political historians to note the close connection between medicine and political espionage in this period, and thus question the 'studied neutrality' so frequently ascribed to medics; ibid., 20.

149. Ostensibly, Butler was granted his Cambridge MD by the King in respect that he had 'practised physic in London with great success, and particularly during the plague, when he gave free access to all, and especially to many hundreds of the meaner sort in a day, and so gained great esteem and experience'. It seems more likely, however, that his degree was some form of down payment for his subsequent activities as 'a quasi-official government agent' with important links to the dissenters in the period from 1670 to 1672. Butler's request in late 1670 that he be granted 'a licence, under the sign manual, for practising physic throughout England' may well have been motivated by a desire to move unimpeded around the country in performance of his duties as a government agent. He had earlier been licensed by the archbishop of Canterbury in 1664 and was later to be made an honorary fellow of the London College of Physicians in September 1680; *CSPD, 1670; Addenda, 1660–1670*, 78–9, 117, 307; Venn, i, 273; Greaves, *Enemies Under His Feet*, 216–22; LPL, Sheldon, fo. 202; Munk, i, 409.

150. Burnett was the brother of the Whig bishop, Gilbert Burnett (1643–1715), and may well have exploited these connections if he was, as Scott alleged, spying on behalf of the government. Five years later, in 1683, he was reported to have conversed with the Scottish insurgent Sir John Cochrane in London; Bodl., Rawlinson MS A 176, fo. 181v; *CSPD, July–September 1683*, 223.

151. See, for example, the letter of a government spy in Utrecht, dated 19/29 February 1686, in which he refers to the recent arrival of a large number of Scots 'lately come over under pretence of students'; BL, Add.MS 41,818, fo. 257.

152. Innes Smith, 60; BL, Add. MS 17,677, fo. 256v. A political refugee from Scotland, the Presbyterian Cummings settled in Ireland after the Glorious Revolution where he played a crucial role in founding the King's and Queen's College of Physicians. Typically, his medical practice was fully informed by his religious beliefs. According to his friend and co-religionist Joseph Boyse (1660–1728), he always combined the use of physical means with prayer and made notes on the outcome. Where patients failed to recover, he ascribed the failure to the 'rebukes of providence to himself'; J. Boyse, *The Works of the Reverend and Learned Mr. Joseph Boyse, of Dublin*, 2 vols (London, 1728), i, 315–16.
153. For Blackadder, see the article by Stuart Handley in *ODNB*. Blackadder's name, along with that of Duncan Cummings and other students and Scottish exiles, appears on a list of men wanted for extradition from the Netherlands in May 1685; BL, Add. MS 17,677, fo. 256v.
154. Innes Smith, 44. Prior to leaving England, Chauncy was widely accused by Bristol's Tories of acting as the main fomenter of sedition in the city. Sir Robert Cann referred to him in July 1683 as 'a pretender to physic', while a government informer claimed that his congregation at the old Castle ruins was the resort of 'all Bristol clubbers'. The latter concluded that 'he is and ever since his coming here has been an incendiary or rather a common pest here, having poisoned more of his Majesty's subjects by sowing amongst them evil principles then he can pretend to have cured by his medicines'. Chauncy's 'pretence' to practise medicine clearly rankled with his political opponents and was almost certainly related to the widespread perception, reported by Chauncy himself, that 'he hath been a great zealot for the factious Party, and by Reason of his Employment of Practising Physick... he hath had very Advantagious Success, in gaining to their cause, and Cherishing in it, very great Numbers of Proselytes'; *CSPD, July–September 1683*, 10, 266; I. Chauncey, *Innocence Vindicated: by a Brief and Impartial Narrative of the Proceedings of the Court of Sessions in Bristol against Ichabod Chauncey, Physician in that City* (London, 1684), 14.
155. For Mrs or Madame Smith, see especially Ashcraft, *Revolutionary Politics*, 420 and n. and *passim*. On the eve of Argyll's ill-fated expedition, she was reported by a government agent to have provided a Scottish minister at Utrecht, one Hogg, with a text from the Psalms, from whence he preached 'a most wicked discourse'; BL, Add. MS 41,812, fos 138v, 222v.
156. For a good summary of Wade's life and career as a radical activist, see the article by Melinda Zook in *ODNB*.
157. BL, Add. MS 41,817, fo. 219r. Ashcraft has described Dare as 'unquestionably the leading English radical in Amsterdam' and his house as 'the focal point for the English radicals in Holland'. John Locke first lodged here on his arrival in Holland; Ashcraft, *Revolutionary Politics*, 378, 411. See also *ODNB*, sub Dare, Thomas.
158. BL, Add. MS 41,818, fos 126r, 283r; *CSPD, 1686–1687*, 78, 89, 138; BL, Add. MS 41,804, fos 212r–v, 241–2. For Hunt, see *ODNB*.
159. Innes Smith, 219; NNkRO, Y/S1/4, fo. 22r. The Spelmans were an important family in Yarmouth and the locus of much opposition to loyalists and Anglicans. In 1667, Samuel's brother George was accused by the bailiffs of the town of speaking 'mutinous and seditious words', for which he was forced to appear before the Privy Council and

issue a groveling apology. Samuel himself may be the same as the nonconformist preacher mentioned by the minister Luke Milbourne in 1683 as practising medicine in the town, who, along with his Presbyterian brother (George?) was accused of possessing 'an inveterate spleen against Sir T[homas] Medowes and the Church of England'. George Spelman, alderman, and Benjamin Spelman, common councilman, were pardoned in June 1688 for not taking the requisite oaths while holding office in the town; TNA, PC 2/59, fo. 279v; *CSPD, 1 January 1683–30 June 1683*, 78; *CSPD, 1687–1689*, 219–20. For Samuel Spelman's nonconformist background, see above note 124.

160. Besse, *Sufferings*, i, 58. Chauncy's fellow signatories were John Griffith, Thomas Bourne and William Turgis. Griffith (see also above 181, 224 n.38) was listed in 1683 as a member of a Whig club in Bristol. In 1680, he, along with Chauncy, supplied letters testimonial on behalf of Nathaniel Blinman of Bridgwater in Somerset, the son of the Bristol congregational minister, Richard Blinman (d.1681), and an applicant for an ecclesiastical medical licence; *CSPD, July–September 1683*, 166; LPL, VX 1A/10/143/1–4; *Cal. Rev.*, 61 [which does not refer to Nathaniel's medical career, but hints at that of his father, who in his will of 1681 left 'bequests of drugs as he had no money']. Bourne (d.1690) was a Quaker and chymical physician, whose father, also Thomas (d.1671), signed the marriage certificate of George Fox and Margaret Fell in 1669; R. Mortimer (ed.), *Minute Book of the Men's Meeting of the Society of Friends in Bristol 1686–1704* (Bristol, Bristol Rec. Soc., vol. 30, 1977), 235 [which errs in ascribing the date of the above petition to 1672]; see also above 167 n.107. I have not been able to trace the religious or political antecedents of Turgis (d.1707), who was probably the Oxford student of that name who received his bachelor's degree of medicine as well as a licence to practise from the university in July 1658; Foster, iv, 1518; Bodl., UOA, NEP/supra/Reg Qa [Register of Congregation, 1647–1659], fo. 144. His dissenting sympathies are strongly suggested by the fact that along with Ichabod Chauncy he witnessed the will of the Quaker John Speed of Bristol in 1675; TNA, PROB 11/348, fo. 11r [will of John Speed of Bristol, Gloucestershire, 12 April 1675, pr. 8 May 1675].

161. Of the sixteen men made honorary fellow on 30 September 1680, at least seven were either nonconformists or Whigs, or sympathetic to the dissenting/Whig interest (William Burnett, Nicholas Butler, Daniel Coxe, Thomas Gibson, Nehemiah Grew, Henry Sampson and Robert Wittie). Five were known royalists/Tories (Francis Barnard, Phineas Fowke, John Garrett, Valentine Oldys and John Windebank). The religious and political affiliations of the other four fellows (John Jones, John Master, Christopher Love Morley and William Stokeham) is either uncertain or unknown. I disagree with Hal Cook, who lists only thirteen honorary fellows, in seeing this series of appointments as essentially non-partisan. The dissenting background of the majority was hugely disproportionate to the ratio of nonconformists within the population at large. It should also be noted that on the same date—30 September 1680—the College granted full licentiate status to the former minister-turned-physician Isaac Chauncy (1632–1712), as well as making Edward Tyson (1651–1708), son of the Cromwellian mayor of Bristol and brother-in-law of Richard Morton, a candidate for membership; H. J. Cook, *The Decline of the Old Medical Regime in Stuart London* (Ithaca & London, 1986), 195 and n; Munk, i, 415–6, 426. For Chauncey and Morton,

see Appendix 2 (a). For Tyson, who was reportedly working with another nonconformist sympathizer, Charles Goodall, in the College's laboratories in the early 1680s, see above 148, 173 n.136.

162. Kirkby's role is alluded to in TNA, PC 2/66, 392 and the diaries of Israel Tonge and Roger Morrice, for which, see I. Tonge, 'Journal of the Plot, 1678', in *Diaries of the Popish Plot*, ed. D. G. Greene (New York, 1977); M. Goldie *et al.* (eds), *The Entring Book of Roger Morrice 1677–1691*, 6 vols (Woodbridge & New York, 2007), ii, 74–5.
163. A good indication of Barker's religious outlook is suggested by the marriage of his daughter Susanna to Sir Francis Bridgeman, the son of Sir Orlando Bridgeman (1609–1674), who as Lord Keeper of the Great Seal promoted various schemes of religious reconciliation in the late 1660s; W. H. Rylands (ed.), *The Visitation of the County of Warwick, 1682–1683* (London, Harleian Soc., vol. 62, 1911), 15; *ODNB*, sub Bridgeman, Sir Orlando. For Tonge's passion for chymistry, ownership of alchemical manuscripts and preference for van Helmont over Paracelsus, see J. Aubrey, *Brief Lives*, ed. A. Clark, 2 vols (Oxford, 1898), ii, 261–2; SUL, HP 26/49/1A–2B; HP 55/4/3A–6B; Oldenburg, *Correspondence*, vii, 23–9 [6 June 1670]. In 1676 Robert Hooke reported that Tonge was associated with a 'Rosicrucian club' in London; H. W. Robinson and W. Adams (eds), *The Diary of Robert Hooke, 1672–1680* (London, 1935), 242.
164. Tonge, 'Journal'. Barker's political views are difficult to divine. His house in the Barbican does appear, however, to have been the focus of proto-Whig activity. In June 1678, for example, an informer named Edmund Everard reported overhearing there one Tobias Cage of Gray's Inn say that Slingsby Bethel had told him that both the King and the duke of York were bastards. Also present was one Dr Cockett, who may have been the same as the John Cockett, licensed by the archbishop of Canterbury in 1663 (among those who signed testimonials on his behalf was the chymical physician Pierre Massonet, for whom see Appendix 1 (a)); *CSPD, 1678*, 239; LPL, VX 1A/10/1; VG 1/1, fo. 171v.
165. Boyle, *Correspondence*, iii, 262; iv, 89–90, 90n, 341, 346, 407; v, 210, 236, 252, 376; vi, 3, 216, 246, 288–9, 392; Oldenburg, *Correspondence*, iv, 581–2; vii, 540–2; viii, 393–5; ix, 20–1, 113–14, 526–7, 646–7; *CSPD, 1667–1668*, 305.
166. I discuss these in more detail above 81.
167. TNA, PC 2/67, 47; PC 2/68, 243.
168. *CSPD, 1678*, 426; TNA, PC 2/67, 131; 2/69, 6.
169. Wakeman was made a royal physician in 1664, probably as a reward for his loyalty to the Stuarts in exile in the 1650s. Like other loyal medics, he engaged in plotting and was involved in an attempt to overthrow Cromwell in 1658. Captured, he remained in prison until the Restoration. Oates and Tonge claimed that Wakeman had been offered a huge sum of money to poison the king. Following his acquittal, he retired to the continent, but returned briefly in 1685 to give evidence against Oates on the occasion of his first trial for perjury. He died the following year; *ODNB*; TNA, LC 3/26, 143.
170. Needham, of North Hallam in Derbyshire, was accused of plotting against the king's life, gathering arms from abroad, and seeking to subvert the Protestant religion, for which he faced a change of high treason. He was pardoned in February 1679, but

remained in custody for at least a year; TNA, PC 2/67, 32, 62, 86; 2/68, 408, 416; Bodl., Carte MS 79, fo. 177 [Philip, Lord Wharton to his son, Thomas, 9 February 1679]; Goldie *et al.* (eds), *Entring Book of Roger Morrice*, ii, 103; Derbyshire Record Office, D 239 M/O 1082 [Henry Hatsell to George Treby, 8 February 1679]; D 239 M/O 1617, 1619, 1637, 1649 [copies of the examination and confession of Needham, February–April 1679].

171. Among those who sought permission to remove themselves and their families from England to the safety of the continent were Andrew Creagh, Henry Titchborne (MD Padua, 1656 and honorary fellow, RCPL, 1664), Peter Vavasor (MD Padua, 1655) and William Waldegrave (MD Padua, 1659 and honorary fellow of the London College of Physicians, 1664); see TNA, PC 2/66, 467 [Creagh]; Munk, i, 334; *CSPD, 1679–1680*, 332 [Titchborne]; TNA, PC 2/68, 160; *CSPD, 1679–1680*, 133 [Waldegrave].

172. Betts was a royal physician who was made a fellow of the London College in October 1664. His Harveian tract *De Ortu et Natura Sanguinis* (London, 1669) was attacked by the Helmontian George Thomson in 1670. He was bound over as a 'Papist recusant' in January 1679; *ODNB*; Munk, i, 318–19; H. Bowler (ed.), *London Sessions Records, 1605–1685* (London, Catholic Rec. Soc., 1934), 214, 220. For Harris (1647–1732), see *ODNB*.

173. *CSPD, 1682*, 546, 547; *CSPD, 1683–1684*, 124, 132.

174. *ODNB*. Interestingly, in the early stages of the Popish Plot, Lower was frequently asked to attend on sick imprisoned Catholics suspected of involvement in the plot. He also attended on the dying Charles II in February 1685, as well as ministering to the rebel, Lord Grey, during his imprisonment in 1685. On the former occasion, one commentator astutely noted that Whig physicians like Lower were asked to attend to dispel any subsequent suggestions of medical foul play; TNA, PC 2/67, 83; 2/68, 98; *CSPD, 1684–1685*, 309; *CSPD, February-December 1685*, 319. Lower also played an important role in contributing to the character assassination of the turncoat-informer Stephen Dugdale in 1681 by diagnosing his sickness as a form of venereal disease. Dugdale's perjured evidence against the 'Protestant joiner' Stephen College was subsequently dismissed as untrustworthy; *CSPD, 1680–1681*, 517–18.

175. Short (1635–1685), a Catholic, had been summoned to appear before the College of Physicians in April 1679 but had bravely opted to remain in London where he worked tirelessly on behalf of his co-religionists, providing medical certificates in order to facilitate their escape to the continent; *ODNB*; Munk, i, 377–9; TNA, PC 2/67, 42, 139, 140; *Historical Manuscripts Commission. Eleventh Report, Appendix, Part II. The Manuscripts of the House of Lords, 1678–1688* (London, 1887), 129–30.

176. *ODNB*. Coxe, whose puritan sympathies and background are well attested (see above 53–4), was widely suspected of engaging in factional politics. In October 1683, for example, a kinsman and dissenting minister named Sampson Wilson wrote to Coxe asking him to intercede on his behalf and so prevent his being called before the Privy Council to answer allegations that he was responsible for circulating pro-Whig newsletters. Eight months later, order was given to search the premises of one Thomas Cox in Bloomsbury Square for treasonable or seditious books, particularly any that might relate to the recent Rye House Plot; *CSPD, 1683–1684*, 3; *CSPD,*

1684–1685, 93. For Wilson, who was admired by Richard Baxter among others, see *Cal. Rev.*, 537.

177. Richard Torlesse (d.1714), for example, was removed from the post of physician to St Thomas' Hospital in 1683 following Quo Warranto proceedings begun by the King. His nonconformist sympathies are suggested by the fact that in the same year the Leiden graduate Charles Morton dedicated his medical thesis to Torlesse, along with the Rev. Charles Morton and Henry Hickman, both leading figures in Anglo-Dutch dissenting circles. Torlesse (MD Oxford, 1666 and fellow of the College of Physicians, 1675) was reinstated after the Glorious Revolution but was permanently removed in 1703 in what looks like a politically motivated act against supporters of the war with France (he was accused of receiving excessive fees for ministering to sick and wounded seamen); F. G. Parsons, *The History of St Thomas's Hospital*, 2 vols (London, 1934), ii, 107, 112, 145, 263; Innes Smith, 165; Foster, iv, 1497; Munk, i, 387; LPL, MS 941, no. 124 [The Case of St Thomas' Hospital, 17 April 1703]. At the same time as Torlesse' dismissal, the crown proposed the royal surgeon John Browne (1642–1702 or 1703) for the vacant place of surgeon at St Thomas'. A political appointment, he was later dismissed in 1691 and continued to argue for reinstatement for the next eight years; *ODNB*; Parsons, *History*, ii, 111–12, 123–4, 127, 130, 265.

178. Bateman was repeatedly arrested in the aftermath of the Rye House Plot for a series of offences. He was finally tried and charged with attempting to seize the King and secure London at the Old Bailey on 9 December 1685, and was executed nine days later. His bodily remains were not interred until May 1689; *CSPD, July–September 1683*, 4, 15, 52, 189, 191, 198, 205, 208, 297; *CSPD, 1683–1684*, 35, 234–5; *CSPD, February-December 1685*, 157, 269, 307; Greaves, *Secrets of the Kingdom*, 250; *CSPD, 1689–1690*, 97. With the connivance of the latitudinarian rector Edward Fowler, Bateman, with fellow Baptist William Kiffin, was made a member of the vestry of the parish of St Giles Cripplegate, London, in the early 1680s. Fowler subsequently came under intense pressure from loyal Tories and hardline Anglicans to present these men in the church courts for a variety of offences, including non-attendance and recusancy, but he steadfastly refused to comply, arguing that 'he was in great hopes of bringing them to the church and to the holy communion'; *CSPD, 1683–1684*, 358; Bowler (ed.), *London Sessions Records*, 373; *ODNB*, sub Fowler, Edward; M. Goldie and J. Spurr, 'Politics and the Restoration Parish: Edward Fowler and the Struggle for St Giles Cripplegate', *English Historical Review*, 109 (1994), 572–96.

179. *ODNB*, sub Ward, Sir Patience; BL, Add. MS 41,818, fo. 185v; *CSPD, 1682*, 572–3; T. Harris, *London Crowds in the Reign of Charles II: Propaganda and Politics from the Restoration to the Exclusion Crisis* (Cambridge, 1987), 187–8.

180. In 1683, Friend was arrested and imprisoned for alleged plotting in Taunton in the wake of the Rye House Plot. He was finally released on bail after claiming to require the constant attention of a physician and apothecary, a claim which the government saw as little more than a standard ruse. A few months later he was arrested at a conventicle in the town by the zealous Tory mayor, Stephen Timewell. He again fell under suspicion after the collapse of Monmouth's Rebellion, but somehow managed to escape the Bloody Assizes and was later made a capital burgess for the town under the new charter issued by James II in September 1688; *CSPD, 1 January–30 June 1683*,

385; *CSPD, July–September 1683*, 77, 321, 332, 338, 367, 385, 389, 391; Goldie *et al.* (eds), *Entring Book of Roger Morrice*, ii, 382, 402; *CSPD, 1683–1684*, 229; Greaves, *Secrets of the Kingdom*, 198; *CSPD, 1687–1689*, 268. Friend's radical career may have had long roots. In the summer of 1656, he was bound over at the assizes for abusing the mayor of the town; TNA, ASSI 24/1, Somerset, Summer 1656.

181. *CSPD, July–September 1683*, 355. I have not been able to identify Hoit (possibly a pseudonym). For Carel, see *Cal. Rev.*, 104.

182. BL, Add. MS 41,803, fo. 320.

183. Henning, i, 709–10; Innes Smith, 10. The medical student Thomas Aylwin was the son of a Chichester gentleman of the same name, who died in 1676. He also dedicated his thesis to another prominent Chichester citizen, John Merlot, a friend and business associate of Braman and Farrington. Alywin's daughter Hannah later married John Eedes (d.1695), the nephew of the third member of our Chichester cabal, Dr Henry Eedes. Nothing is known of Thomas Aylwin's own religious affiliations, but it may be significant that in 1709 he signed letters testimonial in support of the application of the Chichester Quaker and physician, John Bettesworth, an applicant for a Canterbury medical licence; WSxRO, Add. MS 8759; ESxRO, SAS-M/1/692; ESxRO, SAS-WH/201 [will of John Braman, 1703]; Nottinghamshire Archives, DD/N/201/26; *VCH. Sussex. Vol. 3*, ed. L. F. Salzman (London, 1935), 73; LPL, VX 1A/10/432.

184. *VCH. Sussex. Vol. 4*, ed. L. F. Salzman (London, 1953), 62.

185. Foster, ii, 451; Bodl., Tanner MS 148, fo. 47v [Ralph Bridoake to ?, 1677]; MS 38, fos 126–7 [Guy Carleton to William Sancroft, 17 February 1679]; *CSPD, July–September 1683*, 8, 160–1. In February 1686, Eedes was successfully prosecuted for 'commending in discourse at Dr [Samuel] Cradock's table' the work of the parliamentarian political apologist, Philip Hunton; *HMC. Fourteenth Report, Appendix, Part III. MSS of the Duke of Portland, vol. 3* (London, 1894), 394. Cradock was one of the most prominent spokesmen and preachers for the dissenters in Suffolk; *Cal. Rev.*, 140–1.

186. BL, Add. MS 41,803, fo. 273; TNA, PC 2/69, 292; LPL, VX 1A/10/43; VG 1/1, fo. 232; Sheldon, fos 237r–v. Haslen, who received an archiepiscopal licence to practise medicine in January 1673, may have done so under cover of the recent Declaration of Indulgence. Among those who supported his application was Dr Thomas Harrison, an eminent nonconformist minister who was living at Chester in 1672; *Cal. Rev.*, 250–1. Haslen later served as mayor of Chichester in 1687 and 1699, on the former occasion through the direct intervention of James II in his attempt to court support among the dissenting interest. Like others of his ilk who collaborated with James' regime, including Richard Burthogge (below 275), Haslen would appear to have paid a high price for accepting the mayoralty in 1687. Summarily removed from office in the aftermath of the Glorious Revolution, he and fellow collaborators, including Dr Thomas Aylwin (above note 151), brought a case before the assizes in 1691 in an attempt to restore their civic rights and offices. The high steward of the city found against most of the plaintiffs but agreed that Haslen, as a former mayor, should continue as an alderman of the city despite the fact that he was 'not very regularly chosen'; A. Hay, *The History of Chichester* (Chichester & London, 1804), 571; WSxRO, Add. MS 8935.

187. Foster, i, 408; Innes Smith, 69; ESxRO, SAS-M/1/774.

188. R. L'Estrange, *The Accompt Clear'd: In Answer to a Libel Intituled A True Account from Chichester Concerning the Death of Habin the Informer* (London, 1682), 31. Peachey was the father of the medical practitioner, John Peachey or Pechey (1654–1718), who was made a licentiate of the London College of Physicians in December 1684. In the late 1680s, and much to the chagrin of the College, Peachey was responsible with four other licentiates for setting up a joint practice and dispensary in London offering cheap medical advice by return of post. He was also responsible for translating the works of another licentiate, Thomas Sydenham; Venn, iii, 325; Munk, i, 433; *ODNB*, sub Pechey, John. He is not to be confused with the physician of the same name, who, following his ejection as vicar of St Paul's Walden, Hertfordshire, in 1662, took up the practice of medicine and proceeded MD at Caen some time in the early 1680s. He was also made an extra-licentiate of the London College of Physicians in July 1683.
189. *CSPD, July–September 1683*, 369; LPL, VX 1A/10/178/1–2; Sancroft, fo. 244. For a general account of Dale's life and career, particularly in relation to his botanical and antiquarian interests, see the article by Juanita Barmby in *ODNB*. In the light of the earlier discussion, it is worth pointing out that Dale's engagement with the radical scene in London probably dated from his years of apprenticeship there under the apothecary Thomas Wells. Wells, it can safely be assumed, was sympathetic to the Whig cause. He later acted as master to William Tanner, the son of the republican astrologer and physician John Tanner (d.1714) of Amersham, Buckinghamshire, and William Gladman, grandson of the conspirator John Gladman (for whom, see above note 13); SAL, MSS 8200/3 and 4 [court minutes, 1694–1716]. Tanner, licensed in 1674, was yet another radical nonconformist to receive the blessing of the College of Physicians in London; Munk, i, 388.
190. *CSPD, 1661–1662*, 212; Somerset Heritage Centre, Q/SR/99/34; WSA, A1/110, Michaelmas 1661, no. 169; LPL, FII/4/1; F1/C, fo. 133; VX 1A/10/66; VX 1A/10/93/1–3; VX 1A/10/178/1–2. In the last instance, that of George Hammond, a London apothecary who was living in Taunton in 1679, Allen again signed alongside Packe. Allen, who like Dale and Packe (see below) was almost certainly a chymical physician, was able to call on the support of two eminent practitioners, both chymically inclined, John Fryer and Walter Charleton. The fact that the grant of his licence was made through the Faculty Office suggests further evidence of the sympathy shown by the Anglican authorities in London for chymical medicine (above chapter 4).
191. For Benjamin Allen, see J. M. Christy, 'Dr Benjamin Allen (1663–1738) of Braintree: a Forgotten Essex Naturalist', *The Essex Naturalist*, 16 (1911), 145–75; *idem*, 'More about Dr Benjamin Allen (1663- 1738) of Braintree, Naturalist', *The Essex Naturalist*, 17 (1912), 1–14; Venn, i, 16; H. R. French, '"Ingenious and Learned Gentlemen': Social Perceptions and Self-Fashioning among Parish Elites in Essex, 1680–1740', *Social History*, 25 (2000), 50–55. Christy and French differ with regard to Allen's parentage, suggesting that his father was either Benjamin or Thomas Allen, both London physicians. Venn, however, clearly states that he was born in Somerset, the native county of Blaze Allen. The physician Blaze Allen baptized and buried a son called Blaze at Beckington in Somerset in the 1650s. He later referred to another son Benjamin in his will made shortly before his death in 1703; Somerset Heritage Centre,

D\P\BEC/2/1/2 [parish registers of Beckington, Somerset, 1653–1741]; LMA, archdeaconry court of London, will of Blaze Allen, citizen and doctor of physic, of St Botolph Aldgate, London, 2 March 1702/3; pr. 11 June 1703. He was buried at St Botolph Aldgate, 13 June 1703.

192. Both men married the daughters of the Braintree physician Joshua Draper, whose medical connections would have proved invaluable in the early stages of the two men's careers. He may also have shared their religious and political beliefs. An important figure in vestry politics in the town, Draper was probably related to Joseph Draper (or may be the same), one of four elders chosen to govern the Presbyterian church in Braintree in 1648; *ODNB*, sub Dale, Samuel; W. A. Shaw, *A History of the English Church During the Civil Wars and Under the Commonwealth 1640–1660*, 2 vols (London, 1900), ii, 387. Draper had earlier been a student at puritan Emmanuel College, Cambridge, and proceeded to his bachelor's degree in medicine in 1638. He applied for a licence from the bishop of London in 1665; Venn, i, 65; Bloom and James, 47–8.

193. For Packe, see *ODNB*, sub Packe, Christopher, which clearly errs in suggesting that Packe was the son of his namesake, the London commonwealthman and former mayor. In dedicating his translation of Regnier de Graaf's *De Succo Pancreatico; or, A Physical and Anatomical Treatise of the Nature and Office of the Pancreatice Juice* (London, 1676) to Sir Christopher Packe the physician specifically states that 'next to my Parents, I stand more highly engaged to [him] than to any other Person living'. Packe refers to the death of Elizabeth Gaunt in his *Medela Chymica, or, an Account of the Vertues and Uses of a Select Number of Chymical Medicines* (London, 1708), 46. She was tried, convicted and executed, alongside the London alderman Henry Cornish, on 23 October 1685, for her part in conspiring to support Monmouth's rebellion. She was in fact the last woman to be executed for treason (by burning) in England; *ODNB*, sub Gaunt, Elizabeth.

194. TNA, PROB 11/541, fos 267v–272r [will of Christopher Packe, licentiate in physic, of St Giles without Cripplegate, London, 1 April 1714; pr. 9 August 1714]. Packe's will, which provides a great deal of fascinating evidence as to his role as chymical physician to the poor of his local parish as well as his religious proclivities, is not noted in the *ODNB* article of his life. For Asty, see *ODNB*. Other members of Asty's congregation such as the London merchant Nathaniel Huthnance served as pallbearers at Packe's funeral. Implicated in Whig politicking in Norwich, Huthnance later subscribed to Asty's edition of the collected sermons of the celebrated Congregational preacher John Owen. Other subscribers included Packe's son, Edmund, who inherited his father's medical practice; *A Complete Collection of the Sermons of the Reverend and Learned John Owen, D. D.* (London, 1721), 'List of subscribers'.

195. Foster, iv, 1470; *ODNB*, sub Locke, John. For Thomas's voluminous correspondence with Locke, which covers a range of subjects, including the familial (Locke was godson to Thomas's son, John) as well as the medical, see Locke, *Correspondence*, esp. vols i and ii. Thomas also corresponded with the natural philosopher Robert Boyle in the 1660s; Boyle, *Correspondence*, i, 398; ii, 451–3; iv, 435. In 1682, Thomas expressed the wish that Boyle would impart his secret of curing cancers to Locke so that he might employ them in his practice; Locke, *Correspondence*, ii, 477 [Thomas to Locke, 8 February 1682].

196. *ODNB*, sub Goodall, Charles; Innes Smith, 97; Locke, *Correspondence*, ii, 483, 597–8, 696–9, 711–14, 722–3; iii, 530–1. It is feasible that Locke's advice to Clarke to seek out Goodall and speak to him about spas may represent an example of the use of medical discourse as a form of canting language that Richard Ashcraft has seen as a central feature of Locke's correspondence with his old friend in this period; Ashcraft, *Revolutionary Politics*, 384–5, 388, 415, 445–6, 536. For the association of spas with plotting, see above 193–4.
197. TNA, LC 3/26, fo. 58v; Boyle, *Correspondence*, iv, 118–24 [Goodall to Boyle, 29 November 1668]. Goodall's nonconformist sympathies are suggested by an undated letter, written by the ejected minister and physician Edward Warren of Colchester to Goodall, in which he enclosed details of one of his medicines. It was presumably passed on to Goodall's friend Boyle; Royal Society Library, Boyle Letters, vol. 5, fos 117–18.
198. Innes Smith, 37; R. Burthogge, *De Lithiasi et Calculo* (Leiden, 1662) [BL: 1185.g.5 (20)]. It was dedicated to George Hughes and Thomas Martin, both puritan ministers and brothers-in-law, who within a few months would be ejected from their Plymouth livings; *Cal. Rev.*, 281–2, 342.
199. *CSPD, 1687–1689*, 183; M. Goldie, 'John Locke's Circle and James II', *The Historical Journal*, 35 (1992), 579–84; *idem*, 'James II and the Dissenters' Revenge: The Commission of Enquiry of 1688', *Bulletin of the Institute of Historical Research*, 66 (1993), 76–7. Burthogge not only sheltered nonconformist ministers at his house at Bowden in Devon, which was registered in 1672 but, with his wife and sister, was frequently prosecuted in the church courts for failing to attend his parish church. In a diocesan survey of 1665–6, which was particularly concerned to regulate illegal medical practitioners drawn from dissenter ranks, Burthogge was described as 'wholly disaffected to the Government of the Church of England & unlicensed'; *Cal. Rev.*, 58; Bate, *Declaration of Indulgence 1672*, Appendix vii, lxiii; DRO, C 772 [Consistory Court Act Book, 1675–1683], 7 December 1683; LPL, MS 639, fos 307r, 404v.
200. *ODNB*, sub Burthogge, Richard; Locke, *Correspondence*, v. 50–1; vi, 684–6; vii, 709–11, 777–80; viii, 455.
201. R. Burthogge, *Of the Soul of the World, and of Particular Souls. In a Letter to Mr Lock Occasion'd by Mr Keil's Reflections upon an Essay Lately Published concerning Reason* (London, 1699), 32. Coxe had a long-standing interest in the chymical investigation of plants and vegetables, three papers on the subject appearing in the *Philosophical Transactions* in 1674.
202. For Coxe's friendship with Locke, and engagement in the Whig's petitioning campaign of 1679–80, see M. Knights, 'Petitioning and the Political Theorists: John Locke, Algernon Sidney and London's "Monster Petition" of 1680', *Past and Present*, 138 (1993), 105 and n. For Coxe's early passion for Helmontian chymistry and regular communication with Boyle on these and related subjects in the mid-1660s, see Boyle, *Correspondence*, ii, 576–9; iii, 30–44, 51–63, 69–77, 82–90, 132–7, 177–82, 211–17, 250–1, 264–8.
203. Details of the Coxes' relations with Lambert emerge from a series of actions in the Court of Chancery brought by Lambert's dissolute son against his father's allies and kin who had been appointed by Lambert to protect his material interests during his

long imprisonment after 1660; see D. Farr, 'John Blackwell and Daniel Cox: Further Notes on Their Activities in Restoration England and British North America', *Pennsylvania Magazine of History and Biography*, 123 (1999), 227–33; *idem*, *John Lambert, Parliamentary Soldier and Cromwellian Major General, 1619–1684* (Woodbridge, 2003), 224–6. For Coxe's father, see G. E. Aylmer, *The State's Servants: The Civil Service of the English Republic 1649–1660* (London & Boston, 1973), 152–5; *The Mystery of the Good Old Cause Unfolded* (London, 1660), 36. Coxe's radical medico-political connections are further suggested by the fact that his sister Susanna married the physician Thomas Trapham, son of the radical Cromwellian surgeon of the same name, in 1667; Munk, i, 345.

204. Bowler (ed.), *London Sessions Records*, 344. The incident took place at the home of John Coldham, Coxe's father-in-law, at Tooting in Surrey (Coxe married Rebecca Coldham, presumably his second wife, in 1671). Coxe's involvement in radical politics around this time is also suggested by the report of a government spy that one 'D. Coxe', an associate of the radical author Henry Neville and the Whig conspirator John Hampden, had said that the duke of Monmouth was not involved in the Rye House Plot. Coxe may also have provided medical assistance to those hurt in political rioting on the streets of London, as well as helping those arrested and subsequently imprisoned in the Tower; see *CSPD, 1683–1684*, 136; *CSPD, 1682*, 382; TNA, PC 2/69, 326. It is possible that the Dr Coxe mentioned in some of these cases was in fact Dr Thomas Coxe (1615–1685), another friend of Locke who shared his attachment to the Whig cause.

205. Boyle, *Correspondence*, iii, 250–1 [Coxe to Boyle, 14 October 1666], 266–7 [same to same, 7 November 1666].

206. For Goodall and Sydenham, see the article on the former by Hal Cook in the *ODNB*. Further evidence of the close relationship between the two men is suggested by the fact that Goodall was said to have supplied a testimonial for a former servant of Sydenham, one John Fox, in his attempt to secure a licence to practise medicine from the bishop of Winchester some time before 1677. In the latter year, Fox was living at Topsham in Devon where he faced prosecution in the diocesan court for practising physic without a licence. One was subsequently granted thanks to the intervention of the husband of Sydenham's niece, Mary (1632–1701), who was clearly acting on behalf of the London-based physician; DRO, PR 518/Devon/Topsham; Mortimer, 'Index of Medical Licentiates', 113; *ODNB*, sub Chudleigh, Mary.

207. [D. Coxe], *A Discourse, Wherein the Interest of the Patient in Reference to Physick and Physicians is Soberly Debated* (London, 1669). For Coxe's authorship of this work, see F. H. Ellis, 'The Author of Wing C6727: Daniel Coxe, F. R. S., or Thomas Coxe, F. R. S.', *Notes and Records of the Royal Society of London*, 18 (1963), 36–8.

208. The quote is taken from J. R. Milton's summary of Locke's early medical interests in his article on Locke in the *ODNB*. Locke's authorship of these two treatises, written between 1668 and 1669, has been the subject of some debate, most notably following the intervention of Sydenham's biographer Kenneth Dewhurst, who wished to claim them for his subject. For a persuasive attempt to confirm Locke as the author, as well as a detailed account of the close working relationship and shared medical and ideological interests of the two physicians, see P. Romanell, *John Locke and*

Medicine: A New Key to Locke (Buffalo, NY, 1984), 163–5 and *passim*. Locke himself acknowledged his debt to Sydenham when he described him in the preface to his *Essay Concerning Human Understanding* as 'the great Genius of Physick'.

209. We know frustratingly little of Sydenham's movement in dissenting circles after 1660. The nonconformist physician Henry Sampson, however, recorded his presence at a conventicle presided over by Richard Baxter at the Haymarket; BL, Add. MS 4460, fo. 72r.

210. T. Sydenham, *Tractatus de Podagra et Hydrope* (London, 1683), A2r–5r; W. Clagett, *Of the Humanity and Charity of Christians, a Sermon Preached at the Suffolk Feast in St Michael Cornhill, London* [30 November 1686] (London, 1687), unpaginated 'epistle dedicatory'. Clagett, who spent most of the last years of the reign of Charles II attacking the sins of nonconformity and religious disunity, changed his tune after the accession of James II, when he became one of the chief critics of a resurgent Catholicism, even hinting in one sermon at the necessity of armed resistance. It may have been common origins (Clagett was the son of an ejected Suffolk minister) as well as the two men's pronounced anti-Catholicism that led them to cooperate in late 1686 in an organization designed to support the impoverished sons of the clergy from their home county. Examples of such cross-denominational activity were not unknown. Interestingly, Goodall shared the job of stewarding the Suffolk feast with fellow medic and collegiate Andrew Clench (d.1692). Clench's profile suggests that he shared much in common with Goodall. Prior to receiving his Cambridge MD by royal mandate in 1671, he acted as a go-between for the nonconformist physician Nathaniel Fairfax with Henry Oldenburg, secretary of the Royal Society. At roughly the same time, he was writing to Robert Boyle from his native Ipswich about natural curiosities in the course of which correspondence he described Boyle as 'the head of the whole body politick of learninge & Philosophy'. Created a fellow of the London College in 1680, he was later expelled in 1687 for refusing to pay fines for bad behaviour (but reinstalled in February 1688). Cook suggests that his expulsion was probably due to his 'libertarian' instincts (unlike Goodall, he opposed the over-enthusiastic prosecution of illicit practitioners). His problems with the College hierarchy however after 1683 more likely stemmed from his religious and political sympathies which were markedly pro dissent and Whig. In the wake of the Rye House Plot, for example, he sought to facilitate the release of Nathaniel Browne, a dissident surgeon, from imprisonment on the grounds that he was suffering from some form of 'epileptical' disorder; Venn, i, 353; Munk, i, 419; Oldenburg, *Correspondence*, v, 47, 50n; Boyle, *Correspondence*, iii, 322–4 [Clench to Boyle, 1 August 1667]; Cook, *Decline of the Old Medical Regime*, 207–8; *CSPD, July–September 1683*, 404.

211. Foster, ii, 798; Henning, ii, 639. He also took the precaution of securing a licence to practise as a physician in the diocese of Canterbury in April 1662; CCAL, DCb/L/R/17, fo. 148b; DCb/L/B/Box 1, no. 17 [17 April 1662]. In what follows, it is clear, *pace* Henning, that Jacob's 'known connexions' were not restricted to the 'local professional classes'.

212. Locke, *Correspondence*, ii, 80–1 [Sydenham to Locke, 30 August 1679], 95 [same to same, 6 September 1679], 259–60 [Jacob to Locke, *c.*27 September 1680]; BL, Add. MS 15,642, fos 100v–104r. The letter of September 1679 was addressed to Locke at

'Mr Jacobs, an Apothecary in Canterbury'. This was almost certainly William's brother, Israel Jacob, who is frequently referred to as a partner in the probate accounts of William Jacob's patients; see I. Mortimer, *A Directory of Medical Personnel Qualified and Practising in the Diocese of Canterbury,* circa *1560–1730*, www.kentarchaeology.ac, 110–11. Locke was not averse to using medical contacts as safe houses for correspondence. In October 1680 he listed Dr Salanova at Weymouth as one such for the letters of the earl of Shaftesbury; ibid., ii, 272 [Locke to Nicholas Toinard, 4 October 1680]. Sellanova, like Jacob, was a political creature. In 1672–3 Arnold de Salanova served as mayor of the corporation, as well as acting as surgeon to the naval garrison at Weymouth during the Third Dutch War. Like his father, Peter, he provided medical services to the parliamentary armies acting as surgeon to Colonel William Sydenham, Thomas's elder brother, on the Isle of Wight for much of the 1650s. Arnold was resident at Melcombe Regis by the early 1660s, when he was listed on the hearth tax returns; *CSPD, 1672*, 642; *Somerset and Dorset Notes and Queries*, 5 (1896–7), 35; TNA, SP 28/66/III; *CSPD, 1654*, 485; *CSPD, 1659–1660*, 226; C. A. F. Meekings (ed.), *Dorset Hearth Tax Assessments 1662–1664* (Dorchester, 1951), 15.

213. *CSPD, 1682*, 250; ESxRO, FRE 5365 [Jacob to Thomas Markwick, 28 July 1682]. For Markwick, a friend and business associate of Samuel Jeake the elder of Rye, see Hunter and Gregory (eds), *Astrological Diary*, 31, 33, 61 and *passim*.

214. Innes Smith, 20. The other dedicatees, John Durant (1620–1689) and Vincent Denne (*c*.1628–1693), were almost certainly close political confederates of Jacob. Durant, a fiery congregationalist preacher in the city, had fled Canterbury in 1679 and settled temporarily in Holland; *Cal. Rev.*, 173. Denne, who had served as MP for the city in 1656, was re-elected in 1681. A lawyer by profession, he was an exclusionist and Whig collaborator who frequently defended nonconformists from legal prosecution; Henning, ii, 206–7; *CSPD, 1663–1664*, 565–6. Bemister himself was the son of a local surgeon, Richard, who was frequently prosecuted for nonconformity and was a prominent member of Durant's congregation that gathered at the church of St Peter's and St Paul's. Like so many others of his religion, he had taken the precaution of securing a licence to practise surgery from the diocesan authorities before the clampdown against nonconformity in late 1662; *CSPD, 1665–1666*, 42; Cockburn (ed.), *Calendar of Assize Records Charles II 1676–1688*, 146, 156, 210; LPL, MS 639, fo. 154r; CCAL, DCb/L/R/17, fo. 150a; DCb/L/B/Box 1, no. 101 [26 April 1662]. John Bemister's brother, Enoch, was apprenticed to the nonconformist apothecary Jonathan Leigh (for whom, see above 178–9) of London in 1679.

215. Innes Smith, 181. Peters came from a family of medical practitioners based at Canterbury and Dover who, like William Jacob's family, originally came from Flanders.

216. Among those nonconformist students who dedicated their theses to Sylvius were John Durant (d.1683), the son of the ejected Newcastle lecturer William (d.1681) and nephew of John (see note 69 above), and the ejected minister Nathaniel Fairfax. In addition, the dissertation topics of Richard Gilpin and the Quaker Daniel Phillips (1664–1748) were strongly influenced by Sylvius's published writings; Innes Smith, 76, 82; R. Gilpin, *De Hysterica Passione* (Leiden, 1676) [BL: 1185.g.14 (25]; D. Phillips,

A Dissertation of the Small Pox... Translated by T. E. (London, 1702), A4r. The important research of the former minister-turned-physician Richard Morton Snr (1637–1698) was also influenced by his reading of Sylvius; *ODNB*. Samuel Bellingham, a former student of Sylvius at Leiden and the son of the governor of Massachusetts, made profuse notes on his lectures which along with other chymical manuscripts can be found scattered throughout the Sloane MSS in the British Library; Innes Smith, 20.

217. Reynolds praised the work of 'that noble Philosopher... Boyle', citing medical insights from his *Sceptical Chymist* (1661) in a work concerned with the extraordinary feats of fasting of a young Derbyshire maid. In the same work, he also demonstrated a good understanding of current medical research, including recent chymical theories of fermentation and the work of 'moderns' like Thomas Willis and his friend Walter Needham; J. Reynolds, *A Discourse upon Prodigious Abstinence* (London, 1669). Reynolds was ejected as minister at Wolverhampton in 1660. He proceeded to practise medicine at Stourbridge in Worcestershire, but delayed taking his MD at Leiden until August 1682, when he may have been induced to do so following a citation to appear in the consistory court for practising without a licence; *Cal. Rev.*, 409; WRO, 795.02/ BA2302/33/7390.

218. Smith, an Exeter surgeon, wrote to Boyle in 1668, expressing his admiration for his published writings and requesting a medicine to the heal the wounds of a woman that he was treating for breast cancer. He had previously used Boyle's medicines with much success; Boyle, *Correspondence*, iv, 37–9 [Smith to Boyle, 28 February 1668]. Smith was a leading figure in dissenting circles in Exeter after the Restoration. In 1672, his house in the city was licensed for Presbyterian worship. He later moved to Kingston in Surrey where he was repeatedly prosecuted for not attending his parish church. In 1681, he corresponded with Richard Baxter, providing details of a witch-craft case at Honiton in Devon; Bate, *Declaration of Indulgence, 1672*, Appx vii, lxiv; SHC, QR 2/5/Midsummer 1683, 167; ibid., QR 2/5/Michaelmas 1684, 173; R. Baxter, *The Certainty of the Worlds of Spirits* (London, 1691), 65–9 [Smith to Baxter, 4 November 1681]; Elmer, *Witchcraft, Witch-Hunting, and Politics*, 205–6, 213. He may be the same as the Anthony Smith who was granted a licence to practise surgery by the University of Oxford in July 1653; Bodl., UOA, NEP/supra/Reg Qa: Register of Congregation, 1647–1659, fo. 76r.

219. The ejected minister-turned-physician John Peachey was the author of a series of brief and highly formulaic pamphlets on the benefits of imported specifics from the Indies and Asia. Most were published anonymously and, in all likelihood, posthumously between 1693 and 1695. Some are addressed to Boyle, whom the author purportedly claimed to know well, and several cite approvingly from his works, especially those concerned with the virtues of specifics; see for example: *Some Observations Made Upon the Barbado Seeds, Shewing their Admirable Virtue in Curing Dropsies* (London, 1694), 5; *Some Observations Upon the Herb Called Perigua, Imported from the Indies: Shewing Its Admirable Virtue in Curing the Diabetes* (London, 1694), 3–5; *Some Observations upon the Serpent Stones, Imported from the Indies: Shewing Their Admirable Virtues in Curing Malignant Spotted Feavers* (London, 1694), 4–5; *Some Observations Made Upon the Russia Seed. Shewing Its Admirable Virtues in Curing the Rickets in Children. Written by a Doctor of Physick in the Countrey to Esq. Boyle at*

London, 1674 (London, 1694), 3–4; *Some Observations Made Upon the Cyclonian Plant. Shewing Its Admirable Virtues against Deafness. Written by a Physitian to the Honourable Esq.Boyle* (London, 1695), 6; *Some Observations Upon the Herb Cassiny Imported from Carolina. Shewing Its Admirable Virtue in Curing the Small-pox. Written by a Doctor of Physick in the Countrey to Esq. Boyle at London* (London, 1695); It is quite feasible that if, as suggested above (note 188), the minister John Peachey was related to the physician of the same name who was engaged in a prolonged conflict with the College of Physicians in the late 1680s and early 1690s, then the publisher of the vast majority of these tracts may have been his namesake. The two men clearly shared much in common, medically speaking. Peachey the dissenting cleric also eulogized the work of 'the great Dr Sydenham', citing him on numerous occasions alongside Boyle as a proponent of the new clinical medicine based upon observation and experience. Between 1686 and 1698, the other Peachey, prosecuted by the College for contempt, proceeded to translate and publish the complete works of Sydenham. Indeed, it is quite possible that the spate of *Observations* published between 1693 and 1695 (sixteen of the twenty-two appeared at this time), many of which were pointedly addressed to the president of the College, Thomas Burwell, may have been intended as a further act of provocation on behalf of the latter Peachey; *ODNB*, sub Pechey, John; Cook, *Decline of the Old Medical Regime*, 222–6. The contested attribution of the authorship of these tracts to John Peachey the minister is strongly suggested by the fact that the only one to bear a name on the titlepage was the first, which clearly states the author to be John Peachey. It is dedicated to Peachey's patron Sir Jonathan Keate (*c.*1633–1700) and was published by the Presbyterian printer Thomas Parkhurst. Peachey practised medicine at Oxford and Gloucester (this and other tracts in the series refer to patients in both places) and clearly favoured chymically prepared medicines over traditional therapies; John Peachey, *Some Observations Made Upon the Root Cassummuniar Called otherwise Rysagone, Imported from the East Indies. Shewing Its Nature and Virtues, and Its Usefulness... in Apoplexies, Convulsions, Fits of the Mother, the Griping of the Gutts* (London, 1679); Society of Antiquaries Library, London, MS 202, no. 101, fo. 173 [Peachey to anon., Gloucester, 9 July 1684].

220. Among those medical nonconformists or nonconformist sympathizers who wrote to Boyle on a range of medical and natural philosophical subjects were Patrick Adair, Hugh Chamberlen the elder, Andrew Clench, John Durant, Timothy Manlove, Charles Marshall and Samuel Collins. Adair (d.1694 or 1695) was a Presbyterian minister in Ulster who combined the practice of medicine with preaching. He also assisted the botanical researches of Leonard Plukenet (1642–1706); *ODNB* [which fails to mention his medical career]; Boyle, *Correspondence*, vi, 207–9 [Adair to Boyle, 13 January 1687], 276–8 [same to same, 15 November 1688]; L. Plukenet, *Almagestum Botanicum sive Phytographiae* (London, 1696), 45, 115, 136, 156. Chamberlen (for whom see above 207) wrote to Boyle in January 1666 seeking the natural philosopher's support for a series of measures which he hoped the government would adopt in order to combat the plague; ibid., iii, 18–29 [Chamberlen to Boyle, 17 January 1665/6]. For Clench, who as a fellow of the London College was later heavily criticized by his own colleagues for his outspoken defence of empirics, see note 210 above. For Durant, Manlove and

Marshall see above 183, 188, 254 n.216. Manlove may have written to Boyle for advice about his failing eyesight; ibid., vi, 392 [undated letter, now lost]. Marshall was almost certainly the same as 'Marshall, a Quaker', who enquired about phosphorus in 1682; ibid., v, 285 [letter lost]. Collins (1619–1670), who is frequently confused with two other physicians of the same name, was the son of Samuel Collins (d.1667), the puritan minister of Braintree in Essex, who reluctantly conformed after 1660. For his correspondence with Boyle, see Elmer, *Witchcraft, Witch- Hunting, and Politics*, 204–5.

221. Boyle, *Correspondence*, iv, 56 [Sydenham to Boyle, 2 April 1668]; cf. the series of letters addressed to Boyle by John Beale in 1663–4 in which the latter outlined his contempt for orthodox Galenic medicine and preference for the patient-centred approach and well-attested cures of a range of 'empirics' including the chymist Richard Matthews; ibid., ii, 153–66 [Beale to Boyle, 2 November 1663], 170–205 [same to same, 9 November 1663], 236–40 [same to same, 11 January 1664]; 240–7 [same to same, 18 January 1664]; 248–51 [same to same, 21 January 1664]. Beale, like Sydenham, undoubtedly assumed that his prejudices would elicit a sympathetic response from Boyle.

222. W. Westmacott, *Θεολοβοτανολογια: sive, Historia Vegetabilium Sacra: or, A Scripture Herbal* (London, 1694), 6–7. Westmacott was something of an eclectic in his practice, combining respect for Galen and Hippocrates with an interest in Boyle and Sydenham. He was also well versed in the techniques of the iatrochemists; among his early instructors were Valentine Fyge and Abraham Hargrave, for whom see above 162 n.82. For Westmacott, see chapter 4, note 82.

223. *ODNB*; J. Colbatch, *A Physico-Medical Essay, Concerning Alkaly and Acid* (London, 1696), 61, 116, 118, 142. Elsewhere in the same work, Colbatch declared himself a 'Disciple of Helmont' who delighted, above all else, in 'chymical Operations'; ibid., 15. For Colbatch, see especially H. J. Cook, 'Sir John Colbatch and Augustan Medicine: Experimentalism, Character and Entrepreneuralism', *Annals of Science*, 47 (2006), 475–505.

224. Johannes Groenvelt, Richard Browne, Christopher Crell, John Pechey [Peachey] and Philip Guide, *The Oracle for the Sick* (London?, 1687), A5v. The five men were all well-educated physicians and licentiates of the College who may have been acting with the approval of more 'progressive' elements within the College. Shortly after, Pechey or Peachey, the translator of Sydenham (above note 219), Browne and Groenvelt were all hauled before the censors of the College, where they were accused of acting like empirics and bringing the College into disrepute; *ODNB*, sub Browne, Richard. Crell, a Polish-born Socinian with a Leiden MD (1682) and interest in chymistry, was also on friendly terms with Locke and Sydenham; Innes Smith, 219; H. J. McLachlan, *Socinianism in Seventeenth-Century England* (Oxford, 1951), 288–90. For the Dutchman Johannes Groenvelt or John Greenfield, see H. J. Cook, 'Medical Innovation or Medical Malpractice? Or, a Dutch Physician in London: Joannes Groenvelt, 1694–1700', *Tractrix*, 2 (1990), 63–91; *idem*, *Trials of an Ordinary Doctor: Joannes Groenevelt in Seventeenth-Century London* (Baltimore, MD, 1994).

225. C. Merret, *Self-Conviction; or an Enumeration of the Absurdities, Railings, against the College, and Physicians in General* (London, 1670), 20–1. Little is known of Merret's religious convictions. He was, however, a close colleague and admirer of Boyle with

whom he worked closely on numerous projects at the Royal Society in the early 1660s. Merret may also, like Goodall, with whom he shared a strong desire to bolster the authority of a revived, progressive London College of Physicians, have acted as a royal physician; *ODNB*; TNA, LC 3/2, fo. 23v; LC 3/26, fo. 143.

226. Boyle, *Correspondence*, iv, 177 [Stubbe to Boyle, 18 May 1670]. Two weeks later Stubbe claimed that support for his stance was universal in London medical circles, apart from Sydenham and 'young Coxe'; ibid., iv, 179 [same to same, 4 June 1670]. It seems highly likely that Coxe was inspired to write on this subject by Sydenham, the two men sharing a common antipathy for the College of Physicians, of which neither were members. For a good account of the contemporary debate in medical circles over the propriety of physicians compounding their own medicines, and the central role played by Stubbe in arguing for the status quo, see Cook, *Decline of the Old Medical Regime*, 165–80.

227. In 1664, for example, a local physician William Hann appealed to Boyle to act an as arbiter in the case of a monstrous birth at Fisherton Anger in Wiltshire that was reportedly the subject of much fevered speculation in the coffee houses of nearby Salisbury. Hann was especially upset that the parish minister Richard Kent (d.1692) had baptized the conjoined twins with two names since he believed 'the divine must be beholden to the physicians for the determination of it'. What appears on first sight as a dispute over professional territory may instead have arisen from local confessional politics. Hann was a former fellow of New College, Oxford, put in by the parliamentary visitors in 1648 and ejected in 1660. Kent, on the other hand, had been sequestrated as a royalist in the 1640s and was restored to his living in 1660; Boyle, *Correspondence*, ii, 384–5 [Hann to Boyle, 3 November 1664], 423–30 [same to same, 29 November 1664]; Foster, ii, 645; *Wal. Rev.*, 375.

228. For dedications by alchemists and chymical physicians to Boyle, see L. M. Principe, *The Aspiring Adept: Robert Boyle and His Alchemical Quest* (Princeton, NJ, 1998), 112. In addition, Walter Needham dedicated his *Disquisitio Anatomica de Formato Foetu* (London, 1667) to Boyle, with whom he had worked on various experimental projects at Oxford, while Hartlib's son-in-law Frederick Clodius sought to re-ingratiate himself with Boyle in 1670 by promising to dedicate his works to his former friend and associate; Boyle, *Correspondence*, iv, 172 [Clodius to Boyle, 12 March 1670]. Equally interesting in the light of the previous discussion is the dedication to Boyle inserted by John Lancaster in the preface to his translation of Leonardo di Capua's *The Uncertainty of the Art of Physick* (London, 1684). Di Capua (1617–1695), a physician who practised in Naples and taught at the university there, was an enthusiastic proponent of iatrochemistry and the new natural philosophy; see B. M. Dooley (ed.), *Italy in the Baroque: Selected Readings* (New York & London, 1995), 124–5. Boyle was also the subject of a dedication to one of the earliest forays into pediatrics: J. Starsmare, *ΠΑΙΔΩΝ ΝΟΣΗΜΑΤΑ or Children's Diseases Both Outward and Inward* (London, 1664). Nothing is known of the author except that he practised medicine at Oundle in Northamptonshire. Finally, in 1687 John Bishop dedicated a tract on the reform of astrology to Boyle: *The Marrow of Astrology in Two Books* (London, 1687). Bishop described himself on the titlepage as 'a student in astrology and chemistry'. His collaborator Richard Kirby was the author of numerous pro-Whig

and anti-Catholic almanacs as well as a practising physician who specialized in the cure of the bewitched; Elmer, *Witchcraft, Witch-Hunting, and Politics*, 270, 271.

229. Among those whose early medical careers Boyle seems to have taken an active interest are Samuel Colepresse (d.1669?) and Thomas Molyneux (1661–1733). For Colepresse, who corresponded with Boyle prior to his departure for Leiden where he wished 'particularly to be acquainted with the Cartesian way in Chymistry', see Oldenburg, *Correspondence*, iii, 545 [Colepresse to Oldenburg, 28 October 1667]; Boyle, *Correspondence*, iii, 210–11 [Colepresse to Boyle, 28 August 1666], 290–7 [same to same, 1 February 1667], 301–4 [same to same, 19 March 1667], 308–11 [same to same, 26 April 1667]; 317–19 [same to same, 15 June 1667]. Molyneux, a medical student at Trinity College, Dublin, was recommended to Boyle by Narcissus Marsh who hoped that he might be warmly received in London prior to his departure for Leiden, to perfect his studies in medicine, in April 1683. While there, he also corresponded with John Locke; Innes Smith, 161; Boyle, *Correspondence*, v, 406–7 [Marsh to Boyle, 30 April 1683]; Locke, *Correspondence*, ii, 669–70 [Locke to Molyneux, 22 December 1684/1 January 1685]. Other English medical students in Holland such as John Price, who proceeded MD at Harderwyck in 1686, gratefully acknowledged Boyle's encouragement and inspiration; Innes Smith, 186; Boyle, *Correspondence*, vi, 393 [Price to Boyle, undated and no longer extant]. Boyle was also asked to act as a patron and intellectual mentor to two Catholic physicians, Matthew Bacon (MD Padua, 1642) and William Waldegrave (MD Padua, 1659), in 1661; ibid., i, 455 [Robert Southwell to Boyle, 22 May 1661].

230. Examples include William Randolph (*c*.1636–1675), Peter Kennedy and Gustavus Parker. Randolph received his MD from Cambridge in 1668 and later practised at Canterbury in Kent. He wrote from there to Boyle in 1670 with his original thoughts, based on his reading of the great natural philosopher's work on air and respiration, regarding the implications for health of a hypothetical circulation of the air in the body; Venn, iii, 420; Boyle, *Correspondence*, iv, 159–72 [Randolph to Boyle, 25 February 1670]. Kennedy, who proudly described himself as 'chirurgo-medicus' (a title he defended on the grounds that the best doctors practised both arts), shared Randolph's fascination with the Boylean idea of the porosity of bodies which he used as the basis of his novel approach to medicine, claiming that all diseases were curable by external means; P. Kennedy, *An Essay on External Remedies* (London, 1715), 8 and *passim*. Finally Parker, who would appear to have practised some form of occult physic and specialized in the cure of the bewitched, fully utilized Boyle's corpuscularian theories of the air in his own pioneering work on the barometer; G. Parker, *An Account of a Portable Barometer, with Reasons and Rules for the Use of It* (London, 1699), 21, 27, 48–9, 52, 83; Elmer, *Witchcraft, Witch-Hunting, and Politics*, 198, 200, 220–1.

231. The brief accounts of Haworth's life and works in both the *ODNB* and Furdell appear to seriously under-estimate the substantial learning and depth of Haworth's medical thinking. His admiration for Boyle, 'the Mirrour of our Age', is evident in all his writings and in echo of Stubbe, he claimed to owe a particular debt to Boyle's *Usefulness of Natural Philosophy*, which he posited as the foundation of his own emphasis upon the 'Prophylactic or Hygieinal' part of physic; S. Haworth, *A*

Philosophic Discourse Concerning Man (London, 1680); *idem*, *The True Method of Curing Consumptions* (London, 1683); *A Description of the Duke's Bagnio* (London, 1683), 36–7 [citation of Boyle's *Usefulness*]. Haworth's own religious and political predilections are not recorded. His first work (above) was dedicated to his father's patron, Sir John Hartopp (1637–1722), the dissenting Whig and exclusionist MP. Moreover, as an extra-licentiate of the College (1680), he was on close terms with Andrew Clench (for whom, see above). However, he later came under the protection of the duke of York and served as one of James' royal physicians; *Cal. Rev.*, 254; Munk, i, 416–17.

232. For fuller discussion of these issues, see my *Witchcraft, Witch-Hunting, and Politics in Early Modern England*, 197–206.

6
'Every Corporation a Politick Pest-House'
Medicine, Anglicanism and the Tory Reaction, 1660–1688

> As the Natural Body consists of Head and Members, made stable and erect by the Bones, tyed together and curiously interwoven by the Nerves, Ligaments, Tendons, Muscles, and Membranes; pervaded by the nutritious juice, *Lympha* and Blood; irradiated by Natural, Vital, and Animal spirits; animated and enlivened in all its motions by the Energy of a Rational Soul: So in the Political, the Sovereign the Head, and the People the Members, are held together by the strong Sinews and Nerves of Good Laws and Political Constitutions; actuated and enlivened in all their motions by the influence of the Prince and his Government (as the Soul, *Archæus* and Cœlestial fire) whereby every Member performs its Offices in the great Oeconomy, the whole System is kept in regular and orderly Motion, is firmly established and enabled to exert all those beneficial Powers that are admired in a well composed Body Politic. The Body without the Head, being but a Trunk and inanimate Carcase; and the Head without the Body, as a curious piece of Clock-work without Motion.
>
> Nathaniel Johnston, Dr in physick, *The Excellency of Monarchical Government* (London, 1686), 1–2.

Introduction

Writing in the aftermath of the ill-fated expedition of the duke of Monmouth in 1685, the medical student and Tory propagandist John Northleigh (1657–1705) compared the impact of the political events of the previous five years to those of the plague, and the actions of the crown's opponents to 'State Empericks', who had 'poysoned the body politick almost beyond the Antidote of true Medicine and Art' and thus rendered it 'almost incurable'. Northleigh's invocation of the image of a disease-ridden body politic was wholly unexceptional and was echoed in countless sermons by Anglican preachers loyal to traditional conceptions of church and

Medicine in an Age of Revolution. Peter Elmer, Oxford University Press. © Peter Elmer 2023.
DOI: 10.1093/oso/9780198853985.003.0006

state. Equally platitudinous was his conviction that the pestilential politics of the Whigs 'reigned most populously in Towns and Cities' and thus 'turned every Corporation into a politick Pest-House'.[1] The insinuation that disloyalty to the crown was primarily an urban phenomenon has long been recognized by historians as a central feature of political life in late seventeenth-century Britain. What has received much less attention is the growing contribution made by medical practitioners to urban politics in this period, either as defenders of the status quo or as opponents of the crown's religious and political policies, a process that was indicative of the general trend toward the politicization of the medical 'profession' in the second half of the seventeenth century. In the first half of this chapter, I trace the development of this process from the middle decades of the century, reaching its apogee in the 1680s when it coincided with the emergence of the first, embryonic political parties. Two main reasons are suggested for this important development. Firstly, it would appear to reflect a genuine preoccupation among large numbers of medical practitioners with the ideological issues that underpinned political developments in this period. Like other citizens, those engaged in the healing arts were equally concerned to express their religious and political allegiances and have their say in public fora on the pressing issues of the day. And secondly, many who chose to stand for election to local office in this period almost certainly did so because of the material benefits that might accrue, particularly in relation to career progression. In a world that was becoming irredeemably divided along partisan lines, professional advancement often depended upon religious and political allegiance. Medicine was no exception, and many doctors, surgeons, and apothecaries—particularly those among the latter who aspired to the status of physicians—found office-holding an expedient way of advancing their careers at the expense of political rivals. At the same time, loyal medics sought to ingratiate themselves with men of influence, both at the local and national level, by using their privileged positions within local society to inform and spy upon their patients and neighbours.

This process of politicization, however, was not confined to the towns and cities of England. It can also be traced in the government of England's rural populations in the counties, as well as at Westminster and the court, where medics became increasingly engaged in all aspects of judicial and administrative affairs. I explore these developments more fully in the second half of this chapter, where I broaden the discussion to examine the wider contribution that a host of medical practitioners on both sides of the political divide made to the national debate over the future governance of the nation. We have touched on a number of these themes in earlier chapters. Here, the emphasis will fall on the critical role that 'loyal' physicians played in a variety of capacities, including the compilation and publication of political treatises that promoted and upheld the Tory conception of church and state. In the process, it is argued, there emerged something akin to a distinct group of medical men whose support for the high Anglican-Tory cause was forged in the universities both before and after 1660 and was sealed by ties of collegiality and kinship thereafter. In time, large numbers of these men found themselves in conflict with colleagues from across the religious and political divide, representatives of that alternative dissenting-Whig tradition outlined in the previous chapter. While I continue to caution against seeing these developments as over-rigidly defined (after all, as we shall see, there was still evidence of professional cooperation across this divide), the evolution of these two medical cultures was real, manifesting itself in a variety of ways. Earlier attempts by historians to describe and analyse the impact of religious and political developments upon medical practice and belief in this period have tended to portray puritanism and dissent as promoting innovation and reform in the world of medical theory and practice. Conversely, support for Anglicanism and Stuart absolutism has been largely seen as stifling change in the medical sphere. Here, however, I suggest that the two emergent traditions cannot be distinguished in such a dichotomous fashion. Instead, I argue that both were equally open to medical speculation and innovation, the two most readily distinguished by their approach to the diagnosis and cure of specific afflictions rather than their acceptance or rejection of new medical systems. This, I argue in the final chapter is most readily apparent in the contrasting way in which representatives of the two groups responded to a range of ailments that were traditionally envisaged as 'supernatural', or more correctly preternatural, in origin. Before focusing on these developments, however, it is first necessary to trace the origins and development of a separate Anglican-Tory medical culture in Restoration England.

Administering Physic to the Body Politic: Medical Mayors in Restoration England

In 1662, Lord Herbert, a member of the county commission in Gloucestershire charged with implementing the Corporation Act, urged his fellow commissioners to carry out a thorough purge of the troublesome borough of Gloucester by declaring that 'the axiom among physicians, that the body doth every day gather something of ill humour that at length needs to be purged away, is not more true of a natural than a politic body'. They clearly listened to his advice. Within months, over three-quarters of the corporation's membership was removed and replaced by men of seemingly impeccable loyal credentials.[2] Similar developments took place across the country, where the concept of a sanitized body politic was regularly invoked to defend the actions of local governing cliques, many of whom had suffered at the hands of those whom they now sought to displace. Those who refused to conform, either by choice or by legal stricture, were accordingly excluded from participation in corporate governance, and were consequently forced to the margins of society where they struggled to create new networks of mutual support. The process of exclusion, however, was an uneven one, and the official campaign against Dissent unleashed by a hostile Cavalier Parliament was never a complete success. In those towns and cities that chose self-regulation through local purges prior to the passing of the Act, fewer were expelled from aldermanic benches and more survived who had colluded with the various governments of the Interregnum.[3] Consequently, in many corporations it is possible to detect the embryonic stirrings of urban opposition to the religious and political agenda of the restored government from as early as the 1660s. In addition, sympathy for the predicament and plight of moderate nonconformists continued to evoke conciliatory feelings among some in official circles, including the church, court, and municipal corporations. In time, the growing sense of disenchantment with the restored regime would become transformed into a wave of popular antipathy toward what many perceived as the absolutist and pro-Catholic ambitions of the crown, resulting in a concerted attempt to debar Charles' brother, James, duke of York, from succeeding to the throne. While the battle for the hearts and minds of the King's subjects raged throughout the kingdom, it was undoubtedly the case that the most intensive debates and divisions on these issues took place in the incorporated towns and cities of England. And it was here, too, that medical practitioners of diverse religious and political backgrounds became increasingly active in the day-to-day affairs of their divided communities, many aspiring to political office in order to advise how best to cure the various ailments that blighted the body politic.

As we saw in chapter 3, evidence for a politically conscious and active medical profession first became readily discernible in the years immediately after the onset of civil war in 1642, when the organs of an increasingly militarized state required the assistance of men such as physicians who in earlier times were routinely excluded from such functions. In addition to serving as magistrates in town and country, medical practitioners fulfilled a variety of administrative offices within their respective communities, sitting on county militia, assessment, and other committees that were established initially to facilitate the war effort and later to effect a smooth transition from monarchical to republican government. It was not until after the Restoration, however, that medics began to make significant inroads into office-holding at the corporate level, when the return of the King was accompanied by a growing concern in loyalist medical circles with the governance of those 'politick Pest-houses', the towns and boroughs of England. Some of those previously elected or appointed to local, and in some cases national, office survived the purges carried out between 1660 and 1662, though most were new recruits whose religious and political profiles confirm them as dedicated defenders of the restored church and state. One of the most interesting aspects of this process—discussed in more detail below—was the extent to which many of these men also aspired to the leadership of their corporate communities through mayoral election. A very rare phenomenon before 1660, closer inspection of medical office-holding in this period suggests that civic leadership was becoming an increasingly popular option for medical practitioners, including highly qualified physicians, after the Restoration.[4]

Medical men opted to stand for corporate office for a range of reasons, both professional and political in nature. There can be little doubt that for those who did not possess a medical degree or formal qualification to practise medicine the attainment of political office provided one route to professional legitimation. This is evident in the careers of numerous London surgeons and apothecaries who aspired to the status of physicians in this period. The apothecary Thomas Fyge (*c.*1633–1705), for example, whom we have already encountered as an associate and business partner of the chymical 'empiric' Lionel Lockyer (above 137), almost certainly used his election as a common councilman in the city of London as a means of attaining greater medical respectability.[5] In so doing he was following in the footsteps of his father Valentine Fyge (*c.*1600–1685), a prominent figure in the Apothecaries' Company (he served as master in 1662), who served as common councilman for the London ward of Farringdon Without between 1660 and 1662 and was widely referred to by friends and colleagues in later years as 'Dr Fyge'. The Fyges' involvement in London politics, moreover, almost certainly owed as much to the pair's ideological support for Dissent as it did to professional pragmatism. Prior to his election to the common council in 1660, Valentine Fyge was a prominent figure in Presbyterian circles in the capital, serving as a ruling elder and a member of the Grand Committee of the Provincial Assembly in 1655.[6] His son, Valentine, almost certainly shared his father's religious inclinations; he was later a committed supporter of the Whig cause in London in the early 1680s, for which he was removed from office in the Tory backlash of 1683.[7] Other London-based medical practitioners who combined political activism with a career in medicine in this period include the surgeons Thomas Middleton, Thomas Langbridge and Thomas Page, and the apothecary John Garrett. A barber surgeon by training, Middleton (d.1684) acquired something of a reputation as an expert tooth-drawer, an occupation that by itself would have placed him firmly on the lowest rungs of the medical career ladder. He was also an active dissenter and Whig and like Valentine Fyge represented the ward of Farringdon Without, and later St Bride, during the tempestuous debates over Exclusion in 1681–2.[8] Langbridge (1644–1708?) and Page (d.1707), on the other hand, who both served as common councilmen in their respective wards for lengthy periods after the Restoration, were Tory in political orientation.[9] The apothecary, Garrett (d.1683), is a particularly interesting case as he would appear to have secured royal approval for the grant of a Cambridge MD in 1680, in part, it would appear, as a reward for his loyalty to the Tory cause in London in the early years of the Exclusion Crisis.[10]

Outside of the capital, medical practitioners of all ranks, including graduate physicians, were increasingly prominent in civic government in this period. The trend is most notable in the maritime towns and borough ports of England, where a combination of factors conspired to encourage medical practitioners to stand for political office. Dover, Exeter, Faversham, Harwich, Kingston upon Hull, Liverpool, Plymouth, Rochester, Rye, Southampton and Weymouth all elected mayors whose principal occupation lay in medical practice.[11] A common denominator in many of these cases was the fact that the incumbents had served, or continued to serve, the medical services of the royal navy. Like John Conny at Rochester, Robert Seaman (*c.*1627–1695) provided many years of service to the navy in the port of Harwich. A memorial inscription to him set up in the chapel of his local church proudly records his 'steadfast love and reverence to the Church of England' and his 'loyalty to the Government', on whose behalf he almost certainly acted as an informant.[12] This trend is particularly noticeable in the strategically vital maritime boroughs of south-east England and the Cinque Ports. The physician John Golder and the surgeon John Bullack, who both figured prominently in the government of Dover after the Restoration, were equally prominent in the organization and administration of medical services to the naval forces in Dover and the surrounding neighbourhood. Golder, for example, had served as physician to the prisoners and wounded of the first Anglo-Dutch War in 1653, and used his connections in the early years of the Restoration to promote the careers of many former associates, including that of Bullack. Bullack went on to serve as mayor on three separate occasions (1674, 1675 and 1689), becoming increasingly involved in the partisan struggles of the borough initiated by the national debate over Exclusion.[13] Another Cromwellian medic to survive the purges of the early 1660s was the surgeon Arnold Salanova (for whom, see above 254 n.212), who was elected mayor of Weymouth in 1672 and, like Golder and Bullack, was probably sympathetic to the Whigs and dissent. Salanova himself had served as a surgeon to the parliamentary forces in the 1650s alongside his father, Peter, a Channel Islander, who had originally been employed by the duke of Buckingham to attack Spanish shipping in the Channel in the late 1620s but later served as surgeon-general, physician and apothecary to the earl of Bedford in the first civil war.[14]

In addition to sharing a similar political outlook, Golder, Bullack and Salanova also demonstrated another trait in common, namely a propensity to seek political office in order to promote their medical careers. None, for example, possessed formal qualifications to practise as physicians, but all aspired to the status of physician, Golder and Salanova frequently adopting the title 'Doctor', while Bullack, a surgeon by training, was licensed for medical practice. This trend was equally pronounced on the other side of the political divide, where former diehard royalists, many of whose educational and career prospects suffered in the 1650s, were only too eager to aspire to local political office in order to legitimate and promote their medical ambitions. A case in point is suggested by the career of James Welsh (d.1677), who would appear to have possessed no qualifications to practise medicine, but nonetheless established a lucrative medical practice at Rye in Sussex in the early 1660s while at the same time dominating loyalist politics in the borough. Welsh first came to prominence in the autumn of 1662, when he was elected mayor of the corporation in the wake of the mass expulsion of former Cromwellians and nonconformists instigated by the passing of the Corporation Act. At the same time, describing himself as 'medicus', he acquired an ecclesiastical licence to practise physic in the archdeaconry of Lewes.[15] In the years which followed, both as jurat and mayor (1662–4, 1668, 1673), Welsh was to prove an implacable foe to all dissidents opposed to the restored regime. He also set about acquiring further civic posts, including the captaincy of the local trained band as well as the clerkship of the passage, thus enabling him to terrorize his opponents and re-impose traditional standards of governance upon the local populace. Indeed, so great was his dominance of the local political scene that one rival, recently ousted from office by Welsh and his fellow commissioners, fumed at him 'you are Maior and you would be Minister too, Church warden, Survaier, & overseer of the poore, wee will make you Constable too and [then] you shall be all'.[16] Unabashed, Welsh continued the work of purging and restoring the body politic of Rye to its former glory. One of his first acts as mayor in 1662 was to re-impose a strict rule of secrecy upon all members of the town assembly, demanding that its discussions remain private, and a year later, he dutifully offered up the town's charter for renewal in the Quo Warranto proceedings that occupied the last year of his mayoralty.[17] At the same time, he continued to expand his medical practice, often using his civic office to pursue vendettas against men who were both professional as well as political rivals. This is most readily apparent in his harrying of the former town attorney, Philip Frith (d.1670), whom we have already encountered as the nonconformist friend and correspondent of Rye's former minister, John Allin (see above, 136). Frith, who described himself in 1657 as a 'student in Physick and Astrologie', almost certainly practised medicine among his dissenter acquaintances in the borough, and as such represented a rival to Welsh's practice. It comes as no surprise to discover then that Welsh spent much of his first spell as mayor initiating proceedings against the 'contentious and troublesome' Frith, who retaliated by bringing a lawsuit against Welsh for what he perceived as an illegal attempt to force him out of office under the terms of the Corporation Act. Proceedings dragged on for years, but the result was never in much doubt given that Welsh, who was specifically appointed in March 1665 to manage the suit, was provided with the full financial and administrative backing of the borough in pursuit of his objective. Frith died a few years later, a broken man who no longer presented a threat to the ultra-loyal Welsh.[18]

Welsh's value to the restored regime finally led to national recognition when he was asked to act as a government intelligencer in 1667. For the next ten years, he faithfully supplied Secretary Joseph Williamson and others with regular news of maritime and corporate affairs and was rewarded with yet more posts and offices.[19] Rye, of course, like Dover, was an important point of entry for the kingdom which, from the perspective of central government, required vigilant governors to oversee not only the internal affairs of the borough but also the comings and goings of native dissidents who frequently sought refuge on the continent. Medical practitioners like Welsh would appear to have been particularly well placed to carry out this function and were regularly employed by central government to police such places, many of which contained large populations of home-grown dissidents. At Ipswich, for example, where there was a large and well-established nonconformist community, a local physician, Christopher Ludkin, offered to act as a government informant in the borough, which he described in 1668 as infested with conventicles that 'increase in number and boldness daily, having encouragement from examples above'.[20] Further up the Suffolk coast at Aldeburgh, one Dr Richard Browne fulfilled a similar role in the 1660s.[21] On the west coast, the port of Chester, through which goods and people flowed to and from Ireland, was carefully watched, among others, by the Oxford-educated physician Alan Pennington (1622–1696), who was related through marriage to many of the leading figures in local loyalist circles.[22] Meanwhile, in the neighbouring port of Liverpool, municipal affairs were increasingly dominated by the former naval surgeon Silvester Richmond (d.1692), who sat as mayor of the borough in 1672. He, too, probably acted as a government agent; ten years later he corresponded with Secretary Jenkins in London, providing a critical account of the recent visit of the duke of Monmouth to Wallasey and the surrounding neighbourhood.[23] Like other surgeons with naval backgrounds, Richmond sought to use political connections, as well as devotion to the Anglican church, as a means to ascend the medical career ladder. In 1663 he was granted a licence to practise medicine in the province of York, and from the profits of his successful practice he made a fortune by investing in the Atlantic trade. Indeed, so rich and powerful was he by the time of his mayoralty that he was described locally as a 'prince'.[24] Moreover, he may have used his power and influence to promote the medical careers of relatives and former servants. His nephew John Tarleton (1649–1720), for example, followed him into medical practice despite lacking formal qualifications, and later led the Tory faction at Lancaster in the 1680s where he too served as mayor.[25] Likewise, Richmond's former apprentice James Yonge (1647–1721) combined a successful urban medical practice with an active political career following his retirement from naval service in 1668. Building on links made with the admiralty, Yonge was appointed surgeon to the naval hospital at Plymouth and deputy surgeon-general to the navy in 1674. At the same time, he established a lucrative private practice in the town, assisted no doubt by the grant of an episcopal licence to practise surgery and medicine throughout the diocese of Exeter in the same year. Five years later, he entered local politics, serving as a member of the common council in 1679, and afterwards as alderman and finally mayor in 1694–5.[26] Like his former master, Yonge too was an implacable opponent of the Whigs and Dissent. In 1685, at the height of the Tory reaction, he intruded into one of his many medical works a scathing condemnation of the current times as 'an Age of Monsters [and] Prodigees and deformities in all kinds of writing', which had produced traitors, heretics and schismatics in abundance. In particular, he levelled his guns at those who abused the scriptures to defend murder and rebellion, especially those 'Fanatical Covenanters, and other Divines of the faction, both in England and Scotland', and went out of his way to condemn the writings of leading Whigs such as Thomas Hunt.[27]

Occupational insecurity and professional ambition were almost certainly important factors in many of these cases where medics, especially surgeons and apothecaries, actively sought municipal office, but they were certainly not the only ones. For many, probably the majority, a sense of political duty, more often than not a product of sincerely held religious and political beliefs, almost certainly provided the stimulus to enter local politics.[28] This much is clear from the growing numbers of highly educated physicians—men at the top of their profession—who devoted substantial time and effort to the task of securing political and judicial office in order to promote their own brand of partisan political thinking. Typical in this respect were men like John Speed (1628–1711), Anthony Salter (1600–*c.*1668) and Martin Llewellyn (1616–1682), who all possessed Oxford MDs but nonetheless found time amid busy medical practices to serve the interests of Church and King by standing for the office of mayor. All three were demonstrably politicized by the events of the 1640s and 1650s. Speed, who was ejected from his fellowship at Oxford in 1648, deferred the taking of his MD until 1666.[29] Salter (MD 1633) was the son of an Exeter apothecary, whose family suffered financially for their loyalty to Charles I in the first civil war. He first entered corporate politics in the wake of the mass purges of the boroughs in 1662 and became mayor three years later following the death in office of his ultra-loyal brother-in-law, Alan Penny.[30] Finally, Llewellyn (MD 1653), whom we have already encountered as an inveterate opponent of the Quakers in his capacity as mayor of Wycombe in 1671 (above 184), was part of a large body of devoted supporters of church and crown that remained in Oxford after the civil war to pursue medical study while clandestinely promoting the Stuart cause.[31] Despite the fact that there were clear material and professional advantages to be gained from pursuing a political career in local government, physicians such as these were more likely to have been motivated to serve high office by sincerely held political convictions borne from the experience of civil war and its aftermath. All were invariably active and partisan in government. John Speed, for example, whose election as mayor of Southampton in 1681 probably owed much to external influence (itself a mark of the considerable national importance attached to this naval town), was to prove one of the key figures in the government of the town after 1682, particularly in providing strong leadership to the nascent loyalist and Tory faction. As a JP, he was the chief instigator of the persecution of 'fanatics' and plotters in the wake of the Rye House Plot, and, as a regular correspondent with Whitehall, he provided a constant flow of information on the political temperature of the town. He was also the architect of various loyal addresses to both Charles II and James II and played a crucial role in persuading the town to surrender its charter in 1683–4 so as to comply with Charles' somewhat half-hearted attempt to remodel the boroughs following the defeat of the exclusionists.[32]

Corporate Governance and Medical Men: The Case of Restoration Gloucester

Among the many tangible benefits of office-holding in early modern England was the fact that it often facilitated access to important networks of urban patronage and largesse. In many towns and corporations, these were medical in character and thus attracted the attention of ambitious practitioners. An excellent example of how this might work in practice, and encourage factionalism and partisanship in the process, is evident in the machinations that bedevilled the corporate politics of Gloucester after the Restoration. In the summer of 1662, following local enactment of the Corporation Act, the governing body of the city of Gloucester was fundamentally remodelled. Among those newly appointed to the common council and aldermanic bench were two physicians, Robert Fielding (1621 or 1622–1709) and Henry Fowler (*c.*1620–1685), who shared a common social and political background. Both men, for example, were the sons of local Anglican ministers who had suffered at the hands of the puritans in the early 1640s. Fielding, who was ejected from a fellowship at Oxford in 1648 after fighting for the King, joined the growing band of alienated royalists who opted to stay at the university and study medicine in the 1650s, graduating MD in December 1653.[33] Fowler, like Fielding an Oxford alumnus, did not complete his medical studies choosing instead to enrol in the royalist army in the first civil war, during the course of which it was reported that many of his medicaments, including *aurum potabile* and a box full of precious bezoar stones, were smashed to pieces by parliamentarian soldiers.[34] In 1662, both men entered local politics, Fielding as senior alderman, and Fowler as a member of the common council (he was promoted to alderman in the following year), and both set about consolidating their hold on local power by intruding themselves into a variety of corporate posts and offices.[35] Presumably at this stage the two men were motivated by common aims, dedicated as they were to the renunciation of the sectarian agenda of the 1650s and the restoration of the old religious and political order. However, by the late 1660s initial harmony—as in so many reconstituted boroughs—gave way to renewed factional conflict, with the two men emerging as the leaders of opposing groups within the corporation of Gloucester.

While the main reason for the growth of factionalism in the city was related to increasing disenchantment in governing circles, including among some former royalists, with the direction of central government policy on a range of issues concerned with religion, politics, and the conduct of the Second Anglo Dutch War (1665–7), the rift between Fielding and Fowler was, in all probability, a by-product of the competition for lucrative medical posts which lay at the disposal of the corporation. Bad blood between the two would appear to have been sparked by the election in August 1668 for a new physician to the city's hospitals, including St Bartholomew's. Fowler won a resounding success when the chamber voted 23–1 in his favour, despite the fact that the more senior Fielding had served as mayor in 1664 and was currently president of St Bartholomew's hospital.[36] Within a few months of this reverse, Fielding suffered a further rebuff when he was admonished by the common council for entertaining one George Wall in his house, an apothecary and 'foreigner', who sold his wares in the city contrary to the privileges of the mercers' and grocers' company.[37] With his grip on power beginning to slip, Fielding acted swiftly. In August 1669, following the death of the mayor in office, he used his influence among a revitalized 'Presbyterian party' within the corporation to get himself elected as temporary mayor for one month. At the ensuing Michaelmas elections for a new mayor, his opponents, led by Fowler, claimed that Fielding, described in one account as a 'discontented cavalier', was now heading a 'seditious faction' in the chamber intent on promoting the candidacy of a Presbyterian alderman, William Bubb, an apothecary by trade. Fowler countered by putting himself forward for mayor and appealing to the King and Privy Council to disqualify Bubb from office.[38] After much debate, including a personal appearance before the Privy Council, the board found in favour of Fowler. As mayor, he now moved against his political and medical rival, and sought to have him permanently removed from holding any office in the city on the grounds that he continued to employ a 'foreigner' as an apprentice. Following one close vote that went in Fielding's favour, he was finally 'removed and discharged' from his aldermanic and magisterial posts, and 'disfranchised and discharged from being a Burgess & freeman' of Gloucester on 7 August 1671.[39] However, Fowler's success in vanquishing Fielding and his dissenting allies, was largely a pyrrhic victory. As he himself was forced to admit, the failure of the corporation to fill the vacant place left by the removal of Fielding had left the corporation 'a maimed body'. Picking up on the medical analogy, the bishop of Gloucester, William Nicholson, described the condition of the city in October 1671, when Fowler was once again put forward as mayor on the instructions of the King, as 'all mad, Bedlam mad'. By December of that year, things were so bad that Fowler was forced to acknowledge that the day-to-day work of governing the city had been brought to a virtual standstill. The generality of the people, imbued once more with 'the old sullen humour', were refusing to support the city's charitable institutions with the result that the city's hospitals were on the brink of collapse. Cutting an increasingly isolated figure, he concluded: 'I know not what to do, for there is no regard had to me, nor attendance on me as Mayor, so that the authority vested in me by his Majesty's letter is much slighted and contemned'.[40]

Fowler's self-pity was no doubt exacerbated by the fact that he had received little material reward from the King or government in return for his efforts. In September 1671, the dean of Gloucester, Dr Thomas Vyner, had written to Secretary Williamson requesting that 'for the encouragement of the loyal party at Gloucester', the King might move to offer Fowler an Oxford medical degree, he being 'already MB'. Fowler himself followed up a few days later, thanking Williamson for his 'favours and civilities' and requesting further assistance in his pursuit of the royal mandate for MD, but none was forthcoming. The best that Fowler achieved was a university licence to practise medicine, issued in 1678.[41] In time, however, he did manage to exert a stranglehold on the government of the city, creating the nucleus of a loyal caucus that would later evolve into an embryonic Tory party in the city. This he performed with characteristic vigour and vindictiveness. On the day, for example, that his arch-rival Dr Fielding was removed from office, mayor Fowler issued an order that the royal arms and those of the duke of York 'shalbe engraven on the Southgate according as Mr Maior shall see fitt... the same having been defaced for severall yeares past'. His final act as mayor in 1672 was to institute a review of all legislation passed by the common council of the city 'made in the time of the late troubles tending to schisme or Rebellion and to make report to this house of all such Acts that they thinke fitt to be expunged and defaced'. In the years that followed he remained an indefatigable opponent of all forms of dissent. As a JP, he was active throughout the 1670s in suppressing conventicles and hunting down libellers, on one occasion using his medical connections, his own apothecary, to unearth the miscreants.[42] Following another spell as mayor in 1679–80, he was again active throughout the years of the Exclusion Crisis, instigating, composing and signing loyal addresses to Charles II in which he continued to lament the disastrous impact of the civil wars upon the nation, initiated by 'men of seditious principals the dregs of which still remaine'. Equally important, however, from the perspective of his position as one of Gloucester's foremost physicians, he managed at the same time to extend his control over important urban institutions such as the city's hospitals, acting as treasurer and president of St Bartholomew's for much of the 1670s and early 1680s.[43]

In summary, it is probably fair to conclude that Fowler's mission to purge the city of Gloucester of its malignant members was prompted by a combination of factors that included both his deeply held religious and political convictions, as well as a desire to profit from the material benefits that came with office-holding, particularly those relating to his vocation. Indeed, in his eyes and those of his contemporaries the two were understood as largely inseparable. Unsurprisingly, he was not alone in his profession in seeking to promote this dual agenda. In Gloucester itself, the career paths of other medical practitioners followed a similar trajectory, rising and falling with the fortunes of their respective political 'parties' and allies. This is evident, for example, in the careers of two of Fowler's political associates, William Jordan and John Smallwood. Jordan (d.1687), who began life as an apothecary, served the city in various capacities (steward in 1665, sheriff in 1672–3) prior to his appointment as an alderman of the city in 1682. He was subsequently elected, unopposed, as mayor in 1685.[44] A loyal Tory who had earlier supported Fowler in 1671 in his attempt to thwart the mayoral election of fellow apothecary William Bubb, Jordan would appear to have used civic office as a platform from which to advance a medical career. In the same year that he was elected mayor, he thus succeeded Fowler to the post of physician to the city's hospitals.[45] His tenure, however, was short-lived. In November 1687, following the purges instigated by James II, he not only lost his place on the aldermanic bench but was also forced to relinquish his post as civic physician to another apothecary-cum-doctor and common councilman, Nicholas Lane. Thereafter, Jordan spent most of the early years following the Glorious Revolution agitating for the restoration of his post, but following complex and lengthy legal proceedings against the corporation, he finally lost his appeal when the courts ruled that the city was within its rights to displace officials at its hospitals for contravening corporate by-laws (Jordan, it was claimed, not only had been non-resident but had illegally sub-let city property associated with the post of physician).[46] The career of the surgeon John Smallwood (d.1707), who also supported Fowler's efforts to thwart Fielding and his Presbyterian allies in 1671, followed a similar path to that of Jordan. In 1672, he acquired a permanent place on the city's common council as well as the post of surgeon to St Bartholomew's Hospital.[47] Further rewards followed, including the acquisition of hospital lands on an advantageous lease.[48] During the Exclusion Crisis he again performed loyal service on behalf of the corporation's nascent Tory party, signing loyal declarations and addresses, and further preferment followed, culminating in his election as an alderman in 1686.[49] Smallwood's rise, however, came to an abrupt halt in November 1687 when he, along with other diehard Anglican and Tory members, including Jordan, was removed from the corporation. Two weeks later he also lost his post as surgeon to St Bartholomew's and the city's other hospitals, when he was replaced by his long-standing Whig rival, Patrick Clarveato (1629–1694).[50] Like Jordan, his fortunes did not recover after the Revolution, and he spent the last years of his life in apparent destitution. By June 1700 he was reported to be living in 'meane circumstances'. His house, which was leased from the corporation, was described as 'much out of repaire', and he himself was in arrears for his rent. Such were the vicissitudes of political life in late seventeenth-century urban England from which medical men, like others, were no longer exempt.[51]

Medical Men, Civic Governance and Political 'Crisis'

The situation at Gloucester was almost certainly not exceptional. Between 1660 and 1700, the urban boroughs of England witnessed an ever-expanding influx of medical practitioners into the ranks of their governing bodies, encouraged no doubt by a combination of political and professional considerations. Once elected or co-opted, they were able to offer their own distinctive prescription for the ills of the body politic, both local and national. The cyclical nature of this pattern of recruitment is, in fact, quite marked, coinciding with those periods of the most intense religious and political debate—1670–2, 1679–83, 1685–88. The first phase, of course, coincided with the imposition of a new Conventicle Act that radically enhanced the powers of the magistracy to suppress dissent and provoked in the process a heated debate over the merits of an approach to conformity based on force rather than persuasion. It was during this period, for instance, that Henry Fowler was contending with Robert Fielding over the leadership of the borough of Gloucester, Martin Llewellyn was struggling to use his judicial powers as mayor of Wycombe to crush the Quakers, and Silvester Richmond was exerting his grip on the borough of Liverpool. At the same time medical politics came to the fore in Coventry where the mayoral elections in 1671–2 were dogged by partisan controversy engendered by religious divisions. In August 1671 the King had written to the corporation asking that one Abel Brookesby (d.1676), variously described as an apothecary and a 'practitioner in physic and chirurgery', be excused from standing as mayor as it might 'impede him in such charitable exercises of his profession'. It is clear from the King's letter that he was persuaded to write in favour of Brookesby because it was widely reported of him that he had tended sick and wounded royalist soldiers at the battle of Worcester and 'continues the same practice chiefly among the meaner sort of people for charity'. Within a month, however, loyalists within the corporation, including the out-going mayor and two aldermen, petitioned the city's recorder, the earl of Northampton, requesting that the elections should proceed as planned and that Brookesby should serve his turn, as 'it was wounded rebels after Worcester fight that Mr Brookesby attended'. Brookesby was in fact a Congregationalist and partial conformist who was reluctant to swear the requisite oaths of loyalty to Church and state. He was also, as his opponents knew only too well, deeply reluctant to implement the full rigour of the law against those whom he might otherwise have sought to protect—a practice that produced deep unease and exacerbated partisan feeling throughout the towns and boroughs of England at this time.[52]

The crisis induced by the national debate over Exclusion initiated a further influx of medics into corporate politics in the early 1680s, a process that continued into the next reign following the death of Charles II in 1685. We have already noted the presence of medical practitioners in the various political bodies that constituted the government of London, as well as the prominent role of highly qualified physicians such as Henry Fowler and John Speed in the government of boroughs such as Gloucester and Southampton in the early 1680s. Elsewhere, especially in the cathedral cities where senior clergy vied with corporations for power and patronage, loyal and 'well affected' members of the medical profession were encouraged to perform their civic responsibilities. The eminent physician Walter Pope (1628–1714), for example, was almost certainly persuaded to take up his seat as a member of the governing 'thirty' at Salisbury in February 1681 through the auspices of his good friend and neighbour Seth Ward, bishop of Salisbury.[53] Similar motives may have encouraged the physician Peter Parham (1635–1723) to lead the Tory faction in Norwich in 1682. Parham, who studied at Cambridge in the 1650s, was the son-in-law of Anthony Sparrow, bishop of Norwich, one of the most loyal and active members of Charles II's episcopacy, who was widely despised by the dissenters and Whigs.[54] The remodelling of the corporations in the wake of the Quo Warranto proceedings initiated by Charles II and James II proved particularly conducive to attracting new men, including medics, into local government. At Malmesbury, for example, two local physicians, Aquila Smyth (1622–1690) and William Burgess were elected as capital burgesses in 1685,[55] while medical practitioners were similarly intruded at Chichester (Freeman Howse),[56] Chippenham (William Gale),[57] Faversham (Major Michael Greenstreet),[58] Guildford (William Rosewell),[59] Hastings (Peter Fyott)[60] and Hull (Matthew Hardy).[61] Occasionally, some refused office. Samuel Johnston, for example, brother of the prominent Tory physician and propagandist Nathaniel Johnston, declined to serve as an alderman and JP in his native Beverley in 1685.[62] Others, particularly those perceived as disloyal to crown and church, were deliberately kept out of office through the full force of the law. Such a fate seems to have befallen William Cropp at Southampton.[63] Further purges initiated in 1687 in the wake of James's dramatic reversal of policy and his attempt to court the dissenting interest sparked a further influx of medical men into civic office, most notably Richard Burthogge at Totnes, Robert Haslen at Chichester and John Friend at radical Taunton.[64] It is difficult to escape the conclusion that if participation in civic politics is taken as a guide to the changing attitude of medical practitioners to political engagement then the second half of the seventeenth century can be said to have witnessed a truly remarkable watershed in terms of how medical men perceived their wider role in early modern society.

Doctors and the Dispensation of Justice in Restoration England

Office-holding, of course, took many forms in early modern England and was not restricted to the corporate boroughs. Given the concentration of medical services in urban centres, it is not surprising, perhaps, to find the majority of politically ambitious medics active in such places. It would be a mistake, however, to conclude that office-holding at the county, and indeed national, level was beyond the reach of those who made a career from medical practice. The Restoration, in fact, provides numerous examples of medical practitioners actively engaging in county government, most notably by their presence in ever-growing numbers among the ranks of the rural magistracy.[65] A closer analysis of this sample suggests a number of common themes. The vast majority, for example, were highly qualified physicians who either possessed medical degrees from Oxford and Cambridge or were rewarded for their earlier loyalty to king and church with mandated or Lambeth medical degrees granted by Charles II and archbishop Sheldon. Not surprisingly, they were also, by and large, committed royalists and High Church Anglicans, who in most cases were attracted to judicial service through a deep-seated commitment to implementing the legislative agenda of the Cavalier Parliament that was designed to guarantee the Restoration settlement in church and state. Many, for example, were notably assiduous in the judicial campaign to stamp out religious dissent, reserving their particular ire for sects such as the 'anti-magisterial' Quakers. Nathaniel Highmore (1613–1685), who practised at Sherborne in Dorset, Richard Lister of Leicestershire and Robert Thoroton (1623–1678) of Nottinghamshire were all singled out by the Quakers as notorious persecutors of Friends.[66] Others such as Thomas Arris[67] and John Windebank[68] became embroiled in long-running disputes with local dissenters in Hertfordshire and Surrey, respectively, that bear witness to the ideological commitment of these men to the restored government of Charles II. Some, if their opponents are to be believed, even sacrificed their lives in the judicial struggle to crush Dissent. The sudden death of the Lancashire magistrate Dr William Fyfe in 1671, for example, was widely attributed by local nonconformists to his impious behaviour and arrogance in predicting the death of one his patients, the ejected minister Nathaniel Heywood.[69]

Occasionally a combination of factors produced an exceptional concentration of medics serving their local community in a variety of judicial and political functions. In the town and county of Cambridge, for example, physicians were particularly active as office holders in the early years of the Restoration. Here, the presence of the university, with its own unique system of governance and political representation, provided fertile soil for ideologically motivated medical practitioners to enter judicial service in the city of Cambridge and the surrounding countryside. Robert Eade (*c.*1603–1672), John Gostlyn (d.1705), James Jackson (d.1686), Sir Thomas Sclater (1615–1684) and Edward Stoyte (b.*c.*1619) were all products of mid-century Cambridge, whose common profiles and subsequent activities suggest a close ideological bond. All, for example, were committed royalists whose careers suffered to varying degrees during the period of puritan domination of the University and were later rewarded for their loyalty. Many, indeed, rose to prominence within academic circles, Gostlyn and Jackson assuming the presidencies of their respective colleges, Caius and Clare. Not surprisingly, they frequently acted in concert to guarantee law and order in town and county. Sclater and Eade, for example, served as county commissioners overseeing the regulation of the corporations in 1662, while three years later Edward Stoyte worked alongside Sclater in securing the convictions of various local dissenters under the Clarendon Code.[70] Sclater's surviving casebooks testify to his lack of sympathy for the plight of nonconformists, as well as providing firm evidence of his efficiency and industry in all aspects of his work as a county magistrate, including attendance at quarter sessions and the bi-annual assizes.[71] The latter, of course, provided important opportunities for doctors such as Sclater to engage in convivial sociability and to re-affirm and consolidate long-standing social, political and professional relationships. In 1674, for example, Sclater provided entertainment for his fellow JPs at the Lent assizes where the guest list included two fellow physician-magistrates, Gostlyn and Jackson.[72] On occasions such as this, there is little doubt that close political allegiances were formed that would later prove crucial in cementing party bonds in the wake of the Exclusion Crisis. Sclater himself, who had served briefly as MP for the University in 1659, would later occupy the crucial post of sheriff for the county of Cambridgeshire in 1680–1.[73] In this capacity, he, like his dinner guests Gostlyn and Jackson, must also have worked closely with another politically active Cambridge doctor, Robert Brady (*c.*1627–1700), whose role as a leading propagandist for the Tory cause is discussed more fully below. Brady, elected MP for the University in 1681 and again in 1685, was an influential figure in medical circles in Restoration Cambridge who, alongside colleagues like Gostlyn and Jackson, helped to promote the careers of a generation of medical students, the vast majority of whom shared an attachment to the restored government and later supported the Tory cause of 'Church and King'. In 1668, for example, Gostlyn, Jackson and Brady, alongside other politically active medics such as Charles Scarburgh (1615–1694), provided testimonials on behalf of Thomas Short, who sought a royal mandate for his Cambridge MD.[74] Short (1635–1685), the son of a sequestrated Anglican minister, was typical of many medical students of his generation who through a combination of familial poverty and 'small hopes of college preferment' was 'forced to take up the practice of physic' despite the lack of formal qualifications. And like others of his background, he prospered after the Restoration through the support of sympathetic elders within the Cambridge medical faculty. Following the grant of his MD in 1668 (officially an incorporation as he had graduated MD at Padua in 1665), Short set up as a physician in London, converted to Roman Catholicism, and established a lucrative practice among his co-religionists.[75] Temporarily under a cloud during the period of the Popish Plot, when he continued to treat prominent Catholics in prison and provide certificates for others to flee the country (ostensibly for health reasons), Short's career blossomed in the aftermath of the Exclusion Crisis. Not only did he inherit many of the aristocratic clients of the disgraced Whig physician, Richard Lower, but he also found employment ministering to the medical needs of many leading figures in government and at court, including the duchess of Portsmouth, for which he was knighted in 1684.[76] Short's career, in brief, provides a fascinating snapshot of the way in which medicine had become politicized in an age of emerging party divisions, the product in part of physicians like Sclater and Brady who used their political influence, office, and patronage to reconstruct a loyal vision of the body politic in later Stuart England.

Anatomizing the Body Politic: Medical Men, Pamphleteering and Loyal Propaganda

Office-holding at all levels, local and national, provided, as we have seen, medical practitioners with ample opportunity to engage with the political issues and processes that shaped government in seventeenth-century England. Some, like Thomas Arris and Robert Brady, played a dual role, performing vital service as local magistrates while representing their communities in Parliament.[77] Others were content to capitalize on their privileged position in local society by spying on and informing against those whom they perceived as enemies of the regime. Whether acting formally as agents of local and central government, or informally as concerned citizens, it is evident that the Restoration period witnessed the emergence of an ideologically coherent and highly politicized group of medical practitioners committed to upholding traditional notions of order and authority in church and state. Not surprisingly, many later found their way into the ranks of an embryonic Tory party, where they worked tirelessly to undermine their Whig opponents and uphold the established Church and royal authority. Typical in this respect were the actions of doctors like Ralph Ewens, George Neale and Thomas Novell, who, lacking official status to act against their opponents, nonetheless devoted considerable time and energy in promoting the Tory cause. Ewens, who practised at Donyatt in Somerset, supplied the government with details of the activities and opinions of the local Whig grandee George Speke (1623–1689), who was widely suspected of involvement in plotting against Charles II.[78] Neale (d.1691), a medical graduate of Oxford, set up in practice at Leeds in Yorkshire where he was active in the 1670s promoting the prosecution of unlicensed practitioners at the assizes.[79] In the early 1680s, however, he turned his attention to political enemies when he became embroiled in a dispute with the Whig lord mayor of York, Edward Thompson, who had arrested the physician and burned his papers. In November 1683, Neale wrote to the Privy Council in London, complaining that Thompson had obstructed him in the pursuit of his medical labours and was responsible for protecting fanatics and plotters, several of whom he had 'in quest'.[80] Whereas Neale was in all probability politicized while a medical student in Interregnum Oxford, Thomas Novell (d.1686), like fellow Tory activist Peter Parham (above), was a product of Restoration Cambridge, where he was assisted in receiving his mandated medical degree through the intervention of ultra-loyal Anglicans such as Edmund Boldero (1609–1679), master of Jesus College, and Henry Paman (1623–1695). Novell seems to have repaid his superiors by acting as an *agent provocateur* during the fierce debates over Exclusion that took place in the capital. In October 1681 he deposed before London magistrates that he was present in a coffee house on the day of the bitterly contested mayoral elections when, in conversation with Titus Oates and his associate, Captain Spineage, he provoked the former's outrage by claiming that the Tory candidate, Sir John Moore, would attract the moderate dissenting vote. When Oates exploded with rage, the physician Novell calmly suggested that he thought he was suffering from a bout of madness and that 'he ought to bleed', a diagnosis that Oates' companion, Spineage, clearly saw as a ruse designed to infuriate and entrap the infamous 'discoverer' of the Popish Plot.[81]

Evidence of the willingness of medical practitioners from across the political spectrum to engage in the day-to-day affairs of governing the nation, as we have seen, took many forms. The growing aptitude of some, including those of eminence and rank, to take on onerous responsibilities such as public office is merely one indication of the way in which medics were increasingly politicized in the period after 1660. Others played their part by engaging in the often fractious, and sometimes violent, routine of partisan political debate.[82] As the political temperature of the country rose in the late 1670s and early 1680s, medical men on both sides of the 'party' divide also began to engage in another critical aspect of the political process, namely the composition and publication of pamphlets and treatises aimed at persuading the wider populace of the merits of their respective causes. We have already traced the first stirrings of this kind of activity among those medical practitioners writing during the 1650s in support of the new political arrangements associated with the Cromwellian Interregnum. Some, such as Henry Stubbe and Marchamont Nedham, continued to expatiate on public affairs after the Restoration, but with little obvious ideological consistency. Others opted to remain silent in the face of official opprobrium. The Oxford-educated physician Thomas Jeanes (1628–1668), for example, suffered for his youthful indiscretion in co-authoring a pamphlet in defence of the trial and execution of Charles I by the loss of his place as physician at Magdalen College at the Restoration.[83] As the country became increasingly divided in the late 1670s, supporters on both sides drew inspiration from the writings of men whose prime expertise lay in dissecting real bodies but who nonetheless made special claim to anatomize and diagnose the ills of the body politic. On the Whig (or proto-Whig) side, some clearly acted as the mouthpiece for wealthy patrons and patients. John Locke, of course, who served as personal physician to the Whig parliamentary leader the earl of Shaftesbury, is the most famous example, but there were others. In 1677, for instance, the ejected minister-turned-physician Nicholas Cary (d.1697) was fined and imprisoned for his part in the publication the previous year of 'a scandalous and seditious libel' aimed at questioning the legal status of the recently dissolved Parliament. The author was almost certainly his patron and patient Denzil, Lord Holles (1598–1680), but Cary refused to say anything that might incriminate him, opting instead to inform the authorities only that the author was 'an ancient friend, to whom he has been for many years highly obliged'.[84] Cary's prosecution closely paralleled that of another physician, Lewis du Moulin, a few years earlier. In 1673, du Moulin (1606–1680), a noted controversialist who had been ejected from the Camden chair of history at Oxford at the Restoration, was imprisoned for printing and publishing 'a treasonable and seditious book' while working alongside the inveterate plotter, Lord Howard of Escrick (d.1694).[85] Du Moulin was an Erastian Congregationalist, who had previously written in support of the Engagement in 1650 utilizing Hobbesian arguments to back up his pronounced anti-clericalism. He later employed similar thinking in 1678 when, in a work dedicated to Louis XIV's physician, he claimed that medical men were better positioned to pronounce on ecclesiastical matters such as excommunication because they hailed from a profession 'more disinterested and unencumbered by prejudice'.[86] A very similar stance was adopted by the royal physician William Denton (1605–1691), whose political writings after the Restoration, some of which were suppressed, have been compared in tone and nature to those of his more illustrious colleague, John Locke.[87]

A key plank in the armoury of both du Moulin and Denton was their knowledge and understanding of the historical processes that they believed had helped to shape the political world of the late seventeenth century.[88] History, however, as any student of the subject will know, can be highly malleable and easily adapted to suit specific ideological needs. This was equally the case in our period when, if anything, it made even greater appeal to medical defenders of the political status quo. Spurred on no doubt by the admonitions of High Church clerics to dissect and diagnose the diseases afflicting the body politic, loyal physicians like Robert Brady and Nathaniel Johnston readily employed a range of historical arguments and precedents to defend the divinely ordained authority of the Stuarts. We have already charted the distinguished career of Brady as royalist plotter in the 1650s (above 59). Rewarded for his loyalty at the Restoration with the grant of an MD and the mastership of Gonville and Caius College, Cambridge, Brady (*c.*1627–1700) thereafter combined medical practice with political activism, serving the restored government in numerous capacities including as JP, MP and the author of some of the most original works written in defence of divine right monarchy. Political historians, in particular, have observed how his various writings represent 'the development of a new critical historical awareness and method' which he brought to bear on contemporary political issues. Brady, for example, has been credited with being the first 'modern' scholar to study the Domesday Book, and through the close reading of rolls and petitions pioneered new approaches to the origins of Parliament, proving beyond doubt that it was 'a new invention of the thirteenth century'. In later works, he also set out to show—again through close archival research and evidence—that the historical notion of 'community', a concept which lay at the heart of much Whig thinking, denoted the interests of a 'select number' rather than representing the concerns of a whole body of people.[89]

Brady's publications in defence of divine right monarchy and Toryism were mirrored by those of fellow physician, Nathaniel Johnston (1629–1705), who, like Brady, was granted unlimited access to the public records in the Tower of London and other state papers in order to underwrite the claims of his royal master, James II.[90] Like Brady, he too was a product of post-civil war Cambridge and shared Brady's interest in medical research and new approaches in natural philosophy. Brady, for example, had been a student of the celebrated anatomist and physiologist Francis Glisson and an early convert to Harveian notions relating to the circulation of the blood. He subsequently pioneered the use of quinine, or Jesuit's bark, and corresponded with Thomas Sydenham on, among other things, the treatment of rheumatism in the course of which he defended him from the attacks of his medical detractors. Brady finally inherited the Regius chair of medicine at Cambridge on the death of his old mentor, Glisson, in 1677.[91] Brady's colleague, Johnston, may have begun medical practice while a young student at Cambridge in 1651, five years before receiving his MD.[92] His own interests, which extended to botany, mineralogy and chymistry, are evident from his correspondence in the 1670s with the Yorkshire naturalist and physician (and fellow Tory), Martin Lister (1639–1712), during the course of which he referred to the 'many microscopicall observations of the minuter parts of plants' he had undertaken from his home at Pontefract. He would also appear to have possessed a keen interest in strange or difficult births and was clearly practising midwifery with the use of his own instruments.[93]

It is important to stress that Brady and Johnston were not die-in-the-wool traditionalists in terms of their medical and scientific outlooks. Like so many Anglican medical students of their generation, they happily combined a deep-seated respect for religious and political traditions while maintaining an open mind with regard to natural philosophical speculation. At the same time both men showed a remarkable interest in, and aptitude for, historical and antiquarian research, which informed not only their own political writings but also that of many like-minded medical colleagues. Johnston's passion for antiquarianism and local history, for example, was shared by fellow physicians Robert Thoroton and Richard Kuerden (alias Jackson) as well as the royal surgeon John Knight (1622–1680), who was an avid collector of heraldic manuscripts and other historical documents.[94] John Lamphire (1614–1688), who succeeded du Moulin to the chair of the Camden professorship in History at Oxford, combined academic duties with magisterial responsibilities and political ambitions.[95] Henry Knewstub (d.1705), on the other hand, was a clerical physician with a passion for archaeology and numismatics.[96] Some physicians, such as Thomas Skinner (d.1679) and Thomas Frankland (d.1690) developed a special interest in more recent history. Skinner, for example, who wrote to Secretary Williamson in 1677 about his plans to write a biography of General George Monck, the architect of Restoration, was clearly hoping to acquire high-level political patronage for his efforts. In the event, the planned work did not appear in his own lifetime though he did manage to publish a highly partial account of the Restoration and its aftermath that appeared as a separate appendix to an earlier history of the civil wars written by another physician, George Bate (1608–1668).[97] Frankland, widely disparaged as a medical impostor for forging his Oxford MD (for which he was expelled from his fellowship at the College of Physicians), was the author of two historical treatises reflecting positively on the rule of the early Stuarts. Despite his claims to impartiality, both betray his royalist and Anglican sympathies and were published at the height of political tension following the revelations of a Popish plot and the ensuing debate in and outside Parliament over Exclusion.[98] Interestingly, the researches of both Skinner and Frankland would appear to have owed a debt of gratitude to the apothecary-turned-physician Francis Barnard or Bernard (1628–1698), an influential figure in medico-political circles at this time whose loyalty to church and crown was undoubtedly shared by the two doctors.[99]

From the mid 1670s onwards, as the country spiralled toward another bout of internecine, political conflict, medical men thus played their part in putting the case for church and crown. Some, such as the Roman Catholic mountebank Salvator Winter, of whom it was rumoured in 1676 that he was being assisted by 'a great many priests and friers' in writing 'a book about monarchy', probably received official encouragement to write in defence of their beleaguered faith.[100] Others, such as the apothecary-turned-physician Moses Rusden (d.1679), drew inspiration from their daily practice and the natural world (Rusden was also 'beemaster to the king') to write in defence of 'Kingly Government' and patriarchal political thinking.[101] And those who declined to put pen to paper, often assisted in other ways in spreading loyalist propaganda. John Harborough (d.1704), for example, who despite his Cambridge MD had the reputation of a maverick and empiric, actively assisted the antiquarian scholar and ultra-loyal historian Joshua Barnes (1654–1712) in disseminating his pro-Tory account of the reign of Edward III in 1688.[102] A year later, two loyal collegiate physicians, John Elliott (d.1690 or 1691) and Robert Gray, were arrested in Dublin and impeached for high treason for dispersing 'a seditious and treasonable paper' on behalf of the deposed king, James II. Brought before the bar of the House of Lords, both men protested their innocence and denied the authority of Parliament. The charges against them seem to have been dropped.[103] In the years that followed, some Tory diehards in medical circles would appear to have forsaken medicine altogether in order to concentrate on politics and political writing. James Drake (1666–1707), for example, published a number of 'historical' works in the early part of the eighteenth century that were critical of the dual monarchs and their Whig allies, for which he twice faced prosecution before the House of Commons.[104] Jodocus Crull (d.1710) on the other hand, a native of Hamburg who was granted a Cambridge MD at the request of the King in 1681, drifted into a career as an author of politically partisan histories of contemporary Europe following his failure to establish himself as a physician in post-revolutionary England.[105]

It is not, perhaps, surprising that men of a traditionalist mould should turn to the study of the past in an age of political upheaval. But why, one might ask, should physicians, and highly educated ones at that, have played such a prominent and disproportionate part in advancing such pursuits? One obvious answer lies in the classical, humanist education that continued to underpin the medical curricula of Oxford and Cambridge at mid-century. Since the earliest days of the Renaissance classically trained physicians had been attracted, for a variety of reasons, to historical and antiquarian research. To some extent, as Nancy Siraisi has recently suggested, this may have something to do with the nature of medical practice and enquiry itself, dependent as it increasingly was in this period on developments in the field that 'increased emphasis on the recording of particulars, the construction of narrative, and the analysis of past events'.[106] By the middle decades of the seventeenth century, of course, as Siraisi herself acknowledges, the appearance of new understandings of the body, some of which posed a serious challenge to ancient orthodoxies, was beginning to undermine the humanist project. It is a matter of conjecture however as to the precise impact of such developments on the wider cultural interests and intellectual habits of physicians in this period. While medical doctors and natural philosophers were challenging much of the wisdom handed down by the ancients, respect for, and interest in, the literary and intellectual giants of the classical past continued to feature prominently in Restoration culture and university studies. Thus innovative medical research, particularly in the field of human physiology, often proceeded alongside a deep-seated reverence for classical writers like Galen and Hippocrates in medicine, and Aristotle in natural philosophy. Johnston's *magnum opus*, for example, *The Excellency of Monarchical Government* of 1686, which set out to defend divine right monarchy and non-resistance, was largely indebted to classical sources, particularly Aristotle, Cicero, and Tacitus. Brady's historical defence of Tory principles, moreover, may have owed something to the revival of interest in Hippocrates and clinical medicine in the second half of the seventeenth century, a movement spearheaded by Brady's unlikely friend and correspondent, Thomas Sydenham.[107] Sydenham's own medical research, of course, was profoundly indebted to the application of an empirical methodology that emphasized the need to create an accurate and exact history of diseases. Observation, rather than unsubstantiated theorizing, lay at the heart of Sydenham's approach to medicine, an approach that was in many ways mirrored by Brady in his own intensive, first-hand research in the political and legal archives of late Stuart England. Brady, moreover, emphasized the importance of historical context in making sense of past events in much the same way that Sydenham stressed the role of local constitutions in shaping specific diseases. While it is impossible to say for certain that Brady's approach to the collection and investigation of historical facts was definitely indebted to Sydenham's novel clinical methods, there is little doubt that the latter was widely admired in High Church Anglican and Tory medical circles. Brady's Cambridge colleague, Henry Paman (1623–1695), the Roman Catholic Thomas Short (above 277) and the Tory MP and philanthropist Dr John Radcliffe (1650–1714) all expressed admiration for the 'English Hippocrates' and praised his learning and sagacity in developing new empirical treatments for the cure of epidemic diseases.[108] Sydenham's approach to medicine was also popular among Whigs and dissenters, but as I suggest here, recent attempts to depict his methodology as inimical to medical orthodoxy, and by extension political absolutism, simply do not reflect the complexity of medico-political affiliations in the late seventeenth century.[109]

Anglicans, Tories and Medical Innovation

In short, there is no evidence to suggest that the adoption of High Church and Tory values went hand in hand with medical 'conservatism', and, vice versa, that support for the Whigs and moderate Anglicanism or Dissent was synonymous with medical 'progress'. This much is evident not just by reference to what loyalist medical practitioners did and said, but also from the reaction of High Church Anglican clergy to the medical and scientific developments of the post-Restoration period. Indeed, the two groups often forged close bonds and networks which, like their dissenter counterparts, owed much to a common educational background. As previously noted in chapter 4, the medical schools of Oxford and Cambridge offered an attractive refuge for Anglicans in the 1650s. Here, a generation of medical students, many hostile to the prevailing Cromwellian authorities, were exposed to new ideas about medicine and natural philosophy. At the Restoration, a number of these either turned their back on medicine, choosing ordination, or combined medical practice with a career in the restored church. Many, it can safely be assumed, were wholeheartedly antagonistic or unsympathetic to the claims of those whom they displaced. Edmund Cooper, for example, who gained his MD from Clare College, Cambridge, in 1650, and was admitted a candidate of the London College of Physicians in 1653, later defected to the Church, serving as rector of Woodmancote in Sussex from 1666 until his death in 1682. Prior to taking up his new living, Cooper became embroiled in a literary squabble with nonconformists in which he poked fun at those Presbyterians and others ejected after 1660.[110] He also demonstrated his loyalist credentials with verses published to mark the occasion of the recovery of the Queen from a series of ailments in 1664 following her recent arrival in England.[111]

Regardless as to whether such individuals began their university studies before or after 1660, many clearly imbibed medical knowledge as part of their general studies. This is evident from the frequency with which many Interregnum and early Restoration divines cited recent anatomical and physiological developments in their sermons. Harveian circulation and a related interest in respiration, for example, is evident in 1656 in the funeral sermon delivered by Samuel Jacombe (d.1659) on behalf of his Cambridge colleague Edward Bright.[112] Four years later, James Buck (d.1686), in a sermon celebrating the Restoration, cited the work of the Danish anatomist Thomas Bartholin (1616–1680) in order to provide a physiological explanation for the workings of divine grace on the bodies of the faithful.[113] In the same year, Richard Henchman, in a sermon before the lord mayor of London designed to mollify the various warring factions in the restored church, invoked the 'anatomists [who] tell us of an artery, which goes from the Heart to the Tongue: if our Tongue jars, our Hearts cannot make Harmony'.[114] In the heated religious debates that ensued after 1660, Anglican ministers continued to find comforting and exemplary lessons in contemporary anatomical thinking. In 1671, John Torbuck (d.1707), like Henchman, speculated on the anatomy of the heart, in particular 'a Skin called Pericardium, containing in it water, which cools and moistens the heart, lest it should be scorched with continual motion'. Others such as John Warly (1640–1673), a former fellow of Clare College, Cambridge, hoped to convince the 'modern Latitude-Man' among his clerical brethren to avoid 'use of a Petulant Splene in Religious Debates' by citing the example of the physical spleen, which 'some Anatomists' claimed had no certain use and that 'some Creatures may live without'.[115]

Cambridge University, in particular, seems to have provided fertile ground for would-be clerics interested in the most recent developments in medicine and the new philosophy. In an earlier chapter, I noted the widespread interest in chymistry among undergraduates at Interregnum Trinity College, many of whom were Anglican and royalist in orientation. Elsewhere, St John's College, provided a particularly propitious environment for students, both before and after 1660, to engage in medical speculation and scientific experimentation. In the early 1650s, Matthew Robinson (1628–1694), who later became a minister in Yorkshire, was involved in animal vivisection as a medical student at St John's. The physician Thomas Briggs, who completed his MD at Utrecht in 1661, began his studies at St John's in the 1650s and later formed part of a circle of Cambridge-educated medics that included the eminent naturalist Martin Lister (1639–1712).[116] The college remained an important centre of medical education after the Restoration, its impact on students extending to those destined for a career in the church. Robert Grove (1634–1696), for example, who had served as a fellow since the 1650s and was later elevated to the see of Chichester, was also a member of Lister's circle and the author of a lengthy poem in praise of William Harvey. His library of medical works was extensive and probably accounts for his knowledge of more recent developments in anatomy, including Malpighi's discovery of the capillaries.[117] Likewise, Stanford Wolferstan (d.1698), who became vicar of Wootton Wawen in Warwickshire in 1676 following his graduation from St John's, was a medical enthusiast who not only practised medicine but was also an active researcher who employed the microscope in order to investigate the poisonous attributes of the adder. In 1692, he published a tract on medicine which demonstrates that he was fully conversant with the latest iatrochemical and iatromechanical theories of the body, and from which he developed his own highly original speculations as to the origin of most diseases.[118]

Of all Cambridge's colleges, however, it was almost certainly Gonville and Caius that played the prime role in the University as a refuge for loyal, High Church Anglican medics during the Interregnum, and thereafter as the principal centre for the education and training of a new generation of physicians committed to the defence of traditional values in the Restoration church and state. Caius' most celebrated medical alumnus, Francis Glisson (d.1677), who held the regius chair in medicine from 1636 to 1677, was almost certainly responsible for promoting an innovatory approach to the medical curriculum in Cambridge during these years. His work in this respect is well documented. He may also, however, have played a prominent role in attracting and protecting medical students whose loyalty to the various governments of the Interregnum was skin-deep at best. Glisson himself probably harboured royalist sympathies. In 1648, as a Presbyterian elder in Colchester, he was chosen by the royalist leadership of the besieged forces in the town to twice act as a mediator with the parliamentarian leader, General Fairfax.[119] At the same time, in his work as University examiner of candidates for a medical licence, he employed Anglican sympathizers such as fellow Caian Thomas Buckenham (d.1682) to act as assistant.[120] Following the execution of Charles I and the establishment of the Commonwealth, Glisson's role as mentor, teacher and examiner to an influx of medical students, many of whom, like the future archbishop Thomas Tenison (1636–1715), were attracted to medicine 'because of the uncertain times', was crucial in raising the profile of the University's medical school.[121] As regius professor, he also witnessed and may have encouraged the recruitment of former royalists and dissident Anglicans into the medical profession.

Among those who gravitated to Cambridge under the tutelage of Glisson was a young medical student named Robert Brady, who, as we have already seen, was to play an active role in spearheading opposition to the Cromwellian settlement in his native Norfolk and would in due course succeed Glisson in the regius professorship following the latter's death in 1677. Resident at Cambridge in the early 1650s, where he proceeded to his bachelor's degree in medicine in 1653, Brady formed part of a cohort of medical students at Interregnum Caius who shared his antipathy for the religious and political settlement established after 1649. They included Reginald Buckenham, Christopher Ludkin (MD 1653), Thomas Witherley (MD 1655), Edward Gelsthorpe (fellow 1655) and Peter Parham (fellow 1659).[122] Like Brady, all were Norfolk born and bred, and many, again in common with Brady, possessed connections among the royalist gentry of Norfolk, which they used to good effect after the Restoration. Brady himself was able to call on Sir Allen Apsley (1616–1683) and Sir Horatio Townshend (1630–1687)—the latter on more than one occasion—to promote his academic and medical career. In 1660, for example, both men attested to Brady's sufferings on behalf of the royal cause and emphasized his zeal for the restored church and learning.[123] Brady's like-minded colleagues were also to prove highly adept at exploiting ties of kinship and marriage in order to consolidate their grip on social and political power as well as promote their medical careers. The pattern in this respect was set by an earlier graduate of Caius, Robert Eade, whom we have already encountered as a highly active and loyal agent of government in Restoration Cambridge (above 276). Two of Eade's sons-in-law were prominent figures in Anglican circles. Dr Charles Wright (d.1711) was a Cambridge theologian and hebraist, while his brother-in-law Erasmus Warren (d.1718) was a prolific and outspoken apologist for the Church of England after the Restoration. Both men were beneficiaries under Eade's will of 1672, which also included reference to three Cambridge-educated physicians, Ralph Flyer (d.1684), Henry Hogan (d.1684) and Henry Paman. Hogan or Hoogan (MD 1670), who practised at King's Lynn in Norfolk, later married Eade's widow, Anne.[124]

The importance of social networking among this group of doctors, who shared a common commitment to the royal and Anglican cause, was most evident however after 1660. We have already noted the marriage of Peter Parham to the daughter of Anthony Sparrow, bishop of Norwich. Other Caians almost certainly utilized family connections in and outside Norfolk to further their careers. Again, Brady's influence was probably decisive as suggested by the number of medical students recruited from legal backgrounds. Brady himself was the son of a Norfolk attorney, and many of his students at Caius shared a similar background. These included the Tory propagandist James Drake, Robert Howse (B Med 1685) and Ralph Pell, the son of the barrister and town clerk of Great Yarmouth.[125] Brady, of course, remained a keen, amateur student of the law throughout his academic career, his interests underpinning his politically informed research in the nations' legal muniments. Indeed, so great was his repute in this field that it frequently elicited the comment of contemporaries. John Dolben, archbishop of York, for example, noted in 1684 that Brady had 'long since [set himself up] for a great Common Lawyer'. He went on to observe that 'Lawyers and physicians are strangely jumbled at Cambridge', Brady being 'notoriously learned in the Law' while the law professor John Oxinden was 'as well read in Galen and Hippocrates as he is in Corpus J[uris] C[ivilis]'.[126] It is quite conceivable, therefore, that Brady may have used his legal interests to recruit law students to the medical faculty. Robert Schuldam (1653–1705), for example, a fellow of Caius in the late 1670s, was granted dispensation to switch from law to medicine and take his MD in 1681. Ostensibly, the move was authorized and approved by William Sancroft as archbishop of Canterbury, but in all likelihood Brady was the prime mover.

Schuldam later married the daughter of Henry Brady, alderman of Norwich, a kinsman of the regius professor, while two of his daughters married Norfolk clergymen.[127] Brady's influence may also have shaped the future career of another Caius law graduate, John Smith (LL B 1684), the son of a Norfolk cleric, who was licensed to practise medicine by the bishop of Norwich in 1695.[128]

Brady's role as medical and political mentor at Caius was undoubtedly facilitated by the close working relationship which he enjoyed with the president of the College after 1679, John Gostlyn (d.1705), another medic, who had been rewarded for his loyalty to the restored powers by elevation to a fellowship at Caius in 1661 (he proceeded MD in the same year). Gostlyn was a prominent figure in the government of post-Restoration Cambridge.[129] Moreover, like Brady, he supported the use of the royal mandate in the creation of new medical graduates, especially where the crown or a powerful patron sought to reward loyal supporters. He may also have actively encouraged other candidates to proceed along similar lines, including those who found Oxford far less flexible in granting such requests.[130] Nicholas Darrell (d.1679), for example, was fast-tracked in this way when his *alma mater*, Oxford, refused him a royal mandate. The authorities at Caius were equally compliant in 1682, when they happily supported the suspension of the College statutes in order to allow the granting of a mandamus for senior fellow to Edmund Scarburgh (d.1705), medical student and son of the eminent anatomist and royal physician Sir Charles Scarburgh.[131] There is little doubt that the use of the royal prerogative in this way, and the willingness of most college heads to acquiesce, if not fully support, the use of the royal mandate, did cause disquiet in some circles. However, as John Gascoigne has shown, Restoration Cambridge was probably more eager than Oxford to demonstrate its loyal credentials given its 'puritan' past. Under pressure to demonstrate its steadfast support for the crown, it rapidly took on the mantle of chief apologist for High Church Anglicanism and the sanctity of political doctrines incorporating divine right rule and passive obedience. Such aims were of course spearheaded by the clerics who dominated the headships of the various colleges, but they often acted in concert with their like-minded colleagues in the law and medical faculties.[132]

In the process, the medical school at Cambridge fostered the creation of a group of physicians who were united not only by their common interests in the new physiology but also through a shared commitment to the restoration and reinvigoration of the authority of the Anglican church and the regime of the Stuarts. Such links, moreover, were maintained long after graduation. As the correspondence of Cambridge-educated physicians like Simon Blenkerne (d.1688), Thomas Briggs (d.1704), Roger Howman (1640–1705), Peter Parham, John Wright and Martin Lister attests, the bonds established at Cambridge were frequently maintained thereafter, when discussion of medical topics was interspersed with political gossip.[133] As we have seen, the commitment of many of these men to the cause of the restored regime, and later that of Toryism, was often deep-rooted. Both in town and country, university-educated physicians played an increasingly prominent role in the day-to-day government of their communities. That they felt so inclined was in no small part due to the bonds formed at Restoration Oxford and Cambridge, where medical study, like much else, had become inextricably entwined with the wider political and religious currents of the period.

Notes

1. J. Northleigh, *The Triumph of Our Monarchy, over the Plotts and Principles of Our Rebels and Republicans* (London, 1685), B2v. In an earlier work, published anonymously at the height of the Exclusion Crisis, Northleigh's comments on the contemporary scientific scene hinted at a conservatism to match his social, religious and political outlook. There, he sought to conflate the new science with political dissidence. For example, in comparing the loyal Tory to the disobedient Whig, he described how '[t]he Protestant Virtuoso, that views the slips of a government in a Microscope, and so magnifies the biting of a Flea, to the pinching of a Lobster; And for his transubstantiating of Mettals, and Chymical Knacks, exceeds the Dutch van Helmont, or our English Boyle; with a little Panegyrick can sublime a knave to the very Quintessence of honesty; and then with one drop of the venom of his tongue, debase him to the worst of villains'; [J. Northleigh], *The Parallel: Or, The New Specious Association, an Old Rebellious Covenant* (London, 1682), 31. Appearances, however, may be deceptive in this case. In 1696, Northleigh, now living in Exeter, entered into correspondence with Sir Hans Sloane in which it is clear that he was a keen naturalist and observer with a particular penchant for microscopy; BL, Sloane MS 4036, fos 231, 233–4, 257, 274 [Northleigh to Sloane, 17 and 30 March, 23 August and 13 November 1696]. Northleigh was rewarded for his support of James II by the award of a mandated MD from Cambridge in 1687. Wisely, he retired from politics in 1688 and settled at Exeter, where he practised medicine until his death in 1705; Venn, iii, 267; *ODNB*.
2. R. Austin, 'The City of Gloucester and the Regulation of Corporations, 1662-63', *Transactions of the Bristol and Gloucestershire Archaeological Society*, 58 (1936), 265–6. In similar vein, Philip Musgrave, commissioner and magistrate in Cumberland, described himself in September 1662 as 'a state physician' who 'courses about to Kendal, Appleby and Carlisle to purge the corporations'; *CSPD, 1661–1662*, 498.
3. For discussion of the Corporation Act, which stresses its patchy impact and the fact that it did not always produce the desired results, see P. D. Halliday, *Dismembering the Body Politic: Partisan Politics in England's Towns 1650–1730* (Cambridge, 1998), 92–105, especially 100–1. Halliday estimates that three-quarters of those who lost office in 1662–3 were either Presbyterians or Presbyterian sympathizers; ibid., 103, 104–5.
4. While physicians, and especially surgeons, can be found sitting on aldermanic benches in the period between 1640 and 1660 (and indeed earlier), few would appear to have aspired to mayoral office. The one notable exception was Dr John Golder, who officiated as mayor of Dover from 1644 to 1646, and was re-elected in 1661. He was almost

certainly a moderate Presbyterian, who survived the purges of the early 1660s and remained active in local government for the next two decades; BL, Add. MS 28,037, *passim*. For a full list of medical mayors (physicians, apothecaries, and surgeons), 160 in total, who served as mayors in English corporations, see Appendix 3.

5. J. R. Woodhead, *The Rulers of London 1660–1689. A Biographical Record of the Aldermen and Common Councilmen of the City of London* (London, London and Middlesex Archaeological Soc., 1965), 74. Fyge, who practised as a chymical physician and purveyor of pills (above 137), remained an active member of the Apothecaries Company, serving as master in 1690.
6. Woodhead, *Rulers of London*, 74. For Valentine Fyge's religious background and conflict with the College of Physicians in 1640, see above, 71. Following the clampdown on dissenters in the corporation of London, he moved to Stafford, where in September 1663 the nonconformist William Westmacott hoped, at the instigation of the ejected Presbyterian minister John Bryan, to succeed to the practice of 'old Dr Fyge'; FSL, MS V. a. 441 [W. Westmacott, 'Memorabilia'], 16; T. C. Wales and C. P. Hartley (eds), *The Visitation of London Begun in 1687* (London, Harleian Society, vols 16 and 17, 2004), ii, 360. For Westmacott's nonconformist credentials and connection to London iatrochemical circles, see above, 162 n.82.
7. Fyge was restored to office in 1688 and continued to serve as a common councilman for the ward of Bishopsgate Without until 1696; Woodhead, *Rulers of London*, 74.
8. Woodhead, *Rulers of London*, 115. Middleton was arrested, along with the Congregational minister Seth Wood, for attending an illegal conventicle in 1670. Though he appealed against conviction and lost, he was reported the following year to have 'magnified' Lord Chief Justice Vaughan 'for his kindness to him'. His standing among fellow barber surgeons was evidently high as in 1677 he served as warden of their Company; LMA, S[essions] F[ile] 202, loose deposition, indictment and letter of Thomas Middleton, dated 29 June 1670; *CSPD, 1671*, 386.
9. Woodhead, *Rulers of London*, 105, 125. To this list of politically active London surgeons, one might tentatively add the name of Nathaniel Herne (1630–1679), who served as master of the Barber Surgeons' Company in 1674. He represented Coleman Street as a common councilman (1675–6), Billingsgate ward as an alderman (1676–9) and was MP for Dartmouth at the time of his death in 1679. Knighted in 1674, he was serving as sheriff in the same year. However, Herne did not practice as a surgeon, but chose instead to pursue a career as a successful merchant; ibid., 89; Henning, ii, 538–9.
10. Woodhead, *Rulers of London*, 75; Venn, ii, 197. Garrett sat as a common councilman for Tower ward in 1675–80, and as a deputy in 1682. His ascent into the ranks of the established medical profession was sealed through the grant of licentiate status by the London College of Physicians in December 1679, followed less than a year later by his appointment as an honorary fellow; Munk, i, 412–13.
11. Major Michael Greenstreet, who was licensed to practise medicine in the diocese of Canterbury in September 1662, served as mayor of Faversham in 1666, 1673 and 1684. An apothecary by background, he probably used appointment to mayoral office as a means of raising his status in the eyes of patients and fellow practitioners. He was also, in all probability, a staunch royalist. In March 1685, for example, during his third term of office, he attended a special meeting of the guestling at New Romney where the

various Kent corporations met to discuss the composition of a loyal address to the King in the wake of the Rye House Plot; CCAL, DCb/L/R/17, fo. 177b; DCb/L/B/Box 1, no. 188; BL, Add. MS 28,037, fo. 43v. Meanwhile at nearby Rochester, another loyalist, the naval surgeon John Conny (d.1699) twice served as mayor. Conny was a key figure in the administration of the navy's medical services at Chatham and was a frequent correspondent of Secretary Williamson during the second and third Anglo-Dutch Wars. He seems, in the process, to have amassed a fortune, sufficient to educate his son, Robert (*c.*1645–1713), at Oxford, where he graduated MD in 1685; *CSPD, 1659–1660*, 550; *CSPD, 1667*, 187–8 and *passim*; *CSPD, 1671–1672*, 303; *CSPD, 1672*, 115; E. Hasted, *The History and Topographical Survey of the County of Kent*, 12 vols (2nd ed., Canterbury, 1798), iv, 159, 469; Foster, i, 317; Munk, i, 497; *ODNB*, sub Conny, Robert. The surgeon-apothecary Christopher Richardson (1613–1702) served in all the main civic offices of Kingston upon Hull, including as mayor in 1660 and 1678. If not a dissenter, he certainly had puritan-dissenting connections. As a burgess, he had searched the house of John Hotham in Hull in 1643 prior to his defection to the royalists. Many years later, he acted as executor of the will of the ejected minister and schoolmaster, Anthony Stephenson; Bodl., Tanner MS 62A, fo. 235; J. A. R. Bickford and M. E. Bickford (eds), *The Medical Profession in Hull 1400–1900: A Biographical Dictionary* (Kingston upon Hull, 1983), 107–8, 123. The careers of the medical mayors of the other corporations cited here are discussed in more detail elsewhere in this chapter.

12. Seaman had first served as a naval surgeon in the first Anglo-Dutch War in the 1650s. A friend of the Whig astrologer and physician Lancelot Coelson, who dedicated one of his almanacs to him, Seaman was mayor of Harwich on three occasions, in 1672, 1681 and 1690; *CSPD, 1653–1654*, 574; *CSPD, 1657–1658*, 286, 291, 318–9, 558; *CSPD, 1658–1659*, 33; *CSPD, 1659–1660*, 420–1; *CSPD, 1672–3*, 428–9, 439 and *passim*; L. Coelson, *Speculum Perspicuum Uranicum: or, an Almanck* [sic] ... *1678* (London, 1678); S. Dale, *The History and Antiquities of Harwich and Dovercourt* (London, 1730), 38. Many other naval surgeons served as burgesses or aldermen in the port towns. Matthew Hardy, for example, a native of Kingston upon Hull and a former apprentice of Christopher Richardson (above), was admitted as a burgess in May 1660, serving as chamberlain in 1676. He was appointed surgeon to the garrison in March 1685 and was made an alderman under the new charter issued by James II three months later; Bickford and Bickford (eds), *Medical Profession in Hull*, 54; *CSPD, February–December 1685*, 61, 183.
13. *CSPD, 1653–1654*, 178; *CSPD, 1666–1667*, 230, 342–3; *CSPD, 1678*, 364. Bullack was licensed to practise surgery and medicine in the diocese of Canterbury in September 1661 and March 1662, respectively. On the former occasion, he secured eight signatures in support of his application, including that of the current mayor of Dover, Dr John Golder. Among those who provided a certificate in March 1662 was the nonconformist sympathizer, Dr William Jacob, of Canterbury (for whom, see above 214–15); CCAL, DCb/L/R/17, fos 112a, 141a; DCb/L/B/Box 1, nos 43, 44, 74, 75.
14. *CSPD, 1625–1626*, 338, 398, 499; *CSPD, 1627–1628*, 66, 90, 344 and *passim*; *CSPD, 1628–1629*, 501; TNA, SP 28/2B/III, fo. 534; SP 28/36/IV, fo. 432; SP 28/37/VI, fos 658, 659; Peter Salanova would appear to have settled initially at Weymouth and then at

Dorchester, where he was paid by the borough's officers for cures performed on townspeople from the early 1640s onwards. The town also ordered payment to him for his wife's mother, sister, and brother-in-law, who had fled Ireland in February 1642 following the outbreak of the rebellion there; C. H. Mayo (ed.), *The Municipal Records of the Borough of Dorchester, Dorset* (Exeter, 1908), 516, 517, 544, 545. Like many of his comrades in arms, he also sought to cash in on the sale of crown land debentures, which he had been granted in lieu of salary; I. Gentles, 'The Debentures Market and Military Purchases of Crown Land, 1649–1660', Ph. D. (London, 1969), 274.

15. WSxRO, Ep/II/1/1, fo. 43r. I have found no evidence for Welsh's practice before 1662, though he does appear in the probate records of three former patients in Kent for the period between 1663 and 1677; KHLC, PRC 19/3/39; 1/11/41; 2/36/43; 2/37/66.
16. ESxRO, RYE 82/82, 52, 55; RYE 47/169/14. Paul Monod, who cites this incident, nonetheless insists on describing Welsh as a 'moderate'; P. K. Monod, *The Murder of Mr. Grebell: Madness and Civility in an English Town* (New Haven & London, 2003), 90, 108, 109. Welsh served as one of the captains manning the watch in 1665, when he was instructed to carry out the duke of York's recent order to suppress all conventicles in the Cinque Ports. He was subsequently appointed captain of the trained bands and clerk of the passage in 1673 in the wake of the withdrawal of the Second Declaration of Indulgence and in the same year that he was re-appointed as mayor; ESxRO, RYE 1/15, fo. 67v; RYE 19/7.
17. ESxRO, RYE 1/15, fo. 15v and *passim*.
18. ESxRO, FRE MS 606, titlepage; ESxRO, RYE 1/15, fos 5r, 16r, 21r, 57r, 76v, 79v. Welsh's medical aspirations were partially realized by his son, also James, who proceeded to his bachelor's degree in medicine at Cambridge in 1677. He would also appear to have shared his father's deep-seated loyalist convictions. In March 1683, as a jurat of Rye, he informed against the 'pretended' Whig mayor of the borough, Thomas Tournay, for saying that 'sceptres and crowns must tumble down'. Tournay, who refused to hand over the regalia of office to the Tory incumbent, was further accused by Welsh Jnr of hindering the proceedings of justice in the town; Venn, iv, 359; *CSPD, 1 January–30 June 1683*, 147.
19. *CSPD, 1667*, 311. Welsh's voluminous correspondence, which finally came to an end with his death in late 1677, included reference to the election of a new MP for Rye in October 1667 when he expressed his surprise and disappointment at the defeat of the court candidate, Henry Savile; ibid., 539, 543. His recent death is alluded to in a letter dated 29 December 1677. A grateful Williamson later wrote to his son, probably James Jnr, expressing his commiserations and offering to help and support the young physician, as well as the interests of his father's friends in the town; *CSPD, 1677–1678*, 533, 549, 570.
20. *CSPD, 1667–1668*, 522. Ludkin (1615–1677), a native of Norwich, received his MD from Cambridge in 1653 following a brief period as a medical student at Leiden in the early 1640s. It is probably no coincidence that within a few months of offering to act as a government spy, Ludkin was appointed physician in ordinary supernumerary to Charles II; Venn, iii, 115; Innes Smith, 145; TNA, LC 3/26, fo. 141. He may have been put forward as a suitable candidate for a government agent by Charles II's loyal sergeant surgeon, John Knight (1622–1680), who had strong links with the town of

Ipswich. Knight's brother-in-law, Edward Bodham, served a similar role as government correspondent in the port of King's Lynn in this period; *ODNB*, sub Knight, John; *CSPD, 1678*, 349.

21. *CSPD, 1666–1667*, 307, 490. He may be the same as the Richard Browne, surgeon, whose son, also Richard, was born at King's Lynn, Norfolk, and proceeded BA at Cambridge in 1668; Venn, i, 236.
22. Pennington's voluminous correspondence with Secretary Williamson can be found in the state papers for the period. In February 1672, his brother-in-law, Sir Roger Bradshaigh, petitioned on his behalf for the place of physician in ordinary to Charles II in place of the recently deceased Dr Timothy Clarke; *CSPD, 1671–1672*, 145. Chester produced a number of politically active medical men. After the Restoration, the barber surgeon Robert Morrey served as mayor in 1669–70, as well as sheriff on three occasions (1664–5, 1683–4, 1688–9), during which period he signed numerous testimonials for fellow surgeons seeking ecclesiastical licences; W. F. Irvine (ed.), *Marriage Licences Granted Within the Archdeaconry of Chester in the Diocese of Chester*, 4 vols (Lancashire and Cheshire Rec. Soc., vols 65, 69, 73, 77, 1912–24), i, 60; ii, 71, 142, 176, 214; iii, 11, 86, 96. Fellow surgeon Hugh Starkey served two terms as mayor (1687–8, 1700–1), as well as acting as sheriff of the city in 1678–9. He received a licence to practise from the diocesan authorities in 1669, and signed testimonials on behalf of the Chester surgeon Jonathan Whitby in 1677; ibid., ii, 51, 206.
23. *CSPD, 1682*, 410–11.
24. D. Harley, '"Bred Up in the Study of That Faculty": Licensed Physicians in North-West England, 1660–1760', *Medical History*, 38 (1994), 416–17; LPL, FII/4/143; FI/C, fo. 132.
25. Harley, '"Bred Up in the Study of That Faculty", 417; M. Mullett, 'Conflict, Politics and Elections in Lancaster, 1660–1688', *Northern History*, 19 (1983), 75, 79.
26. *ODNB*; DRO, Chanter MS 45, 314 [9 June 1674].
27. J. Yonge, *Medicaster Medicatus, or a Remedy for the Itch of Scribling. The First Part* (London, 1685), 5, 6. In 1708 the Anglican clergyman John Agate of Exeter thanked Yonge for providing him with details of events in Plymouth in the 1650s, materials which Agate used in his on-going pamphlet dispute with the dissenters of Exeter; J. Agate, *The Plain Truth: Or, An Answer to Mr Withers His Defense, &c. Part 1* (Exeter, 1708), 66. Yonge, it should be noted, was sympathetic to medical progress, though uncomfortable with aspects of reform mooted by some within the profession. He engaged in original research, using the microscope to promote a 'mechanical account' of the body's operation, and was a keen proponent of observational and clinical techniques derived from his practice in the naval hospital at Plymouth. He reacted ambivalently, however, to the claims of the iatrochemists preferring instead the insights of Boyle and Glisson. In particular, he was scathing in his condemnation of the pretensions of van Helmont 'and all the little Chymists that pretend to be his followers ... in their ranting and opprobrious way', whom he denigrated as empirics and unlearned pillmongers, 'Phanaticks in Physick', whose writings he placed on a par with the 'Enthusiasticall' ravings of Jacob Boehme and the Rosicrucians; see e.g. Yonge, *Currus Triumphalis, è Terebinthô ... Or an Account of the Many Admirable Vertues of Oleum Terebinthinae* (London, 1679), A7r; 12, 46, 58–9; *idem*, *Wounds of the Brain proved Curable* (London, 1682), 51 and *passim*; *idem*, *Medicaster Medicatus*, 3–4.

28. Other medics lacking formal, academic qualifications to practise medicine, who may have profited from holding mayoral office after the Restoration, especially if loyal to the crown, include Thomas Archer (Hertford, 1681, 1694), Sampson Birch (Stafford, 1682), Moses Bruch (Windsor, deputy mayor 1686–8; mayor 1690), Robert Norman (Beverley, 1664, 1668) and Thomas Tiddeman (Dover, 1684). For Archer (d.1699), who would appear to have favoured chymical medicine, see Sir H. Chauncy, *The Historical Antiquities of Hertfordshire*, 2 vols (Bishop's Stortford, 1836), i, 493, 503, 504; J. R. Glauber, *The Works... Translated into English... by Christopher Packe* (London, 1689), list of subscribers; TNA, PROB 11/452, fos 188v–189r [will of Thomas Archer, physitian, of Hertford, 7 October 1699; pr. 23 October 1699]. Birch (d.1713) was an apothecary who corresponded with Leoline Jenkins as mayor of Stafford in 1682 describing the recent visit of the duke of Monmouth; *CSPD, 1682*, 427–9. Bruch (d.1701) was a loyal Tory who presided as deputy mayor and mayor over a tumultuous period in the politics of the borough of Windsor. An apothecary by upbringing, he became established 'in a long and skilfull Practise of Physick' in the town following the award of a licence to practise by archbishop Sheldon in 1675, a fact pointedly recorded on his gravestone; LPL, FII/16/14; F1/D, fo. 118v; E. Ashmole, *The Antiquities of Berkshire*, 3 vols (London, 1719), iii, 92. His long career as a common councilman (1673), bailiff (1679), alderman (1683–1701), deputy mayor and mayor, and chamberlain (1688–9, 1691–3) can be traced in the minutes of the borough; Berkshire RO, W1/AC1/1/1, fos 32r–262. For Norman, see J. Dennett (ed.), *Beverley Borough Records 1575–1821* (Wakefield, Yorkshire Archaeological Soc., vol. 84, 1932), 129, 134–8, 144. Tiddeman was a surgeon, who possessed a diocesan licence to practise, issued in 1662. In 1682, while serving as a jurat in Dover, he, the mayor and other jurats exhibited articles against their political rival and former mayor, Nicholas Cullen. Two years later, Tiddeman was elected mayor in the wake of the Tory reaction in the port town; CCAL, DCb/L/R/17, fo. 160a; TNA, PC 2/69, fo. 276r; BL, Add. MS 28,037, fo. 34r.
29. Speed was the grandson of the celebrated cartographer of the same name. The former's father, also John (1595–1640), was the first anatomy lecturer at Oxford. He was granted the reversion of the place of physic professor at the university by Charles I, but predeceased the incumbent, Thomas Clayton; *ODNB*, sub Speed, John.
30. Foster, iv, 1303; Green, *CPCC*, ii, 1397–8; *Commons' Journal*, vii (1802), 198; DRO, ECA 10, fo. 166v; R. Izacke, *Remarkable Antiquities of the City of Exeter* (London, 1723), 170. In early 1643, the parliamentarian defenders of Exeter ordered that Dr Salter and other known delinquents 'who came lately in' should be secured or expelled; DRO, DD 36995B. In office, he also advised the corporation on the care and cure of sick petitioners among the town's poor and, opportunely, was able to provide professional advice to prevent the spread of plague in the city in 1665; DRO, ECA 11, 38, 56, 60, 62, 63, 64, 66; ECA, File 1/6 [petitions for relief].
31. For Llewellyn, who may well have been tempted to use corporate office as a way of suppressing medical rivals in the town, see above 184.
32. *CSPD, January 1683-June 1683*, 361; *CSPD, July–September 1683*, 391; *CSPD, 1683–1684*, 105–6, 107; Southampton City Archives, SC2/1/9, 66, 71, 72–3, 90, 97 and *passim*; BL, Add. MS 41,803, fos 89, 100, 138. Speed served a second term as mayor in 1694–5.

33. Foster, ii, 490; *Wal. Rev.*, 23, 173. Fielding was shot in the eye with a musket bullet at the first battle of Newbury. He subsequently suffered from partial deafness and other complications, and underwent surgery to have the bullet removed some thirty years later, at the height of his troubles with the corporation of Gloucester; BL, Sloane MS 1968, fo. 202. For the suggestion that Fielding may have been attracted to the ideas of van Helmont and Francis Glisson while studying at Oxford, see above 74.
34. Foster, ii, 524; B. Ryves, *Mercurius Rusticus* (Oxford?, 1646), 158. Given Fowler's predilection for chymical medicines, he is probably the same as the Dr Fowler who was involved with fellow royalist Dud Dudley in a scheme to smelt iron with coal in the Forest of Dean in the early 1650s; D. Dudley, *Dud Dudley's Metallum Martis* (London, 1665), 39. For Dudley, see above 171 n.129.
35. Fielding was resident in Gloucester before the Restoration as the minute book of the corporation records that in March 1659 he was asked to procure a copy of the recently published polyglot bible for the city's library. He also baptized and buried several children in the parish of St Michael's from 1656 onwards. Fielding first appears as an alderman of the city in October 1662, having been put in as senior alderman by the Corporation Act commissioners. Within a month of his appointment, he was rewarded with the post of president of the city's hospitals and served in the same capacity in 1667. His medical authority in the city may also have grown in the wake of the decision of the London College of Physicians to make him an honorary fellow of that body in December 1664; GRO, GBR B3/3, 97, 246, 248, 345; Munk, i, 346–7. Fowler was admitted to the common council in July 1662, and a few weeks later was made a freeman, by gift. In quick succession he was empowered under the provisions of the Corporation Act to serve as a city bailiff, was appointed almoner of the city's hospitals, and was made an alderman (in March 1663); GRO, GBR B3/3, 236, 239–40, 244, 253; J. Juřica (ed.), *A Calendar of the Freemen of the City of Gloucester 1641–1838* (Bristol, Gloucestershire Record Series, vol. 4, 1991), 20.
36. GRO, GBR B3/4, 25.
37. GRO, GBR B3/4, 91. It seems likely that a further cause of contention between Fielding and Fowler related to the former's attempt to encourage and foster the fledgling medical careers of some of the city's apothecaries. In 1672 for example, Thomas Wall was granted a Canterbury medical licence, his application stating that he had been educated under an apothecary (his father, George, above?) and 'for some yeares under Dr Fielding, an able and learned physician'; LPL, FII/13/88a–b. Fielding was also responsible for signing testimonials on behalf of two other Gloucester medics, John Deighton (d.1676) and David Williams (*c*.1651–1703), in 1673 and 1678, respectively; LPL, VX 1A/10/49/1–4; FII/19/100a–d.
38. *CSPD, 1670, with Addenda 1660–1670*, 419–20, 428, 431, 448, 455; *CSPD, 1671*, 411–2, 419 and *passim*; TNA, PC 2/63, fos 53r–v, 55v. The struggle between the two factions is well documented and has been fully discussed by numerous historians concerned with charting the political divisions in English urban life after 1660. See for example A. Warmington, '"Madd, Bedlam Madd": An Incident in Gloucester's Seventeenth-Century Municipal History Reconsidered', *Transactions of the Bristol and Gloucestershire Archaeological Society*, 111 (1993), 165–73; Halliday, *Dismembering*

the Body Politic, 178–82; J. Miller, *Politics and Religion in English Provincial Towns 1660–1722* (Oxford, 2007), 169–72.

39. GRO, GBR 3/4, 196, 446, 449–50, 481. At this point Fielding would appear to have retired from active politics and to have concentrated on his medical practice. He was widely esteemed. The royal surgeon Richard Wiseman, for example, who described him as 'an eminent Physician of the city of Gloucester', consulted with him over a case. By 1684, he was living in the wealthy Middlesex parish of St Paul's, Covent Garden, but retired to Withington in Gloucestershire sometime before his death in 1709; R. Wiseman, *Severall Chirurgicall Treatises* (London, 1676), 270; *CSPD, 1680–1681*, 157–8; TNA, PROB 11/510, fos 116r–v [will of Robert Fielding, doctor of physic, of Withington, Gloucestershire, 5 October 1704; pr. 12 August 1709]. For his wife, family and pedigree, see G. D. Squibb (ed.), *The Visitation of Somerset and the City of Bristol 1672* (London, Harleian Society, vol. 11, 1992), 186–7.
40. *CSPD, 1671*, 429, 521; *CSPD, 1671–1672*, 24, 41.
41. *CSPD, 1671*, 507, 513; Foster, ii, 524.
42. GRO, GBR B3/3. 446, 449–50, 478, 481, 503; GBR B3/6, fo. 280v [reversed]; *CSPD, 1675–1676*, 567; *CSPD, 1676–1677*, 19, 23, 51, 56, 182, 189, 259–60, 274–5, 319. While Fowler's medical ambitions were thwarted, he nonetheless continued to seek reward for his loyal retainer, the apothecary Mr Rogers, whom he described as having 'hazarded his life and fortune for his Majesty in the late unnatural war to the utter ruin of a considerable estate'; ibid., 182.
43. GRO, GBR B3/3, 789, 840, 842–3. Fowler was elected president of the city's hospitals in 1672–3, 1677–8, 1680–1, and served as treasurer to the same in 1676 and 1683–5; ibid., 534, 667, 684, 686, 742, 772, 773, 851, 871, 901. For Fowler's family background, marriage, and children, see T. F. Fenwick and W. C. Metcalfe (eds), *The Visitation of the County of Gloucester, 1682–1683* (Exeter, 1884), 62–3.
44. J. Barlow (ed.), *A Calendar of the Registers of Apprentices of the City of Gloucester 1595–1700* (Gloucestershire Rec. Soc., vol. 14, 2001), 138, 148, 166, 173, 184, 192, 223; GRO, GBR B3/3, 219, 312, 524, 789, 825, 826, 894; GBR B3/6, fos 19r, 113v.
45. GRO, GBR B3/3, 902; B3/4, 308; B3/6, fo. 124v. Jordan described himself as a medical licentiate in 1681, when he signed letters testimonial on behalf of the Gloucestershire medical practitioner and candidate for a Canterbury medical licence, James Stansfield.
46. GRO, GBR B3/6, fos 257v, 265v; B3/7, fos 8r, 19v, 55v; K1/31. Jordan's successor Nicholas Lane (1634–1719) obtained a licence to practise medicine from the archbishop of Canterbury in June 1671. Among those who signed testimonials on his behalf was the royal physician and future Whig, Hugh Chamberlen. Two years later he repaid the compliment when, alongside Robert Fielding, he provided letters on behalf of another medical candidate and fellow citizen, John Deighton. However, the exact nature of Lane's political inclinations is obscure. As a common councilman in 1671 he had voted with Fowler against the proto-Whig faction led by Fielding, and while he retained his post as physician to St Bartholomew's and the other city hospitals after 1688, he was repeatedly overlooked for alderman, despite his seniority. His son, Nicholas (1672–1728), however, did succeed as Whig mayor of the city in 1703; LPL, VX 1A/10/35, 49/1–4; VG 1/1, fo. 228; Sheldon, fo. 235v; GRO, GBR 3/7, fo. 246v;

N. M. Herbert (ed.), *VCH. Gloucestershire, vol.4* (London, 1988), 115, 379; GRO, B3/8, 110, 113.

47. GRO, GBR B3/4, 177, 308, 328; GBR B3/3, 502–3, 521–2.
48. GRO, D 3117/151, 153. Smallwood was also paid by the city to minister to sick prisoners; see, for example, GRO, Q/SO 1, fo. 106a. He was temporarily displaced as surgeon to the city's hospitals in 1675, but was appointed one of the two scrutineers to these institutions in 1677. At the Michaelmas elections in the autumn of 1678 Smallwood was fined £20 for 'voluntarily' absenting himself from the electoral process to avoid appointment to one of the two vacant offices of town sheriff. He did take up the role, however, the following year when he was appointed senior sheriff for 1679–80; GBR B3/3, 628, 687, 707, 742.
49. GRO, GBR B3/3, 789, 839, 884, 887; GBR B3/6, fos 97r, 99r, 101r, 137r. In the period of Tory ascendancy, Smallwood was appointed surveyor to the hospitals and overseer of the poor. He was also granted a new lease, on favourable terms, to various city properties; GRO, GBR B3/3, 852, 885; GBR, B3/6, fo. 132r.
50. GRO, GBR B3/6, fos 174v, 176v; GBR K1/31. Clarveato, who was referred to in 1681 as Dr Clarveato, when he was paid by the corporation for 'salves and medicines for the boyes in the blew coat Hospitall', was removed as surgeon in May 1685 for 'his insufficiency and his insolent carriage towards the maior and Aldermen'. He was reinstated in December 1687, when the reconstituted city chamber declared itself 'not satisfied in the Causes of his Removall'. He was dead by September 1694 when William Fowler was appointed in his place; GRO, GBR B3/3, 628, 884, 885; GBR B3/6, fos 95v, 97r, 176v; K1/31; GBR B3/7, fo. 108r. Clarveato was the son of the Lichfield physician, William Clarveato (d.1656), a client of the astrologer Elias Ashmole. He was resident in Gloucester by 1661, and was made a freeman (through marriage to a freeman's daughter) in 1667. A year later, he received no votes in the election for a new physician to the city's hospitals. In 1671, he was described as a freeman and 'person of quality', when his name was added to those eligible to vote under the new charter of 1672; TNA, PROB 11/260, fos 297r–v [will of William Clarvetto, doctor of physic, of Lichfield, Staffordshire, 11 November 1656; pr. 23 December 1656]; Josten, *Ashmole*, ii, 509; iii, 898; Juřica, *Calendar of Freemen of Gloucester*, 24; GRO, GBR 3/4, 25; Bodl., Add. MS C 303, fos 225–6.
51. GRO, GBR B3/7, fos 8r, 239r.
52. *CSPD, 1671*, 444, 472, 474; Staffordshire RO, B/V/1/72, 17 November 1665. For the strength of dissent in Restoration Coventry, see J. J. Hurwich, '"A Fanatick Town": The Political Influence of Dissenters in Coventry, 1660–1720', *Midland History*, 4 (1977–8), 15–47.
53. WSA, G23/1/4, fo. 244v and *passim*. Pope (MD Oxford, 1661) was a regular attender of council meetings until May 1689, when he presumably fell victim to the purge of Tories in the new reign. He was made 'free' of the city shortly after his appointment to the corporation along with his close friend and medical colleague, Daubeny Turberville (1612–1696), who almost certainly shared his religious and political sympathies; ibid., fo. 247r. For a general account of Pope's life, career, and scientific and medical interests, which fails to note his residence in Salisbury from about 1676 to 1689, nor his involvement in the corporate affairs of the city, see *ODNB*.

54. Parham was described as the bishop's son-in-law in an anonymous account of the city's bitter religious and political divisions in February 1682; *CSPD, 1682*, 54. Parham married Susan, the daughter of Anthony Sparrow, in the chapel belonging to the bishop's palace, Norwich, on 13 August 1679. He would go on to wield ecclesiastical patronage in favour of his father-in-law's acolytes. In 1689, for example, he presented Charles Wells (d.1691), formerly principal registrar to Sparrow, to the rectory of Garboldisham in Norfolk; see NNkRO, PD 499/2 [parish registers of St Mary in the Marsh, Norwich, i.e., Cathedral Close, 1667–1724]; F. Blomefield, *An Essay Towards a Topographical History of the County of Norfolk*, 11 vols (London, 1805–1811), i, 272. For Parham, who proceeded MD from Caius College, Cambridge, in 1679, having been a fellow of the college for twenty years, see Venn, iii, 304.
55. In September 1669, Smyth, who styled himself MD of Cork in Ireland, wrote a commendatory poem appended to James Wolveridge's *Speculum Matricis Hybernicum* (London, 1670). He had earlier supplicated for a royal mandate for his MD at Oxford in 1660, but no record of such a grant survives. By 1675 he was living at Malmesbury in Wiltshire where, describing himself as MA of Queen's College, Oxford, he was licensed to practise medicine by the archbishop of Canterbury. He was named as a capital burgess in the new charter for Malmesbury in March 1685, alongside fellow medic, William Burgess, whose application for a medical licence from the bishop of Salisbury Smyth had supported in August 1677. A year later, Smyth was appointed 'alderman' or mayor of the borough. Nothing else is known of Burgess, other than that he married the widow of Abia Qui (below); Foster, iv, 1369; *CSPD, 1660–1661*, 147; LPL, VX 1A/10/81; VG 1/1, fo. 177; Sheldon, fo. 259; WSA, D1/14/1/1e; *CSPD, February–December 1685*, 65; Malmesbury Borough Archives, Malmesbury, Corporation Minute Book, 1600–1721, fo. 190r. Malmesbury would appear to have attracted a disproportionate number of medics into civic government. The career of Abia Qui (d.1675), for example, set the pattern for politically ambitious medics in the town. A former surgeon in the royalist army, he settled at Malmesbury after the civil war and steadily rose to prominence in the town's government, serving as deputy high steward in 1659 and high steward from 1660 to 1670. Thereafter, he was chosen as an assistant burgess and capital burgess (1671), acquiring the most senior position of 'alderman' or mayor in 1672–3. Towards the end of his career he was regularly referred to as Dr Qui or 'medicus'; WSA, A1/110, Michaelmas 1659, no. 120; Easter 1669, no. 99; Malmesbury Borough Archives, Corporation Minute Book, 1600–1721, fos 117r, 123r, 135v, 136r, 156v; TNA, PROB 11/350, f.431v [will of Abia Qui of Malmesbury, Wiltshire, 17 July 1675; pr. 10 May 1676]. Other Malmesbury medics who likewise obtained the office of alderman or mayor include Elias Ferris (1688–9) and Nicholas Hayes (1698–9). Both men acted as overseers to Dr Qui's will and probably owed their promotion in the town to his influence. I am particularly grateful to a number of people for facilitating access to the Malmesbury archives. In particular, I would like to thank Elisabeth Snell, town archivist, and the Warden and Freemen of Malmesbury for allowing permission to see the originals records of the corporation. I would also like to thank Mr Donald Box for sharing his wide knowledge of seventeenth-century Malmesbury's records and its people. I would particularly like to pay special thanks to Steven Hobbs, archivist at the Wiltshire Archives, for various illuminating discussions over Malmesbury's very own 'Doctor Who'.

56. Howse (d.1699), who was licensed to practise medicine and surgery at Rye in Sussex in 1679, was appointed comptroller of the customs at Chichester in 1674, a post he clung on to until 1691. He was made a common councilman of the city in 1685. Medically, he was a committed advocate of chymical medicines and frequently wrote to the Helmontian physician Christopher Packe (for whom, see above) in the 1690s, commending his pills. He also witnessed the will of the Helmontian clergyman Edmund Yalden; LPL, VX 1A/10/132; Sancroft, fo. 223v; *Calendar of Treasury Books*, vol.9 [1689–1692] (London, 1931), 1252, 1253, 2009; A. Hay, *The History of Chichester* (Chichester and London, 1804), 589; C. Packe, *Medela Chymica* (London, 1708), 126–7, 131–3, 142, 142–5; *idem*, *Mineralogia* (London, 1693), 38–40; SHC, SW/25/730 [will of Edmund Yalden, clerk and rector, of Compton, Surrey, 25 December 1684, pr. 27 May 1685].
57. Gale, who was appointed a capital burgess in February 1685, had practised medicine in Chippenham since at least 1667, when he signed a testimonial on behalf of Henry Palmer, surgeon in the town; *CSPD, February–December 1685*, 39; WSA, D1/14/1/1b, no. 97.
58. KHLC, Fa/I/12. For Greenstreet, see above note 11.
59. William Rosewell (d.1691), formerly a fellow of All Souls College, Oxford, was granted a Lambeth MD in 1675. His father, Colonel William Rosewell (1603–1680), was a London apothecary who was wounded and imprisoned while fighting for the King in the Civil War. Rosewell Jnr was active as an alderman in Guildford in 1686, but may have been elected at an earlier date; Foster, iii, 1281; SHC, K174/6/2; TNA, PC 2/71, fo. 164r.
60. Originally from the Channel Islands, Fyott was an Oxford MD (1657) who was accused in 1659 of acting as an accomplice of the Baptist governor of Jersey, Colonel Mason. Some time after the Restoration, he seems to have settled at Hastings in Sussex, where he was made a jurat of the corporation under the new charter of October 1685. At the same time, he would appear to have undergone a political conversion for two years earlier, at the height of the Tory reaction, he laid informations against Joseph Turton, minister of St Clement's, Hastings, for speaking scandalous words against the duke of York; Foster, ii, 498; T. Aston, *Satan in Samuels Mantle, or the Cruelty of Germany Acted in Jersey* (London, 1659), 25; *CSPD, July–September 1683*, p.283; *CSPD, February–December 1685*, 347.
61. For Hardy, see above note 12.
62. Dennett (ed.), *Beverley Borough Records*, 111, 155. For Nathaniel Johnston, see above 281.
63. Cropp, an apothecary-cum-physician, was originally licensed to practise medicine by the archbishop of Canterbury in 1672. Ten years later he was made a burgess of Southampton, but his admission would appear to have provoked widespread opposition. He was not re-admitted until November 1685, when he was also made a junior bailiff and common councilman. He later served as mayor in 1696, following a disputed election, and was frequently referred to thereafter in the town minutes as Dr Cropp—another example, in all probability, of the process whereby the occupation of high civic office helped to bestow medical legitimacy; LPL, VX 1A/10/41; VG 1/1, fo. 237v; Sheldon, fo. 239v; Southampton City Archives, SC3/1/1, fo. 239v; SC2/1/9, 54, 66, 106, 231, 248 and *passim*.

64. For Burthogge, Haslen and Friend, see chapter 5.
65. An initial survey has located twenty-four medical practitioners active as JPs in their respective shires between 1660 and 1688. A more methodical search would undoubtedly unearth further examples. They are: Thomas Arris (Hertfordshire, 1660–*c*.1684); Sir John Baber (Middlesex, *c*.1662–*c*.1668); Edward Beaucock (Essex, post-1660); John Bidgood (Devon, 1662); Robert Brady (Middlesex and Westminster, 1687–9); Richard Burthogge (Devon, 1688); Robert Deane (Hertfordshire, *c*.1664–1669); George Dodsworth (Somerset, 1683); Robert Eade (Cambridgeshire, post-1660); Walter Everenden (Sussex, 1674); William Fyfe (Lancashire, post-1660); John Gostlyn (Cambridgeshire, 1674); Griffith or Griffin Hatley (Kent, post-1660); Nathaniel Highmore (Hampshire and Dorset, post-1660); James Jackson (Cambridgeshire, 1674); John Lamphire (Oxfordshire, post-1660); Richard Lister (Leicestershire, post-1660); Thomas Sclater (Cambridgeshire, post-1660); Edward Stoyte (Cambridgeshire, *c*.1660–1670s); Edward Sturton (Lincolnshire, 1680); Robert Thoroton (Nottinghamshire, 1660–1678); John Windebank (Surrey, *c*.1665–1679?); John Yardley (Hertfordshire, 1685–1697). NB: dates in brackets indicate periods when known to be active.
66. Besse, i, 169, 170 [Highmore], 342–3, 344 [Lister], 554, 556, 558 and *passim* [Thoroton]. Highmore, better known for his work with Harvey and other Oxford physiologists in the 1640s and 1650s, was an active participant in all aspects of local government, both in church and state. As well as serving as a JP and county treasurer, he played an active role in church affairs in Sherborne, where he also served as governor of the local school and almshouse. In July 1669 he was investigating claims of an intended uprising in neighbouring Hampshire; *ODNB*; TNA, ASSI 24/22, fo.164v. Lister, like Highmore, was also prominent in other areas of county government. A former royalist soldier, he served as a colonel of the trained bands as well as deputy lieutenant in Leicestershire in the 1670s and 1680s; Venn, iii, 90; Bodl., MS Eng. hist. c. 478, fos 215, 219, 222. Thoroton, too, served his county loyally in other capacities, most notably as a local commissioner involved in the imposition and collection of royal aids and subsidies. A close friend of archbishop Sheldon, to whom he dedicated his famous work, *The Antiquities of Nottinghamshire* (London, 1677), he was rewarded with the grant of a Lambeth MD in 1663.
67. Arris (MD Oxford, 1651), who also served as MP for his native St Albans in the Cavalier Parliament, was active throughout the Restoration as a government informer and zealous persecutor of Quakers, Anabaptists and others suspected of seditious activity; *CSPD, 1661–1662*, 529; W. J. Hardy (ed.), *Hertford County Records. Notes and Extracts from the Sessions Rolls 1581 to 1698* (Hertford, 1905), 148, 157, 223; W. Le Hardy (ed.), *Hertfordshire County Records. Calendar to the Sessions Books and Sessions Minute Books . . . 1658 to 1700*, 6 vols (Hertford, 1930), vi, 206. He was rewarded for his loyalty in 1675 with the grant of the office of comptroller of customs at Exeter; *Calendar of Treasury Books*, iv, 715; *CSPD, 1677–1678*, 91. For a good summary of his political career, see Henning, i, 548.
68. Windebank (1618–1704), a long-standing JP in Restoration Surrey, became involved in a heated controversy in 1670–1 over his handling of the prosecution of a group of conventiclers in his hometown of Guildford. In particular, he sought to punish several

local officers for failing to act against and distrain the goods of various offenders prosecuted under the new Conventicle Act. The case was ultimately referred to the adjudication of two assize judges; SHC, QS 2/1/2, 481, 484; QS 2/1/3, 18–19; QS 2/5/ Easter 1671, 41, 42, 43–7, 210–11. For Windebank's earlier career and later grant of a mandated MD in 1677, see above 57–8. His Anglican credentials are strongly suggested by the fact that he was a business partner of the restored cleric and Helmontian physician Edmund Yalden of Compton, Surrey; Somerset Heritage Centre, DD\S/BT 30/3/9, 30/6/11, 15.

69. [O. Heywood], *Some Remarks upon the Life of... Mr. Nathanael Heywood, Minister of the Gospel of Christ at Ormeskirk in Lancashire* (London, 1695), 23–4. Fyfe, previously a student at Trinity College, Oxford, was granted a Lambeth MD in 1663. His loyalty to the new regime suggests that he is the same as the physician named Fife who was created physician in extraordinary to Charles II on 25 March 1662; LPL, F1/C, fo. 124; Foster, ii, 541; TNA, LC3/26, fo. 143. If so, then he may have been granted these rewards in partial recompense for the circumstances surrounding his failure to secure a seat in the House of Commons for his native town of Preston in 1661. In that year, his election was overturned in favour of a rival medical practitioner and member of the corporation, Jeffrey Rishton (d.1667). Any professional and political rivalry between the two men may well have been exacerbated by the fact that Rishton was the son of a prominent, local Presbyterian, who probably used his additional powers as a commissioner for corporations to protect fellow dissenters. For Rishton, see Henning, iii, 335. Preston's divisions in the wake of the Restoration are discussed in M. Mullett, '"To Dwell Together in Unity": The Search for Agreement in Preston Politics, 1660–1690', *Transactions of the Historic Society of Lancashire and Cheshire*, 125 (1974), 64–5.

70. For Eade, see Venn, ii, 80, 402; W. M. Palmer, 'The Reformation of the Corporation of Cambridge, July 1662', *Proceedings of the Cambridgeshire Antiquarian Society*, 17 (1912–13), 78, 80, 105, 116–17. Eade's loyalty to Charles I may account for the professional rivalry and unpleasantness which characterized his relationship with the puritan doctor, John Symcotts, in 1647; F. N. L. Poynter and W. J. Bishop, *A Seventeenth-Century Doctor and His Patients: John Symcotts, 1592?–1662* (Bedfordshire Historical Records Society, vol. 31, 1951), 79, 83. For Stoyte, see Venn, iv, 172; Palmer, 'Reformation of the Corporation of Cambridge', 111, 115, 116–17, 119. Stoyte's antipathy for the puritan authorities in interregnum Cambridge is suggested by the fact that in 1651, the year of his graduation as MD, he signed the petition in favour of the reinstatement of the royalist Charles Hotham, recently deposed from his fellowship at Peterhouse by the machinations of the ultra-puritan Master, Lazarus Seaman; C. Hotham, *A True State of the Case of Mr. Hotham* (London, 1651), 14–15. For this incident, see above 118 n.203.

71. Two volumes of Sclater's legal casebooks survive, extracts from which appear in Palmer, 'Reformation of the Corporation of Cambridge', 75–136. For the original manuscript volumes, see Bodl., Rawlinson MSS C 948 and D 1137.

72. Palmer, 'Reformation of the Corporation of Cambridge', 90. Gostlyn, who was denied a fellowship at Caius through the opposition of the puritan master William Dell, was subsequently made fellow and MD by Charles II in 1661. Thereafter, he remained at Caius for the rest of his career, where he combined medical practice with college duties

(bursar, steward, and president) and wrote a continuation of the college's annals from 1660 to 1679; Venn, ii, 243; *ODNB*, sub Gostlin, John. Jackson, who served as a fellow of Clare College for 55 years, was awarded his MD in 1657. He would appear to have possessed a particular interest in botany. In the year of his graduation, Elias Ashmole described him as searching the Fens for plants; Venn, ii, 455; C. H. Josten (ed.), *Elias Ashmole (1617–1692): His Autobiographical and Historical Notes, His Correspondence, and Other Contemporary Sources Relating to his Life and Work*, 5 vols (Oxford, 1966), ii, 721. Both Gostlyn and Jackson were remembered in Sclater's will; TNA, PROB 11/379, fos 85v-89r [will of Sir Thomas Slater of Cambridge, 21 November 1681 and numerous codicils; pr. 27 January 1684/5].

73. Despite Sclater's pronounced Anglican and royalist leanings, he was none the less widely admired as a 'moderate' in interregnum Cambridge. Elected as MP for the university in 1659, he elicited strong support from the Cambridge Platonist, Ralph Cudworth, who warmly recommended him to Secretary Thurloe in January 1660. His academic conservatism (and possible motive for seeking election?) is suggested by the fact that in April 1659 he signed a University petition opposing the recent establishment of a new college at Durham; Thurloe, *State Papers*, vii, 587, 595; CUL, CUA, Grace Book H, 1645–1668, 200. Sclater's alchemical interests, and those of fellow interregnum Cambridge Anglicans and royalists are discussed above, 79.

74. *CSPD, 1667–1668*, 452, 460. The eminent physiologist Scarburgh (1615–1694), like Highmore, was a member of William Harvey's circle at royalist Oxford in the 1640s. In 1664 he signed a petition addressed to the Privy Council from the parish of Blackfriars in London, complaining that many in the parish were of 'factious Principles, & dangerous Practices, tending to sedition & hazard of the publique Peace'. A creature of the duke of York, he finally accepted political office as a court dependent in 1685 when he was elected MP for Camelford in Cornwall. He was subsequently ordered to stand for Grampound in the same county in the aborted election of 1688; *ODNB*; TNA, PC 2/57, 174; Henning, iii, 403–4.

75. For a brief overview of Short's career, which fails to mention his MD from Padua, see *ODNB*. Short was inscribed at the medical faculty at Padua on 30 May 1664, graduating MD on 26 September 1665. In the spring of 1663, an English traveller Philip Skippon noted that Short, along with another Englishman John Constable (*fl.*1663–1690), was enrolled as a medical student at Louvain. Constable, a Lincolnshire Catholic, graduated MD at Padua on the same day as Short, prompting speculation that the latter was already reconciled to the Roman Catholic faith; Royal College of Physicians of Edinburgh, Innes Smith MSS: www.rcpe.ac.uk/library/history/english-students/index, sub Padua; P. Skippon, 'An Account of a Journey Made Thru' Part of the Low Countries, Germany, Italy, and France [1663–1666]' in *A Collection of Voyages and Travels... in Six Volumes* (London, 1732), vi, 377.

76. Munk, i, 377–9; TNA, PC 2/67, 42, 139, 140; *HMC. Eleventh Report, Appendix, Part II. The Manuscripts of the House of Lords, 1678–1688* (London, 1887), 129–30; *CSPD, 1 January–30 June 1683*, 276; *CSPD, 1684–1685*, 177, 180. Short died on 28 September 1685 amid rumours spread by his enemies that he had been poisoned, an appropriate fate perhaps given that he was alleged to have gossiped that Charles II had died in a similar fashion. He is probably the 'Dr Shorter', 'a libertine and a Papist', who was

reported to have said that he had been converted from his evil ways by witnessing the death throes of the notorious Restoration rake and poet, John Wilmot, earl of Rochester; J. Redwood, *Reason, Ridicule and Religion: The Age of Enlightenment in England, 1660–1750* (London,1976), 43.

77. For the Hertfordshire physician and magistrate Arris, who sat as MP for St Albans from 1661 to 1678, see above note 67. As well as standing as an MP for Cambridge University, Brady sat as a magistrate in Westminster and Middlesex throughout the reign of James II. As a friend of secretary of state, Leoline Jenkins, he also played an active, if informal, role in the examination of various suspects in the wake of the Rye House Plot in 1683; *ODNB*; TNA, PC 2/71, fo. 188v; *CSPD, 1 January–30 June 1683*, 350–1.

78. *CSPD, 1683–1684*, 1–2. Ewens (d.1697 or 1698) does not appear to have held any formal medical qualifications. He may be the same as the student of that name who matriculated at Exeter College, Oxford, in 1658, but failed to graduate; Foster, ii, 476; TNA, PROB 11/448, ff.61v-62r [will of Ralph Ewens, physician, of Donyatt, Somerset, 20 December 1697; pr. 19 November 1698]. He was a close neighbour of Speke, whose house at nearby White Lackington was a major centre of Whig intrigue and nonconformist gatherings. Speke himself went into exile in Holland shortly after Ewens' intervention. For Speke, see *ODNB*.

79. Foster, iii, 1053; R. Thoresby, *Ducatus Leodiensis: or, the Topography of the Ancient and Populous Town and Parish of Leedes* (London, 1715), 21; TNA, ASSI 44/25. In referring to Neale's role in the prosecution of five unlicensed practitioners at the Yorkshire assizes in 1677, David Harley mistranscribes his name as 'Heale'; Harley, '"Bred Up in the Study of That Faculty"', 401n. Neale was also proposed as a potential arbitrator by the Helmontian Dr George Tonstall (*c.*1617–1682) in his dispute with the Galenist (and Presbyterian) Robert Wittie over the merits of the spa waters at Scarborough in 1672; G. Tonstall, *A New-Years-Gift for Doctor Witty* (London, 1672), 76, 99 and unpaginated Appendix.

80. *CSPD, 1683–1684*, 118–19. While lacking official status as a JP, Neale claimed to be acting as 'physician extraordinary to both the King and Queen'. His name, however, does not appear on any official list of royal physicians. For another contemporary account of Thompson's 'disloyalty' and attempts by the ecclesiastical authorities to conciliate with him, see Bodl., Tanner MS 32, fo. 182 [John Dolben, archbishop of York, to William Sancroft, archbishop of Canterbury, 26 November 1683].

81. Novell, who lived in the parish of Little Eastcheap, London, was made a fellow of the London College in April 1680. He was earlier granted a royal mandate for his MD because a speech impediment rendered him 'incapable the exercises required by the statutes'; Venn, iii, 261; Munk, i, 402; *CSPD, 1675–1676*, 181, 244; H. Bowler (ed.), *London Sessions Records* (London, Catholic Rec. Soc., 1934), 344–5. Shortly before his death in a debtor's prison in 1686, Novell was present at the interrogation of the suspected Rye House plotter, Richard Raw; BL, Add. MS 41,804, fo. 139.

82. In Exeter, for example, the apothecary-cum-physician, John Somers was sent to prison in August 1688 for assaulting William Shapcott, a political rival. Somers' long-standing loyalist credentials are suggested by the fact that in 1671 his apprentice, John Cove, was prosecuted for assaulting a local merchant and accusing him of formerly being in arms

against the King; DRO, ECA, C/1/65, fos 365r–v; C/1/66, fo. 206v [mispaginated in original; should read 212v]. Somers' son, also John, attended Leiden as a medical student in 1682 (but did not graduate); Innes Smith, 218. On the other side of the political divide, Somers' competitors in Exeter's medical marketplace were equally active in promoting the Whig cause. The apothecary Charles Cunningham (d.1686), for example, who acquired an archiepiscopal licence to practise medicine in 1681 with the support of leading local Whigs such as William Glyde and Thomas Jefford, was prosecuted at quarter sessions two years later for dispersing 'a scandalous letter' in the coffee houses of the city. In his will of 1686, he named Glyde and Jefford as executors. The chief beneficiary was his nephew Richard, son of his brother and fellow Whig Richard Cunningham, who was arrested after the Revolution for collaborating with the regime of James II. Richard the younger attended Leiden to study philosophy in 1687; LPL, VX 1A/10/163/1–3; Sancroft, fo. 240; DRO, ECA C/1/66, fo. 21v; TNA, PROB 11/382, fo. 304v [will of Charles Cunningham, apothecary, of Exeter, 3 March 1685/6; pr. 30 April 1686]; *CSPD, 1690–1691*, 31; Leiden University Archives, ASF 12, 317.

83. While an undergraduate at Trinity College, Cambridge, Jeanes wrote with two others *The Parliament Justified in Their Late Proceedings Against Charles Stuart* (London, 1649), a short but devastating critique of Charles' reign, 'it being apparent he degenerated from a King unto a Tyrant' (15). It also contains a brief discussion of the various forms of government, in which aristocratic is preferred over monarchical, in part by recourse to the example of the Dutch and the states of Holland (8–9). Jeanes was rewarded with a fellowship at Magdalen College, Oxford, where he proceeded B. Med in 1655 and MD in 1659. At the Restoration he became embroiled in a dispute with the loyalist Dr Henry Yerbury (d.1686), who had previously been ejected from his place as physician in the College. Jeanes subsequently retired to the continent, taking the grand tour in 1664–5, before settling into medical practice at Peterborough; Venn, ii, 464; Foster, ii, 804; *CSPD, 1660–1661*, 202–3; *CSPD, 1661–1662*, 190; P. Skippon, 'An Account of a Journey Made' in *A Collection of Voyages and Travels*, vi, 650, 704, 714, 732.

84. [D. Holles], *Some Considerations upon the Question, Whether the Parliament is Dissolved by It's Prorogation for 15 Months* (London?, 1676); *CSPD, 1675–1676*, 547; *CSPD, 1676–1677*, 543, 544, 555, 565; *CSPD, 1677–1678*, 47, 135, 188. According to Calamy, Cary had notable success in curing those with eye and ear complaints. His later political loyalties are strongly suggested by the letter which he wrote to the Whig MP and exclusionist George Treby (d.1700) in early 1681 congratulating him on his recent knighthood; *Cal. Rev.*, 103; Derbyshire Record Office, D 239 M/O 1121 [Cary to Treby, 22 January 1680/1].

85. *Cal. Rev.*, 172; *CSPD, 1673*, 380; BL, Add. MS 35,104, fo. 21r [William Blathwayte to William Carr, August 1681]. For du Moulin's life and career, including reference to his medical activities, see the excellent article by Vivienne Larminie in the *ODNB*, supplemented by additional information on du Moulin's wife and family in G. C. R. Morris, 'On the Identity of Jaques du Moulin, F.R.S., 1667', *Notes and Records of the Royal Society*, 45 (1991), 1–10, especially 3.

86. L. du Moulin, *La Tyrannie des Prejugez, ou, Reflexions sur le Fragment d'une Lettre de Mademoiselle Marie du Moulin* (London, 1678), a3r ['d'une profession plus

disinterestée & degagée de tout prejugé']. The work was dedicated to fellow Huguenot Antoine Menjot (d.1696).

87. For Denton, see *ODNB*. His *Jus Regiminis* of 1689 has been described by Mark Knights as a tract that 'employed thoroughly Lockean arguments' and, like Locke's *Two Treatises*, had, according to Denton, 'been written several years and kept close, because the government would not bear such prints'; M. Knights, *Representation and Misrepresentation in Later Stuart Britain: Partisanship and Political Culture* (Oxford & New York, 2005), 96n; Denton, *Jus Regiminis: Being a Justification of Defensive Arms in General and Consequently of Our Late Revolutions and Transactions to be the Just Right of the Kingdom* (London 1689), 'Advertisement to the Reader'.

88. Du Moulin's role as a history don in Cromwellian Oxford has already been noted. For Denton's passion for history in general and his specific debt to the Venetian historian Paolo Sarpi (1552–1623) in his political works, see *ODNB* and J. A. I. Champion, *The Pillars of Priestcraft Shaken: The Church of England and Its Enemies, 1660–1730* (Cambridge, 1992), 94–7.

89. For positive assessments of Brady as a historian, see J. G. A. Pocock, 'Robert Brady, 1627–1700: A Cambridge Historian of the Restoration', *Cambridge Historical Journal*, 10 (1950–2), 186–204; V. Morgan, *A History of the University of Cambridge. Volume II 1546–1750* (Cambridge, 2004), 487–94, especially 488–9; Knights, *Representation and Misrepresentation*, 104. Brady first mooted his design to write a history of England, in an effort to boost the morale of fellow loyalists, in 1675 in a letter to Secretary Williamson. Government support followed in the wake of the Exclusion Crisis when he was granted access to the public records in the Tower. He was rewarded for his loyal services with the grant of the office of royal physician in November 1682 following the dismissal of his Whig rival, Hugh Chamberlen (for whom, see above 206, 241 n.140), and continued to work closely alongside key government figures in the years that followed, playing an active, though informal role, in the examination of suspects arrested after the discovery of the Rye House Plot. His medical post at court was confirmed by the new king, James II, in 1685, to whom in the same year a grateful Brady dedicated the first part of his *Complete History of England*. He remained loyal to James throughout his short reign, confirming on oath in October 1688 that the king's new-born son was genuinely his progeny and, remarkably perhaps, survived the Revolution by retaining his post as master of Gonville and Caius. He was, however, prosecuted by a group of Collegiate physicians in 1693, ostensibly on the grounds of medical negligence in killing one of his patients. It is highly likely that the accusations were politically motivated, a response in all probability to his publication of works such as his *Treatise of Cities and Boroughs* (1690) which had been written in order to justify Charles II's controversial policy regarding the reversion of charters; *CSPD, Addenda 1660–1685*, 448; *CSPD, 1675–1676*, 53–4; *CSPD, 1682*, 546, 547; TNA, LC 3/24, fo. 16; LC 3/56, 11; *CSPD, 1 January–30 June 1683*, 350–1; *CSPD, 1686–1687*, 147; *CSPD, 1687–1689*, 327; Munk, i, 418.

90. *CSPD, 1686–1687*, 367; *CSPD, 1687–1689*, 14, 99. Johnston's defence of the absolutist Stuarts was published as *The Excellency of Monarchical Government* (London, 1686). His admiration for Brady is evident throughout this work, where he repeatedly cites his published writings and refers to the 'judicious', 'profoundly learned', most industrious'

and 'ingenious' labours of his colleague and political ally; ibid., 150, 154, 155, 186, 188–9, 198, 203, 205, 209, 210, 213–14, 216, 226, 228–9, 261, 264, 277, 279, 325–6. For an excellent overview of Johnston's career and publications, see the entry by Mark Goldie in the *ODNB*.

91. R. G. Frank Jnr, The Physician as Virtuoso in Seventeenth-Century England', in B. Shapiro and R. G. Frank (eds.), *English Scientific Virtuosi in the Sixteenth and Seventeenth Centuries* (Los Angeles, 1979), 74; J. Gascoigne, *Cambridge in the Age of Enlightenment: Science, Religion and Politics from the Restoration to the French Revolution* (Cambridge, 1989), 61. Brady appended a prefatory letter, dated 30 December 1679, to Sydenham's *Epistolae Responsoriae* (London, 1680), which recorded discussions between the two men on the natural history of epidemics.
92. Venn, ii, 480. He is presumably the same as the Nathaniel Johnson who was awarded a licence to practise medicine by the University of Cambridge in 1651; CUL, CUA, Grace Book H (1645–1668), 81 [but not found in Venn].
93. Bodl., Lister MS 35, fos 9–20 [Johnston to Lister, 22 April 1672, 13 May 1672, 3 June 1672, 25 June 1672, 21 January 1672/3, 30 December 1673], 36 [same to same, 10 March 1674/5], 39 [same to same, 22 January 1675/6]. As a friend of the Yorkshire physician Robert Wittie, Johnston subscribed to the articles to establish an association of graduate physicians in Yorkshire in 1672; BL, Sloane MS 1393, fo. 13. He was also on familiar terms with the various disputants in the controversy over the merits of the spa waters at Scarborough, opining at one point that if Dr Tonstall should continue to 'write long in this manner he will write himself out of repute'; Bodl., Lister MS 35, fo. 17 [Johnston to Lister, 25 June 1672]. According to Michael Hunter, Johnston's associate and fellow naturalist, Martin Lister, was 'a stiff and conservative figure' and 'a strong champion of hierarchic values who mistrusted innovations both within medicine and without'; M. Hunter, *Science and Society in Restoration England* (London & New York, 1981), 116, 206. For a revised evaluation of Lister's worth as an original natural philosopher whose interest in chymistry spilled over into his work as a physician, see A. M. Roos, 'Lodestones and Gallstones: The Magnetic Iatrochemistry of Martin Lister (1639–1712)', *History of Science*, 46 (2008), 343–64 and *idem*, *Web of Nature: Martin Lister (1639–1712)* (Leiden, 2011).
94. Johnston himself planned a history of Yorkshire, which was never completed. His collection of old coins was noted by Elias Ashmole, who visited the doctor at Pontefract in 1657; Josten, *Ashmole*, ii, 271. For Thoroton, see above 276, 300 n.66. Kuerden, who may have come under Helmontian influence at Oxford in the 1650s, practised medicine at Preston after the Restoration. Like Thoroton, he was on friendly terms with the country's leading antiquarian, Sir William Dugdale (1605–1686), but unlike his Nottinghamshire colleague he never managed to publish his own county-based researches. For Kuerden, see especially W. D. Shannon, *Seventeenth-Century Lancashire Restored: The Life and Work of Dr Richard Kuerden, Antiquaryand Topographer, 1623–1702* (Manchester, Chetham Soc., vol. 54, 2020); *ODNB*, sub Jackson, Richard; G. Ormerod (ed.), *Epistolary Relics of Lancashire and Cheshire Antiquaries, 1653–1673* (Manchester, Chetham Soc., vol. 24, 1850), 8. Knight's exploits on behalf of the exiled court in the interregnum are detailed above, 56. He was rewarded at the Restoration with various posts, including that of sergeant surgeon,

surgeon-general to the armed forces in England and Wales, and a nomination to a mandated MD from the University of Cambridge in 1669 (which he may not have taken up). Knight possessed an extensive collection of heraldic manuscripts which he probably inherited from his grandfather, Edmund (d.1593), Norroy King of Arms, and which he later bequeathed to Gonville and Caius College, Cambridge. His large collection of topographical books and maps was willed to Ipswich town library; *ODNB*; J. Blatchly, *The Town Library of Ipswich* (Woodbridge, 1989), 40–4.

95. Lamphire, who had something of a reputation as a royalist wit and literary scholar, served as a JP for Restoration Oxfordshire in which capacity he helped to improve the counties' roads and drainage. His patient, Anthony Wood, described him as 'public spirited', though 'not fit to govern' as he was 'much given to his pleasures'. In 1679, he unsuccessfully stood for election to Parliament as prospective MP for the University; *ODNB*; Foster, iii, 872; Wood, *Life and Times*, ii, 440–3.

96. Venn, iii, 28; J. Nichols, *The History and Antiquities of the County of Leicester*, 4 vols (London, 1795–1815), ii, 289–90. In 1677, Knewstub was issued with a licence from the archbishop of Canterbury, supported among others by Thomas Briggs (MD Utrecht, 1661), a close friend and correspondent of Martin Lister and other Anglican medics; LPL, VX 1A/10/102/1–3; Sheldon, fo. 266; Bodl., Lister MS 3, fos 19–30 [Briggs to Lister, 22 August 1655, 28 April 1668, 20 May 1668, 27 April 1673, 14 July 1673, 8 May 1675, 5 February 1675/6, Good Friday, 1676?]. Other contemporary physicians who combined medical practice with a deep-seated interested in antiquarianism and Romano-British history include Thomas Guidott (d.1706), Christopher Hunter (1675–1757) and William Musgrave (1655–1721), for whom see their respective entries in *ODNB*.

97. *ODNB*; T. Skinner, *Elenchi Motuum Nuperorum in Anglia, Pars III. Sive, Motus Compositi* (London, 1676), dedicated to Williamson. In his letter to Williamson, Skinner (MD Oxford, 1672), who was then practising at Colchester in Essex, recounted how his writing had undermined his local reputation, the town being 'a factious and ill-natured place, where the little seditious teachers in conventicles are the only oracles to the people and the sole arbitrators among them of other mens fame or infamy'; Foster, iv, 1362; *CSPD, 1676–1677*, 525–6 [Skinner to Williamson, 31 January 1676/7]. He was still seeking Williamson's patronage and support six months later, when he mentioned his intention of removing to London; *CSPD, 1677–1678*, 189–90 [same to same, 12 June 1677]. For the royal apologist Bate, see *ODNB*.

98. *ODNB*; Munk, i, 382–7. In his first work, *The Honours of the Lords Spiritual Asserted: and Their Priviledges to Vote in Capital Cases in Parliament* (London, 1679), Frankland claimed to have based his findings upon original manuscripts and records in the Tower of London (cf. Brady and Johnston, above). His medico-political aims are made clear at the outset, where he issues a warning that 'in our English Israel... there are yet here amongst us some Remainders of the Men of 42 and that the disease itself sticks as close to them... as the Leprosie did under the Law... and it seems to be as hardly removed as that levitical distemper, which some Naturalists and Physicians say cannot be done but only by Blood'; ibid., unpaginated 'To the Reader'. Two years later, in *The Annals of King James and King Charles the First* (London, 1681), he attempted to use the recent machinations of the Catholics as a spur to encourage the dissenters to return to the Anglican fold; ibid., a2r–v.

99. Barnard appended a congratulatory poem to Skinner's *Elenchi Motuum* (A6r), while Frankland acknowledged the help of his 'good friend' Dr Barnard, physician to St Bartholomew's, for lending him a collection of manuscripts of the speeches, resolutions and debates of Charles I's parliaments in 1628–9; Frankland, *Annals of King James*, A3r. Barnard began his career as an apothecary to St Bartholomew's, but rose rapidly in London medical circles largely through the support of powerful patrons within the Anglican hierarchy (he himself was the son of the sequestrated vicar of Croydon, Samuel Barnard, who died in 1657). In 1678 he was granted a Lambeth MD by archbishop Sancroft, his sponsor John Finch alluding to his father's lament that he was unable to give his son, Francis, a university education. Seventeen years earlier, Finch had successfully interceded with the government and governors of St Bartholomew's in securing Barnard's appointment as apothecary to that institution. Barnard's meteoric rise continued after 1678 in which year his Lambeth MD was incorporated at Cambridge and he was made assistant physician at St Bartholomew's. In September 1680, he became an honorary fellow of the London College and was appointed physician in ordinary to James II in 1685. As a full fellow of the College from 1687, he consistently opposed all attempts by the College's Whig hierarchy to bring the apothecaries to submission, and he was equally committed to supporting recalcitrant colleagues such as Johannes Groenvelt and John Badger. Like his younger brother Charles (1652–1710), a barber-surgeon turned physician, he was a committed Tory and high churchman who seems to have placed his vast collection of books and manuscripts at the disposal of those who shared his religious and political beliefs; *ODNB*, sub Bernard, Francis; Bernard, Charles; *Wal. Rev.*, 349; CUL, Collect.Admin.8, 587; LPL, F1/D, fos 183, 214; Bodl., Tanner MS 40, fos 98, 134 [Heneage Finch to John Tillotson, dean of Canterbury, 2 January 1677/8]; *CSPD, 1660–1661*, 533; Munk, i, 449–50.

100. *HMC. Eleventh Report, Appendix, Part VII* (London, 1888), 17. Winter was a Neapolitan quack, who had resided in England since the civil war in which he fought on the side of the King. In one of his handbills, he referred to having served under Sir Charles Lucas at Colchester [in 1648]. His son, also Salvador, was granted an archiepiscopal licence to practise medicine and surgery in the province of Canterbury in 1679; S. Winter, *Directions for the Use of My Elixir, My Philosophical Petza or Plaister, and My Balsam* (London, 1664?); LPL, VX 1A/10/142/1–2; Sancroft, fo. 223v. Some Catholic medics played a more militant role in the political controversies of the late 1670s and early 1680s. Antoine or Anthony Choqueux, for example, who was suspected of involvement in the Popish Plot, acted as Roger L'Estrange's agent in 1681 in an attempt to get the son of one of the main conspirators, Israel Tonge, to turn king's evidence and provide proof that the plot was a fabrication; *HMC. Eleventh Report, Appendix, Part II. The Manuscripts of the House of Lords, 1678–1688*, 1, 18, 19, 246–50; *Lords' Journal*, vol.13, 343, 346, 348, 358; S. Tonge, *The Narrative and Case of Simson Tonge, Gent* (London, 1681). Choqueux had a long, colourful and distinguished career in the service of the Stuarts. He first came to England in 1634, served as a surgeon in the Bishops' Wars and English civil wars as well as personal surgeon to Prince Rupert and Charles II and was implicated in an attempt to assassinate Cromwell in 1654. He was prosecuted for recusancy in 1674

and 1679; *CSPD, 1660–1661*, 284; *CSPD, 1664–1665*, 241, 263; TNA, LC 3/26, fo. 145; Thurloe, *State Papers*, ii, 336, 512.

101. M. Rusden, *A Further Discovery of Bees, Treating of the Nature, Government, Generation and Preservation of the Bee* (London, 1679; 2nd ed., 1685), epistle dedicatory to King Charles II. Rusden was living in London at the time of publication, but had previously been licensed to practise medicine and surgery at Wallingford in Berkshire by archbishop Sheldon, in 1672; LPL, VX 1A/10/45; VG 1/1, fo. 236v; Sheldon, fo. 239.
102. The work in question was Barnes' *The History of the Most Victorious Monarch Edward III* (Cambridge, 1688); S. L. C. Clapp, 'Subscription Publishers Prior to Jacob Tonson', *The Library*, 19 (1932), 168 [citing adverts in the *Gazette* directing would-be subscribers to Harborough]; Venn, ii, 300. Harborough was described by one anonymous source in 1689 as a 'quack-doctor, living by Doctors Commons'. He was later prosecuted by the College of Physicians in 1702 for illicit practice. Part of the College's animus against Harborough undoubtedly stemmed from the fact that he was probably the most prolific signatory of testimonials for archiepiscopal licences in the post-Restoration period. Between 1679 and 1704, he put his name to thirty-two such applications. His loyal credentials are further suggested by his marriage to a daughter of Thomas Strickland of Westmorland, 'a Captain in the service of King Charles the First'; *CSPD, 1689–1690*, 376; RCPL, LEGAC/ENV 79, 244; Wales and Hartley (eds), *Visitation of London, 1687*, i, 61–2.
103. *ODNB*, sub Elliott, John; Cook, *Decline of the Old Medical Regime*, 217; *CSPD,1689–1690*, 145, 165; Venn, ii, 95; Munk, i, 454, 474.
104. *ODNB*; Venn, ii, 63. Drake, the son of a Cambridge attorney, may have possessed Catholic connections. He and his father were remembered in the will of the Catholic physician and iatrochemist John Fryer (d.1672); TNA, PROB 11/340, ff.163r–165r [will of John Fryer, doctor of phisick, of Little Brittaine, 1 September 1672; pr. 21 November 1672].
105. *ODNB*; *CSPD, 1680–1681*, 253. Crull, who probably studied at Leiden before coming to England in 1681, seems to have been another loyal Anglican who benefited from the patronage of archbishop Sancroft; see Bodl., Tanner MS 36, fo. 64 [Paman to Sancroft, 2 July 1681].
106. N. Siraisi, *History, Medicine, and the Traditions of Renaissance Learning* (Ann Arbor, MICH, 2007), 19.
107. For the Hippocratic revival in England, and Sydenham's central role in that process, see A. Cunningham, 'The Transformation of Hippocrates in Seventeenth-Century Britain', in D. Cantor (ed.), *Reinventing Hippocrates* (Aldershot, 2002), 91–115.
108. Paman praised Sydenham's work on the history and treatment of venereal disease in the former's *Epistolae Responsoriae* [Paman to Sydenham, 12 February 1679/80]. Henry Paman, another product of interregnum Cambridge (MD 1658), held High Church views and was a close friend of archbishop Sancroft with whom he lived after 1677 at Lambeth Palace. He was appointed Master of the Faculties by Sancroft in 1684, thus increasing his powers of medical patronage within the province of Canterbury; *ODNB*; Munk, i, 446 [honorary fellow, 1664; full fellow 1687]. Sydenham dedicated his *Treatise on Gout and Dropsy* to his friend, Thomas Short;

see above, 277. The 'confirmed Jacobite and violent Tory' John Radcliffe, who despised much traditional medical learning, gained a particular fame for his cure of smallpox in which he recommended the 'cooling treatments' prescribed by Sydenham; *ODNB*; A. Sakula, 'Dr John Radcliffe, Court Physician, and the Death of Queen Anne', *Journal of the Royal College of Physicians of London*, 19 (1985), 256. Like Brady, Radcliffe entered national politics, serving as MP for Bramber in Sussex in the 1690s and later as MP for Buckingham in 1713 as part of the Tory revival at the end of the reign of Queen Anne.

109. For an attempt to equate Sydenham's medical empiricism and distaste for anatomical and physiological enquiry with an emergent Whig political culture, see especially R. L. Martensen, 'Hippocrates and the Politics of Medical Knowledge in Early Modern England', in Cantor (ed.), *Reinventing Hippocrates*, 121–4.

110. Venn, i, 390; Munk, i, 267, 348; E. Cooper, *The Asse Beaten for Bawling; or, A Replie from the Citie, to the Crie of the Country* (London, 1661). Munk suggests that in May 1659 Cooper stated his intentions of no longer seeking membership of the College. However, in December 1664 (as 'Edward Cooper'), he was made an honorary fellow of the College, part of an attempt by the puritan leadership of the College to ingratiate themselves with the government (see above, 131). His membership, as Edmund Cooper, is confirmed in a later subscription book, where he is described as 'Medicinae Dr. Coll: Lond.'; Munk, i, 267; WSA, D1/22/4, fo. 18v. Following presentation to the living of Woodmancote, Cooper continued to practise among his parishioners with whom he would appear to have had a fractious and difficult relationship; see WSxRO, Par/214/1/1/1, 32–4; H. Sykes-McLean (ed.), *The Registers of Woodmancote, 1582–1812* (Brighton, 1932); R. W. Blencowe, 'Extracts from the Parish Registers and Other Parochial Documents of East Sussex', *Sussex Archaeological Collections*, 4 (1851), 280–3.

111. E. C[ooper], *On the Recovery of Our Most Gracious Queen Katherine from Her Late Grievous and Deplorable Fit of Sicknesse* (London, 1664).

112. S. Jacombe, *Moses His Death: Opened and Applied, in a Sermon at Christ-Church in London at the Funeral of Mr Edward Bright* [23 December 1656] (London, 1657), 43. It may be no coincidence that among those who supplied further elegies to the deceased was William Croone (1633–1684), a fellow of Emmanuel, who would later achieve fame as a founder member of the Royal Society and an eminent anatomist. His pioneering work on the muscles, in which he proposed that nerve juice from the brain mixes and reacts chemically with the spirits of the blood in the muscles, was first published anonymously in 1664 alongside Thomas Willis' *Cerebri Anatome* (London, 1664). More importantly, in the light of Jacombe's reference to the role of air in cooling the heart's blood, he was one of the first to carry out experiments in the mechanics of respiration at the Royal Society in the early 1660s. For Croone, who received his mandated MD in 1662, see *ODNB*.

113. J. Buck, *St Paul's Thanksgiving set forth in a Sermon Preached before the Right Honorable House of Peers* [10 May 1660] ... *Being the Day of Solemn Thanksgiving to Almighty God for His Late Blessings upon this Kingdom* (London, 1660), 4–5. For Buck, a product of pre-civil war Cambridge and an acolyte of bishop Matthew Wren, see Venn, i, 245; *Wal. Rev.*, 330.

114. R. Henchman, *A Peace-Offering in the Temple; Or, A Seasonable Plea for Unity among Dissenting Brethren* [14 October 1660] (London, 1661), 9. The sermon was dedicated to Henchman's kinsman, Humphrey Henchman, bishop of Salisbury [for whose medical interests, see Appendix 1b].

115. J. Torbuck, *Ημέως παρ Ημέως. Extraordinary Dayes, Or, Sermons on the Most Solemn Feasts* (Oxford, 1671), 73; J. Warly, *The Reasoning Apostate: or Modern Latitude-Man Considered, as He Opposeth the Authority of the King and Church* (London, 1677), 13–14. Warly was more than happy to promote new discoveries in natural philosophy (at one point he invokes the *tria prima* of the Paracelsians), but he was insistent that scientific innovation or natural theology, as promoted by the latitudinarians, should not be used to justify 'new creeds in divinity'; ibid., 82–3, 86–7. Elsewhere, he lauded the discovery of the telescope and microscope, as well as the work of Galileo and Descartes, while remaining committed to the fundamental separation of matters of faith and reason; *idem*, *The Natural Fanatick, or, Reason Consider'd in its Extravagancy in Religion* (London, 1676), 12–13 and *passim*.

116. For Robinson, vicar of Burneston in Yorkshire, who was himself prosecuted for practising without a licence in 1676, see Venn, iii, 472; *ODNB*. For Briggs, see Innes Smith, 30. For Briggs' correspondence with Lister between 1665 and 1676, see Bodl., Lister MS 3, fos 19–30.

117. For Grove's educational and clerical career, see *ODNB* (which unfortunately fails to note his medical interests, poetry, or library); Venn, ii, p.271; L. R. C. Agnew, 'De Sanguine Episcopoque: A Discussion of Bishop Robert Grove [1634–1696] and his *Carmen de Sanguinis Circuitu, &c* (1685)', *Bulletin of the History of Medicine*, 34 (1960), 318–30. For Grove's correspondence with Lister, see Bodl., Lister MSS 3, fos 112–17; 35, fo. 82. His imminent commencement as DD was noted in a letter by a colleague, John Peck, to Lister in April 1681; ibid., fo. 47.

118. Venn, iv, 447; S. Wolferstan, *An Enquiry into the Causes of Diseases in General, and the Disturbances of the Humors in Mans Body* (London, 1692). Wolferstan's speculations surrounding the role of bad air in health echo the earlier thoughts of another student of St John's, William Randolph (d.1675), who graduated MD in 1668. Inspired by Boyle's *Spring of the Air* (1660), Randolph wrote to the author in 1670 to explain how he believed the air and respiration held the key to life and good health. Citing the recent physiological discoveries of Walter Needham, Thomas Willis and Richard Lower, he argued that the air was able to penetrate all parts of the body, including the brain, heart, and muscles, and that it circulated through the body in a way reminiscent of the movement of the blood; Venn, iii, 420; Boyle, *Correspondence*, iv, 159–72.

119. P. Morant, *The History and Antiquities of the County of Essex*, 2 vols (London, 1768), i, 67, 110. For Glisson's Presbyterianism, see above 48, 85 n.23.

120. CUL, CUA, Grace Book H (1645–1668), 21, 37, 63. Buckenham's Anglican sympathies are suggested by the comment of the deposed bishop, Ralph Brownrigg, who records the 'good company' and 'kind and courteous welcome' afforded to him by the doctor at his home at Bury St Edmunds in 1653; Bodl., Tanner MS 52, fo. 11 [Brownrigg to William Sancroft, 21 May 1653]. During the early stages of the civil war, Buckenham was a medical student at Leiden and Padua. He later returned to

Cambridge, where he received his MD in 1646; Venn, i, 247; Innes Smith, 35; Worthington, *Diary*, i, 26.

121. For Tenison's short-lived indulgence of medical study, see E. Carpenter, *Thomas Tenison, Archbishop of Canterbury: His Life and Times* (London, 1948), 7. Tenison later corresponded with Henry Oldenburg of the Royal Society, supplying him with detailed descriptions of the local springs at Holywell-cum-Needingworth, Huntingdonshire (where he served as rector), as well as providing important information on the agriculture and topography of the area. These suggest a keen interest in chymistry and a Baconian desire to promote any cause that might assist 'the deposing of Aristotle from his Popedome'; Oldenburg, *Correspondence*, vii, 494–5 [4 March 1670/1], 552–9 [6 April 1671]; viii, 344–9 [7 November 1671].
122. For Ludkin, Gelsthorpe and Parham, see above 101 n.104, 275, 286, 293 n.20, 298 n.54. Buckenham was a fellow of Caius from 1646–52. Having briefly enrolled as a medical student at Leiden in 1641, he later practised medicine at Great Yarmouth. His religious sensibilities are suggested by the fact that in 1672 he penned an epitaph on behalf of the Anglican apologist and Norfolk cleric, Edward Boys (1599–1667); Venn, i, 247; Innes Smith, 35; E. Boys, *Sixteen Sermons* (London, 1672). Witherley (1618–1694), who was made an honorary fellow of the London College of Physicians in December 1664, would later serve as personal physician to both Charles II and James II as well as president of the College of Physicians from 1684 to 1687. His loyalty to James was acknowledged with a knighthood; Venn, iv, 444; Munk, i, 394; TNA, LC 3/26, fos 141, 143; 3/24, fo.1 6; 3/56, 9.
123. NNkRO, MC 1/17 386x5 [Sir Allen Apsley to Humphrey Henchman, 1660]; *CSPD, 1671*, 78.
124. TNA, PROB 11/340, fos 18r–19r [will of Robert Eade, doctor of phisicke, of Cambridge, Cambridgeshire, 20 April 1672, pr. 10 September 1672].
125. For Drake's activities as a Tory pamphleteer and historian, see above ???. For Howse and Pell, see Venn, ii, 419; iii, 337. Pell, who later practised medicine at Fakenham in Norfolk, did not graduate from Caius with any medical qualifications.
126. *HMC. Reports on the Manuscripts of the Marquess of Downshire... Vol.1... Part 1* (London, 1924), 25. Dolben also commented on the promotion by royal mandate of Henry Paman (MD St John's, Cambridge, 1658) to his doctorate in law at Cambridge in the same year. Paman almost certainly acted as a crucial intermediary between Sancroft and Brady in these years, and was particularly instrumental in promoting the interests of the church and other loyalists in the medical profession in his various capacities as Master of the Faculties (1684) and through his membership of the London College of Physicians (1687).
127. Venn, iv, 70; *CSPD, 1680–1681*, 291–2; A. W. Hughes Clarke and A. Campling (eds), *The Visitation of Norfolk... 1664* (London, Harleian Soc., vol. 86, 1934), 174, 194–5.
128. Venn, iv, 103.
129. For Gostlyn, see above 288 and note 72. Like fellow Caian and medic, Peter Parham, Gostlyn wielded ecclesiastical patronage, holding the advowson of Hethersett in Norfolk. He bequeathed the right of presentation to the College in his will of 1702; TNA, PROB 11/481, ff.40r–41v [will of John Gostlyn, doctor of physic and fellow of Gonville and Caius College, Cambridge, 16 September 1702; pr. 15 March 1704/5].

130. For disquiet caused by this policy, see especially J. Twigg, *The University of Cambridge and the English Revolution 1625–1688* (Woodbridge, 1990), 268–74. The difficulty of gaining mandated medical degrees from Oxford is amply demonstrated by the case of Samuel Jackson (d.1675). In 1671, he was awarded his MD after much arm-twisting at the behest of the loyal cleric and vice chancellor Peter Mews, a former colleague in arms. It was granted by convocation, however, only on the express condition that no precedent was being established; Foster, ii, 796; *CSPD, 1671*, 330, 334–5.
131. For Darrell, see Foster, i, 373; Venn, ii, 12; Munk, i, 398; *CSPD, 1677–1678*, 212, 216, 392. For Scarburgh, see Venn, iv, 28; *CSPD, 1682*, 241. Scarburgh subsequently switched to a career in the church, serving as prebend of Salisbury from 1687 to 1705.
132. Gascoigne, *Cambridge in the Age of Enlightenment*, 27–39.
133. Blenkerne, Howman and Parham were all products of Caius. Briggs and Lister were alumni of interregnum St John's, while Wright, a former fellow, graduated from the same college as MD in 1684. For Blenkerne (MD 1676), who practised at King's Lynn in Norfolk, see Venn, i, 167; *CSPD, 1676–1677*, 41; B. Mackerell, *The History and Antiquities of... King's Lynn in the County of Norfolk* (London, 1738), 52; BL, Sloane MS 123, fos 7v, 10r. For Briggs and Lister, former students of interregnum St John's, see above 285 and note 96. Briggs also corresponded with Blenkerne (above), Parham and Howman; BL, Sloane MS 123, fos 2, 6, 7r, 7v, 10; TCD, MS 889, fo. 167. Howman (MD 1674) was the son of a Norfolk clergyman and practised medicine at Norwich; Venn, ii, 420–1. Wright, who corresponded with Briggs in 1681, was provided with a lengthy commendation by Humphrey Gower in 1675 in a letter to the Yorkshire naturalist and physician Martin Lister; Venn, iv, 474; BL, Sloane MS 123, fos 2r, 7r; Bodl., Lister MS 3, fos 107r–v.

7
Conclusions
Medicine in an Age of Revolution

> Destructive times, distractive muzings yeeld
> Expect not therefore method now of me.
>
> George Wither, *Campo-Musae* (London, 1643), 3.

As the last two chapters have shown, the religious and political divisions and controversies that blighted the body politic of Restoration England were reflected in the fragmented and politicized condition of the medical 'profession'. The emergence of a dissenting medical tradition, forged in the furnace of religious persecution and political exclusion, and consolidated through study abroad, had its parallel in the creation of a High Church, Anglican medical establishment which first took shape at Oxford and Cambridge in the 1650s and subsequently held sway throughout much of the kingdom (though not, as I have suggested in London, where the College of Physicians acted as a moderating influence for much of the period). I have also suggested that an important symptom of this process of medical politicization was the growing attraction of political and judicial office-holding for medical practitioners, a process that had its roots in the 1640s and 1650s and continued apace at the Restoration, when loyal medics, the majority located in the towns and boroughs of England, began to appear in ever greater numbers among the ranks of the governing classes. While for some, the pragmatic search for patronage, patients and hospital posts may have dictated such actions, ideological commitment also played its part. This is most evident, perhaps, in the willingness of physicians to engage in public debate and openly declare their political allegiance through the printing press—again, a process that had its roots in the middle decades of the century. But it is equally probable that for many educated medical practitioners, the temptation to analyse and debate the causes and likely outcomes of the various diseases afflicting the body politic was too great to pass up. The 'corporate' nature of British politics, focused on those miniature bodies politic, the boroughs, may have accentuated this process. Physicians naturally gravitated to the towns and cities because that was where the best qualified were most likely to make their mark. Apothecaries and surgeons, on the other hand, were embedded in corporate structures through companies, apprenticeship and the grant of freedom which in turn enabled them to participate in corporate politics. While university-educated physicians may have lacked

Medicine in an Age of Revolution. Peter Elmer, Oxford University Press. © Peter Elmer 2023.
DOI: 10.1093/oso/9780198853985.003.0007

such routes to civic respectability, it should be remembered that many, nonetheless, were the sons of leading townsmen and possessed first-hand experience in their youth of corporate politics.[1] When consensus evaporated in the heat of partisan debate, it was perhaps only natural therefore that medical experts on the human body should feel compelled to comment upon and suggest remedies for the ailments afflicting the towns and cities that constituted the wider body politic.

A politicized medical profession, of course, implies a politicized medical system and body of knowledge, though here it is more difficult to say with certainty how exactly the political controversies of the day impacted upon medical practice and theory. Doctors, of course, had always needed to tread carefully when tending to the medical concerns of politically eminent patients, be they kings and princes, prisoners or enemies of the state. Certainly, there is no evidence to suggest that party affiliation or religious orientation was a critical factor in determining what medical theories physicians chose to inform their daily practice. As should be clear from earlier chapters, interest in the iatrochemical principles and practices promoted by Paracelsus, van Helmont, and their followers was widespread and extended to the court of Charles II, despite the attempt by some contemporaries to depict the chymical physicians as the agents of sectarian discord who sought to destabilize the body politic. It is equally the case that subscription to specific religious and political agendas, be they puritan, parliamentarian, Whig, royalist, Anglican or Tory, does not appear to have dictated how medical practitioners responded to the issue of regulation in the medical marketplace. The cause of empiricism or the freedom to practise unhindered by legal restriction was never the exclusive concern of a single religious or political faction. Politics and religious orientation did, however, intrude into the daily lives of medical practitioners in other ways. Proponents of astrological medicine were, for obvious reasons, deeply divided on political grounds, as the verbal jousting of John Gadbury and John Partridge suggests. In 1687, Gadbury thus invoked the image of the body politic as a stick to beat his radical opponent, claiming that '[i]f God had intended a Man should have been in Love with a Commonwealth, he would have Created him with a Head on each Shoulder [for] [i]f Government… like the Body Natural, should have many Heads, 'tis a Monster, and we know it ever bodes Ill'. In response, Partridge tersely noted that heads were often 'too big for the body', concluding that 'a single Head may be a Monster as well as two Heads'.[2]

Political considerations may also have shaped attitudes to specific complaints or ailments. As previously discussed, there seems little doubt that interest in the appearance of 'new diseases', a popular conceit in medical discourse after 1640, carried political connotations. Initially conceived as a specifically puritan project, the 'discovery' of the rickets, for example, was later adopted by Anglican apologists as a weapon in the polemical debate against dissent.[3] Rickets, of course, was just one of many 'new diseases' identified by medical practitioners in the seventeenth century.[4] It was widely mooted in medical circles that 'modern' diseases were more complex and intractable than in the days of the ancients. Proponents of medical innovation, such as those who favoured iatrochemical methods, were quick to seize on such suggestions. The Helmontian William Johnson, for example, claimed in 1692 that diabetes was far more common now than in the age of Galen, a fact that he put down to the 'Debaucheries of our Times'.[5] The moral decline of the nation, hinted at here in the enfeebled 'constitutions' of modern bodies, clearly carried a contemporary political resonance. It was a commonplace among many observers that the political and religious upheavals of the middle decades of the seventeenth century had induced such a decline. A willingness to concede the existence of new diseases, and by extension new therapies, may well then have proceeded from the wider debate in political circles as to the ailments currently afflicting the body politic. The point was well made by Charles II at the opening of Parliament in November 1661, when he told his auditors that he found 'the general Temper and Affections of the Nation ... not so well composed' and went on to advise that 'if you find new Diseases you must study new Remedies'—an interesting aside given the King's support for chymical medicine.[6]

The political awakening of the medical profession in the aftermath of the British civil wars was thus manifest in a number of ways both great and small. Individual medical practitioners frequently nailed their political colours to the mast in a range of actions. On occasion, this even extended to the naming of their children. Shortly after the battle of Marston Moor in 1644, the militant parliamentarian astrologer John Booker christened his daughter Victory. Five years later, on 2 February 1649, the royalist physician Thomas Horsington poignantly opted to name his son Charles, born on the day of the regicide, in memory of the royal martyr.[7] Personal actions of this kind clearly reflected a wider process of politicization among the communities in which medical men lived and worked, one in which the annual calendar of commemoration could no longer be relied upon to generate communal consensus. On a grander scale, however, I think it is possible to see the political events of the 1640s, culminating in the abolition of the monarchy, as an important turning-point, even a revolutionary moment, in British medicine. The mood of optimism is neatly captured in the correspondence of two disaffected royalist physicians in the early 1650s, Reuben Robinson and Henry Power, who, despite their political conservatism, were convinced of the fact that they were witnessing the onset of a golden age in medicine. The two men met while students at Cambridge in the 1640s, when both became attracted to medical study. Initially drawn to the study of anatomy, both men subsequently took a keen interest in chymistry and its potential application to medicine. On 5 March 1650, Robinson (*c.*1628–1665), the son of an apothecary who settled in his native Maldon, wrote to Power (1625–1668) waxing lyrical with respect to recent medical advances. In particular, he commented upon the widespread enthusiasm for the writings of van Helmont, who 'is much adored every where & extreamely read not only in London but in both ye universities', and concluded by noting that 'the world is in great expectation [for] truly, if my confidence betrays mee not this age will have newe knowledge in physic then all ye preceding'.[8]

The two friends continued to correspond for over a decade, during which time their commitment to medical and natural philosophical innovation never faltered. Both engaged in experimentation with the assistance of new instruments such as microscopes and telescopes, making a range of observations that they were keen to promote and publicize. Power, who prospered under the guidance of powerful mentors such as Sir Thomas Browne and Francis Glisson, graduated MD from Cambridge in 1655 and went on to become a figure of national significance, publishing the first work in English on microscopy in 1664.[9] The career of Robinson, who remained a largely obscure figure, nonetheless demonstrates the importance of provincial practitioners in creating local networks of like-minded virtuosi (he was, for example, on friendly terms with fellow Maldon practitioner, James Thickens (d.1666), who, as we have seen was himself lauded as a pioneer of Helmontianism in 1650). Like Thickens, moreover, Robinson was a committed royalist and defender of the Anglican Church. He served as an alderman and bailiff in the borough of Maldon, often intervening in corporate affairs as in April 1660 when he was 'the chief agent & witness' to the 'factious' designs of Colonel Mildmay, prospective parliamentary candidate for the borough. Robinson was also active in prosecuting nonconformists after the Restoration, his reverence for the restored church evident in his will of 1665 in which he asked to be buried according to 'the liturgie of the church of England in whose peace and communion I thanke God it is my great happinesse always to have lived and in the same by Gods blessing to dye'.[10]

The enthusiastic reception afforded to medical innovation, particularly Helmontian chymistry, by practitioners such as Reuben Robinson highlights a number of important issues raised in earlier chapters. Robinson, first and foremost, was a member of a group of like-minded physicians and natural philosophers who shared a common religious and political identity. In addition to his friendship with men like James Thickens and Henry Power, Robinson moved almost exclusively in Anglican and royalist circles. In October 1650, for example, he describes an encounter with 'Horsington ye Chymist', whose royalist credentials we have previously noted above. Four years later, he was engaged with Thickens and a fellow Essex physician, Mr Thompson—almost certainly the future leader of the Society of Chymical Physicians, George Thomson—in anatomizing the cadaver of a local horse thief executed at Chelmsford assizes.[11] The actions and associations of this group of medical researchers underscores once more the extent to which it is inconceivable to envisage support for medical change in this period as the sole preserve of a particular religious or political grouping. At the same time, Robinson's correspondence with Henry Power, who graduated MD at Cambridge in 1655, provides further evidence of the key role that the universities played in promoting such change. This, it should be stressed, was largely despite rather than because of the zeal of the puritan authorities that oversaw the 'reform' of the academies in the 1650s. As the case of Trinity College, Cambridge, discussed in chapter 3 suggests, many scholars, often from Anglican and royalist backgrounds, were attracted to the 'new philosophy' and medical innovation precisely because it offered a meaningful and attractive diversion from the stultifying banalities of the orthodox curriculum favoured by the 'usurpers'.[12]

Rather than fixate on the ideological origins of the 'medical revolution' of the mid-seventeenth century, which would appear to have no firm foundation in any specific religious or political outlook, we might perhaps speculate more fruitfully on the wider causes that helped to generate a burgeoning enthusiasm for medicine, both within and outside the universities, from the 1650s onwards. Within elite medicine, as Robert Frank has shown, there was an exponential growth in the numbers of men graduating with medical degrees in the seventeenth century, the numbers peaking in the 1650s. Frank partly explains the growth of medical graduates as a function of increased demand for the services of educated physicians among the wealthy, both in London and the provinces. However, it is equally noteworthy that more recent research has revealed that such demand was mirrored within the wider population.[13] Again, the 1650s would appear to represent a watershed in this development, as it was during this decade that demand for vernacular medical publications witnessed an unprecedented explosion. Cheap pamphlets and single sheet advertisements enabled practitioners to reach a wide audience, and undoubtedly encouraged many who lacked the traditional educational qualifications to pursue medicine as a viable and attractive career option.

Such developments were part and parcel of wider changes taking place in British society at this time. The growth in medical publishing almost certainly reflected the growing value placed on literacy in the commercial marketplace of early modern England. More and more people were better educated and thus able to access the knowledge economy, including medicine, of the period. At the same time, Britain was experiencing rapid economic and commercial growth, much of it dependent upon the expansion of the country as a global and colonial power. This in turn placed increasing emphasis upon naval power, and a growing role for the state in supporting such enterprise through the mercantilist policies pursued by consecutive governments of various ideological flavours. All these interdependent developments were 'good' for medicine. There is insufficient space here to discuss all aspects of this process, but it is important to note that the emergence of Britain as a military and naval power, competing on the world stage, helped to facilitate an enormous growth in demand for medical services in order to enable the state to function effectively as a defender and promoter of the nation's trading interests. This process began in earnest in the 1640s as a by-product of the internecine disputes that erupted throughout the British Isles in the wake of rebellion and civil war. It continued throughout the 1650s, when the Cromwellian state first began to establish an embryonic system of health care for its soldiers and sailors, and continued to evolve in the second half of the seventeenth century against a backdrop of almost unbroken foreign warfare and conflict. The huge increase in the numbers of men entering the profession of surgery by about 1700 was in large part a reflection of such developments and may well have spurred the growing status and authority wielded by surgeons in the early eighteenth century.

Understanding of the role of the state in early modern medicine in Britain is in its infancy. There is still a great deal of work to be undertaken in order to understand precisely how successive governments interacted with the medical profession, and how this in turn created an increasingly politicized atmosphere in which medical practitioners pursued their chosen careers. Two examples follow in order to suggest potential areas of future research. In the first instance, it is becoming increasingly clear that the appointment of doctors, surgeons and apothecaries to prestigious posts within the London medical establishment, as well as its military and naval wing, was frequently shaped by political partisanship. This was particularly evident in periods of acute political conflict such as the Exclusion Crisis, when, as Craig Rose has convincingly demonstrated, party allegiances, both of hospital governors and medical men, informed decision-making including the forced resignation and appointment of new medical personnel. All five London hospitals were thus affected leaving a legacy of bitter conflict that often lingered for decades. In the case of the Tory loyalist John Browne, surgeon at St Thomas' Hospital, the dispute over his appointment and subsequent dismissal in the aftermath of the Glorious Revolution was still ongoing in 1699.[14] Elsewhere, similar disputes divided the medical community, frequently exacerbating political tension in bodies such as the College of Physicians. The case of Dr John Downes (1627–1694), who sought the vacant post as physician to Christ's Hospital in 1682, was to prove particularly troublesome for the College. Determined to promote the appointment of Nathaniel Hodges following the death of the previous incumbent, Dr John Micklethwaite, an old puritan, Downes was consistently overlooked for the post despite his exceptional religious and political credentials.[15] He nonetheless acquired the support of powerful supporters, including Judge George Jeffreys and James II, who in 1685 ordered the College to reimburse Downes for lost salary. The College refused to relent, however, and in 1693 reopened the case against Downes in an attempt to foreclose once and for all this long-running and damaging dispute.[16]

In the eighteenth century, with the emergence of new voluntary hospitals in provincial England, political factors frequently impinged upon procedures for the admission of patients. Loyalty to the Whig authorities was widely expected as a token of a patient's deservedness to receive medical assistance.[17] In the previous century, political factors may also have played a prominent, if somewhat more sinister, role in admissions to the country's only specialist hospital for the cure of the mad, Bedlam. As a 'state institution', answerable jointly to the crown and civic authorities in London, Bedlam's governors often acceded to the demands of the powers-that-be in incarcerating lunatics like Richard Stafford, who were seen as endangering the political status quo. In this way, Jonathan Andrews has claimed that Bedlam operated, in part, as a space of 'political quarantine', and that as a result 'lunacy itself was being politicised'.[18] Such a view can, I think, be corroborated in other ways, though there is insufficient space here to examine this process in full. Politics and religion intruded into the discussion of a range of diseases linked to contemporary understandings of the relationship between mind and body in early modern Europe and may even have helped to re-shape the medical landscape with respect to attitudes to mental illness. As disputed terrain, physicians and clergymen constantly debated the origins and nomenclature of such complaints, their views often informed by partisan attachments to specific religious and political aims and beliefs. Elsewhere, I have tried to show how such conflicting attitudes helped to shape distinctively different approaches among medical men to one category of diseases, namely those induced by witchcraft.[19] Here, I would like to suggest that such developments were symptomatic of wider changes in British society that had their origin in the breakdown of political consensus contingent upon the outbreak of civil war in England in 1642.

In my study of the Irish miracle healer Valentine Greatrakes and those who sought his help, I intimated that on one level Greatrakes was acting as a therapist to a generation of men and women whose illnesses might be seen as an expression of wider dysfunction in the social, religious and political world of Restoration Britain. In the wake of the return of Charles II in 1660 and the various attempts that were made to restore order and stability to the body politic, certain groups and individuals, particularly those exposed to legal prohibitions, became increasingly prone to a range of illnesses, many of which involved the symptoms of mental sickness. Of course, the source of all such contention and division was the period of the civil wars itself, which created unprecedented divisions and in the process traumatized a generation.[20] In the process, it may also have encouraged a trend that had its roots in the pre–civil war period whereby specialist medical care for the mad was often provided by men who inhabited and served those religious and political communities that were most prone to marginalization and persecution. Roman Catholic physicians in particular would appear to have claimed a special skill in the cure of the mad and melancholic. Prior to 1640, the recusant John Bartlett, who was frequently in trouble with the College of Physicians in London, was described by Bulstrode Whitelocke as 'famous for the cure of such distempers'.[21] Over twenty years later, it was another Catholic physician, Dr Thomas Lentall (1612–1673), who was chosen to attempt the cure of the mad courtier Sir John Denham following the failure of Greatrakes' stroking. Lentall, a former clergyman who converted to Catholicism in the 1640s, clearly had aspirations to succeed in this particular field of medicine. In 1667, he unsuccessfully sought election to the post of physician to Bedlam Hospital.[22]

Interestingly, colleagues on the opposite side of the confessional divide, most notably pre–civil war puritans and their Restoration nonconformist heirs shared the sensitivity of Roman Catholic physicians to mental afflictions. In the period immediately prior to the outbreak of the civil war, the Huntingdonshire gentleman and advocate of godly reform, John Spencer, for example, offered refuge to the mad and melancholic at his home in Great Staughton. In 1641, he published a passionate defence of puritanism in which he alluded to his role as a local peacemaker and spiritual counsellor and added a brief discourse on melancholy that owed much to both Galenic and Paracelsian principles.[23] Likewise, the Sussex physician John Panton (d.1654), who belonged to a family long associated with puritanism and dissent in his native Lewes, would appear to have specialized in the cure of the mad. Among his patients was Henry Sackville, the second son of Lord Buckhurst, who suffered a 'distraction of his senses' and died at Dr Panton's house in 1635.[24] After the Restoration, Richard Panton (d.1684), probably a relation, set himself up as a specialist in the cure of the mad. Despite lacking formal qualifications, Panton, of Batheaston, Somerset, was licensed to 'practise and only to administer Phisick to persons distracted and troubled with a Lunasie or madnesse'.[25] Other nonconformists who committed to the cure of the mad may also include the celebrated botanist James Newton (1639–1718) who established one of the first private madhouses in London. His practice in Clerkenwell, which he later bequeathed to his son, also James (*c.*1664–1750), attracted a fair amount of notoriety, much of it no doubt in part due to Newton's role as a self-publicist and the bold claims which he made for his methods in print.[26]

We should not perhaps be surprised to discover Catholic, puritan, and dissenting medical practitioners so fully engaged with the care and cure of the mad, for, as Michael MacDonald pointed out in 1981, those communities in which religious conflict was most marked were always more likely to produce patients suffering from a range of mental afflictions.[27] Given that it was common for physicians to practise among their co-religionists, it would appear to follow that such medical men also witnessed higher levels of mental anxiety caused, in part, by the persecution inflicted on such groups by the state. Again, the key moment here is surely the breakdown of political consensus and unity incident upon the outbreak of civil war in 1642 that culminated in regicide, religious fragmentation and the demise of the unitary state. By the end of the seventeenth century, the 'age of party' saw religious and political pluralism enshrined in the 'constitution'. The toll on the body politic was mirrored in the impact upon individual bodies as contemporaries struggled to make sense of a world that was now permanently out of joint. In order to contain or treat such sicknesses, physicians of all party stripes and religious affiliations were called upon to proffer diagnoses and cures. By 1700, the role of the doctor as political commentator was now commonplace in ways that would have been considered inconceivable before 1640. And in taking on such a role, it was impossible to avoid party strife and religious controversy. Some, such as the Whig James Welwood (1652–1727), opted to nail their political colours to the mast, producing openly propagandistic material in support of the Glorious Revolution.[28] Others, like Peter Paxton (*c.*1657–1707), a prolific author of both medical and political texts, tried to project the figure of the disinterested observer, akin to the experimental natural philosopher, who was above all parties and disputes and rejected all systems or theories, be they medical or political.[29] In the feverish environment of the late seventeenth and early eighteenth centuries, however, it was largely impossible for medics to escape the shackles of political partisanship. In practice, party politics began to intrude into all areas of practice, including forensic medicine, as for example in the case of the high-profile prosecution of Spencer Cowper for the murder of the Quaker maid Sarah Stout at Hertford in 1699.[30] On this occasion, Cowper's defence was able to call upon some of the most prominent Whig physicians in London while the prosecution relied exclusively on the input of Tory-minded doctors. Thirteen years later, in a case with distinct echoes of the Cowper case, similar battle lines were drawn in the trial of Jane Wenham for witchcraft at Hertford assizes.[31]

In conclusion then, medicine and its practitioners, were to prove no more immune to the all-encompassing effects of political debate and division incident upon the outbreak of civil war in 1642 than other groups in English society. Politics helped to shape the way in which medical practitioners worked and thought, while at the same time, the latter were equally engaged with politics, contributing in a variety of ways to daily political life as both commentators and exponents. The two processes were to all intents and purposes complementary and mutually reinforcing. With the collapse of political consensus after 1642, medical men, in particular, were well positioned to proffer advice on the state of the body politic and in the process became more open to new ways of understanding the operation and dysfunction of individual bodies. Political historians are, at last, becoming increasingly sensitive to these developments. Mark Knights, for example, has noted the prominence of natural philosophers and doctors in the emerging public sphere of later seventeenth-century England, a polity characterized by increasing political ambiguity and misrepresentation of factual knowledge.[32] In like fashion, medical historians too are becoming attuned to such developments.[33] We may not have all the answers as yet, but this work is written in the hope that it might serve as a starting point for further investigation of the relationship between medicine and politics in a period characterized by some as a splenetic age in which opponents were routinely assigned to one 'dangerous kidney' or another.

Notes

1. Examples of medical students at Cambridge and Oxford after 1660 who were the sons of civic dignitaries and aldermen include from the former: William Briggs (MD 1677; son of Tory mayor of Norwich), James Drake (B Med and MD, 1690, 1694; son of Cambridge alderman), Henry Loades (B Med and MD, 1691, 1697; son of London alderman and Tory); James Welsh (B Med, 1677; son of mayor of Rye). Examples from Oxford: Robert Conny (MD 1685; son of mayor of Rochester), Phineas Ellwood (MD 1682; son of mayor of Sandwich), Edward Exton (MD 1666; son of mayor of Chichester). Many others married into the families of urban patricians, or were otherwise closely related to leading urban political figures. Sandford Arthington (B Med Oxford, 1690), for example, was the son-in-law of the Tory mayor of Leeds, Marmaduke Hickes. Francis Geers (B Med Cambridge, 1682) was the brother of Thomas Geers, recorder of Hereford and Tory MP for the city, 1685–7.
2. For the debate between Gadbury and Partridge, forged in the aftermath of the Exclusion Crisis and the reign of James II, see D. R. Woodcraft, 'A "Politick Engine": Astrology and Politics 1678–1715', Ph. D. (Warwick, 1997), 133–4. It is interesting to note that in terms of the two men's approach to astrology, the Tory Gadbury proved to be an advocate of reform while the Whig Partridge was much more conservative in his approach to the subject.
3. In 1678, the loyal preacher Robert Neville, for example, described the current fad for preaching as 'the Epidemical Disease of this Age, being the Rickets of Religion', its proponents 'having the great Heads, Heads swell'd... but their Legs weak and impotent, not able to walk in the ways of God's commandments'; R. Neville, *The Necessity of Receiving the Holy Sacrament... Declared in a Sermon* [Ware, 28 August 1678] (London, 1679), 14–15. Like many clergy educated at Cambridge after the Restoration, Neville (BD 1671) frequently invoked or alluded to medical themes. As a youthful fellow of King's College, he was the author of a play in which he cited the opinions of anatomists on ligatures and their effect on the heart. In later sermons, he invoked, among others, the Paracelsian Oswald Croll (*c.*1563–1609) in defence of the idea of petrification in the womb, invoked the authority of Hippocrates and the 'Greek physicians', and disparaged chymists, comparing them and their utopian, misguided labours to the aims of Arians and Pelagians. Neville's medical wisdom may have owed a debt to his kinsman, Dr James Wilmot or Willimot (1621–1702), to whom he dedicated one of his published sermons. Wilmot (MD Padua 1645) was an active servant of the restored regime, serving as a JP in his native Hertfordshire from 1662 to 1698 and, in 1683, as high sheriff of the county; *idem*, *The Poor Scholar. A Comedy* (London, 1662), I.II.ll. 36–44; *idem*, *The Nature and Causes of Hardness of Heart, Together with the Remedies Against It. Discovered in a Sermon* [St Mary's, Cambridge, n.d.] (London, 1683), 3, 4, 15, 16; *idem*, *An English Inquisition for a Heretick Or, The Punishment due to Hereticks* [visitation sermon, Ware, 19 April 1672] (London, 1673), 7; *idem*, *TA ANΩ. The Things Above Proved to be the Most Proper Objects of the Mind and Affections, in a Sermon Preached before the University in Great St Maries Church in Cambridge* (London, 1683). For Neville, see Venn, iii, 244; *ODNB*. For Wilmot, see

Innes Smith MSS; Venn, iv, 421; Le Hardy (ed.), *Hertfordshire County Records*, vi, 154, 526.

4. For scurvy as a 'new disease', see R. Elwyn-Hughes, 'The Rise and Fall of the "Antiscorbutics": Some Notes on the Traditional Cures for "Land Scurvy"', *Medical History*, 34 (1990), 52–64. For the propensity of late seventeenth-century Englishmen to think in terms of new diseases, even when discussing conventional distempers or maladies, see J. L., *The New Disease or a Rational Account of the Great Colds and Coughs now Raging Amongst Us* (London, 1676).
5. C. Packe, *Mineralogia: or, An Account of the Preparation, Manifold Vertues and Uses of a Mineral Salt* (London, 1693), 27 [Johnson to Packe, Warwick, 11 March 1692]. Johnson (d.1725), who practised at Warwick, was a medical graduate of Anjou who incorporated his degree at Cambridge in 1682. He would appear to have acted as physician to Lord and Lady Conway at Ragley, where he may have met van Helmont Jnr in person. Packe, for whom Johnson supplied a testimonial in 1674, was responsible for translating many of F. M. van Helmont's writings; Venn, ii, 483; Innes Smith, 129; *CSPD, 1677–1678*, 219, 289, 305–6, 335; *CSPD, 1679–1680*, 621; *CSPD, 1680–1681*, 121; LPL, VX 1A/10/66. For other examples of chymical physicians advocating the need to use novel remedies to cure diseases that were no longer 'singular', see A. Colley, *Nature's Champion, Sounding a Challenge to Her Stoutest Assailants: Or, a More Ample Explanation of the Virtue and Use of My Pillulae Aureae Purgantes* (London, 1670); A. Hargrave, *Reason in Season: Or, A Word on the Behalf of the Non-Collegiate Physicians* (London, 1676), 3–4. For the latter, see above 162 n.82. Colley, who lived in the parish of St Leonard's, Shoreditch, was appointed chymist in ordinary to Charles II in November 1670. Like many of his chymical colleagues, he too was granted a licence to practise medicine by the bishop of London in 1669; TNA, LC 3/26, fo. 142; Bloom and James, 44.
6. Cited in J. L. Malcolm, 'Charles II and the Reconstruction of Royal Power', *The Historical Journal*, 35 (1992), 325. For Charles II and iatrochemistry, see chapter 4. Medical terminology was frequently voiced in Charles' earliest parliaments. Recalling the debates of earlier, pre-civil war sessions, MPs were regularly addressed as the 'great Physicians of the Kingdom' and admonished to administer a range of remedies for their 'distempered Patients'; *Lords' Journal*, vol. 11 (1660–1666), 242. In December 1661, they were also reminded by the Speaker of the demonstrable truth of Harveian circulation in the 'experimental' blushes exhibited on their bodies following the King's speech to Parliament requesting money!; ibid., 357.
7. LMA, P69/AND4/A/001/MS04107/002 [parish registers of St Andrew Undershaft, London, 1634–1692, baptisms, *sub* 19 July 1644]; J. L. Chester (ed), *The Parish Registers of St Thomas the Apostle, London, 1558 to 1754* (London, Harleian Soc., 1881), 57.
8. BL, Sloane MS 1326, fos 94v–96r [Robinson to Power, 5 March 1649/50].
9. For Power, see *ODNB*; C. Webster, 'Henry Power's Experimental Philosophy', *Ambix*, 14 (1967), 150–78. For Sir Thomas Browne's encouragement of both Power and Robinson, and the close relationship between the three men, see C. Webster, *The Great Instauration: Science, Medicine and Reform 1626–1660* (London, 1975), 137–8; S. Wilkin (ed.), *Sir Thomas Browne's Works. Including his Life and Correspondence*, 4 vols (London & Norwich, 1836), i, 421–4 [Robinson to Browne, 12 December 1659].

10. For Robinson, see Venn, iii, 473; J. J. Howard (ed.), *A Visitation of the County of Essex. Begun 1664, Finished 1668* (London, 1888), 75; BL, Sloane MS 1326, fo. 102v [Robinson to Power, 30 April 1660]; TNA, ASSI 35/104/1/20 [Chelmsford assizes, 23 March 1663]; ERO, D/ABW 63/61 [will of Reuben Robinson, gent, of Maldon, 3 February 1664/5 and 6 April 1665, pr. 5 June 1665]. Robinson's will mentions his 'loving friend' James Thickens and 'learned friend' Henry Power, to whom he gave 'two or three of the best' of his books. Mr Reuben Robinson, alderman and professor of physick, was buried at All Saints, Maldon, on 10 April 1665; Essex RO, D/P 201/1/1.
11. BL, Sloane MS 1326, fos 76r–77v [Robinson to Power, 7 October 1650], 98r–99v [same to same, 20 October 1654].
12. Robinson was a frequent visitor to Cambridge in these years, often praising his friend Power for raising 'new heterodox questions [which] very well suite with ye Genius of ye University which if I am rightly informed runs altogether in this new way of Philosophy'; BL, Sloane MS 3515, fo. 95r [Robinson to Power, 15 October 1653].
13. I. Mortimer, *The Dying and the Doctors: The Medical Revolution in Seventeenth-Century England* (London, 2009).
14. C. Rose, 'Politics and the London Royal Hospitals, 1683–1692', in L. Granshaw and R. Porter (eds), *The Hospital in History* (London & New York, 1989), 123–48.
15. For a recent assessment of Downes' deep-seated Anglican convictions, see S. Mann, 'Physic and Divinity; the Case of Dr John Downes, M.D. (1627–1694)', *The Seventeenth Century*, 31 (2016), 451–70. The certificates demonstrating Downes' exceptional devotion to the Anglican cause, cited by Mann, were in fact produced as part of Downes' concerted campaign to secure the appointment of physician to Christ's Hospital. For various papers amassed by Downes in pursuit of this goal, see especially BL, Sloane MS 3299, fos 56–7, 62–4, 66–73. For testimonials attesting to his exceptional piety and loyalty to the Anglican church, see BL, Sloane MS 203, fos 145–6.
16. *CSPD, February–December 1685*, 312; RCPL, Annals, v, 43; vi, 85.
17. M. Fissell, *Patients, Power, and the Poor in Eighteenth-Century Bristol* (Cambridge, 1991).
18. J. Andrews, 'The Politics of Committal to Early Modern Bethlem', in R. Porter (ed.), *Medicine in the Enlightenment* (Amsterdam, 1995), 6–63 [quote at 26].
19. P. Elmer, *Witchcraft, Witch-Hunting, and Politics in Early Modern England* (Oxford, 2016), esp. 251–63.
20. For an original and groundbreaking attempt to demonstrate how the collapse of the body politic after 1642 triggered mental breakdown among individual sufferers, especially those engaged in the fighting, see E. Peters, 'Trauma Narratives of the English Civil War', *Journal for Early Modern Cultural Studies*, 16 (2016), 78–94.
21. Bartlett, who had no official medical credentials, resided at Bow where he kept a private madhouse and charged £200 plus fifty shillings a week for board to cure Whitelocke's wife Rebecca; R. Spalding (ed.), *The Diary of Bulstrode Whitelocke 1605–1675* (Oxford, 1990), 76–7, 81. For Bartlett's recusancy, see J. C. Jeaffreson, *Middlesex County Records*, 6 vols (London, 1888–1892), iii, *passim*. For frequent complaints made about Bartlett's practice (and recusancy) before the College of Physicians between 1613 and 1626, see RCPL, Annals, 1613–1626.
22. Lentall, a former fellow of Pembroke College, Cambridge, was licensed to practise medicine by the College of Physicians in London in 1649; Venn, iii, 74; *Wal. Rev.*, 38;

Munk, i, 248. Practising from a house in the Charterhouse, London, he was described in 1666 as 'one that pretends to cure those in [Sir John Denham's] condition'; *HMC. Sixth Report, Part 1, Report & Appendix* (London, 1877), 339. For his recusancy, see H. Bowler, *London Sessions Records 1605–1685* (London, Catholic Rec. Soc., 1934), 131, 137, 151. For Bedlam, see J. Andrews, 'Bedlam Revisited: A History of Bethlem Hospital, *c.*1634–*c.*1770', Ph. D. (Queen Mary & Westfield College, London, 1991), 253n.

23. J. Spencer, *A Discourse of Divers Petitions of High Government, and Great Consequence, delivered by the Authour into the Hands of King James... and King Charles... A Treatise of Melancholie* (London, 1641), including 'A Treatise of Melancholie' (89–99). Spencer's son, also John, was created MD at Cambridge in 1650 and practised at Bedford; Venn, iv, 132.
24. C. Brent, *Pre-Georgian Lewes* c.*690–1714; The Emergence of a County Town* (2004), 221, 274. Panton was educated at Oxford, where he graduated as a bachelor of medicine with a university licence to practise on 20 November 1626; Foster, iii, 1112. He was also the author of a brief manuscript treatise on the cure of the mad; BL, Sloane MS 3505, fos 99v–100r. Panton's two sons, John (d.1688) and Henry (1632–1688), the former ejected from his fellowship at All Souls, Oxford, in 1660, both practised medicine after the Restoration and were prominent supporters of Dissent.
25. Somerset Heritage Centre, D\D/bs/39, *sub* 5 June 1668. Eight years later, in 1676, Panton was issued with a full licence allowing him to practise both medicine and surgery throughout the diocese of Bath and Wells; Somerset Heritage Centre, D\D/bs/42. Charles Panton (1662–1711), an Oxford graduate, succeeded to his father's practice at Batheaston and was made an extra licentiate of the College of Physicians in London in 1686; Foster, iii, 1112; Munk, i, 438.
26. Newton's nonconformity is inferred from two pieces of evidence. Firstly, in April 1704 he, alongside James Watson, dissenting minister at Harrow, Middlesex, took the oath of allegiance. And secondly, in his will of 1716 Newton left £5 to the 'poor of the congregation I belong to', a common form of shorthand used in wills at this time to indicate membership of a dissenting church; W. J. Hardy (ed.), *Middlesex County Records. Calendar of Sessions Books, 1689–1709* (1905), 271; TNA, PROB 11/565, fos 64r–65r [will of James Newton of St James Clerkenwell, Middlesex, 1 September 1716; pr. 5 August 1718]. Some time around 1674, Newton issued a handbill in which he provided evidence of his many successes in healing the mad, including one poor soul who laboured under the delusion that he was Charles II. He concluded by offering to take three patients from nearby Bedlam Hospital and to cure them at no cost; BL, c.112 f.9 (72). I hope to discuss Newton's practice, including frequent confrontations with the law and College of Physicians, in future publications.
27. M. MacDonald, *Mystical Bedlam: Madness, Anxiety, and Healing in Seventeenth-Century England* (Cambridge, 1981), 68–9.
28. *ODNB*, sub Welwood, John; E. L. Furdell, *James Welwood: Physician to the Glorious Revolution* (Conshohocken, PA, 1998).
29. *ODNB*, sub Paxton, Peter; J. A. W. Gunn, 'The *Civil Polity* of Peter Paxton', *Past and Present*, 40 (1968), 42–57. Paxton, who practised medicine at Buckingham, was admitted to his Cambridge MD by royal mandate in 1687; Venn, iii, 322; *CSPD, 1686–1687*,

351. For Paxton's dispassionate and undogmatic approach to medicine, in line with his espousal of Locke and moderate Whiggism, see his *An Essay Concerning the Body of Man, Wherein Its Changes or Diseases are Consider'd, and the Operations of Medicines Observ'd* (London, 1701), preface. Typically, he argued that most diseases were the product of human idleness, luxury and folly, an approach he extended to account for the illness and subsequent death of the religious enthusiast John Mason of neighbouring Water Stratford in 1693; P. Paxton, *A Directory Physico-Medical, Composed for the Benefit of all Such as Deign to Study and Practise the Art of Physick* (London, 1707), xiv; *Bedfordshire Notes and Queries*, 1 (1886), 26; B. Willis, *The History and Antiquities of the Town, Hundred, and Deanery of Buckingham* (London, 1755), 344–5.

30. M. Knights, *The Devil in Disguise: Deception, Delusion, and Fanaticism in the Early English Enlightenment* (Oxford, 2011), 10–24; A. Rosenberg, 'The Sarah Stout Murder Case: An Early Example of the Doctor as an Expert Witness', *Journal of the History of Medicine and Allied Sciences*, 12 (1957), 61–70.

31. Elmer, *Witchcraft, Witch-Hunting, and Politics*, 278.

32. M. Knights, *Representation and Misrepresentation in Later Stuart Britain* (Oxford, 2005), 57–62.

33. For an excellent recent example, see L. Caron, 'Thomas Willis, the Restoration and the First Works of Neurology', *Medical History*, 59 (2015), 525–53. There, Caron attempts to read Willis's pioneering work on the brain as a contribution to the debate on the correctness of Anglican liturgical practices after 1660. Unfortunately, I was not able to cite Caron's work in my earlier book on witchcraft, where I likewise argue for a 'political' reading of the impact of Willis's medical work. There, I suggest that Willis's writings had a profound effect upon Anglican understanding of witchcraft, encouraging an incipient scepticism. For another example of that process in action, see the work of the Kent physician-turned-clergyman Thomas Curtis (1662–1747), who claimed to have prevented a witch from being hanged following his intervention in the case of a boy suffering from an affliction brought on by worms and a faulty nervous system; see T. Curtis, *Essays on the Preservation and Recovery of Health* (London, 1704), 210–17.

APPENDIX 1 (A)

Biographical index of medical signatories in favour of the creation of a Society of Chymical Physicians (1665)

Jeremiah ASTEL (d.1675)

Astel signed a letter of support in favour of the creation of a Society of Chymical Physicians in 1665 as a 'chymical student and practitioner'. He was also an enthusiastic supporter of the miraculous claims of the miracle healer Valentine Greatrakes. Astel was active as a physician in London during the plague, for which he was rewarded by the King with the gift of a piece of plate valued at £10. In 1675, he was responsible for publishing the work of fellow iatrochemist, **George Starkey**, entitled *Liquor Alcahest* (London, 1675), which he dedicated to his friend, the natural philosopher Robert Boyle. A letter to Boyle, written in 1664, is now lost. Astel was also engaged, with other chymical physicians, in writing testimonials for candidates for ecclesiastical licences to practise medicine. In April 1665, he signed a certificate on behalf of John Dabbs, MA, who was seeking a medical licence from the bishop of London. Other signatories included the Helmontian John Collop and R. Barker, probably **Richard Barker**. In 1668, when he described himself as MD, he signed letters in support of the application of Henry Bingham, of Mitcham, Surrey, for a licence to practise medicine from the archbishop of Canterbury. He himself was licensed to practise medicine in the diocese of London on 12 March 1663, letters testimonial being supplied by fellow iatrochemist and signatory of the chymists' petition, **John Fryer**, MD. He is probably the 'Dr Astall' who was consulted by Ann Savile in March 1666, when she claimed to see images in a crystal ball owned by the doctor. In the same year, he visited **Sir Edmund Warcup**, then a prisoner in Oxford. The two men may have worked closely together in London during the plague (Warcup, as a serving JP in the capital, also received a gift of plate from a grateful monarch).

Little is known of his origins or private life. He may have been the Jeremiah Astel, the son of Edward Astel, citizen and farrier, of London, who was apprenticed to William Wright as a bookseller in 1657. He petitioned for non-enrolment and was discharged three years later. The London surgeon Henry Bryers (d.1665) refers to him as 'brother' in his will of 1665, where he also named Astel as sole executor. Astel was married to a woman named Grisell, and the couple had one son, Jeremiah, who was baptised at Stepney in 1673. He was buried the following year at St Sepulchre, London. Astel himself was buried at St Clement Danes, Middlesex, on 8 March 1675.

Thomson, *Loimologia*, 17; TNA, PC 2/59, fo. 17r; Boyle, *Correspondence*, ii, 235; Bloom and James, 45; LPL, VX 1A/10/14; Wellcome Library, MS 5334, *sub nominum*; *HMC. Leybourne-Popham Manuscripts*, 197 [Ann Savile to William Shippen, 30 March 1666]; Bodl., Rawlinson MS D 384, fo. 70; Scott (ed.), *Apprenticeship Disputes in the Lord Mayor's Court of London 1573–1723*, 115; TNA, PROB 11/318, fos 331r–v [will of Henry Bryers, chirurgion, of St Thomas the Apostle, London, 24 September 1665, pr. 25 September 1665]; LMA, P93/DUN/258 [parish registers of St Dunstan's, Stepney,

Middlesex, 1656–1710]; P69/SEP/A/001/MS07219/001 [parish registers of St Sepulchre, London, 1662–1679]; City of Westminster Archives, STC/PR/7/4 [parish registers of St Clement Danes, Middlesex, 1673–1700].

(Sir) Richard BARKER (*c.*1622–1686)

A physician, Barker was practising in London in 1656 when he was fined £50 by the College of Physicians for illegal practice. At the time, he was resident in the parish of St John the Baptist, Dowgate. At the Restoration, his practice prospered, and he moved to a new home in the Barbican. He would appear to have been on friendly terms with the former Leveller-turned-Ranter, Captain William Rainsborough of Stepney, for whom he provided a bond of £500 for good behaviour in February 1661. Rainsborough had been charged in December 1660 with selling arms in his charge to civilians.

Barker was the author of numerous works concerned with the theory and practice of chymical medicine. He seems to have stayed in London during the plague, when he published *Consilium Anti-Pestilentiale* (London, 1665), dedicated to the Lord Mayor, Sir John Lawrence. In it, Barker proposed chymical remedies for the disease and claimed to have been practising in London for about fifteen years. Barker's frequent altercations with the College of Physicians probably inclined him to speak fondly of the celebrated empiric William Trigge, whose lucrative practice he may have inherited. In 1665, he was employing Trigge's kinsman, Timothy Woodfield, to prepare his medicines. He is probably the R. Barker and Ri. Barker, sometimes described as licentiate, who provided testimonials for William Williams (1664), John Dabbs (1665) and Francis Dye (1683), all candidates for ecclesiastical medical licences. Given the reference to himself as 'licentiate', he is probably the same as the Richard Barke, who was licensed to practise medicine in November 1663. Barker was, according to his colleague **William Goddard**, a founder member of the Society of Chymical Physicians, which first began meeting in London in May 1664. In addition to chymistry, Barker was praised, among others, for his love of astrology by John Gadbury and William Salmon.

On 31 December 1673, Barker was appointed physician in ordinary, probably without fee, to Charles II. In 1678 he facilitated the meeting of Israel Tonge and Titus Oates at his house in the Barbican where the two men hatched the Popish Plot. Tonge shared Barker's passion for chymistry as well as his detestation for Catholics, mutual interests that probably prompted Barker to finance and encourage the two men's crusade. In 1678, for example, as patron of the living of Avon Dassett in Warwickshire, Barker sought to present Tonge as rector. Barker's royal position and links with the chymical community at court probably helped to smooth the way for Tonge to meet the King and warn him of the threat to his life from a supposed Catholic conspiracy in 1678.

Barker was well connected. He married Theodosia (*c.*1631–1678), the daughter of Sir John Wray of Glentworth, Lincolnshire, and MP in the Long Parliament. Wray had favoured the abolition of episcopacy. He was succeeded to the baronetcy by his son John, who sat in the 1654 Parliament. In 1666–7 Barker and his wife became involved in a legal battle over the custody of Theodosia's lunatic brother, Sir Bethel Wray. Their daughter, Susanna, married Sir Francis Bridgeman, the son of Sir Orlando Bridgeman (d.1674), a prominent figure in Restoration legal circles who, as Lord Keeper of the Great Seal, actively promoted schemes of religious moderation and reconciliation in the late 1660s.

Barker was too sick to attend the trial of Titus Oates in May 1685. A servant deposed that he was then 'a crazy man, and ancient', and that he was recuperating at his daughter's house in Putney, Surrey. He died of dropsy in the parish of St Giles Cripplegate on 1 April 1686 and was carried away to be buried at Helmdon in Northamptonshire on 8 April 1686. A tomb monument, no longer extant, recorded that he died aged 64, and was interred at Helmdon 'in obedience to his command'. Helmdon may have been the parish of his birth, but no entry survives in the parish register. Following his death, Barker's only surviving child, Susanna was the main beneficiary of his will.

ODNB, new article by the author, April 2016; Cook, *Decline of the Old Medical Regime in Stuart London*, 129; *CSPD, 1660–1661*, 505; Barker, *Consilium Anti-Pestilentiale*, A5r; 5; Bloom and James, 45, 74; LPL, VX 1A/10/192/1–2; Wellcome Library, MS 5334, *sub nominum*; TNA, C 10/477/110; TNA, LC3/27, fo. 46v; Gadbury, *Ephemeris... 1672*; Salmon, *Horae Mathematicae*, sigs A3r–v; Tonge, 'Journal of the Plot, 1678', in Greene (ed.), *Diaries of the Popish Plot*; *ODNB*, *sub* Tonge, Israel; TNA, PC 2/68, 272; *CSPD, 1679–1680*, 176; *Law Reports of Sir Edmund Saunders... Court of King's Bench*, 3 vols (London, 1799–1802), vol. 1, case 8, Hilary Ch. II 18 & 19, Barker v. Thorold; Rylands (ed.), *The Visitation of the County of Warwick, 1682–1683* (London, Harleian Soc., vol. 62, 1911), 15; LMA, P69/GIS/A/002/MS06419/010 [parish registers of St Giles Cripplegate, London, 1680–1688]; Northamptonshire RO, 162P/1 [parish registers of Helmdon, Northamptonshire, 1572–1705]; Baker, *The History and Antiquities of Northamptonshire*, 5 vols (London, 1822–41), i, 633; TNA, PROB 11/383, fos 194v–195v [will of Richard Barker, undated, pr. 1 June 1686].

Thomas BARKER

Barker was a signatory to the 'engagement' of chymical physicians. He may be the same as the Thomas Barker (d.1701) of St Saviour's, Southwark, Surrey, a surgeon, who signed various letters testimonial on behalf of candidates for archiepiscopal medical licences in 1683 and 1685. On the former occasion, he signed alongside one 'Ri. Barker', probably **Richard Barker** above.

LPL, VX 1A/10/192/1–2; VX 1A/10/223/1–4.

William BARKLEY or BERKELEY

Barkley was a signatory to the 'engagement' of chymical physicians. He was in all probability the same as the Dr Berkeley, whom Samuel Hartlib described in a letter to John Evelyn in April 1660. Hartlib refers to 'some amazing and in a manner miraculous cures lately performed' by him, whom he describes as 'lately come from Bermudas or N[ew] England'. He seems to have struck up a rapport with Hartlib's son-in-law, the chymist, Frederick Clodius, with whom he was lodging in Axe Yard. Hartlib's description echoes the comments of John Ward, who noted his meeting in 1662 with one 'Dr Bartly'. The two men discussed the philosopher's stone. According to Ward, 'Bartly' had spent sixteen years in the East Indies [*sic*], returning to London in about 1658. Here, he is said to have performed 'great cures with his powder and pils', so much so, that 'the phisitians beginne to be troublesome'.

One William Berckley was licensed to practise medicine and surgery throughout the province of Canterbury, 31 October 1665. He may have been attracted to England by fellow Bermudan adept, **George Starkey**. He was named by **William Goddard** as one of the founder members of the Society in May 1664 and was still alive in October 1666 when

Goddard sought reimbursement from Barkley and others in order to pay the Society's attorney, Thomas Dangerfield.

He may be the same as the William Berkeley, who described himself in his will of 1704 as 'aged' and a 'practitioner in medicine' in the parish of St Mary's, Whitechapel. Unfortunately, there are few other clues in this will to his identity. Alternatively, he may be the Quaker physician of the same name, living 'without Bishopsgate Street', who died on 7 July 1674, aged about 70, and was interred at the Friends burial ground at Chequer's Alley.

Newman, *Gehennical Fire*, 40–1; BL, Add. MS 15,948, fos 98A–98B; FSL, V.a.292, fos 3v, 66r; LPL, VG 1/1, fo. 185; Sheldon, fo. 210; TNA, C 10/477/110; TNA, PROB 11/488, fos 128v–129r [will of William Berkeley, practitioner in medicine, of St Mary's, Whitechapel, Middlesex, 6 June 1704, pr. 6 May 1706]; TNA, RG6/499 [quarterly meeting of Friends, London and Middlesex, burials, 1661–1700].

Robert BATHURST

Bathurst was a signatory to the 'engagement' of chymical physicians. According to the Yorkshire antiquary Ralph Thoresby, Bathurst was the son of Robert Bathurst and was born at Bandon in Ireland. In 1673, he was employed as a chymist by **George Villiers, duke of Buckingham**, who may have been a distant relative (George, the youngest son of Lancelot Bathurst, married Elizabeth Villiers, a relation of the duke). He was also the brother-in-law of another of Buckingham's protégés, **Edward Bolnest**. Some time around 1662, Bathurst, describing himself as a physician, signed a testimonial on behalf of William Bruton Jnr, of Alwington, Devon, who was seeking a licence to practise medicine in the diocese of Exeter. Bruton's application was also signed by five other physicians, three of whom, **Edward Bolnest**, **William Burman** and **Robert Turner**, were also signatories of the petition to establish a Society of Chymical Physicians in London in 1665. He did the same, along with his brother-in-law Bolnest, on behalf of John Powell (1664) and **Thomas O'Dowde** (1665).

Robert Bathurst of Kingston upon Thames, Surrey, was licensed to practise medicine and surgery in the diocese of Winchester on 18 July 1664, the same day as fellow chemist and protégé of the duke of Buckingham, **Thomas Tillison**. Bathurst, like his brother-in-law Bolnest, was a founder member of the Society which first began to meet in May 1664.

DRO, PR 518, *sub* Allington [*sic*]; Thoresby, *Ducatus Leodiensis*, 13; Wellcome Library, MS 5334, *sub nominum*; Bax, 'Marriage and Other Licences in the Commissary Court of Surrey', 226, 238; TNA, C 10/477/110.

Edward BOLNEST (1627–1703)

Bolnest was a signatory to the *Advertisement* in 1665, when he gave his address as Jewen Street, in the parish of St Giles, Cripplegate. In residence here since the autumn of the previous year, according to his new landlord Bolnest and unnamed friends (presumably his fellow chymists) made numerous modifications to the property, including the construction of 'severall furnaces of bricke in the upper roomes', which threatened to destroy the house. As a founder member of the Society of Chymical Physicians, which first began to meet in May 1664, the property at Jewen Street may well have served as one of the Society's main centres of chymical research and investigation. It subsequently became the focus of a legal dispute in which it was alleged that Bolnest had refused to enter into and sign a counterlease on the property. Under pressure, he was initially willing to quit the property in the spring of

1666, partly on the grounds that he was proferred a place as physician to the duke of Buckingham's household, but he later changed his mind as property in London became scarce after the Great Fire.

Edward Bolnest was the son of Edward Bolnest, merchant tailor, and his wife Mary, and was baptised at St Mary Aldermary, London, 14 October 1627. Bolnest was apprenticed to Hammond Ward, mercer, of London, the brother of the mystic Jane Leade, on 18 July 1645. He may have met and married his wife Mildred while a soldier in Ireland in the 1650s. She was the sister of fellow chymist and signatory, **Robert Bathurst**, who, like Bolnest, was a client of **George Villiers, duke of Buckingham**. In 1665, Bolnest was chosen by **Thomas O'Dowde**, at the request of the King, to attend on the victims of plague in Southampton. However, he failed to take up his post, choosing to remain in London, where two daughters, Isabella and Mary, died of the disease. Bolnest was the author of *Medicina Instaurata*, dedicated to his patron, the duke of Buckingham. It contained a lengthy 'epistolary discourse' by fellow chymist, **Marchamont Nedham**. In October and November 1666, he was recommended to Robert Boyle as a potential collaborator by another keen iatrochemist, Daniel Coxe, who claimed that Bolnest 'hath great misteries to reveal which none excepting your selfe are worthy to bee acquainted withall'. He is almost certainly the same as the 'Edward Boldnesse' who was appointed chymical physician in ordinary to Charles II in November 1670. In 1672, he published a second work, *Aurora Chymica*, in which he described himself on the titlepage as physician in ordinary to the King. The work itself was dedicated, like his first published work, to Buckingham and gives his new address as Queen Street, near the Guildhall. In it, he alludes to the imminent publication of a work called *Fontina Salutis*, available from his printer John Starkey, which does not appear to have survived. He was still living at Queen Street, in the parish of St Mary-le-Bow, in December 1678, when he put up sureties for Michael Warton, 'a distiller of Waters', who was accused of being a 'recusant' and refusing to take the oaths of allegiance and supremacy. In September 1687, Bolnest was summoned (but did not appear) before the heraldic visitation of the city of London, where he is described as living in the parish of St Pancras, Soper Lane.

Like many of his chymical colleagues, Bolnest frequently provided testimonials for fellow medics seeking episcopal or archiepiscopal licences to practise. In around 1662, he wrote one on behalf of William Bruton Jnr, of Alwington, Devon, where he described himself as 'doctor and student of medicine, of King's College, Cambridge' (no record of his attendance survives in the college annals). He did the same in 1684 for one George Penhellick, of Kidderminster in Worcestershire. On both occasions, he signed alongside fellow chymist **William Burman**. Bolnest may also have supplemented his income as a physician by instructing students in the art of chymistry. William Thraster, the author of *The Marrow of Chymical Physick* (1669), claimed to have been taught the art of chymistry by Bolnest. Bolnest, like **Richard Barker**, was also on cordial terms with the astrologer John Gadbury.

One of the earliest recorded references to Bolnest relates to his dispute with the alchemist and natural philosopher Thomas Vaughan, alias Eugenius Philalethes. According to a deposition taken in 1661, Vaughan claimed that Bolnest had approached him in about 1656–7 offering to pay £300 for instruction in 'naturall philosophy and Chimicall physicke', but paid less than a tenth. Bolnest subsequently brought soldiers to plunder Vaughan's house and arrest him (Vaughan claimed that Bolnest was using connections at the Cromwellian court, having served under Cromwell in Ireland). Vaughan offered a bond from which Bolnest offered release in return for 'a certain physicall receipt of great value', to which Vaughan agreed. Bolnest later counter-sued for £150. Vaughan retaliated by subpoenaeing Bolnest, who denied all Vaughan's charges. Bolnest claimed he had lent

Vaughan £250 to make the philosopher's stone, which he had failed to accomplish. He also categorically denied any suggestion that he had sought instruction from Vaughan or that he was a former associate of 'that late Traytor and Tyrant' Cromwell, but he did admit to serving the army in Ireland in the 1650s. The outcome of the case is unknown.

Edward Bolnest was almost certainly related to William Bolnest, of Whitechapel, who applied for a medical licence from the bishop of London in 1674 (one of his referees was Edward Bolnest's student, William Thrasher or Thraster). Edward Bolnest was also a minor beneficiary under the will of the widow of his former colleague **Thomas O'Dowde** in 1665. Another son Edward followed his father into medical practice. Bolnest himself, described as an 'aged chymist', was buried at St Giles Cripplegate, London, on 24 September 1703.

ODNB; TNA, C10/489/83; C10/477/110; Chester (ed.), *The Parish Registers of St Mary Aldermary, London 1558 to 1754*, 80; Records of London's Livery Companies Online, admissions and freemen; www.londonroll.org [accessed 24 January 2017]; Thoresby, *Ducatus Leodiensis*, 13; Thomson, *Loimologia*, 15; O'Dowde, *Two Letters Concerning the Cure of the Plague*; Bell, *The Great Plague of London in 1665*, 147; Boyle, *Correspondence*, iii, 250–1, 268; TNA, LC3/26, fo. 142; Bowler (ed.), *London Sessions Records 1605–1685*, 207–8; Wales and Hartley (eds), *The Visitation of London Begun in 1687*, ii, 604, 651, 652; DRO, PR 518, *sub* Allington [*sic*]; LPL, VX 1A/10/212/1–4; Thraster, *The Marrow of Chymical Physick*, A2r; Gadbury, *London's Deliverance Predicted: In A Short Discourse Shewing the Causes of Plagues in General*, 39; TNA, C7/354/45; Bloom and James, 39; TNA, PROB 11/319, fos 239r–v [will of Jane O'Dowde, widow, of St Clement Danes, Middlesex, 24 August 1665, pr. 12 February 1665/6]; LMA, P69/GIS/A/002/MS06419/013 [parish registers of St Giles Cripplegate, London, 1702–1711].

William BOREMAN or BURMAN (d.1707)

William Burman or Boreman, of Wilmington, Kent, practised medicine throughout much of southeastern England in the second half of the seventeenth century. He first appears in about 1662, when he signed a testimonial (as 'med. lic') on behalf of William Bruton Jnr, of Alwington, Devon, a candidate for a licence to practise medicine in the diocese of Exeter. He did the same for George Penhellick of Kidderminster, Worcestershire, in 1684, and for John Rallett of Braintree, Essex, in 1688. In the former, he described himself as a 'royal physician', though no record exists of his appointment to the court. He may, like his friend, John Pordage, have been appointed by the Board of Greencloth to minister to plague victims in London in 1665. In a case brought before the Court of Arches in 1683–4, Burman insisted that he was no 'pretended doctor of physick' but was approved and licensed by Sir Richard Chaworth on 10 October 1661 to practise medicine throughout the province of Canterbury.

Burman seems to have specialized in diagnosing witchcraft or other preternatural ills. He twice appeared as an assize witness at witchcraft trials in Kent in 1681 and 1690. In addition, he was almost certainly the Dr Boreman who sought to exorcise a young maid at Orpington in Kent in 1679. Further evidence of his practice, in particular his specialization in cases of diabolical possession, is provided by the detailed records of a case brought before the Court of Arches in 1683–4 in which he sought to defend his reputation from a charge, possibly politically motivated, of adultery with one of his possessed patients. According to the nonconformist physician Henry Sampson, Burman was widely reputed to be a conjuror, many of whose cures were likened to a form of white witchcraft. Sampson added that he was a frequent visitor to London, keeping a chamber in Walbrooke, and grew rich from his London practice. His fame and reputation led Daniel Defoe to describe his practice in some depth in his *A System of Magick*. Burman's view of witchcraft was highly politicized. He himself appeared before the Kent assizes in 1684 charged with asserting that the duke of York was a wizard, who rode about at night 'in fiery charriotts to torment soules' and predicted that 'his witchcraft will lay the nation in blood and Popish slavery'. On another occasion, he recommended that the duke of Monmouth 'make an interest in every county of England to be his friends' to carry on his designs. In the aftermath of the duke's failed rebellion in 1685, a government spy in Amsterdam reported that two of the duke's sisters had lately arrived from Germany with a magical sword that contained 'a Potent Talismanicall Spell' before which all their brother's enemies would flee. They would appear to have received the sword from 'one Dr Boreman in or about London' with whom they had consulted on other matters as 'they both pretended to magicall Sciences, and something to the Philosophicall Stone'. Burman's radical past is further attested by an earlier informant who in 1678 testified that Burman had told him at Sandwich in Kent that he was 'for no king in England nor for any head of the Church but Jesus Christ' and that he had formerly been acquainted with John Lilburne 'and was privy to all his affairs and undertakings'.

Burman was an early associate of the Behmenist and Philadelphian, Jane Leade (1624–1704), and was responsible for funding and assisting the publication of the posthumous works of Lead's chief inspiration, John Pordage (d.1681). Dr Edward Hooker (d.1707), who assisted Burman and Leade in this task, was one of Burman's fellow witnesses at the witchcraft trial of Thomas Whiteing of How in Kent in 1681. Various publications appeared under his name (or variant thereupon) in the 1690s, possibly capitalizing on his fame. In 1696, he was credited as the author of a collection of anti-Catholic and anti-French prophecies extolling the virtues of William III as a Protestant saviour. Three years later various translations were attributed to Boreman under the title *Aristotle's Legacy*, which promoted the merits of palmistry and other occult sciences.

William Boreman, *medicus*, married Sarai Maundy of Sandridge, Kent, at Eltham in the same county in 1662. The couple were residents of Bexley, where they baptised and buried several children, from 1662 until about 1682. Shortly after this date, Boreman removed to Wilmington, near Dartford, in Kent, where he was buried on 28 December 1707.

Elmer, *Witchcraft, Witch-Hunting, and Politics*, 198–200, 272–4; DRO, PR 518, *sub* Allington [*sic*]; LPL, VX 1A/10/212/1–4; VX 1A/10/250/1–3; LPL, Court of Arches, A16, fos 426v, 442v–443r; B10/217; D324B; *Witch Hunting and Witch Trials*, 261, 263; *Strange News from Arpington near Bexly in Kent*; BL, Add. MS 4460, fos 47v–48r; Defoe, *A System of Magick*, ii, ch. 3; TNA, ASSI 35/127/7, 203 [Cockburn (ed.), *Calendar of Assize Records: Kent Indictments 1676–1688*, 190]; *CSPD, 1684–1685*, 268; BL, Add. MS 41,812, fos 236r, 236v; *CSPD, 1678*, 394, 396, 401; TNA, SP 29/406/102, 122; Pordage, *Theologia Mystica*; [Dr Bouram], *Strange and Wonderful Prophesies Foretelling the Alterations of the Time*; [Dr Borman], *Aristotle's Legacy, or His Golden Cabinet of Secrets Opened*; LMA, P97/JNB2/A/01/001 [parish registers of Eltham, Kent, 1583–1685]; Bexley Local Studies & Archive Centre, Bexleyheath, parish registers of Bexley; Medway Archives & Local Studies Centre, Rochester, P397/1/1 [parish registers of Wilmington, 1683–1793]; TNA, PROB 11/584, fos 173v–174r [will of William Burman, gent, 5 April 1704, pr. 19 April 1722].

Edward COKE or COOKE

Coke's name appears as one of the 'Chymical Students and Practitioners' who pledged support for Thomson's scheme to create a Society of Chymical Physicians. Along with

Marchamont Nedham and **William Goddard**, Coke testified to the medical competence of **Thomas O'Dowde** in 1665. According to Goddard, Coke was a founder member of the Society, which first began to meet in May 1664. A surgeon of this name was active ministering to sick and wounded soldiers at Dover in 1658. He may be the same as the Edward Cooke (d.1689), surgeon, who practised at Stepney after the Restoration. If so, then he was connected to radical circles. His second wife Rebecca was the widow of the fifth monarchist propagandist John Rye of Stoke Newington. At her death in 1683, she left bequests to the poor of the congregation of another fifth monarchist, Colonel Henry Danvers, of the same place.

Thomson, *Loimologia*, 17; Thomson, *A Gag for Johnson*, 30–1; TNA, C 10/477/110; *CSPD, 1658–1659*, 67, 79, 126–7; LMA, P69/A/002/MS07894/001 [parish registers of St James, Duke's Place, London, 1664–1692]; P93/DUN/279 and 280 [parish registers of St Dunstan's, Stepney, Middlesex, 1666–1684; 1684–1694]; Capp, *Fifth Monarchy Men*, 261; Greaves, 'Henry Danvers and the Radical Underground', 157–78; TNA, PROB 11/374, fos 77v–81r [will of Rebecca Cooke, wife of Edward Cooke, surgeon, of Stepney, 14 July 1683, pr. 30 October 1683].

William CURRER (1617–1668)

William Currer was the son of Henry Currer of Stainton Cotes, Gargrave, Yorkshire, and was baptised at Gargrave on 21 September 1617. He graduated MD at Leiden in 1643 (incorporated at Oxford, 1646). In 1646, he was serving as physician to the army in Ireland, a post he reacquired at the Restoration, possibly through the intercession of his patron, **James Butler, duke of Ormond**. In 1646, and again in 1652, he appeared before the London College of Physicians, being gently admonished on the latter occasion to submit himself to an examination if he wished to continue practising in the city. A year earlier, he compounded 'for adhering to the King, not being sequestered'. Samuel Hartlib sheds a little more light on Currer's activities prior to this date when he reported of him that he was 'Inchiquin's Physitian before hee wheeled about' (the earl of Inchiquin commanded the parliamentary forces in Munster in southern Ireland before reaffirming his allegiance to the King in 1648). While in Ireland, Currer had made a collection of Irish medicines as well as composing a natural history of the island, but these papers were seized in the early 1650s by his political enemies.

Back in England, he seems to have devoted himself to two objectives: the pursuit of his career as a chymist and physician, and the attempt to recover his financial situation. With regard to the former, Hartlib's correspondent Robert Child reported in 1652 that Currer, described as thriving in London, was a 'reall and honest… and a very good Chymist'. He recommended him as a companion to the mercurial newcomer, **George Starkey**. The two men do seem to have worked closely together, though in 1658 Starkey published a stinging rebuke of Currer, whose abilities as a spagyrist were unimpugned, but who was said to 'hath his dark Intervals'. Using 'unworthy malicious tricks', Starkey accused Currer of perverting the course of justice in a law suit that Currer would appear to have brought against Starkey in 1657, and which led to the latter's imprisonment. Currer was also a close friend of the alchemist Elias Ashmole, whom he first met in 1650. In August 1653, Ashmole accompanied Currer on a visit to Cornwall, 'he going thither to open a myne for the Lord Moone' [i.e. Warwick Mohun of Boconnoe, second Baron Mohun of Okehampton]. Currer's financial situation would appear to have been alleviated through the success of his practice supplemented by the purchase of former crown lands in his native Yorkshire in 1653. He also owned property in Dublin and Barnoldswick, Yorkshire. At the same time, he engaged in financial dealings with fellow royalist Richard Boyle, second earl of Cork, in relation to property and coal mines at Giggleswick in Yorkshire.

In addition to his chymical interests and medical practice, Currer was actively engaged in lexicographical work. In 1658, he assisted Edward Phillips in compiling his *The New World of English Words: or a Generall Dictionary* (London, 1658), and a year later contributed towards the cost of printing William Somner's *Dictionarium Saxonico-Latino-Anglicum* (Oxford, 1659). Writing in 1662, John Ward claimed that Currer was the greatest physician in London, who 'keeps an operator or two under him'. He was also named as one of the founder members of the Irish College of Physicians in 1667. In that year, he was accused by three other physicians of killing a servant of the duke of Ormond with one of his pills. Currer died in London on 16 September 1668, and was buried in the chancel of St Clement Danes, Westminster, on 1 October 1668. In his will, he bequeathed all his books, medicines and chymical glasses to his friend and fellow chymist, Nathaniel Henshaw.

ODNB; North Yorkshire RO, N/PR/GGV1/1 [parish registers of Gargrave, Yorkshire]; Innes Smith, 61; *HMC. Fourteenth Report, Appendix, Part VII. The Manuscripts of the Marquis of Ormonde, Preserved at the Castle, Kilkenny. Volume 1* (London, HMSO, 1895), 257; Green, *CPCC*, iv, 2780; SUL, HP 28/2/12A; 15/5/18B; Starkey, *Pyrotechny Asserted and Illustrated*, 161–4; Josten (ed.), *Elias Ashmole*, ii, 542, 654; Bodl., Rawlinson MS D 864, fo. 221; Ashmole MS 1459, ii, 32; Gentles, 'The Debentures Market and Military Purchases of Crown Land', 272; Bodl., Carte MS 154, fos 158v–159r; Lancashire Record Office, DDB/62/92; Chatsworth House, Lismore MS 29, 27 December 1650, 29 December 1650, 28 January 1650/1 and *passim*; Lismore MS 30, no. 46 [Currer to Cork, 1 December 1658]; *CSP Ireland, 1660–1662*, 11; *CSP Ireland, 1663–1665*, 93, 106; FSL, V.a.293, fo. 109r; V.a.296, fo. 16r; Bodl., Carte MS 49, fo. 263; TNA, PROB 11/328, fo. 79v [will of William Currer, doctor in physic, of St Clement Danes, Middlesex, September 1668, pr. 12 October 1668].

Joseph DEY (1615–1665)

A chymical physician, Dey was the son of Robert Dey (d.1651), apothecary, and was baptised at St Peter Mancroft, Norwich, on 27 April 1615. He was educated at Caius College, Cambridge (BA 1633, MA 1636) and proceeded MD at Padua in 1642. He subsequently became a licentiate of the London College of Physicians in 1645. Dey died of the plague in 1665. Of him, his fellow chymist **George Thomson** wrote that he 'eviscerated and spent himself in toilsome Manual Operations, leaving the way of Riches [and] Honour his Colleagues trod in…whom he deserted…for Conscience-sake, abominating their indirect and destructive manner of Practice, knowing the Professors thereof…to be quite out of the Way of Curing Diseases'. In the early 1660s, he signed a certificate along with four other chymical physicians, including **George Thomson** and **John Fryer**, testifying to the expertise and experience of fellow chymist, **Thomas Horsington**, who was seeking a royal mandate for a Cambridge MD. In February 1662, he also signed letters testimonial on behalf of John Bale of Canterbury, a candidate for an episcopal licence in the diocese of Canterbury. Dey may have been related to Samuel Dey, a medical practitioner, who approved the practice of John Boothe of Norwich, a candidate for a Canterbury medical licence, in 1670. Among the other signatories was Lionel Lockier, a well-known associate of many of those chymists who signed the petition for the creation of a Society of Chymical Physicians in 1665.

Dey was living in the parish of St Olave, Hart Street, London, when he married Margaret Keighley of St Dunstan in the West at St James Garlickhithe on 10 April 1662. The couple had one son, Benjamin, who was baptised at St Olave's on 4 March 1663/4. Edward Browne, son of the celebrated Norwich physician Sir Thomas Browne, records trying to visit Dr Dey at his house in Crutched Friars in March 1664. No record of Dr Dey's burial survives.

NNkRO, PD 26/1 [parish registers of St Peter Mancroft, Norwich, 1538–1737]; Munk, i, 243; Venn, ii, 23; Thomson, *ΛΟΙΜΟΤΟΜΙΑ or the Pest Anatomized*, 84, 96, 98–99; TNA, SP 29/66/27; Canterbury Cathedral Archives and Library, Canterbury, Liber P [1644–64], fo. 190b; LPL, VX 1A/10/22/1–4; LMA, P69/JS2/A/002/MS09140 [parish registers of St James Garlickhithe, London, 1535–1693]; Bannerman (ed.), *The Parish Registers of St Olave's, Hart Street, London, 1563–1700*, 71; Wilkin (ed.), *Sir Thomas Browne's Works. Including His Life and Correspondence*, i, 52.

Sir Kenelm DIGBY (1603–1665)

Digby's interest in chymistry and its medical applications was long-standing and pre-dated the civil war. During the 1630s, he practised chymical experiments at Gresham College in London and was taught in the art by the Hungarian adept, Johannes Banff Hunyades. Later in the 1650s he attended the chymistry lectures of **Nicholas Le Fèvre** in Paris. He was also involved with the planned sponsorship of the design to create a 'chemical council' in interregnum England. At the Restoration, he was living in Covent Garden, where he had his own chymical laboratory. A member of the council of the Royal Society, of which he was a founder member, he left at his death in 1665 two volumes of chymical preparations which were subsequently published by his steward and laboratory assistant, George Hartmann. Digby was a Roman Catholic, who actively sought to obtain relief for his co-religionists in England in the 1650s.

ODNB; Petersson, *Sir Kenelm Digby: the Ornament of England 1603–1665*; Webster, *Great Instauration*, 303–4; Aubrey, *Brief Lives*, ed. A. Clark, i, 227; Digby, *Choice and Experimented Receipts in Physick and Chyrurgery*; *idem*, *A Choice Collection of Rare Chymical Secrets and Experiments in Philosophy*; Janacek, 'Catholic Natural Philosophy: Alchemy and the Revivification of Sir Kenelm Digby', 89–118; Hedrick, 'Romancing the Salve: Sir Kenelm Digby and the Powder of Sympathy', 161–86.

John FLOYD

Floyd was a signatory to the 'engagement' of the chymical physicians. Possibly the same as the Mr Floyd, described in 1650 by Samuel Hartlib as surgeon to Oliver Cromwell, who claimed that there was 'more reality in Paracelsus works then in Carte's Philosophies'. Otherwise unidentified.

SUL, HP 28/1/44B–45A.

John FRYER (d.1672)

Fryer was a signatory to the 'engagement' to create a Society of Chymical Physicians in 1665. He was the son of the physician Thomas Fryer (d.1623), who disinherited his son for unspecified misdemeanours committed against his mother and siblings. Fryer graduated MD at Padua in 1610. A Roman Catholic, he became a candidate for membership of the

London College of Physicians in 1612, but was never elected a fellow, probably because of his religion. In 1633, he was reproved by the College for using mercurial medicines and rebuked for making agreements with patients 'which was not permitted to a physician'. In 1636, along with fellow doctors Thomas Cadyman, Robert Fludd and Piers Roche, he approved a manuscript treatise in defence of the legitimacy of the weapon salve written by a London doctor and fellow Catholic, Mark Bellwood (d.1647). He was living in Little Britain in 1662, when John Ward recorded that he was worth £20,000. In 1663 and 1664, John Fryer MD supplied letters testimonial on behalf of two applicants for a Canterbury medical licence. He also signed a certificate on behalf of fellow chymist **Thomas Horsington**, who was seeking a Cambridge MD, as well as supplying a testimonial for **Jeremiah Astel** in March 1663. His recent death is referred to in a letter to the Yorkshire physician and naturalist Martin Lister, in November 1672. According to Richard Smyth, old Doctor John Frier of Little Britain died on 12 November 1672, aged 96, and was buried seven days later.

His wealth, as alluded to by Ward, was substantial. In his will, he left a series of generous bequests, made possible according to Fryer through large sums of money and investments in the Grocers and Goldsmiths companies in the city of London. He also owned various properties in Little Britain, many of them occupied by booksellers, as well as the manor of Harleton in Cambridgeshire.

ODNB; BL, Sloane MS 172 [Fryer's Padua MD diploma, 1610]; Gee, *The Foot Out of the Snare*, Xr; RCPL, Annals, iii, fos 128b, 129b; Munk, i, 319–21; CUL, Dd. VI. 10; FSL, V. a.292, fos 24r, 69r, 87r; LPL, FII/4/1; FII/4/110a-b; TNA, SP 29/66/27; Bodl., Lister MS 34, fo. 70r [John Brooke to Lister, 14 November 1672]; Wellcome Library, MS 5334, *sub nominum*; *The Obituary of Richard Smyth* (London, Camden Soc., 1849), 97; TNA, PROB 11/340, fos 163v–165r [will of John Fryer, doctor in phisick, of Little Brittaine, 1 September 1672, pr. 21 November 1672].

William GODDARD (d.1670)

Goddard was the son of Thomas Goddard (d.1628) of Rudham, Norfolk, and was educated at Caius College, Cambridge, which he left without graduating. He was awarded his MD from Padua in 1627, incorporated at Oxford in 1634. Goddard became a fellow of the London College of Physicians in 1634, serving as censor in 1638, 1641 and 1644. He was dismissed from his fellowship, however, in November 1649, and subsequently appealed his case, unsuccessfully, to the Court of King's Bench. At about the same time, he told Samuel Hartlib that he intended to 'perfect himself and those studies that tend to the perfection of Medicina and Chymistry in a true Experimental Way [and] for which purpose he is about erecting of an excellent Laboratorie'. At the Restoration, he once again sought to be restored to his college fellowship, but after a lengthy court battle, failed in his mission. In February 1662, John Ward reported that Goddard had earlier lived with a kinsman, Lodowick Dyer, before going to Holland, ostensibly because of the poor quality of glass for distilling to be found in England. At the time, he was practising medicine in Westminster. In 1665, he gave his address as St John's Close, near Clerkenwell. Goddard was a founder member of the Society of Chymical Physicians. In October 1666 he was forced to go to law in order to seek reimbursement from his former colleagues who were being sued by one Thomas Dangerfield, an attorney in the Court of King's Bench, for moneys spent on behalf of the group in their efforts to become incorporated. The outcome of the suit is not known.

Goddard married Mary Matthews at St Mary Woolnoth, London, on 23 November 1629. The couple had eight children, all baptised at St Andrew Holborn, where Goddard lived for much of the early part of his life. He subsequently moved to St James Clerkenwell, where he was buried on 13 January 1670. Fellow chymist **George Thomson** claimed that he 'lost his own life to save his patients'. At his death he owned a small property in Teversham, Kent, which he had purchased from his son-in-law Michael Pemberton of Gray's Inn. In addition to a few small bequests, he made his widow Mary sole executrix.

Venn, ii, 226; Munk, i, 216; Cook, *Decline of the Old Medical Regime in Stuart London*, 116, 135; SUL, HP 28/1/27B; FSL, V.a.291, fo. 161r; V.a.292, fo.11v; *An Advertisement for the Society of Chemical Physitians*; Thomson, *A Letter Sent to Mr Henry Stubbe*, 21, 26; TNA, C 10/477/110; Brooke and Hallen (eds), *The Transcript of the Registers of St Mary Woolnoth, London, 1538 to 1760*, 145; LMA, P82/AND/A/001/MS06667/002 and 003 [parish register of St Andrew Holborn, London/Middlesex, baptisms, 1623–1642; 1642–1654]; P82/AND2/A/010/MS06673/003 [parish registers of St Andrew Holborn, London/Middlesex, burials, 1642–1653]; Hovenden (ed.), *Parish Registers of St James Clerkenwell, Burials, 1666–1719*, 18; TNA, PROB 11/332, fos 288v–289r [will of William Goddard, doctor of physic, of St James, Clerkenwell, Middlesex, 20 November 1667, pr. 9 March 1669/70].

Thomas HORSINGTON (1619–1666)

Missing from O'Dowde's original list of chymical physicians, Dr Horsington was included in a subsequent list compiled by **George Thomson**. He was the son of Simon Horsington, variously described as a tailor, chymist or alchemist, of St Saviour's, Southwark, where he was born and baptised on 20 May 1619. Horsington entered Leiden as a medical student in December 1642 but does not appear to have graduated. He finally proceeded MD at Cambridge in 1663 on the recommendation of the King. His elevation probably owed a debt to **George Thomson**, who with four other physicians attested to Horsington's fitness for medical practice a year earlier. In February 1662, he was said to be living in Cloke Lane, London, where he had a shop 'at the signe of Paracelsus'. In June 1663, he signed letters testimonial on behalf of the staunch royalist surgeon-physician, Silvester Richmond (d.1692), of Liverpool, who was seeking a Canterbury medical licence. Horsington may have served with Richmond, a naval surgeon, in the navy, as the other testimonial was signed by a naval veteran, Dr Thomas Wilson, physician to General Penn's fleet in the West Indies in 1655.

Intriguingly, Horsington's passion for iatrochemistry was shared by his wife Sarah, who compiled a brief manuscript treatise entitled 'Arcana or Mysteries, in the Theory of Physiology and Chemistry' in 1666. These include a number of her husband's medical receipts and prescriptions, as well as directions for making remedies taken from Robert Boyle. Thomas and Sarah were residents of the parish of St Thomas Apostle in London, where they baptised six children between 1649 and 1663. They also make clear Thomas' political affiliations. His first child, born on 30 January 1649 (the day of the regicide) was christened Charles. Horsington died on 13 June 1666 and was buried the following day. His widow Sarah married John Hodder at St James' Duke's Place the following year.

Thomas may have been the brother of the surgeon, Captain Giles Horsington, of Westminster, who promised to obtain for James Long, FRS, 'the relation of the killing by a brother of his and the discription of a flying serpent about one foote long, and as bigg as a ratt in the body. All under his Brothers hand'. Unlike Thomas, Giles would appear to have been disaffected to the restored regime of Charles II. In December 1660, he was accused of saying that General Monck had fomented the White Plot in order to precipitate another conflict. He was nonetheless commissioned as a captain in the earl of Manchester's regiment of foot in 1667. He had earlier served the parliamentary forces in Munster, in southern Ireland, and in 1653 was involved in the sale of traitors' lands.

Interestingly, there were others in London named Horsington who were clearly engaged in the same business as Thomas. William Horsington, a druggist of St Botolph Aldgate, was also described as an alchemist in the entry for his burial in 1655. Both men may have been related to Samuel Horsington, alias 'Paracelsus', of Dublin who, with others, petitioned the duke of Ormond in 1663 for a licence to distil and sell strong waters in Ireland (one of the same name, a distiller, was serving as churchwarden of Kingston upon Thames, Surrey, in 1671).

Thomson, *Loimologia*, 17; LMA, parish registers of St Saviour's, Southwark, Surrey, 1609–1659; BL, Sloane MS 1708, fo. 113; Innes Smith, 121; Venn, ii, 410; BL, Sloane MS 1708, fo. 113; *CSPD, 1661–1662*, 612 [TNA, SP 29/66/27]; *CSPD, 1663–1664*, 151; FSL, V. a.291, fos 154v, 155r, 156v; LPL, FII/4/143; William Andrews Clark Memorial Library, MS H817Z A668; Hunter, 'Sisters of the Royal Society: The Circle of Katherine Jones, Lady Ranelagh', 191–4; Chester (ed.), *The Parish Registers of St Thomas the Apostle, London 1558 to 1754*, 56, 38, 60, 61, 62, 64, 129, 133, 135, 136, 139; LMA, P69/JS1/A/002/MS07894/001 [parish registers of St James, Duke's Place, London, 1664–1692]; Oldenburg, *Correspondence*, ii, 121–2; *CSPD, 1660–1661*, 418; *Commons Journal* (1648–51), vi, 282; *CSPD, 1653–1654*, 314; LMA, P69/BOT2/A/015/MS09222/002 [parish registers of St Botolph Aldgate, London, burials 1625–65]; Bodl., Carte MS 159, fo. 80v; SHC, QS 2/5/ Michaelmas 1671.

Mr HORSNEL

Horsnel's name appeared in a list of 'chymical students and practitioners' compiled by **George Thomson** in 1665, all of whom, according to Thomson, were in favour of the creation of a Society of Chymical Physicians. He may be the same as the H. Horsdeznell who appended a prefatory poem to the work of his friend, the astrological physician William Ramesay, in 1651. In the same year, one Henry Horsnell informed against enemies of the Commonwealth. In 1657, Sir Miles Hobart petitioned that Horsnell might be allowed to stay in England for a further three months (suggesting he was foreign, or perhaps French as in 'Horsdeznell'?). In July 1663, **James Compton, the earl of Northampton**, signed a certificate on behalf of one Lt. Col. Henry Horzdesnell, attesting that he had loyally served the late King and had been imprisoned on several occasions by Cromwell.

Two further possibilities are: Thomas Horsnell, who was appointed sewer of the chamber in extraordinary to Charles II, 10 October 1662; and George Horsnell (*c.*1632–1697), a barber surgeon, living in the parish of St Andrew Holborn. The latter served as warden of the Barber Surgeon's Company in 1685 and was described as 'a master anatomist' by the eminent London physician Sir Charles Scarburgh. He was also a close friend of the naturalist John Ray.

Thomson, *Loimologia*, 17; Ramesay, *Vox Stellarum, or the Voice of the Starres*; *CSPD, 1651*, 93, 424; *CSPD, 1657–1658*, 61, 158, 281; *CSPD, 1663–1664*, 208; TNA, LC 3/26, fo. 120; Rider, *New Practical Observations in Surgery*, 55; BL, Sloane MS 1601 [C. Scarburgh, *Syllabus Musculorum*, 1663]; Ray, *Synopsis Methodica Stirpium Britannicarum*, 96. Roos (ed.), *The Correspondence of Dr Martin Lister (1639–1712). Volume One: 1662–1677*, 122n.

James JOLLY (b.1627)

Jolly's name appears on a list of chymical physicians appended to Thomas O'Dowde's *The Poor Man's Physician* (1665). He was baptised at Gorton Chapel near Manchester on 17 June 1627 and was the eldest son of Major James Jolly (1610–1666), a retired clothier of Chester, who fought for Parliament in the civil war and was a staunch Independent in religion. He remained a committed dissenter after the Restoration and was seized at a conventicle in Chester in July 1665, dying the following year. His son James studied at Cambridge and was made a fellow of Trinity College in 1649. There, he seems to have formed an attachment to the vice-master of the college, Alexander Akehurst. When Akehurst was accused in 1654 of a variety of offences, including blasphemy and atheism, Jolly wrote an impassioned defence of his mentor, claiming that he was suffering from some form of mental breakdown brought on by a spiritual crisis.

The two men would appear to have shared a passion for chymistry and religious mysticism. Akehurst may well have introduced Jolly to chymistry as he had a furnace built in his college lodgings and was described by Samuel Hartlib as 'chymically given'. In 1653, Samuel Hartlib referred to Jolly as 'a kind of Rosicrucian or Adepti' and three years later recorded a visit from Jolly, who came to enquire about Gabriel Plattes and his 'Transmutation of Metals'. Jolly also shared Akehurst's radical leanings. In 1654, after the arrival of the first Quakers in Cambridge, Jolly came close to joining the sect and resigning his fellowship. Following a change of heart, he nonetheless signed a profession of faith in which he rejected the University's role as a seminary for priests and defended the mission of the Quakers. His mentor Akehurst did, briefly, join the Friends; after the Restoration he chose to practise medicine at Leatherhead in Surrey. The nonconformist minister Oliver Heywood (1630–1702), who studied with Thomas and James Jolly at Trinity, was almost certainly referring to the latter when he cited him as an example of one who had become a 'degenerate plant of a strange vine', who had turned Quaker 'and a licentious creature at this day'. His brothers Thomas and John later became prominent nonconformist ministers in the north of England. James Jolly was still alive at the time of his father's death but was dead before October 1684. He may be the James Jolly, who was buried at St Margaret's, Westminster, on 26 January 1672.

Manchester Archives and Local Studies, parish registers of Manchester, Lancashire, 1616–1653; Fishwick (ed.), *The Note Book of the Rev. Thomas Jolly, 1671–93*, iii–vi; BL, Harleian MS 2161, 200; Cooper, *Annals of Cambridge*, iii, 457–8; Thurloe, *State Papers*, ii, 464; SUL, HP 28/2/53A [Ephemerides, 1 January–1 March 1653], 28/2/62A [March–May 1653], 29/5/104B [23 December 1656]; Friends House Library, Portfolio 36, fo. 154 [transcription in *Journal of the Friends Historical Society*, 125 (1928), 54–5]; LPL, VG 1/1, fo. 183; Sheldon, fo. 203; Horsfall Turner (ed.), *The Rev. Oliver Heywood, B.A. 1630–1702; His Autobiography*, i, 161; City of Westminster Archives, parish registers of St Margaret's, Westminster.

Johann Sibertus KÜFFELER (1595–1677)

Kűffeler was the eldest son of Jacob and Margaret Kuffeler and was born at Cologne on 5 July 1595. He became a student of the celebrated encyclopaedist Johann Heinrich Alsted at Herborn where he wrote a thesis on the physics of natural bodies in 1615. After graduating MD at Padua in 1618, he married Catherina, the daughter of the Flemish inventor Cornelius Drebbel (1572–1633). He first arrived in England in the 1630s, returning in

1656, probably at the instigation of his mentor Johann Moriaen (*c*.1591–1668) in the Netherlands and Samuel Hartlib in London, who were both keen to promote his invention of the torpedo with the Cromwellian administration. He was assisted in moving from Arnhem to London through the grant of a loan of £100 made by one of Hartlib's correspondents, Israel Tonge, who shared Küffeler's passion for chymistry. Küffeler was later designated as one of the teaching staff at the new college at Durham in the 1650s and briefly served after the Restoration as physician to James, duke of York. In 1663, Robert Hooke reported that Kuffeler's wife Catherina had recently enquired of him about 'an engine for distilling waters'. Küffeler's projects were many and various. In England in the late 1650s, in addition to promoting the torpedo, he also sought to patent a new oven and promoted new methods of water distillation (both potentially of great use to both the army and navy). He was also an admirer of the alchemical adept Isaac Hollandus. In April 1659, Samuel Hartlib was busy promoting his cause as potential physician to Roger Boyle, lord Broghill. In 1666, he was again linked with the Boyle family when his old associate Tonge sought to push his candidacy as chymical assistant to Robert Boyle. He is probably the 'Mr Cuffly', whom John Ward tried to visit at Bow in 1662 on the recommendation of **George Starkey**.

Identification of Kuffeler is often confusing as he had a brother Abraham who shared his flare for inventions and also married another daughter of Cornelius Drebbel. Both men were also involved, with their father-in-law, in the establishment of a new dye works at Bow just outside London. Abraham had been active in England since the late 1620s during which time he met John Winthrop Jnr, who shared Abraham's interest in chymistry. Kuffeler also worked closely with his nephew Augustus Kuffeler, an associate of the iatrochemist Dr Thomas Ridgley and operative at the Bow dyeworks. In 1675 Augustus, who described himself as 'professor of surgery', signed letters testimonial on behalf of Honoratus Le Beg of Canterbury, Kent, a candidate for an archiepiscopal licence. He left behind a collection of remedies, many chymical, including one related to him by Dr Tonge (above). Earlier reports of Johann Sibertus' death in 1666 proved erroneous. He was in fact buried at St Margaret's, Westminster, on 28 March 1677.

Nieuw Nederlandsch Biografisch Woordenboek (Leiden, 1912); Young, *Faith, Medical Alchemy and Natural Philosophy*, 53–7; Webster, *Great Instauration*, 387–91, 530; Greenfield, *A Perfect Red*, 126–42; Boyle, *Correspondence*, i, 285–6, 334; ii, 84, 101; iii, 116–7; Oldenburg, *Correspondence*, xiii, 330–4; FSL, V.a.292, fo. 10v; Woodward, *Prospero's America*, 32; SUL, HP 18/1/1A–2B; 29/5/72B; 29/7/6A; 53/5A–5B; 53/41/4A–5B; 66/18/1; LPL, VX 1A/10/76/1–2; CUL, MS LI.v.8, 319; City of Westminster Archives, parish registers of St Margaret's, Westminster.

Nicolas or Nicaise LE FÉVRE (d.1669)

A chymist, of French origin, Le Févre (or Febure) studied at the University of Sedan prior to his appointment as demonstrator of chymistry at the Jardin du Roi in Paris in the 1650s. He was appointed professor of chymistry to Charles II in November 1660, as well as apothecary in ordinary to the royal household in which capacity he managed a laboratory at St James' Palace. He became FRS in 1661. His *Traicté de la Chymie* (2 vols, Paris, 1660) was translated into English by P. D. C. Esq, 'one of the gent[lemen] of the privy chamber' as *A Compendious Body of Chymistry*. The translator was probably the French-born merchant Pierre de Cardonnel (1614–1667), an important and well-connected member of royalist circles in London and Paris in the 1640s and 1650s. It was republished in 1670 and also appeared in German and Latin translations. The work itself was largely derivative of other chymists, particularly Paracelsus, van Helmont and Glauber. In 1664 he also published his *Discours sur le Grand Cordial de Sir Walter Rawleigh*, which was translated into English by Peter Belon in the same year. Le Févre died in the parish of St Martin-in-the-Fields, London, in the spring of 1669.

ODNB, *sub* Le Févre, Nicaise; Hunter, *The Royal Society and Its Fellows*, 152–3; Malcolm, *Aspects of Hobbes*, 259–316, especially 281–4, 301, 314; FSL, V.a.287, fo. 79r; V.a.293, fo. 117v; V.a.294, fo. 1v; V.a.296, fo. 2v.

Pierre MASSONET

Originally a French Protestant from Geneva, Massonet was awarded his MD at Oxford by Charles I on 9 April 1646, on which occasion he was described as second, or under-tutor, to James, duke of York. Later that year, in August, on petitioning the House of Lords, it was agreed that Massonet should be paid to leave for France. He may well have been back in England a year later, however, as in 1647 he subscribed an epistolary poem to his friend, physician and fellow countryman, Theophilus Garencières' *Angliae Flagellum*. During the 1650s, he seems to have spied for John Thurloe, though he may have been acting as a 'double agent' (possibly the royalist spy, 'Mr Marsenat', active in 1659). Some time between 1657 and 1658, he was living in Maastricht, where he became acquainted with Sir Robert Moray (1609–1673). The two men shared a passion for chymistry including the work of van Helmont and Glauber. Later they would both sign testimonials on behalf of fellow iatro-chemist John Cockett in 1663.

In 1663, he described himself as physician in ordinary to the duke of York. He does not appear, however, to have profited from the Restoration. Frequently requesting payment of arrears, by 1668 he was seemingly in dire financial straits. In that year, he petitioned Arlington, describing himself as 'the saddest object of pity of all the King's servants'. He claimed to have attended on the royal household as French tutor and writing master for thirty-two years, as well as holding the posts of clerk of the patents and foreign secretary. At the Restoration, however, he lost all but the former and was over £800 in arrears. His wife was acting as a royal laundress. Some reward finally did follow. In October 1672, Charles II appointed Massonet physician in ordinary, probably without fee, so it is doubtful the position was much more than honorific.

Massonet married Agnes Taylor at St Gregory's, London, on 28 January 1636. The couple baptised a son, Robert, at Oxford in June 1643. Dr Petrus Massonet was buried in the church of St Martin in the Fields, Middlesex, on 9 October 1674.

Foster, iii, 985; *Lords Journal*, viii, 463 [13 August 1646]; Thurloe, *State Papers*, ii, 328, 610; iii, 493; Stevenson (ed.), *Letters of Sir Robert Moray to the Earl of Kincardine, 1657–1673*, 102, 112, 114 130 and *passim*; LPL, VX 1A/10/1; VG 1/1, fo. 171v; *CSPD, 1659–1660*, 22; *CSPD, 1661–1662*, 292; LPL, VX 1A/10/1; *CSPD, 1663–1664*, p384, 526–7; *CSPD, 1667*, 439; *CSPD, 1667–1668*, 444–5; *CSPD, 1668–1669*, 129; *Calendar of Treasury Books*, vol.2, 346, 365, 589; vol.3, 62, 217, 739; vol.4, 63; TNA, LC3/27, fo. 46v; Firth, 'Cromwell and the Insurrection of 1655', 323–50; LMA, P69/GRE/A/002/MS10232 [parish registers of St Gregory's by St Paul's, London, 1627–1659]; ORO, registers of Christ Church, Oxford; City of Westminster Archives, STM/PR/6/48 [parish registers of St Martin in the Fields, Middlesex, 1667–1683].

Everard MAYNWARING (*c.*1629–1713)

An extremely prolific author of iatrochemical works after the Restoration, Maynwaring was a signatory to the chymist's petition in 1665. He was the son of Kenelm Maynwaring (d.1661), the sequestrated rector of Gravesend in Kent, and was educated at St John's College, Cambridge, where he proceeded B Med in 1652. From 1653 to 1660, he seems to have practised in Chester, though at some time during this period he visited America, where he developed a lasting friendship with Christopher Lawrence, MD, of Dublin. Maynwaring was created MD at Trinity College, Dublin, in 1655. By 1663 he was living in London and dedicated his first two works to prominent patrons of Helmontian medicine, Prince Rupert and **George Villiers, second duke of Buckingham**. During the plague, he was placed in charge of the pesthouse in Middlesex, where he claimed to have cured an exceptionally large number of patients by using chymical medicines. He seems to have been on friendly terms with fellow chymical physicians, **George Thomson** and **George Starkey**. In other respects, he would appear to have been a more moderate supporter of the aims of the chymists who, despite his attachment to van Helmont, was reluctant to condemn completely academic or Galenic medicine. His *Morbus Polyrhizos et Polymorphaeus* (1665) was dedicated to another aristocratic supporter of the Society of Chemical Physicians, **Montague Bertie, second earl of Lindsey**.

Maynwaring continued to practice for over four decades following the collapse of the chymists' Society. He was buried at St Andrew Holborn, Middlesex, on 21 February 1713.

ODNB; *Wal. Rev.*, 221; J. Barry, '"The Compleat Physician" and Experimentation in Medicines: Everard Maynwaring (*c.*1629–1713) and the Restoration Debate on Medical Reform in London', 155–76; LMA, P69/AND2/A/010/MS06673/007 [parish registers of St Andrew Holborn, Middlesex, burials 1698–1716].

Marchamont NEDHAM (1620–1678)

Best known as a political pamphleteer and journalist, who changed sides with alarming regularity throughout his writing career, Nedham seems to have possessed a lifelong interest in medicine, which he first began studying and practising in the 1640s. He was an early convert to the new chymical medicine, and became a consistent and outspoken advocate of its therapeutic benefits. According to **William Goddard**, he was a founder member of the Society of Chymical Physicians, which first began to meet in May 1664. In 1665, he published *Medela Medicinae*, dedicated to the Marquis of Dorchester, in which he claimed to have been practising medicine for about twenty years. In it, he defended the claims of the iatrochemists over their Galenic and collegiate rivals and repeated these views in a lengthy 'epistolary discourse' appended to **Edward Bolnest**'s *Medicina Instaurata* (1665). In 1675, he also contributed a preface to the English edition of Franciscus de la Boë Sylvius' *New Idea of the Practice of Physic*. A year earlier, with other chymical physicians, he supplied letters testimonial on behalf of John Langford of London, a candidate for a Canterbury medical licence. Given Nedham's long-standing interest in iatrochemistry, it is just possible that his friend James Thompson, 'attorney and fellow wit', was the man of the same name who published a defence of Helmontian medicine in 1657. Marchamont's son, Temple Nedham (b.1664), a surgeon by training was similarly critical of the over-reliance of university-trained physicians upon formal learning and argued that they would benefit immeasurably from working alongside an apothecary in order to better understand how to make medicines.

Attempts to locate any consistency in Marchamont's religious and political views have proved both elusive and controversial, though he does seem to have retained a consistent animus against Presbyterianism. At the Restoration, he was reported by government spies to have largely turned his back on political activism and radical sectarianism and to be concerned purely with seeking the King's good grace. By 1676, however, he was enticed by the government to once again enter the political fray, and over the next three years produced three pamphlets designed to tarnish the reputation of the earl of Shaftesbury.

Nedham, like **Bolnest**, was a minor beneficiary under the will of the widow of former colleague **Thomas O'Dowde** in 1665.

Little is known of Nedham's private life. He and his first wife Lucy (d.1659) baptised ten children at several London parishes between 1645 and 1659. In April 1663, Nedham married Elizabeth Thompson, a widow, at St Faith's in Fleet Street, who may have been the widow of his close friend James Thompson (above). They had a son Temple (above). In the same year, Nedham alleged the marriage of Sir John Russell (1640–1669) and Frances Rich (1638–1720), the youngest daughter of Oliver Cromwell and widow of Robert Rich, suggesting in the process that he was still walking in elevated political circles. Nedham was buried at St Clement Danes, Middlesex, on 25 November 1678 (and not 29 as recorded by Anthony Wood).

ODNB; TNA, C 10/477/110; Worden, *Literature and Politics in Cromwellian England*, 17, 48n, 77; Thompson, *Helmont Disguised* (London, 1657); Lyon Turner, 'Williamson's Spy Book', 253; Wood, *Ath. Ox.*, ii, 626; Boyle, *Correspondence*, iii, 11–14; LPL, VX 1A/10/60; Nedham, *A Treatise of Consumption*, 'To the Reader'; TNA, PROB 11/319, ff.239r–v [will of Jane O'Dowde, widow, of St Clement Danes, Middlesex, 24 August 1665, pr. 12 February 1665/6]; LMA, P69/AND/A/001/MS06667/003 [parish registers of St Andrew Holborn, Middlesex 1642–54];

P69/DUN2/A/005/MS010346 [parish registers of St Dunstan in the West, London, 1645–1656]; Burke (ed.), *Memorials of St Margaret's Church Westminster... Parish Registers 1539–1660*, 223, 228, 233, 240, 251, 258, 657; LMA, P69/BRI/A/005/MS06540/001 [parish registers of St Faith, Fleet Street, London, 1653–1699]; Foster (ed.), *London Marriage Licences, 1521–1869*, 961, 1168; LMA, P69/TRI3/A/002/MS09156 [parish registers of Holy Trinity the Less, London, 1653–1730]; CWA, STC/PR/7/4 [parish registers of St Clement Danes, Middlesex, 1673–1700].

Thomas NORTON (d.1669)

A Mr Thomas Norton is listed as one of the 'Chymical Students and Practitioners' supportive of the attempt to create a Society of Chemical Physicians in George Thomson's *Loimologia* (1665). He is probably the same as the Thomas Norton who was appointed physician in extraordinary to Charles II on 18 March 1668. Thomas Norton, 'phisican', was buried at St Olave's, Southwark, Surrey, on 5 April 1669.

TNA, LC 3/26, fo. 143; LMA, P71/OLA/011 [parish registers of St Olave's, Southwark, Surrey, 1665–1685].

Thomas O'DOWDE (d.1665)

O'Dowde was a leading figure in the attempt to establish a Society of Chemical Physicians in 1665. Like many of his colleagues, he succumbed to the plague in the same year. The fullest account of his life is provided by his daughter Mary Trye, who inherited his practice. According to Trye, following the death of his Irish father, Thomas O'Dowde lost his inheritance following the Catholic rebellion of 1641. Thereafter, he became a servant of Charles I, frequently undertaking spying missions to England which led to numerous terms of imprisonment and exposure to other dangers. Banished from England by Cromwell, he once again returned and was imprisoned at Nottingham some time around September 1658. He seems to have taken up medicine around this time, having an 'inclination leading him from his Childhood to medicinal Scrutinies and Chymical Curiosities'. O'Dowde himself added some further details in the various editions of his *The Poor Man's Physician*. Here, he describes his practice at Langley in Derbyshire, where he went under the name of Dr Brown for about four and a half years. Immediately prior to this, he claimed to have lost his employment as an agent for the King's maritime affairs at the port of Dunkirk. It also mentions cures performed on, and witnessed by, several of his acquaintances and friends, including **Colonel Robert Werden**, **Henry Peck** and **Ralph Whitfield**. In addition to these gentlemen, O'Dowde was probably involved in a scheme to search out concealed lands in Surrey in 1663 with fellow groom of the bedchamber, **Edward Progers**.

Further evidence of his role in espionage, and links with future signatories of the chemists' petition, can be found in the examination of the royalist turncoat Thomas Coke in 1651. According to Coke, O'Dowde (or Doud/Dowd as he commonly refers to him) was acting in 1650 as a go-between for the exiled heir to the throne in Scotland, Charles, with Sir George Booth and his royalist friends in Cheshire. Here, he almost certainly encountered **Robert Werden** and **Geoffrey Shakerley**. In the same year—1651—O'Dowde, described as a delinquent surgeon, lost all his estates near St Clement's church to the sequestrators.

At the Restoration, O'Dowde was appointed groom of the great chamber. At the same time, he petitioned for the office of Assay Master, or Comptroller of the Mint, a post then held by another chymical physician, the Helmontian Aaron Gurdon. In 1663 sought restitution of his father's estates in Ireland, and in 1665 he gave his address as next to St Clement's church in the Strand, where he had a laboratory. His own status as a medical practitioner was guaranteed by the grant of a licence to practise medicine in the diocese of Winchester, dated 8 June 1665. In the same year, O'Dowde published *Two Letters Concerning the Cure of the Plague* in which he explained his decision to decline the King's offer to undertake the role of physician to the plague-ridden town of Southampton. The rest consists largely of a diatribe aimed at 'those Learned Runaway Dutchmen of Amen Corner', the collegiate physicians and the 'heathenish authors' on whom they rely for medicines. He ends by referring to a new book preparing in the press entitled, *A Whip for Gallianism*, which, because of O'Dowde's sudden death, never appeared.

Thomas O'Dowde was buried in the parish of St Clement Danes on 28 August 1665. His wife Jane was buried there on 3 October 1665. In her will, she named **Colonel Robert Werden** as joint executor. He and his two sons, Robert and John, were also beneficiaries. O'Dowde's friendship with Colonel Werden is also evident from Jane's statement that it was 'my deare husbands [*sic*] intentions and will' that she bequeathed 'all my husbands [*sic*] Turneing Engines and Tooles' to him. Other recipients of small legacies included O'Dowde's two colleagues, **Edward Bolnest** and **Marchamont Nedham**.

Trye, *Medicatrix*, 26–31; Linden, 'Mrs Mary Trye, Medicatrix: Chemistry and Controversy in Restoration England', *Women's Writing*, 341–53; O'Dowde, *The Poor Man's Physician*; *CSPD, 1663–1664*, 101; *HMC. Thirteenth Report, Appendix, Part 1: MSS of the Duke of Portland, vol. 1*, 577, 579, 580, 582–3, 585, 590, 592; Green (ed.), *CPCC*,

1643–60, iv, 2766; TNA, LC 3/24, fo. 11; *CSPD, 1660–1661*, 11; Bodl., Carte MS 67, fos 36v, 46r, 46v; Bax, 'Marriage and Other Licences in the Commissary Court of Surrey', 238; CWA, HTK/PR/4/3 [parish registers of St Clement Danes, Middlesex, 1653–1675]; TNA, PROB 11/319, fos 239r–v [will of Jane O'Dowde, widow, of St Clement Danes, Middlesex, 24 August 1665, pr. 12 February 1665/6].

Thomas SMART

Chymist and signatory to the chymical physicians' petition in 1665, Smart first came to prominence in the 1650s as chymical assistant to the marquis of Dorchester at his laboratories in Vauxhall. In 1655, Samuel Hartlib reported that he had performed 'a very strange and wonderful cure of one that was to bee cut of the stone in the bladder by Spirit of Salt'. In 1657, he also noted the recent appearance of an advert for Smart and his medicines in the *Publick Adviser*. After the Restoration, he was reported to be living with one 'Molter' near Clerkenwell, and later in the house of Duke Hamilton (possibly **Sir George Hamilton**) near Mill Bank. In a letter to Robert Boyle in 1663, the physician Samuel Collins referred to Smart as 'a drudging operator' from whom he purchased supplies of arsenic and 'a striking sulphurous balsam, that I have used with miraculous success in sore eyes'. Boyle himself recorded in his work diaries for the 1650s numerous medical recipes attributed to Smart. In February 1664, he wrote a short, printed pamphlet (unpublished), addressed to Sir John Lawson, commander in chief of the navy, in which he extolled the merits of his *auram purgans* and advocated its use for naval surgeons. He probably perished in the plague.

Webster, *Great Instauration*, 304 and n.; SUL, HP 29/5/17A, 18B; Boyle, *Correspondence*, i, 230; ii, 106–7, 108; Royal Society Library, B[oyle] P[apers] 8, fos 140r–v, 143v, 147v; B[oyle] P[apers] 25, 347–57; FSL, V.a.292, fos 46r–v, 111v, 118v; Hampshire Record Office, 18M51/636/22.

John SPRANGER (1625–1685)

Probably the Dr Spranger appended to a list of 'chymical doctors' in favour of the creation of a Society of Chymical Physicians in 1665. Educated at Cambridge in the 1640s, where he proceeded B Med in 1649, Spranger was the son of Richard Spranger of North Weald, near Epping, in Essex, where he was baptised on 6 February 1625. He graduated MD at Leiden in 1656, writing a thesis on diseases of the lungs. A resident of Hailey Hall, near Amwell, Hertfordshire, Spranger and his wife Mary, née Searle, baptised four sons at All Saints, Hertford, between 1655 and 1661. In the latter year, he was probably the doctor 'Spraynger' who was appointed physician in extraordinary to Charles II. He may also have been the Johannes Spranger, who was ordained deacon by bishop **Humphrey Henchman** in September 1671. Spranger was buried at Epping, Essex, on 18 September 1685.

Thomson, *Loimologia*, 17; Venn, iv, 137; ERO, D/P 84/1/1 [parish registers of North Weald, Essex]; *CSPD, 1655–1656*, 581; Innes Smith, 220; Foster (ed.), London Marriage Licences, 1521–1869, 1270; HALS, parish registers of All Saints, Hertford, Hertfordshire, 1653–1675 [transcript made by William Harrison Andrews, churchwarden of All Saints, 1893, after fire of 1891 had caused substantial damage to original registers]; TNA, LC 3/26, fo. 143; Guildhall Library, MS 9531/16; Chauncy, *The Historical Antiquities of Hertfordshire*, 2 vols (London, 1720), i, 555; ERO, D/P 302/1/4 [parish registers of Epping, Essex].

George STARKEY (1628–1665)

Probably the most well-known of the various chymical physicians who supported the plan to create a Society of Chymical Physicians in 1665, Starkey was born in Bermuda and educated at Harvard College in Massachusetts. He emigrated to England in 1650, where he was enthusiastically received as a young adept in alchemical circles. During the 1650s, he published two major works espousing the virtues of Helmontian medicine and became a fierce critic of the Galenists. Closely associated with the circle of scholars and educational reformers surrounding Samuel Hartlib, Starkey played an important role in encouraging Robert Boyle's early interest in chymistry. He seems to have fallen out of favour with Hartlib and many of his supporters by the middle of the 1650s, when he fell into debt, was imprisoned, and was accused by some of excessive drinking and loose morals. He lived and worked briefly in Bristol between 1655 and 1656, but returned to London, where he lived until his death in 1665.

At the Restoration, he wrote several pamphlets celebrating the return of Charles II and, as a Presbyterian, advocated an alliance with moderate episcopalians. He also became engaged in prolonged disputes with other physicians and empirics such as Richard Matthews and Lionel Lockyer over the provenance and merits of their pills and chymical potions. The chymically inclined Restoration clergyman John Ward recorded numerous conversations or 'chymical discourse' with him in 1662, but ultimately concluded that he was 'a careless idle fellow [and] one that is given to tipling and spending too as I hear'. Starkey died in the plague of 1665, his death attributed by his friend **George Thomson** to his consumption of excessive quantities of beer that counteracted the effect of his own medicines. In an alternative version, fellow chymist John Allin claimed that Starkey had become infected with six other chymical physicians after carrying out dissections on the bodies of plague victims. Others to repeat the latter version of events included the respected Yorkshire physician and chymical enthusiast, Dr Henry Power. He is almost certainly the same as the 'Dockter Starke', who was buried at St Peter Poer, London, on 23 September 1665.

Starkey also wrote under various pseudonyms, including Eirenaeus Philalethes, in which guise he may have performed chymical experiments before Charles II. However, most of these works of alchemical scholarship were not published until after his death in 1665. Starkey's private life is a cause of some conjecture, particularly regarding his marriage or marriages. It is usually assumed that Starkey married Susanna, the daughter of Colonel Israel Stoughton of Dorchester, Massachusetts, before he set off for England in 1650. However, the parish registers of St Dunstan's, Stepney, state that Elizabeth, the wife of George Starkey, physician, of Ratcliffe Highway was buried at Stepney in September 1654. And one Susanna, the wife of George Stirkey, was buried at St Thomas Apostle, London, on 21 February 1662.

ODNB; Newman, *Gehennical Fire*; Newman and Principe, *Alchemy Tried in the Fire*; SUL, HP 28/1/58A, 80A, 82B; 28/2/6A; 29/5/47B, 86A-B; McGrath (ed.), *Merchants and Merchandise in Seventeenth-Century Bristol*, 114–15; Bristol Archives, Bristol Deposition Book, 1654–7, fo. 58r; ESxRO, FRE 5466 [John Allin to Philip Frith, 14 September 1665]; BL, Sloane MS 1326, fo. 150v; FSL, V.a.292, fos 2v, 3r, 4r, 5v, 10r–v, 11r, 12r, 13v, 58r–v, 59v, 62r, 65r, 69v, 72v, 73r, 75r; V.a.295, fo. 17r; V.a.296, fo. 16r; LMA, P69/PET2/A/001/MS04093/001 [parish registers of St Peter Poer, London, 1561–1723]; P93/DUN/278 [parish registers of St Dunstan's, Stepney, Middlesex, 1622–1666]; Chester (ed), *The Parish Registers of St Thomas the Apostle, London... 1558 to 1754*, 134.

George THOMSON (*c.*1620–1677)

Like his medical mentor, the apothecary-cum-physician Job Weale (1600–1668), Thomson was active in the royal cause during the civil war and suffered a brief period of imprisonment after his capture at the battle of Newbury in 1644. After receiving an MA from Edinburgh University, he was examined by the College of Physicians in London in December 1647 and January 1648, but was rejected because he was unable, or unwilling, to pay the requisite fees. On his third appearance in February 1648, the censors advised him 'to employ himself studiously in reading the books of physicians'. He subsequently went to study medicine at Leiden, where he graduated MD in 1648. During the 1650s, he practised medicine in Essex and became a convert to the medical philosophy of van Helmont. In 1654, for example, he was collaborating with two early (royalist) converts to Helmontianism, Reuben Robinson (d.1665) and James Thickens or Thickness (d.1666), in conducting anatomical research upon the body of a convicted criminal. By 1659, he was living in London, where he had established a medical practice based on strict Helmontian principles. During the plague, he remained in London, where with like-minded friends he treated the sick poor as well as performing autopsies on plague victims (an able anatomist, he claimed to have performed the first splenectomy in the previous decade). He was clearly on close terms with fellow Helmontian **George Starkey**, and was largely responsible, along with the court empiric, **Thomas O'Dowde**, for fostering support for the embryonic Society of Chymical Physicians in 1665 (he was a founder member of the group). Thomson subsequently became an inveterate opponent of the London College of Physicians, and its domination by Galenists, and wrote numerous polemical works attacking the College's monopoly. Thomson subsequently became involved in a war of words with the College chymist William Johnson, and later with Henry Stubbe. Thomson died in London in 1677, and some of his unpublished works appeared in the press in 1680 under the imprimatur of his pupil, Richard Hope.

The current *ODNB* entry errs in stating that Thompson never married. He married twice: firstly to Abigail, the daughter of Hugh Nettleship, salter, of London (d.1668) in 1667; and secondly to Martha (b.1648), the daughter of William Bathurst and his wife Elizabeth, in 1672. Thompson was buried at St Mary-le-Bow on 17 March 1677. In his will, Thomson stipulated that Hope should receive £20 if within six months of his death he attempted to instruct his brother, Edward Thomson, in the art of making his 'true Stomack spirit and Pyle Polychrest'. In the event, it does not appear that Edward took up the offer. Hope, however, did continue in practice as a chymical physician as did his son, also Richard (d.1725), for whom he provided a testimonial for a diocesan licence to practise at Cranbrook in Kent in 1685.

ODNB; Thomson, *A Letter Sent to Mr Henry Stubbe*, 4–5; RCPL, Annals, iv, fos 11a, 12a; Innes Smith, 232; Oldenburg, *Correspondence*, ii, 578–9 [Oldenburg to Boyle, 24 October 1665]; BL, Sloane MS 1326, fo. 98v [Reuben Robinson to Henry Power, 20 October 1654]; TNA, C 10/477/110; *An Elegy upon the Death of Doctor Thomson*; LPL, VM 1/5, 2 November 1667; Foster (ed.), *London Marriage Licences, 1521–1869*, 1331; TNA, PROB 11/353, fos 271v–272v [will of George Thomson, doctor in physic, of London, 30 December 1676, pr. 16 March 1676/7]; CCAL, DCb/L/B/361 [6 April 1685]; Allan, 'The Coming of the Doctor', 1–15.

George THORNLY (d.1665)

Thornly's name appears on a list of 'chymical students and practitioners' supportive of the attempt to create a Society of Chymical Physicians in 1665. He was probably Doctor George

Thornley, otherwise unidentified, who died of the plague and was buried at St Antholin's, London, on 4 September 1665.

Thomson, *Loimologia*, 17; Chester and Armytage (eds), *The Parish Registers of St Antholin, Budge Row, London, 1538 to 1754*, 91.

Thomas TILLISON or TILSON

Tillison was a signatory to the petition seeking to create a Society of Chymical Physicians in 1665. He is probably identical with the Thomas Tillion, who described himself as 'a Philosopher by fire to the Duke of Buckingham' in prefatory verses addressed to the duke's astrologer, John Heydon. Tillison was licensed to practise medicine and surgery in the diocese of Winchester on 18 July 1664, the same day as **Robert Bathurst**, another chemist and protégé of **George Villiers, duke of Buckingham**.

In April 1661, Tillison wrote to the Yorkshire physician and natural philosopher Dr Henry Power (d.1668), providing details of his attempt to use the most up-to-date telescopes to observe with Christian Huygens and others the transit of mercury in London. At the same time, he acted as a go-between for Power with the anatomist William Croone (1633–1684), then registrar at Gresham College. Two years later, in 1663, he was communicating with Richard Towneley in Lancashire and providing news of 'a strange and new magneticall phenomenon' that he claimed would produce much new knowledge and innovations. Elsewhere, he described himself as a merchant. He probably came into the duke of Buckingham's circle as a result of his involvement in the duke's glassworks and his attempt to patent a new method for the construction of glass. In 1663, he received the patent previously granted to the duke's two servants (and co-signatories of the Society of Chymical Physicians), **Martin Clifford** and **Thomas Paulden**. Tillison was specifically exempted from the jurisdiction of the Glass Sellers Company in their charter of 1664.

Nothing is known of Tillison's fate after 1665. He may be the same as the Thomas Tillison, who made his will in February 1668. Unfortunately, it is very brief and lacking in detail, mentioning only a brother John and friend Katherine Bradford.

O'Dowde, *The Poor Man's Physician* (3rd ed., 1665), unpaginated appendix; Thomson, *Loimologia*, 17; Heydon, *The Wise-Mans Crown*; Wellcome Library, London, MS 5339; Bax, 'Marriage and Other Licenses in the Commissary Court of Surrey', 226; BL, Sloane MS 1326, fo. 22v–23r, 24v, 26v, 27v, 121r; MacLeod, *Inventing the Industrial Revolution: The English Patent System, 1660–1800*, 25, 228n; TNA, PROB 11/345, fos 194v–195r [will of Thomas Tillison, 4 February 1667/8, pr. 6 June 1674].

John TROUTBECK (1612–1684)

John Troutbeck was the son of Edmund Troutbeck (d.1659), surgeon, of Hope Hall, Bramham, Yorkshire, and was baptised at Bramham on 23 February 1611/12. He spent a brief spell at Cambridge without graduating in the early 1630s. Troutbeck may be the same as the John Troutbeck, who in June 1642 was prosecuted for speaking contemptuous words of the King at Knaresborough, Yorkshire. He almost certainly served as a surgeon to the Parliamentarian forces in the north during the civil wars and was attending to wounded troops at the siege of Pontefract Castle in 1648. During the 1650s, when Troutbeck served as surgeon to the parliamentary forces in Scotland and the north, he began accumulating leases to the estates of sequestered royalists in Yorkshire. Having served under the command of John Lambert, he joined Monck in Scotland in 1659 having heard that the King 'would restore the people to their former liberties'. He was clearly a close and trusted associate of **George Monck, later duke of Albemarle**. Pepys described the two men as drinking companions, and Troutbeck later served under the latter's command in the second Dutch War. For his services in promoting the Restoration as a member of the Coldstream regiment, he was appointed surgeon in ordinary supernumerary, without fee or allowance, to Charles II in July 1660, this as compensation for the loss of £2,000 of crown lands that he had acquired in Yorkshire in 1653 (when he described himself as of York, esquire). He was also made physician general to the fleet in 1666. However, as various petitions dating from 1666 suggest, Troutbeck gained little from such appointments. As surgeon to the King, he complained that no moneys had been paid him on account of his inability 'to procure the passing of his warrant' for the post. He was finally granted a pension of £200 a year in 1667, paid for out of the tenths of the clergy in the diocese of Lincoln. In 1672, he was included in a list of officers proposed for the duke of Buckingham's regiment. His pension, however, was in arrears by July 1676.

As further reward for his services in promoting the Restoration, Troutbeck was granted a Cambridge MD by royal dispensation in 1661. He was later granted a licence to practise medicine by the bishop of London on 9 March 1678. His interest in chymistry is attested by the fact that in 1672 the nonconformist Charles Hotham bequeathed all his chemical iron tools to Troutbeck. He also supplied three plates, depicting his own designs for furnaces and chemical vessels, to the revised and enlarged second edition of the *Medulla Chymiae* (1683) written by his friend John Francis Vigani (d.1712). In the preface to this work, a mutual friend T.R. (probably Thomas Robson, a former army colleague of Troutbeck and fellow surgeon) applauded Troutbeck as the equal of the celebrated German chemist Otto Tachenius (1610–1680). He would also appear to have been well thought of as an anatomist. In 1672, his Yorkshire friend, the Presbyterian physician Robert Wittie (1613–1684), referred to his presence at the autopsy of an unidentified 'Noble Peer of this Realm' (possibly his old friend, Albemarle), and he was likewise employed, along with his brother, Joseph, to embalm a member of the Cavendish family in 1680.

Troutbeck was also responsible for the translation into English of Thomas Erastus' *The Nullity of Church Censures*. The translator, probably Troutbeck's young nephew and clerical controversialist Edmund Hickeringill (1631–1708), dedicated the work to his patron, John Troutbeck of Hope, 'late Chyrurgion-Generall in the Northern Army', which, he claims, 'was done at your Direction, and in your Service received its Birth'. Hickeringill, who shared his uncle's Erastianism and hatred of the overweening power of the bishops, later referred to the fact that Troutbeck had altered the terms of his will 'lest any of the lawn-sleeves [i.e. bishops] should lay their fingers on't'. The rebarbative tone and outspoken nature of Hickeringill's assault on the clerical establishment, however, may have been too excessive even for Troutbeck for in May 1683 Hickeringill wrote to him apologizing for any offence caused by his ungovernable temper, and disowning all his scandalous principles to be found in his published writings.

Troutbeck died in the parish of St Martins-in-the-Fields in London on 19 June 1684 and was buried in the same parish three days later. He may have been related to **John** and **Robert Werden** as he mentions a sister, Dame Isabella Werden of Preston, in his will. Though his will was altered, I have found no ostensible evidence to support Hickeringill's assertion that this was done as an affront to the dignity of the Church. Troutbeck's son Thomas, who entered Cambridge in 1661, may have been a co-signatory of the chemists' petition in 1665 (see below).

ODNB, new article by the author [April 2016]; Borthwick Institute, York, MF 647 [parish registers of Bramham]; Venn, iv, 268; TNA, ASSI 45/1/4/57–8; TNA, SP 28/250/II, fo. 261 [petition of Henry Smith of York, 23 November 1648]; Green *CPCC*, iii, 2229–30, 2242–3; WSxRO, PHA/682 [Troutbeck to Capt John Phips, March 1656]; *CSPD, 1657–1658*, 85; TNA, LR2/266/29–30; C54/3749/32; C54/3751/8; E121/5/5/30; LC 3/26, fo. 144; LC 3/2, fo. 24; Latham and Matthews (eds), *Diary of Samuel Pepys*, vii, 79, 354; viii, 52, 198; *CSPD, 1665–1666*, 386; *CSPD, 1666–1667*, 156, 355, 475, 579; *CSPD, 1667*, 474–5; *CSPD, 1670, with Addenda 1660–1670*, 339; *CSPD, 1672*, 252; *CSPD, 1676–1677*, 236; Lincolnshire Archives, MON/7/11/62; Bloom and James, 32; *Cal. Rev.*, 279; R. Wittie, *Scarbroughs Spagyrical Anatomizer Dissected* (London, 1672), 51; Nottinghamshire Archives, DD/4P/36/7; Hickeringill, *Works*, iii, 117; LPL, MS 930, nos 158, 184 [Hickeringill to Troutbeck, 8 May 1683]; CWA, STM/PR/6/32 [parish registers of St Martin in the Fields, Middlesex, 1681–1692]; TNA, PROB 11/377, fos 320v–321v [will of John Troutbeck, doctor in physic, of St Martin in the Fields, Middlesex, 15 June 1684, pr. 28 June 1684]; 11/378, fos 276v–277v [sentence of will of John Troutbeck, doctor of medicine, 10 July 1684].

Thomas TROUTBECK

Dr Thomas Troutbeck was listed as one of the 'chymical doctors' in favour of the creation of a Society of Chymical Physicians in 1665. This was probably an error on George Thomson's part for John above. Alternatively, this may be Thomas Troutbeck, the son of John, who entered Cambridge in 1661 but does not appear to have graduated, or to have been awarded a medical degree. A third possibility is that this is an error for John's brother, Joseph Troutbeck, a surgeon to the duke of Buckingham's regiment in 1673, and later a surgeon in the Coldstream Guards in the 1680s. As surgeon of Lord Craven's regiment of the King's guard, Joseph provided a testimonial on behalf of the Helmontian physician Albertus Otto Faber in 1677.

Thomas was originally bequeathed an annuity of £12 for life in his father's will, but this was altered shortly before his death, and a new bond issued allowing him £40 for life.

Thomson, *Loimologia*, 17; Venn, iv, 268; Dalton (ed.), *English Army Lists and Commission Registers, 1661–1714*, i, 160, 272, 318; *CSPD, 1673*, 568; *CSPD, 1679–1680*, 426; Faber, *De Auro Potabili*, 8; TNA, PROB 11/377, fos 320v–321v [will of John Troutbeck, doctor in physic, of St Martin in the Fields, Middlesex, 15 June 1684, pr. 28 June 1684]; 11/378, fos 276v–277v [sentence of will of John Troutbeck, doctor of medicine, 10 July 1684].

Robert TURNER (1626–1665/6?)

Robert Turner, *pace* ODNB, was a native of Holshot in the parish of Heckfield, Hampshire, which he frequently mentions in his published works and where he was probably residing for much of the 1650s. He was the son of Henry Turner and was baptised at Heckfield on 30 July 1626 (Turner's friend, the astrologer John Gadbury, states that he was born the previous day). A chymical physician and hermetic philosopher, Turner was a prolific translator of works of occult natural philosophy and medicine, including several works by Paracelsus. His translation of *Ars Notoria* in 1657 became the subject of complaint in Parliament in January 1657, when some MPs sought to ban it on the grounds that it contained 'witchcraft and blasphemy and free will'.

Many of his publications are laced with anti-puritan or more specifically anti-presbyterian rhetoric suggesting that he was probably a royalist at heart. He certainly walked in loyalist circles. In 1658, he provided lexicographical help with magical words in Edward Phillips' new dictionary, alongside other royalists with similar interests including Elias Ashmole, **William Currer** and the royal physician and iatrochemist Dr Peter Mark Sparcke (*c.*1608–1676). Another patron, the alchemist William Backhouse (1593–1662), an associate of Ashmole and Currer, was a near neighbour at Swallowfield, just across, the border from Holshot. Loyalist sympathies probably ran in the family as he counted amongst his kinsmen Thomas Turner (1592–1672), a native of Heckfield and staunch defender of the monarchy and Anglican Church.

He was licensed to practise medicine by the bishop of London in March 1661, and subsequently provided testimonials for other candidates for episcopal licences in July 1661, 1662 (with fellow chemists and co-signatories **Edward Bolnest**, **William Boreman** and **Robert Bathurst**), 1663 and in June 1666 (on the latter occasion on behalf of fellow iatrochemist, Abraham Hargrave). He dedicated one of his last works, *BOTANOΛO'TIA, or The Brittish Physician* (1664), to Sir Richard Chaworth, vicar general to the province of Canterbury and chancellor of the diocese of London. In the same year, he supplied an 'advertisement to the reader' to John Heydon's *Theomagia* (1664). In 1665, he advertised a cure for the plague, to be sold at the shop of the bookseller Samuel Speed in London. In all probability, Turner, who was living in Christopher Alley in the parish of St Martin in the Fields from the late 1650s onwards, perished in the plague of 1665–6.

ODNB; Hampshire RO, Winchester, 27M79 PR3 [parish registers of Heckfield, 1605–1663]; Gadbury, *Collectio Geniturarum*, 134; Venn, iv, 276 [who identifies Turner, in error, as the student who proceeded BA at Cambridge in 1639]; *The New World of English Words*, a2r; Rutt (ed.), *Diary of Thomas Burton, 1656–1659*, i, 305–7; *ODNB*, sub Turner, Thomas; Bloom and James, 29, 54, 71, 70, 82–3; DRO, PR 518, *sub* Allington [*sic*]; Wellcome Library, MS 5337, *sub* Minors, Thomas [not included in Bloom and James]; Kephale, *Medela Pestilentiae*, advertisement appended at rear.

Edward WARNER (1612–1691)

Signatory of the chymist's petition, Warner was the son of Edmund Warner of Parham, where he was baptised on 19 August 1612. He was educated at Cambridge and Padua, proceeding MD from the latter in 1648. On the morning of 12 October 1660, Warner's friend Elias Ashmole showed the King two young children that Warner had preserved in a special liquid. Later the same day, Ashmole presented Warner before the King, who rewarded him with an antique gold ring. Ashmole records that Charles 'commended very much his Invention of the Liquour' that had preserved the children. Warner was presumably already known to the King for in September 1660 he had been appointed physician in ordinary supernumerary, though Warner was consistently overlooked when vacancies arose. In 1664, he was made an honorary fellow of the London College of Physicians, an appointment that must have jarred with his support for the chymists in the following year. From 1664 to June 1683, Warner also held the post of physician to Colonel John Russell's regiment of guards and was made physician to the general of the armed forces in May 1678. It was presumably in the former capacity that Warner was able to recommend the radical Behmenist John Pordage (d.1688) for a Canterbury medical licence in 1669. In his testimonial, Warner attested that the latter provided medical care to the royal household as well as the regiment of foot guards under the command of Colonel Russell during the late plague. Pordage undoubtedly shared Warner's chymical interests, as did another of his associates, the Helmontian Major John Chalk or Choke, whose teething bracelet for children was approved by Warner in September 1675. Four years later, in 1679, he provided a testimonial for the royalist projector, ironmaster and chymist, Dud Dudley (d.1684), a friend of Ashmole, who was seeking a Canterbury medical licence.

Warner's links at court may also have extended to Prince Rupert for in 1676 Warner was involved in a scheme to empower the Prince and others to prosecute the forgers of debentures and public faith bills issued under the Commonwealth. In June 1682, he was described as still eager 'to drive on that interest of false bills and debentures'. In 1678, he also used his court connections to claim sanctuary from arrest and to escape the attentions of various creditors. On this occasion, he was ultimately unsuccessful as the King ordered him to be forcibly removed from the court by the Lord Chamberlain, the earl of Arlington, and to appear before a judge to answer the charges brought against him. By 1682, he may have been in dire financial straits for in July of that year he petitioned the King 'showing that he was sworn and admitted physician in ordinary to his Majesty in August 1660 but without fee, to come in with fee on the first vacancy and, having received no benefit thereof, praying that his Majesty would take his age and low condition into consideration'.

Warner married Sarah Champante (d.1698), the widow of Thomas Penruddock, youngest brother of John Penruddock (d.1655) the plotter, in 1652. The couple lived in the parish of St Paul, Covent Garden, where they baptised five children between 1656 and 1664. Dr Edmund Warner, physician, was buried at St Pancras, Middlesex, 2 July 1691.

Venn, iv, 338; Munk, i, 332; Josten (ed.), *Elias Ashmole*, ii, 795–6 [Bodl., Ashmole MS 826, fo. 75]; TNA, 3/25, fo. 51; 3/26, fo. 141; *CSPD, 1667–1668*, 135, 395; Dalton (ed.), *English Army Lists*, 46, 236; *CSPD, 1663–1664*, 668; *CSPD, 1678*, 149; LPL, VX 1A/10/243; VX 1A/10/126/1–3; *CSPD, 1675–1676*, 300; TNA, SP 29/390/23; TNA, PC 2/66, 324, 339, 342; *CSPD, 1682*, 241, 312; WSA, 487/1 [parish registers of Compton Chamberlaine, Wiltshire, 1538–1746]; Hunt (ed.), *The Parish Registers of St Paul's Church, Covent Garden, London. Vol. I Christenings, 1653–1752*, 6, 8, 18; Hunt (ed), *The Registers of St Paul's Church, Covent Garden, London. Vol. IV Burials, 1653–1752*, 7, 16, 17, 24, 29; LMA, P90/PAN1/003 [parish registers of St Pancras, Middlesex, burials, 1688–1730].

John WILKINSON

Signatory (as John Wilkisson) to the engagement of the Society of Chymical Physicians, 1665. In all probability, this is John Wilkinson of Yorkshire, who graduated MD from Leiden in 1662. His thesis, on military fevers, was dedicated to his cousin John Topham. He was the son of Christopher Wilkinson of Burnsall, Yorkshire, and spent a brief period at Cambridge in 1652 without graduating. Given the nature of his doctoral thesis, he may be the same as the John Wilkinson who was appointed surgeon to Colonel Roger Alsop's regiment in August 1659.

Innes Smith, 249; Venn, iv, 411; *CSPD, 1659–1660*, 151.

Sir Thomas WILLIAMS (*c.*1621–1712)

Signatory to the chymists' petition, Williams, a founder member, would appear to have played a central role in the counsels of the fledgling Society of Chymical Physicians. In correspondence with the otherwise unknown chymist John Read, Williams asked Read to consider becoming an 'operator' for the Society, as well as acting as a go-between with Robert Boyle. He also wanted Read to share some of his chymical secrets with him. In a later letter, Read refers to Williams' role in the Society, and his compilation of a catalogue of fifty-three chymical medicines purveyed by the Society. At the time, Williams was living at Two Cranes Court in Fleet Street, and was a kinsman of fellow Helmontian Thomas Sherley, who was created physician in ordinary to Charles II in 1675.

Prior to the Restoration, Williams was practising medicine at Elham, Kent. He was admitted a licentiate of the College of Physicians in London in February 1660 (despite the sarcastic undertones of the censors, who noted his deficiency in Latin). His career, both as physician and speculator, really took off in the late 1660s, when he came into royal favour. In 1667, he was appointed chymical physician to Charles II, as well as physician in ordinary supernumerary. He was clearly highly valued by the King, the warrant for his appointment (not confirmed until 7 May 1669) referring to Charles' wish to 'encourage so important an art... hearing of the extraordinary learning and skill which he shows in compounding and inventing medicines, some of which have been prepared in the royal presence'. Accordingly, Williams was given the right to 'make experiments in all his Majesty's laboratories'. By 1674, he was drawing £1,000 a year for laboratory equipment. In November 1668, he was granted the reversion of the office of Assay Master of all coinages of tin in Devon and Cornwall, and in March 1669, he was jointly granted the office of the examiners and registrars to the Commissioners of Bankrupts in London. In the same month, the King recommended that Williams should be awarded a Cambridge MD, dispensing with all the normal requirements.

Around the same time, Williams began plans for a political career, establishing a base in Herefordshire and his native Breconshire. In 1670, he prepared to contest Leominster and finally prevailed at nearby Weobley in a by-election in 1675. Initially, he seems to have been on friendly terms with **George Villiers, duke of Buckingham**, who shared Williams' passion for chymistry. By 1674, however, it was widely reported that Williams had overheard the duke say that the King was an 'arrant knave' and 'unfit to govern'. Moderately active in Parliament, he was seen as court voting fodder and marked as 'thrice vile' by Shaftesbury. An anonymous opposition pamphlet described him in 1677 as 'a poor quack chemist, now the king's chemist, [who] has got at least £40,000 by making provocatives for lechery; and yet at this time all his land is under extent, and his protection only keeps him out of prison'. He eventually lost his seat in 1678. Williams's garrulity got him into further trouble in 1678, when three witnesses attested that he had carried false messages between Titus Oates and the duke of York. Another reported of him that he had said that 'he knew enough of the Plot to breake the Dukes Neck and his whole partie, & that if the said Duke should anger him he... would declare all in due time'. 'It was plain', commented Sir Robert Southwell, that he 'had been blowing other coals than what concerned him in the profession of a chemist'. Despite attempts to revive his political career, he did not stand again for election to Parliament and was removed from the commission of the peace in 1680. He did, however, retain his place at court, and was reappointed to his post as chymical physician to James II in 1685. It is possible that he now converted to Roman Catholicism. Following the Revolution, he lost all his offices and obtained protection from creditors only by describing himself as the menial servant of the earl of Suffolk.

Williams married Anne Hogben (d.1665) at St Mary Bredin, Canterbury, Kent, on 16 August 1653. The couple baptised five children at Elham between 1653 and 1662. Sir Thomas Williams, baronet, died on 12 September 1712 and was buried at Glasbury, Breconshire, on 20 September 1712. He was succeeded to the baronetcy by his son John (1653–1723), who had been appointed joint chemical physician to Charles II in 1679.

ODNB, entry by author [April 2016]; Henning, iii, 726–7; TNA, C 10/477/110; Boyle, *Correspondence*, iii, 2–14; *CSPD, 1673–1675*, 605; *Munk*, i, 297; RCPL, Annals, iv, fo. 74b; TNA, LC 3/24, fo. 16; 3/26, fo. 145; 3/30, fo. 42; Timbers, *Magic and Masculinity: Ritual Magic and Gender in the Early Modern Era*, 133; BL, Sloane MS 2566; *CSPD, 1668–1669*, 73, 98, 224, 245, 315; Harris, 'Lady Sophia's Visions: Sir Robert Moray, the earl of Lauderdale and the Restoration Government of Scotland', 144, 146; Venn, iv, 418; *A Seasonable Argument* (Amsterdam, 1677), 10; TNA, PC 2/68, 231, 237; Canterbury Cathedral Archives and Library, parish registers of St Mary Bredin, Canterbury, Kent; Kent History Centre, Maidstone, parish registers of Elham, Kent; T. Wood (ed.), *The Registers of Glasbury, Breconshire, 1660–1836*, 72.

Mr [George?] WILSON

Mr Wilson signed as one of the 'chymical students and practitioners' listed by George Thomson in his *Loimologia*. In all probability, this is George Wilson (*c*.1631–1711), chemist, of whose origins little is known. By his own account, he lacked 'the great blessings of academical education' save what he 'fetched out of the fire' in his laboratory. Shortly before 1665, he was established in London at the sign of Hermes Trismegistus in Watling Street, where he made and sold chemical medicines. He and his wife Mary baptised two children and buried a third at St Giles Cripplegate between 1665 and 1669. During the plague of 1665, he was busy supplying potions to doctors, among them **George Starkey**, from whom he acquired the recipe for his famous 'compound soap pills'. In the 1670s, Wilson developed a popular 'anti-rheumatick tincture', and with these two nostrums he began to acquire wealthy and well-connected patrons such as William Paston, second earl of Yarmouth (himself an amateur chymist) and James, duke of York, later James II. Because of his connection with James, his laboratory was destroyed by a mob in December 1688, the crowd believing that it was being used to prepare 'the Devils' Fireworks, purposely to burn the City and Whitehall'. His customers also included the political activist and philosopher, John Locke, who in 1679 was asked by his friend, physician and fellow chymical enthusiast, David Thomas (d.1694), to get 'Mr Willson' of Watling Street to send him 'Bezoard mineral'.

In the 1690s, he moved to an address in West Smithfield, where he began to give courses of lectures in chymistry, mainly to physicians and medical students. As a complement to this activity, in 1691 he published *A Compleat Course of Chymistry*, which was illustrated with engravings of chymical apparatus. The third edition of 1709 gives his age as 78. He died in 1711 and was buried in the parish of St Bartholomew the Less, London.

ODNB; Thomson, *Loimologia*, 17; *ODNB*; Gibbs, 'George Wilson, 1631–1711', *Encounter*, 12 (1953), 182–5; LMA, P69/GIS/A/002/MS06419/007 [parish registers of St Giles Cripplegate, London, 1662–1673]; Locke, *Correspondence*, ii, 128 and n [where De Beer mistakenly suggests that this is the chemist, Thomas Wilson]; Wigelsworth, *Selling Science in the Age of Newton*, 55 and *passim*; St Bartholomew's Hospital, London, parish registers of St Bartholomew the Less, London.

Thomas YARDLEY

Signatory to the 'engagement' of the chemical physicians in 1665. Otherwise unidentified.

APPENDIX 1 (B)

Biographical index of non-medical signatories in favour of the creation of a Society of Chemical Physicians (1665)

Arthur ANNESLEY, first earl of Anglesey (1614–1686)

Born in Dublin, Annesley was instrumental in helping to effect a relatively bloodless restoration of the Stuarts in 1660. He was a member of Charles II's privy council and president of the Council of State (1660) and was later appointed treasurer to the navy (1667–8). Annesley was a cousin of **George Villiers, duke of Buckingham**, and shared his tolerance of religious dissent and patronage of nonconformists. Anthony Wood described him as 'a great Calvinist', whose support for 'Persons of very different persuasions in matters of Religion' made it difficult to determine 'among what sort of men, as to point of Religion, he himself... ought to be ranked'. He was also known to Samuel Hartlib, who described him as 'my very special good lord'. Hartlib and other members of his circle were hopeful that Annesley might provide funding to finance a new hospital scheme in 1661. He was also used by Hartlib to expedite payments of collected funds to the troubled Protestants of Bohemia. He was made a fellow of the Royal Society in 1668 but was not a regular attender of meetings.

ODNB; Wood, *Ath. Ox.*, ii, 789–90; Whiting, *Studies in English Puritanism from the Restoration to the Revolution, 1666–1688*, 415; Worthington, *Diary*, i, 270, 312; ii, 80, 92, 99; Hunter, *The Royal Society and Its Fellows 1660–1700*, 182–3.

Goring BALLE (d.1683)

Balle was the son of Sir Peter Balle (1598–1680) of Mamhead, Devon, a staunch royalist who served as recorder of Exeter after the Restoration. Goring was admitted to the Middle Temple, 4 February 1652 and was subsequently appointed as counsel for the city of Exeter in September 1663. Goring's brothers Peter (*c.*1638–1675) and William (1627–1690) were both early and active members of the Royal Society. The former practised as a physician, having graduated MD at Padua in 1660. In the minutes of the Royal Society, it is recorded that at their meeting on 19 December 1678, Sir John Hoskyns presented to the Society for their repository a branch of white coral, which he had received from Mr Goring Ball.

Goring Ball, esquire, of the Middle Temple, was buried in the Temple church, 21 April 1683.

DRO, ECA 11, 9; Sturgess, *Register of Admissions to the Middle Temple*, i, 151; *ODNB*, Ball, Sir Peter (1598–1680) and Ball, Peter (*c.*1638–1675); Hunter, *The Royal Society and Its Fellows, 1660–1700*, 134–5, 160–1; Birch, *History of the Royal Society*, iii, 449; Woods (ed.), *Register of Burials at the Temple Church, 1628–1853*, 25.

Montague BERTIE, second earl of Lindsey (1607 or 1608–1666)

Bertie was a loyal royalist in the civil war, fighting at all the major battles of the various campaigns. Following the defeat of the King, he suffered huge financial losses and retired to the ancestral estates at Grimethorpe, Lincolnshire, where he seems to have retreated from political engagement and plotting. At the Restoration, he was restored to the Privy Council and in 1661 received the order of the Garter as well as being given back his post as Lord High Chamberlain of England. He died at London on 25 July 1666. The chymical physician **Everard Maynwaring** dedicated his *Morbus Polyrhizos et Polymorphaeus. A Treatise of the Scurvy* (1665) to Bertie, in which he praised the earl for his steadfast defence of the 'truth of Royal Interest, and a Kingdoms safety'.

ODNB; Maynwaring, *Morbus Polyrhizos*, A2r–A3v.

Henry BISHOP (1611–1691)

An intransigent royalist in the 1650s, Colonel Henry Bishop of Henfield, Sussex, was nonetheless in contact with the Levellers for much of the 1650s with whom he engaged in plotting against the various governments of the interregnum. Bishop was also an intimate acquaintance of fellow conspirator John Wildman (d.1693), who possessed connections with both radical and royalist opponents of the Cromwellian regime. At the Restoration, Bishop obtained the office of Post-master General, which he was forced to relinquish in 1663, probably as a result of his predilection for 'continuing disaffected persons in the management of the post'. Some opponents were of the opinion that he was under the influence of Wildman, to whom he was financially indebted. He is widely credited with having invented the modern post-mark.

He would also appear to have been on close terms with fellow royalist conspirator and signatory, **Robert Werden**, whom he entrusted with various estates at Waddon in Surrey.

Underdown, *Royalist Conspiracy in England, 1649–1660*, 123–4, 166, 176, 210–11; Thurloe, *State Papers*, iv, 151, 160, 190, 281, 344, 673; vii, 80; Ashley, *John Wildman: Plotter and Postmaster*, 86, 119–20, 156, 168–71, 176–7, 196, 283; TNA, PC 2/56, 123; *CSPD, 1663–1664*, 157; Johnson, 'Post-Restoration Nonconformity and Plotting, 1660–1675', MA (Manchester, 1967), 32–3; Greaves, *Deliver Us From Evil*, 78, 84; TNA, PROB 11/408 [will of Henry Bishop, 16 March 1690/1, pr. 21 March 1691/2].

Richard BRETT

Unidentified. Possibly Major Richard Brett (d.1689), later of Richmond, esq, who would appear to have made a fortune as a victualler to the royal navy, as well as lending large sums to the crown. At the time of his death, one of his properties in Little Queen Street in St Giles in the Fields was occupied by the former plotter Major John Wildman.

Calendar of Treasury Books, vol. 8, 394; TNA, PROB 11/397, fos 88r–90r [will of Richard Brett, esquire, of Richmond, Surrey, 15 June 1689, pr. 18 November 1689].

Robert BRUCE, second earl of Elgin and first earl of Ailesbury (1626–1685)

Known in later years for his intellectual curiosity and collection of antiquities and manuscripts, Bruce was an early member of the fledgling Royal Society. His father, Thomas, was a moderate Parliamentarian, but Robert became an active royalist conspirator in the 1650s and was rewarded at the Restoration with the post of joint Lord Lieutenant of Bedfordshire. Elevated to the Scottish peerage in December 1663, he was created earl of Ailesbury in March 1664 and sat in the English House of Lords.

ODNB; Hunter, *The Royal Society and Its Fellows, 1660–1700*, 144–5.

Edmund BUTLER, fourth viscount Mountgarett (d.1679)

Butler served as a captain in the exiled army of Charles II. He was also a Roman Catholic whose father had played a prominent role in the armies of the Irish Confederation in the revolt of the 1640s. In 1663, he petitioned the restored king on behalf of the Catholic cause.

Doubleday and Lord Howard de Walden (eds), *The Complete Peerage or a History of the House of Lords and all Its Members*, ix, 323–4.

James BUTLER, twelfth earl and first duke of Ormond (1610–1688)

Butler remained loyal to the royal cause in Ireland throughout the civil war and ultimately shared Prince Charles' exile on the continent in the 1650s. In 1660, he was placed on the commission for the treasury and navy, appointed lord steward of the King's household, privy councillor, lord lieutenant of Somerset, and held various other high-ranking offices of state. In 1661, he was further rewarded with the title of duke of Ormond and lord high steward of England. Ormond seems to have had a general interest in medical matters, and in chymical medicine and alchemy in particular. In 1667, he oversaw the incorporation of the first Irish College of Physicians. Two of his personal physicians had strong interests in iatrochemistry and alchemy. In 1652 William Fogarty, an Irish Catholic, was reported by Hartlib's son-in-law, Frederick Clodius, to have recently discovered the medical, chymical and alchemical papers of one Higgins, servant to the famed Dr Butler, which Fogarty promised to give Clodius 'upon condition that he should explain the doubtful and enigmaticall passages unto him'. Another member of the Hartlib circle and signatory of the chymists in 1665, **William Currer**, acted as Ormond's personal physician after the Restoration. In addition, Ormond used his powers as Lord Lieutenant to promote the cause of another chymical physician, John Archer, who was seeking an MD from Trinity College, Dublin, in 1664. Archer, who was appointed chymical physician in ordinary to the King in 1670, was repeatedly in trouble with the College of Physicians in London, which accused him of practising illicitly and without sufficient medical knowledge. In 1662 the astrologer and occult physician John Heydon dedicated one of his Rosicrucian tracts to Ormond. Towards the end of his life, Ormond attracted the chymical physician Peter Belon to Dublin, where he hoped to establish a successful medical spa at Chapelizod.

ODNB; SUL, HP 28/2/27B–28A, 29A; *ODNB*, sub Currer, William; Bodl., Carte MS 144, fos 44r–v; *ODNB*, *sub* Archer, John [which fails to mention the link with Ormond]; TNA, LC3/26, fo. 142; Heydon, *The Harmony of the World*; Elmer, 'Promoting Medical Change in

Restoration Ireland: The Chemical Revolution and the Patronage of James Butler, duke of Ormond (1610–1688), 84–101.

Henry CAVENDISH, Lord Mansfield (1630–1691)

Cavendish, like his father, the first duke of Newcastle, was a staunch royalist. At the Restoration, he was appointed Master of the Robes, 5 June 1660 (vacant by 9 May 1662) and also served as a gentleman of the bedchamber from either 1661 or 1662 until Charles II's death in 1685. On the death of his father, he was created second duke of Newcastle, 25 December 1676. In 1661, he was elected MP for Northumberland in the Cavalier Parliament, where he loyally served the court interest. He was later a committed opponent of exclusion.

ODNB; TNA, LC3/24, fos 2, 21; LC3/25, fo. 7; *CSPD, 1661–1662*, 367.

Martin CLIFFORD (*c*.1624–1677)

Probably the same as 'Mat. Clifford', who signed O'Dowde's engagement. Clifford was a creature of **George Villiers, second duke of Buckingham**, who was instrumental in securing the post of master of the Charterhouse for Clifford in 1671. Little is known of Clifford's early life, though he probably followed the court into exile in the 1650s. At the Restoration, he gained a reputation as a wit and a poet and was also widely suspected of holding deist beliefs. Clifford was reputedly the author of *A Treatise of Humane Reason* (1674), of which bishop Laney is said to have claimed that 'it made every man's private Fancy judge of Religion'. He was involved in a scheme with **Thomas Paulden** to manufacture and sell crystal glass, Paulden having been granted the patent for the invention of the process in 1662.

ODNB; Wood, *Ath. Ox*, iii, 999; *CSPD, 1661–1662*, 536; *CSPD, 1663–1664*, 229.

Colonel Thomas COLEPEPER (1637–1708)

Colepeper was a member of the royalist underground in the 1650s and was arrested and imprisoned in 1659 on suspicion of plotting on behalf of the King. At the Restoration, he was scantly rewarded for his loyalty, and, financially desperate, threw himself into various schemes and projects. These included a land reclamation scheme in Lancashire, in which he was jointly concerned with **Edward Progers** in 1665. In the same year, he entered the royal service as a gunfounder, and was later appointed (in 1675) as an engineer to the Ordinance Office. Forced, in the words of his biographer, 'to live by his wits and the exercise of his scientific imagination' (he was elected FRS in 1668), he consistently failed to profit from his ingenuity and fell deeper into debt. Nonetheless, he continued to develop new ideas to alleviate his plight, including various projects designed for the improvement of the army, navy and the collection of the revenue. He also became entangled, disastrously, with William Cavendish, the fourth duke of Newcastle, and was disgraced for fighting with the duke in full view of the King in 1685. He had earlier eloped and married Frances, the youngest daughter of Lord Frescheville.

ODNB; *CSPD, 1660–1661*, 90; *CSPD, 1664–1665*, 222; Hunter, *The Royal Society and Its* Fellows, 184–5.

James COMPTON, third earl of Northampton (1622–1681)

Educated at Eton College and Cambridge, Compton was heavily fined for fighting against the parliamentary forces during the civil war. He also suffered frequent arrests and terms of imprisonment during the 1650s. At the Restoration, he was made lord lieutenant of Warwickshire and recorder of Coventry. He was also a frequent attender at the House of Lords and was responsible for introducing the bill demanding the perpetual banishment of the earl of Clarendon in 1667. Elected a fellow of the Royal Society in the early 1660s, he is best remembered today for his translations of classical and contemporary literature as well as his patronage of actors and dramatists.

ODNB; Doubleday and Lord Howard de Walden (eds), *The Complete Peerage*, ix, 681–2; Hunter, *The Royal Society and Its Fellows*, 138–9.

John CREW, first baron Crewe of Stene (1598–1679)

Crew supported the Parliamentarian cause in the civil war but was always moderately inclined and supported accommodation with the King. He was an enthusiastic proponent of the Restoration, meeting the King at The Hague in 1660, and was subsequently rewarded with the title of baron Crew of Stene. Elected MP for Northamptonshire, Crew represented the interests of the 'political Presbyterians' and sought to mollify the excesses of the more militant Anglican members. Little is known of his scientific or medical interests, but he was involved in drawing up the statutes for the new college at Durham in 1656.

ODNB.

Aubrey DE VERE, twentieth earl of Oxford (1627–1703)

De Vere, who may have fought for the King in the civil war, was certainly a dedicated royalist conspirator in the 1650s. He was frequently detained and imprisoned (1654, 1659) for his activities and suffered financially for his royalism. He was richly rewarded at the Restoration with several offices and appointments. In 1660 (invested 1661) he was granted the Order of the Garter and served as lord lieutenant of Essex from 1660 to 1703 (with only a very brief intermission in 1688). He was also given command of the King's regiment of horse (the 'Oxford Blues') in 1660, which later helped to suppress Venner's Rising (1661). According to his biographer, he 'lived riotously on the Piazza at Covent Garden' in the 1660s and was politically supportive of the court throughout this period. He was made a Privy Councillor in 1670 and a Gentleman of the Bedchamber in 1678, but suffered a temporary eclipse under James II. Following the Revolution, he rapidly sided with William III and fought alongside the new king at the battle of the Boyne.

The royalist astrologer and occult philosopher, John Heydon, referred to him as a patron in 1665.

ODNB; J. Heydon, *El Havarevna or the English Physitians Tutor*, A3v.

Sir John ERNLE (*c.*1620–1697)

Of Whetham, near Calne, in Wiltshire, Ernle served as a JP in his native county for almost forty years, as well as sitting as an MP for five different constituencies between 1654 and

1690. Despite his service to the Commonwealth (he was appointed commissioner of assessments in 1657), at the Restoration he petitioned the King for the place of Clerk of the Pells on the grounds that he had expended his fortune in promoting the King's return. Re-elected MP for Wiltshire for the Convention Parliament in 1660, he was also appointed captain of militia horse in the same year and deputy lieutenant for the county in 1661. He served as MP for Cricklade in the Cavalier Parliament (1661). Knighted some time before 1664, shortly thereafter he entered the naval service and steadily rose through the ranks of government administrators. In 1671, he was appointed to the Navy Board as comptroller of naval stores, and in 1677 became an Admiralty Lord. He was also a member of the Privy Council (1676) and a follower of Danby. In February 1681, he was elected MP for Great Bedwyn, probably through the patronage of **Robert Bruce, earl of Ailesbury**. Loyal to James II, he subsequently made his peace with the government of William III but was stripped of his naval posts. He died in 1697.

ODNB; Henning, ii, 271–4; De Beer (ed.), *Diary of John Evelyn*, iv, 533 and n; *CSPD, 1660–1661*, 447; Baxter, *The Development of the Treasury, 1660–1702.*

Charles GORING, second earl of Norwich (1615–1671)

Along with his father, the first earl, Goring fought for the King in the civil war, and suffered huge financial losses as a result. He was created clerk of the Council of Wales in 1661.

Doubleday and Lord H. de Walden (eds), *The Complete Peerage*, ix, 776–7; *ODNB, sub* Goring, George, first earl of Norwich.

Sir George HAMILTON (*c*.1608–1679)

An Irish Roman Catholic, Hamilton served Charles I in Scotland as well as in Ireland in the 1640s, in association with his brother-in-law, **James Butler, twelfth earl and first duke of Ormond**. In 1649, he was made governor of Nenagh Castle, but following its capture by Ireton, Hamilton went into exile in France. At the Restoration, he was fully compensated for his earlier losses. An act was passed restoring Sir George to his full estates, and in 1662 he was granted all the penalties and forfeitures that the crown might receive through the violation of acts of Parliament concerning agricultural practices. In 1661, he gained the royal warrant to dig mines north of the river Trent and in Wales. His son, also Sir George, married Francis Jennings, maid of honour to the duchess of York (1664–6) and was killed in battle in 1676.

ODNB, sub Hamilton, James, first earl of Abercorn; *CSPD, 1660–1661*, 504.

Sir Charles HARBORD (1596–1679)

Harbord was re-appointed to the post of surveyor-general of crown lands in 1660, a position he had lost at the outbreak of the civil war. There seems little doubt that it would have brought him into close contact with many other signatories of the chymists' petition, particularly those who specialized in land speculation and mining operations. For example, **Sir George Hamilton** enlisted the support of Harbord to smooth the way for the purchase of Moor Park on behalf of his brother-in-law, **James Butler, the duke of Ormond**. He was described by the political opposition in 1677 as having profiteered as a solicitor of

Staples Inn to the tune of £100,000, 'till his lewdness and poverty brought him to Court'. Harbord sat as MP for Launceston in Cornwall from 1661 to 1679, as well as serving as a JP in Norfolk and Middlesex after the Restoration.

Henning, ii, 477–88; Bodl., Carte MS 32, fos 167, 279; *A Seasonable Argument* (Amsterdam, 1677), 5.

Humphrey HENCHMAN, bishop of London (1592–1675)

An ardent royalist, Henchman lost all his ecclesiastical preferments during the civil war as well as suffering sequestration of his considerable personal estates. He retired to Salisbury, where he was in touch with royalist exiles and helped to secure the escape of Charles II after the battle of Worcester. He was also on friendly terms with several high-ranking and excluded Anglican clergymen, including **Gilbert Sheldon**. At the Restoration, he was rewarded with the diocese of Salisbury. Following Sheldon's appointment as archbishop of Canterbury in 1663, Henchman was promoted to the diocese of London. Here, he gained a reputation as a moderate and charitable churchman, indulgent to 'sober' nonconformists such as Thomas Manton (1620–1677), who was widely praised in 1665 for remaining at his post during the plague while many of his junior colleagues fled the city. He was also held in high esteem by the King, who admired his fiercely independent frame of mind.

Henchman's interest in 'alternative' medicine is suggested by the fact that he was the subject of a dedication by **Robert Turner** to his *The Brittish Physician*. He was also a supporter and sponsor of the royal chymist, Major John Cheke (alternatively Choke or Chalk), who claimed to be related to van Helmont. Choke was granted a licence to practise medicine in the diocese of London by Henchman in July 1667. A month later, Henchman testified to his personal knowledge of 'the wonderful cures, which he has wrought on many desperate cases'.

ODNB; Williams, 'The Church of England and Protestant Nonconformity in Wiltshire, 1645–1665', M. Litt (Bristol, 1971), 148; Bloom and James, 43; TNA, LC3/26, fo. 142; *CSPD, 1667*, 352.

Philip HERBERT, fifth earl of Pembroke (1621–1669)

As Lord Herbert, he sat as MP for Wiltshire in the Short Parliament, and for Glamorgan in the Long Parliament. Like his father, he sided with the Parliamentarians in the civil war. Following his father's death in 1650, he took over his seat for Berkshire in the Rump Parliament. Elected a member of the Council of State in December 1651, he was briefly president in 1652 and thereafter served the Cromwellian state in various guises throughout the 1650s. His interest in radical religion probably dates from this period. Some time in the mid-1650s he was rumoured to have paid for the publication of various Quaker pamphlets, though the embryonic leadership of the sect were suspicious of his intentions. At the Restoration, he made his peace with Charles II and was appointed a councillor for trade and navigation in November 1660. He acted as cupbearer at Charles' coronation on 23 April 1661. Pembroke possessed no taste for public life and soon after retired to Wilton, where he died in December 1669. According to Aubrey, he possessed 'an admirable witt, and was contemplative', but his chief interest lay in 'Chymistrie, which [he] did understand very well and he made Medicines, that did great cures'. His early interest in medical unorthodoxy and the occult is suggested by his cure at the hands of the eirenic miracle healer Matthew Coker in London in 1654, as well as his willingness to publicly subscribe to Coker's other successes.

Herbert seems to have learned chymistry at the hands of the Bohemian exile and chymist, Johannes Banff Hunyades (1576–1646), who may have been introduced to him by his father-in-law, Sir Robert Naunton, an active supporter of the cause of Frederick, the deposed Elector Palatine and King of Bohemia. In the early 1660s, Hunyades' son apparently lived in Pembroke's household for a brief period where he made chymical and medical preparations. In 1662, John Ward reported that Pembroke was 'a pretender to Chymistrie, and often comes to a refiner in Wood Street [one Wilmot] to doe things for him'. Little is known, however, of Pembroke's precise scientific or religious beliefs though it was reported of him by Charles II, no less, that he held 'pretty notions' of the first chapter of Genesis for which he was mocked at court. His interest in hermeticism and related beliefs was probably long-standing. In 1651, the radical sectary and Paracelsian Henry Pinnell dedicated his *Five Treatises of the Philosophers Stone* to Herbert. Sixteen years later, John Evelyn claimed that he was trying the patience of his son's tutor, Milton's nephew and amanuensis Edward Phillips, 'in interpreting some of the late Teutonic philosophers, to whose Mystic Theology [he] is not a little addicted'. A year later, the virtuoso John Beale confirmed Pembroke's addiction to 'Teutonic Oracles'. He may well have been receiving advice about this time from various members of the Pordage circle, a group of mystical Behmenists who gathered at Bradfield and London under the tutelage of John Pordage and Thomas Bromley. Bromley was reported to have visited Wilton in late 1666, 'where he had not beene for many yeares'. He may have been encouraged by John Pordage's eldest son Samuel, who served as the earl's steward for much of the 1660s and shared his father's passion for alchemical and Behmenist thinking. In all probability, the earl was bankrolling Pordage's activities as well as assisting in the publication of Behmenist texts.

ODNB; Lever, *The Herberts of Wilton*, 118–19; Webster, *Great Instauration*, 301; FHL, MS S 81 [formerly Caton MS 3], fo. 184r [Francis Howgill to Margaret Fell, 10 August ?]; Latham and Matthews (eds), *Diary of Samuel Pepys*, ix, 150–1; Dick (ed.), *Aubrey's Brief Lives*, 146; *Conway Letters*, 99 [Robert Gell to Lady Conway, 26 May 1654], 280; FSL, V. a.292, fos 33r, 84v; H. P[innell], *Five Treatises of the Philosophers Stone* (London, 1652); BL, Add. MS 78,298, fo. 166r [John Evelyn to Sir James Langley, 31 July 1667]; BL, Add. MS 78,312, fo. 81v [John Beale to Evelyn, 9 May 1668]; *ODNB, sub* Phillips, Edward; Bodl., Rawlinson MS D 833, fo. 64r; DWL, 186.18 (1), a, Epistle I [Francis Lee to Pierre Poiret, c.1701]; Hessayon, *'Gold Tried in the Fire': The Prophet Theauraujohn Tany and the English Revolution*, 320–3; Clark (ed.), *Brief Lives by John Aubrey*, ii, 160.

Sir Frescheville HOLLES (1642–1672)

Holles was a naval officer and son of the royalist antiquarian and civil war veteran, Gervase Holles (d.1675), who lived in exile from 1649 to 1660 and subsequently played an active part in the Restoration of Charles II. Frescheville Holles was appointed a major in the Westminster militia, serving from 1664 to 1667. As a successful commander of the privateer *Panther* in 1665, he came to the notice of **George Monck, duke of Albermarle**, who helped to secure a naval commission for Holles. In October 1665 he was appointed captain of the *Antelope*. He was knighted for gallantry following a naval engagement in June 1666 during the second Anglo-Dutch War. He subsequently sat as MP for Great Grimsby in 1667 and used the House of Commons to launch an attack on the naval administration's misconduct of the war. At this time, he would appear to have been an ally of **George Villiers, duke of**

Buckingham and spoke in favour of religious toleration. As a result, he became unpopular with the court and lost various military posts and offices, including his place as a gentleman of the privy chamber, which he had held since 1664. He subsequently made his peace with the court, regained his naval posts, and was killed at the battle of Solebay on 28 May 1672. Though praised by some for his bravery, Samuel Pepys did not have a good word to say for Holles, whom he depicted as 'a conceited, idle, prating, lying fellow'. Nothing is known of his intellectual and scientific interests, though he did employ the astrologer John Gadbury. He was also made a fellow of the Royal Society shortly before his death and may have been the 'person of Qualitie and witt, who had his arm shott off', whom Robert Boyle interviewed in relation to enquiries about phantom pains. He was certainly on good terms with Boyle's brother, Roger, earl of Orrery, who described him variously as 'his true and worthy friend' and 'faithful creature'.

ODNB; Henning, ii, 564–5; Thomas, *Religion and the Decline of Magic*, 310; Hunter, *The Royal Society and Its Fellows*, 188–9; Royal Society Library, B[oyle] P[apers], 75, no. 413; *HMC. Calendar of the Manuscripts of the Marquis of Bath*, ii, 152 [Orrery to Col. Gervase Holles, 17 October 1670]; *CSP Ireland, 1669–1670.Addenda 1625–1670*, 292.

Charles HOWARD, first earl of Carlisle (1628–1685)

Howard was probably a royalist in the civil war, who accepted local office in the 1650s. In 1650, for example, he served as High Sheriff of Cumberland, despite the fact that he was charged with disaffection to the government in that year. He subsequently fought on the side of Parliament at the battle of Worcester in 1651 and sat as MP for Westmorland in the Barebone's Parliament of 1653. He also became a member of the Council of State in that year and later captain of the Lord Protector's bodyguard. For this and other services to the Cromwellian state, he was rewarded by promotion to Cromwell's 'other house' in 1657. During the course of 1659 he sided with the moderates and eventually welcomed the Restoration. He was soon appointed as a privy councillor, *custos rotulorum* of Essex, and lord lieutenant of Cumberland and Westmorland. He was created earl of Carlisle on 20 April 1661. Further offices followed, and in 1663–4 he served as an ambassador to Russia, Sweden and Denmark. On his return to England, he was rewarded with numerous military and political dignities. Initially a supporter of Shaftesbury and sympathetic to exclusion, he seems to have changed his mind by 1684 and died the following year.

ODNB.

Henry JERMYN, earl of St Albans (*c.*1605–1684)

A long-standing and loyal member of the royal household, Jermyn was particularly attached to Charles I's queen, Henrietta Maria, whose retinue he first joined as a gentleman usher in 1627. During the civil war he fought for the King, though spending much of his time in the entourage of the queen with whom he left for France and exile in April 1644. Following the King's execution, he continued to advise Henrietta Maria as well as Prince Charles and, much to Hyde's chagrin, played a leading role in the royalist government in exile, frequently negotiating with foreign princes and potential allies. He was created earl of St Albans by Charles in December 1659. However, at the Restoration Edward Hyde, now earl of Clarendon, succeeded in excluding Jermyn from the King's councils. Instead, he became ambassador to France in 1661, where he helped to promote the King's marriage to the Catholic Catherine of Braganza. In return for his former loyalty and the vast debts he accrued in the royal cause, Charles rewarded Jermyn with numerous posts and offices. In 1660, he was appointed joint registrar of the court of Chancery. In 1662 he became keeper of Greenwich House and Park and served as Lord Chamberlain to Charles II from 1672 to 1674. Despite all these preferments and offices, he still died heavily in debt in 1684. He supported a policy of religious toleration, largely in order to allow Roman Catholics the right to worship freely in England.

ODNB.

Sir William KILLIGREW (1606–1695)

Dramatist and courtier, Killigrew was knighted in 1626 by Charles I. He served Charles as a gentleman usher and attended him throughout the civil war. Killigrew suffered for his royalism and was forced to scheme in order to avoid complete impoverishment in the 1650s. In 1654, for example, he was involved in fen drainage. Active behind the scenes in 1659–60 promoting the Restoration, Killigrew was rewarded by being reappointed gentleman usher of the privy chamber in the summer of 1660. By February 1664, he was also serving as the queen's vice-chamberlain. Further grants and offices followed for himself and his family. In 1661, he was awarded the profits of 'certain concealed waste lands', and in the following year was granted a joint share of 'certain bonds for sequestration moneys in Lancashire'. He was also active politically, being returned as MP for Richmond in April 1664. He was later an energetic member of the court party and would appear to have played an important role in devising Charles' financial policies and plans to raise further revenues. He is best known today, however, as a playwright, many of whose plays, first performed in the 1660s, were concerned with topical political themes such as succession, usurpation and royal authority.

ODNB; *CSPD, 1654*, 152.

Sir John MENNES (1599–1671)

A naval officer, he was knighted by Charles I in February 1642 for safely conveying Queen Henrietta Maria to France and was soon after rewarded with the office of rear admiral in the navy. At the outbreak of civil war, he transferred to the army and fought loyally for the King throughout the conflict. By 1648, he was back at sea in the King's service and soon joined the exiled court abroad. During the 1650s, he was principally active as a secret agent, though he also served as medical adviser to the exiled cavaliers, claiming a special gift in the cure of venereal diseases. At the Restoration, he was appointed a gentleman of the privy chamber and received other minor rewards. In 1661, he was appointed comptroller of the navy, an office for which he was ill equipped. He was also made a member of the council for foreign plantations (1661), master of Trinity House (1662), a member of the Tangier Company (1662) and a founder assistant of the Royal Fishery Company (1664). According to Anthony Wood, Mennes was 'well skill'd in Physic and Chymistry', a judgement shared by his naval associate Samuel Pepys. It seems likely, therefore, that he was a competent judge of the claims made by the chymists in 1665. He is perhaps better known today for his poetry and contribution to royalist genres of writing such as 'drollery'.

ODNB; Wood, *Ath. Ox.*, ii, 350–1; Latham and Matthews (eds), *Diary of Samuel Pepys*, iv, 218, 334; v, 241–2; Raylor, *Cavaliers, Clubs, and Literary Culture: Sir John Mennes, James Smith, and the Order of Fancy.*

Sir William MEYRICK (d.1669)

A civil lawyer and judge, Meyrick was appointed judge of the prerogative court of Canterbury in September 1641 by William Laud. After joining the King at Oxford in 1643, he was replaced by the Parliamentarian Sir Nathaniel Brent, but was reinstated at the Restoration. He was knighted on 8 November 1661. He made his will in 1665 and died in 1669.

ODNB; Green, *The Re-Establishment of the Church of England 1660–1663*, 124, 132.

George MONCK, first duke of Albemarle (1608–1670)

The principal architect of the Restoration, the Devonian Monck was knighted by Charles II in 1660, as well as being inducted into the Order of the Garter. In 1665, he deputized for the duke of York as lord high admiral to the fleet. During the plague, he stayed in London and superintended the necessary measures to check the spread of the disease. A moderate in religion, Monck was acquainted with the chymical physician **John Troutbeck**, and may have been a kinsman of **Edmund Warcup**. His preference for unorthodox medical ideas is suggested by Christopher Irvine's dedication of his *Medicina Magnetica* to Monck, as commander-in-chief of the forces in Scotland, in 1656, as well as the fact that in 1669 he was treated for the dropsy by the empiric, William Sermon.

ODNB.

Thomas PAULDEN (b.1625)

Originally from Yorkshire, after a brief sojourn at Cambridge Paulden enlisted with the royalist army and may have fought at the battle of Naseby. He was partly responsible for capturing Pontefract castle in the second civil war, during the siege of which he was accused of murdering the Parliamentarian officer Colonel William Rainsborough. Refusing terms, Paulden finally fled into exile and the court of Prince Charles in March 1649. During the 1650s, he frequently engaged in spying missions to England, was caught and escaped, and did not return for good until 1660, when he renewed intimacy with his former patron, **George Villiers, second duke of Buckingham**. In November 1660, he sought to benefit from his former loyalty by petitioning the crown for lands near Holy Island, which he wished to improve. In 1662, he was granted the patent for an invention to manufacture crystal glass, a scheme that led him into collaboration with another of Buckingham's servants, **Martin Clifford**. At the same time, he was also an associate of the poet, Abraham Cowley (1618–1667). In 1668, he was recommended by the King for the post of commissioner of excise upon the first vacancy. In 1678, Paulden played a minor role in the drama surrounding the murder of Sir Edmund Berry Godfrey, when he gave evidence as to his being in Duke's Coffee House at the time it was first reported that Godfrey's body had been found. He seems to have died in poverty some time between 1702 and 1710.

ODNB; Underdown, *Royalist Conspiracy in England*, 9, 86n, 145, 207–8; Thurloe, *State Papers*, i, 714, 719; iii, 240–2, 264; *Calendar of Treasury Books, 1660–1667*, 34; *CSPD, 1663–1664*, 229; Pritchard, 'Six Letters by Cowley', *Review of English Studies*, 18 (1967), 261; Marshall, *Strange Death of Edmund Godfrey: Plots and Politics in Restoration London* (Stroud, 1999), 95, 104.

Henry PECK (d.1675)

Thomas O'Dowde described Peck as 'my very loving friend, Justice Peck', who lived near the new chapel in Tuttle Street, Westminster. In April 1661, Henry Peck, 'one of the Gentlemen of the Privy Chamber in Extraordinary', was ordered to be paid over £3,400 'in consideration, as by a vote of Parliament of 10 December last, of an estate taken from him and disposed by some of the late usurping powers'. His appointment at court is not noted by Bucholz in his database of court officers.

He is almost certainly the Captain Henry Peck, who petitioned Cromwell in April 1654 seeking reimbursement of over £4,000, moneys that he claimed were owed to his father 'in recompense of an estate disposed of by Parliament to Col. Massey'. The land in question was a lease on an ironworks in the Forest of Dean. A stop was placed on payment of the money in December 1648. Peck begged, 'for the sake of my fathers wounds and expenses in the service, and the multitude of his children, that the stay be removed'. Peck served as a JP for Middlesex after the Restoration. He was buried at St Margaret's, Westminster, on 2 December 1675.

O'Dowde, *The Poor Man's Physician* (3rd ed., 1665), 68–9; *Calendar of Treasury Books, 1660–1667*, 236; *CSPD, 1654*, 96, 329; TNA, PROB 11/350, fos 173r–v [will of Henry Peck, esquire, of Westminster, 1 April 1675, pr. 21 February 1675/6]; City of Westminster Archives, parish registers of St Margaret's, Westminster.

Edward PROGERS (1621–1713)

A life-time servant of the Stuart court, Progers was appointed at a young age as a page of honour to Charles I and spent the civil war with the court at Oxford. On joining Henrietta Maria in Paris in 1646, he was sent to Jersey, where he was appointed one of the grooms of the bedchamber by Prince Charles in November of that year. Thereafter, Progers or 'Poge' was one of Charles' closest confidantes and was frequently trusted to undertake sensitive missions on behalf of the King in exile. He also suffered imprisonment for these activities and was not surprisingly entrusted to carry out further such missions on the eve of the Restoration. He was subsequently confirmed as groom of the bedchamber on 3 February 1661. Throughout the 1660s, he repeatedly importuned the King for office and favours, both for himself and his family. He was also involved in numerous money-making schemes, including land reclamation in Lancashire with **Colonel Thomas Colepeper**, attempts to secure tithes in Hatfield Chase, and improvements to the farming of the customs. By 1663, he was acting as deputy to **George Monck, duke of Albemarle** as ranger of Bushy Park at Hampton Court and succeeded as ranger on the duke's death in 1670. As MP for Brecknockshire from 1662 until 1679, he supported the court, but did not stand for election in 1679 on account of his royal duties. He was also appointed deputy lieutenant for the county in 1674. Progers retired to Hampton after losing his post as groom of the bedchamber at the accession of James II in 1685 and died there in 1713. He was probably responsible for the appointment of his brother, **Henry** to various royal positions after 1660.

ODNB; Hervey, *West Stow Parish Registers*, 191–222; *CSPD, 1652–1653*, 94; *CSPD, 1655*, 204; Thurloe, *State Papers*, iii, 339; TNA, LC 3/24, fo. 3; *Calendar of Treasury Books, 1660–1667*, 125, 172; *CSPD, 1663–1664*, 101; *CSPD, 1664–1665*, 222, 370 and *passim*; TNA, PC 2/60, 25; Copinger, *The Manors of Suffolk*, i, 408–10.

Henry PROGERS (d.1687)

Henry was the younger brother of **Edward** (above). Like his brother, Henry was a staunch royalist, who, as a servant of Lord Cottington and Edward Hyde, was implicated in the murder of the parliamentary envoy and political apologist Anthony Ascham in Madrid in 1650. Progers was appointed king's equerry in ordinary and groom of the bedchamber at the Restoration (though no official record of his appointment as the latter has survived). During the 1660s, he was involved in numerous schemes and profit-making ventures with his brother Edward, including one designed to regulate the sedan-chair men in 1665. In 1681, he was appointed sergeant porter at court.

ODNB, *sub* Ascham, Anthony; TNA, LS 13/252, fo. 44v; LS 13/253, fo. 88; LS 13/9, fo. 15A; LS 13/255, fos 3v, 21v; *CSPD, 1660–1661*, 320; *CSPD, 1661–1662*, 500; *CSPD, 1665–1666*, 160 and *passim*.

Sir Geoffrey SHAKERLEY (1619–1696)

A committed royalist in the civil war and plotter in the 1650s, Sir Geoffrey Shakerley of Hulme was made one of the commissioners for corporations in 1662. A year later, in August 1663, he was appointed governor of Chester Castle, probably at the instigation of **Colonel Robert Werden**, among whose papers the petition to install Shakerley was found. He was elected MP for Wigan in 1661, where his brother-in-law Roger Bradshaigh had the strongest interest. Moderately active at Westminster, he spent little time in London following his appointment at Chester. He did, however, maintain a regular correspondence with Joseph Williamson, whom he supplied with a constant flow of information relating to the activities of local felons, traitors and sectaries. He was particularly zealous in prosecuting dissenters during the Second Anglo-Dutch War, at the outset of which he was appointed deputy-lieutenant of Cheshire (1665). At the same time, he was noticeably more lenient to Catholics, many of whom had loyally served the King during the years of civil war and interregnum. Accounted a friend of **James Butler, duke of Ormond**, he continued to persecute nonconformists in the 1670s, and was not surprisingly a Tory supporter in the following decade. He died on 17 October 1696 and was buried at Nether Peover, Cheshire. His son Peter sat as the Tory MP for Wigan, 1690–8, and for Chester, 1698–1715.

He may have known **Thomas O'Dowde** from the early 1650s, when both men moved in the same royalist circles in Cheshire. An interest in chymistry is suggested by his involvement with his brother-in-law, the loyalist physician Allan Pennington (1622–1696), in a scheme to extract silver from lead ore in north Wales in 1670. He was also active in seeking royal grants of land and favour after the Restoration. In September 1660, he petitioned for a lease of meadows in Lambeth, Surrey.

Henning, iii, 426–7; Green, *CPCC*, ii, 1446; Cheshire and Chester Archives and Local Studies, Chester, ZA/B/2, fo. 137v; *CSPD, 1663–1664*, 205, 248, 303, 431; *CSPD, 1664–1665*, 461, 478 and *passim*; *CSPD, 1670, with Addenda 1660–1670*, 148 and *passim*; Manchester Central Library, L1/48/6/1, 57, 216; *Calendar of Treasury Books, 1660–1667*, 22.

Gilbert SHELDON, archbishop of Canterbury (1598–1677)

Appointed bishop of London in 1660 and archbishop of Canterbury in 1663, Sheldon exercised an important role in dispensing medical patronage in the early Restoration church through control of the machinery to grant medical licences to practise, both in London and throughout the province of Canterbury. There is every reason to suspect that he was personally agreeable to the new methods of the iatrochemists; many were certainly licensed during his period of office. Indeed, his interest in chymical medicine may date from the 1650s when Henry More reported that 'Dr Shelden of Oxford' was conversant with the maker of a medicinal 'powder' that he was eager to recommend to Lady Conway. He was also able to grant Lambeth B. Meds and MDs as well as licence medical books. The surgeon Edmund King, who first came to Charles II's notice as an experimental chymist in the early years of the Restoration, was awarded a Lambeth B. Med by Sheldon in 1663. Moreover, the Helmontian Albertus Otto Faber claimed to have cured Sheldon with his aurum potabile. At the height of the controversy between the chymists and Galenists, the former's leader, **George Thomson**, dedicated his *Galeno-Pale* to Sheldon, whom he thanked for his encouragement and support. Perhaps the most significant evidence of Sheldon's support for the chymists, and his antagonism towards the college Galenists, is evident in his patronage of the would-be medical reformer and apothecary Adrian Huyberts, who actively canvassed for the creation of a new college of physicians in 1675 under the protection of Sheldon. Huyberts, who claimed that medicine in the capital would be in better hands if overall control of licensing were placed in the hands of the church, was clearly echoing the views of his patron.

ODNB; *Conway Letters*, 106; Furdell, *The Royal Doctors 1485–1714*, 171–2; LPL, FII/4/58; F1/C, fos 121v, 126v; Faber, *De Auro Potabili Medicinali*, 'Of Some Cures more, done since the former were published', 5–8; Huyberts, *A Corner-Stone Laid Towards the Building of a New Colledge*, 34–8; LPL, VX 1A/10/74/1–4.

George VILLIERS, second duke of Buckingham (1628–1687)

Buckingham received the Order of the Garter in 1649 for services rendered to the royalist cause during the civil war. He spent much of the 1650s abroad at the court of the exiled Charles II and seems to have engaged in a bewildering variety of insurrectionary schemes and alliances aimed at overthrowing the Cromwellian government. Nonetheless, he returned to England in 1657 and sought to make peace with the powers-that-be. At the Restoration, residual uncertainty surrounding Buckingham's loyalties and motives meant that rewards came slowly. He was belatedly appointed a gentleman of the King's bedchamber in 1661 and in the following year was restored to his membership of the Privy Council. From 1661 to 1667, he served as lord lieutenant for the West Riding of Yorkshire, in which capacity he was instrumental in putting down a rising of religious and political dissidents in that county in 1663. In April 1665, he joined the fleet but soon fell out with the duke of York and the earl of Sandwich and was ordered ashore.

He now retired briefly from political life and may have used this time to pursue one of his great hobbies, experimental chymistry. A member of the Royal Society since 1661, he was an active chymist and, like the King, possessed his own laboratory at Wallingford House. Some even considered that he was close to discovering the much sought-after philosopher's stone. A number of medical receipts attributed to him, including a pill for the pox, can be found in a collection of chymical remedies attributed to Augustus Küffeler, probably the nephew of **Johann Sibertus Küffeler**. He was also, like so many of the patrons of the chymical physicians, a projector interested in money-making schemes that were often linked to chymistry and metallurgy. In 1663, for example, he sought a patent for the manufacture of crystal glasses, working alongside his secretary, **Martin Clifford** and former royalist **Thomas Paulden**. His efforts resulted in the construction of a successful glass-making factory at Vauxhall. His chymical and occult interests might account for the accusation levelled against him by his political opponents in 1667 that he had employed John Heydon to calculate Charles II's horoscope. Heydon, who claimed Buckingham as a patron, dedicated a Rosicrucian tract to the duke in 1664. From 1668 onward, he was a firm proponent of the principle of religious toleration, which he consistently promoted in Parliament. His commitment to the cause of religious freedom may, however, have been prompted as much by pragmatic political concerns as ideological conviction. Richard Baxter claimed that he was a man of 'no Religion but notoriously and professedly lustful', though he added that he was known to countenance 'fanatics and sectaries'. He died in 1687.

Robert Bathurst, **Edward Bolnest** and **Thomas Tillison** were all employed by the duke for their chymical expertise, while he was the subject of an effusive dedication from another chymical physician and signatory, **Everard Maynwaring**. He was also on close terms in the 1670s with another leading figure in the abortive Society of Chemical Physicians, **Thomas Williams**. The duke's interest almost certainly pre-dated the Restoration. In 1664 Philip Skippon reported meeting one Regio in Padua, 'a Fleming born' and a 'chymist, who had formerly lived in England with the duke of Bucks'.

ODNB; *CSPD, 1663–1664*, 186–7; Hunter, *The Royal Society and Its Fellows 1660–1700*, 148–9; CUL, MS Ll.V.8, 172, 386; Heydon, *Theomagia* (London, 1664); Yardley, 'George Villiers, Second Duke of Buckingham, and the Politics of Toleration', 317–37; Baxter, *Reliquiae Baxterianae*, iii, 21; Skippon, 'An Account of a Journey Made Thru' Part of the Low Countries, Germany, Italy, and France [1663–1666]' in *A Collection of Voyages and Travels*, vi, 534.

Sir Edmund WARCUP (1627–1712)

Warcup first came to political prominence in 1648, when, through the influence of his uncle William Lenthall, speaker of the Long Parliament, he became secretary to the parliamentary commissioners on the Isle of Wight. In 1651, he was at Lincoln's Inn and during the course of the next decade was involved in Welsh land deals and coal mining schemes. With regard to the latter, he was involved in a project to propagate a new method of smelting coal in the Forest of Dean, in which capacity he may have come into contact with **George Starkey**. Warcup may have been related to **George Monck** for whom he worked in the 1660s. In 1660, possibly at Monck's instigation, he drafted a bill setting out terms for the restoration of Charles II. At about the same time, he became associated with the earl of Shaftesbury, a connection that grew after 1660 when Warcup was appointed farmer of the excise in Wiltshire and Dorset under Shaftesbury as Chancellor of the Exchequer. In 1664, he succeeded his father as bailiff of Southwark and became a magistrate in London. During the plague, he helped to supervise plans to contain the disease in London and was consequently rewarded for his troubles with a royal gift of plate. In 1665–6, he was again working for Monck in the disposal of naval prizes. He also officiated as cupbearer to James, duke of York.

After a brief fall from grace in 1666, during which time he was briefly imprisoned at Oxford where he was visited by the chymical physician **Jeremiah Astel**, he resumed his career as a magistrate and was active in local and national politics, largely as a supporter of the earl of Shaftesbury. During the Popish Plot, he took an active part, probably at the instigation of Shaftesbury, in examining witnesses. However, by 1681, he had switched political allegiances and was acting for the King and the Tories in prosecuting the earl for treason. In the aftermath of Shaftesbury's acquittal, Warcup was vilified by the Whigs and withdrew to his Oxfordshire estates. He was finally knighted by a grateful king in 1684 and initially welcomed the accession of James II, though he later applauded the revolution of 1688 and became a church Tory under William and Mary and Queen Anne.

The physician Jodocus Crull (d.1710) dedicated his *The Antient and Present State of Muscovy* (1698) to his friend Warcup, in which he expresses admiration for the latter's account of his travels in Italy published at London in 1660. Crull also provides a flattering and uncritical biography of Warcup.

ODNB; Feiling and Needham (eds), 'The Journals of Edmund Warcupp, 1676–84', 235–60; TNA, PC 2/59, 23, 104, 121, 131; PC 2/68, 92, 283, 403; 2/69, 235; Webster, *Great Instauration*, 401 and n.; Thurloe, *State Papers*, iii, 496; *CSPD, 1655*, 171, 191; Rees, *Industry Before the Industrial Revolution*, i, 294–5n; Wood, *Fasti Oxonienses*, 184; Bodl., Rawlinson MS D 384, fo. 70.

Sir John WERDEN (1640–1716)

Diplomat and politician, Sir John Werden was the son and heir of **Robert Werden** who, like his father, signed both the 'engagement' of the chymists and subscribed to the list of eminent patrons of the proposed Society of Chymical Physicians in 1665. Called to the bar in 1660, he became a baron of the exchequer for Cheshire in November 1664, a position he probably owed to his father's close connections with James, duke of York. During the second Anglo-Dutch War he served on diplomatic missions to Copenhagen, Madrid and Lisbon. He continued in the diplomatic service at the end of the war, and in 1672 was granted a baronetcy. He served as the duke of York's secretary from 1673 to 1683 and was returned as MP for Reigate on the duke's interest in 1673. Denounced by Shaftesbury and in Whig propaganda as a supporter of popery, he was one of the MPs named to investigate the Popish Plot in 1678. Defeated in the election of 1679, he returned to Parliament as MP for Reigate in 1685. During the reign of his former patron, he was appointed commissioner for customs and lieutenant for the city of London, and not surprisingly, was excluded by William III from those he was willing to pardon. Though he continued to hold, intermittently, his customs' posts, he was widely suspected of colluding with the supporters of James in exile. He died on 29 October 1716 and was buried at St Martin-in-the-Fields, London.

In 1665, he was named as a minor beneficiary, along with his father and brother Robert, in the will of Jane, the wife of **Thomas O'Dowde**. The various letters that he wrote to Henry Oldenburg while serving as a diplomat in Sweden in 1671 attest to his genuine interest in the new science. There, he refers to reading the recent works of Boyle on cold and the air, and records various measurements taken with an early thermometer. He was also evidently an avid reader and collector of the Royal Society's *Philosophical Transactions*.

ODNB; Henning, iii, 688–9; Green, *CPCC*, ii, 1154–6; TNA, PROB 11/319, fos 239r–v [will of Jane O'Dowde, widow, of St Clement Danes, Middlesex, 24 August 1665, pr. 12 February 1665/6]; Oldenburg, *Correspondence*, viii, 30–2, 117–19.

Robert WERDEN (*c*.1622–1690)

Werden, of Burton Hall, Cheshire, like his son, **John**, signed both the engagement of the chymists and subscribed to the list of eminent patrons of the newly proposed Society in

1665. A royalist colonel of horse in the civil war, he compounded with his father, John, in 1646 for £600. He was subsequently involved throughout the 1650s in royalist conspiracies, including an ambitious scheme to capture Chester Castle, but the failure of this and other plans led to some suspicions in royalist circles as to the sincerity of his devotion to the cause. His activities in Cheshire at this time probably brought him into early contact with **Thomas O'Dowde**, with whom Werden was on familiar terms in 1665. In that year, O'Dowde's widow, on her husband's instructions, bequeathed 'all my husbands [*sic*] Turneing Engines and Tooles' to Werden, as well as granting smaller legacies to his two sons, Robert and **John** (above). Doubts surrounding Werden's loyalty to the Stuart cause continued following his recruitment to the secret service of the Protectorate by Thomas Scott. He nonetheless participated in Booth's rising in 1659, and was reprieved after 1660, though some royalists remained unconvinced by Werden's actions. During the 1660s, he became attached to the household of the duke of York, who appointed him groom to his bedchamber (1661–1675), and through whose influence he was commissioned as a lieutenant in the duke's regiment of guards (1665), later major (1667) and lieutenant-colonel (1672–1685). He was elected as MP for Chester, on the duke's interest, in 1673, though he was inactive in Parliament. Shaftesbury nonetheless marked him as 'thrice vile' and other opponents labelled him 'a betrayer of the old Cavaliers' and 'the Duke of York's creature'. Loyalists such as Roger North, however, preferred to remember him as 'an incomparable courtier, Cavalier, and a most faithful servant in the royal family'. Prepared to fight against William of Orange, he never accepted the new regime though his death in 1690 prevented a show of active opposition.

ODNB; Henning, iii, 689–90; O'Dowde, *The Poor Man's Physician* (3rd ed., 1665), 2; TNA, PROB 11/319, fos 239r–v [will of Jane O'Dowde, widow, of St Clement Danes, Middlesex, 24 August 1665, pr. 12 February 1665/6]; *CSPD, 1660–1661*, 9; *CSPD, 1661–1662*, 218; Underdown, *Royalist Conspiracy in England*, 148–9, 288–9, 319; Thurloe, *State Papers*, iii, 337, iv, 315–16; Morrill, *County Government and Society During the English Revolution*, 255 and *passim*.

Sir Ralph WHITFIELD (b.1621)

Probably the son of Sir Ralph Whitfield (d.1645), sergeant at law to Charles I (appointed 1639) and later an active Parliamentarian. In addition to supporting the cause of the chymists at court, Whitfield was described by **Thomas O'Dowde** as a witness to the cure of one Richard Rawlinson.

Prest, *The Rise of the Barristers: A Social History of the English Bar, 1590–1640*, 402; O'Dowde, *The Poor Man's Physician* (3rd ed., 1665), 6.

APPENDIX 2 (A)

Ejected ministers practising medicine after 1660 (those not noted by Birken are marked with an asterisk)

Name	When and where ejected	Notes
John ALLIN	Vicar of Rye, 1662	Friend of Helmontian George Starkey; *Cal. Rev.*, 5–6.
Nathaniel BANNE	ejection uncertain?	MD Cambridge, 1690. Nonconformist sympathizer, who practised mainly among low church Anglicans and nonconformists in Cheshire; *Cal. Rev.*, 27; Harley, 'Licensed Physicians', 410, 414.
Andrew BARNETT	Rodington, Salop, 1662	*Cal. Rev.*, 29.
Stephen BAXTER	Harvington, Worcs, 1662	Practised medicine after ejection according to Richard Baxter. Licensed diocese of Worcester, 1663; *Cal. Rev.*, 39; WRO, 795.02/ BA 2302/8/1752.
John BEEBIE (BEEBY)	Tideswell, Derbys, 1660	Combined preaching with medicine; *Cal. Rev.*, 44–5.
Samuel BERESFORD	St Werburgh's, Derby, 1660	Limited medical practice to particular friends; *Cal. Rev.*, 51.
Robert BIRCH	Birch, Manchester	*Cal. Rev.*, 56.
Tobias BOUCHER	Creed, Cornwall, 1660	Practising medicine at Helston, 1665; *Cal. Rev.*, 66; DRO, PR 362–364/33/25.
John BRETT	Magdalen Coll., Oxford, 1661	Combined preaching with medicine; *Cal. Rev.*, 71.
Robert BRINSLEY	Emmanuel Coll., Cambridge, fellow, 1662	MD Leiden, 1668; extra-lic RCPL 1664; Innes Smith, 30; Munk, i, 315. Son of John Brinsley, ejected Yarmouth, 1662; *Cal. Rev.*, 75.
Patrick BROMFIELD	Ellington, Northumberland, 1661	*Cal. Rev.*, 77.
John BULKLEY	Fordham, Essex, 1660	Practised medicine and ministered to a congregation at Wapping; *Cal. Rev.*, 85; Calamy, *Abridgment*, ii, 311–12.

Continued

Name	When and where ejected	Notes
William BURNET(T)	Enstone, Oxon, 1660	MD Anjou, 1663; Hon Fell RCPL, 1680; *Cal. Rev.*, 90; Munk, i, 410.
Thomas CARTER	Chatham, Kent	Practised medicine at Newington Butts; licensed in archbishop of Canterbury's peculiar of the Arches, 1666; *Cal. Rev.*, 102; LPL, VH 1/1, fo. 4.
Nicholas CARY	Monmouth, 1662	Imprisoned for publishing libel in 1677. Specialized in cure of eye and ear complaints; *Cal. Rev.*, 103.
Ichabod CHAUNCY	Not ejected	Military chaplain and nonconformist. Extra-lic, RCPL, 1666; established medical practice at Bristol. Later medical student at Leiden, 1684, where engaged in seditious activity; *Cal. Rev.*, 112; Munk, i, 354–5; Innes Smith, 44.
Isaac CHAUNCY	Woodborough, Wilts, 1662	Extra-lic RCPL, 1669; full lic 1680. Presented at assizes for sedition, 1669 *Cal. Rev.*, 112; Munk, i, 415.
John CHESTER Snr	Witherley, Leics, 1660	He or son of same name, of Ewell, Surrey, licensed to practise medicine in diocese and province of Canterbury, 1683; *Cal. Rev.*, 113–4; LPL, FII/24/15; CCAL, DCb/L/R/23, fo. 203b; DCb/L/B/473.
John CLARK*	Cotgrave, Notts, 1662	Practised physick after 1662, but not for money. He was licensed to practise medicine in the diocese of Canterbury the same day as Chester (above) in 1683; Calamy, *Abridgment*, ii, 529; CCAL, DCb/L/R/23, fo. 203b; DCb/L/B/473.
Joseph CLARK	Master of Grantham School	Died 1690, as of Grantham, MD. Licensed diocese of Lincoln 1662; archdeaconry of Leicester 1679; LAO, Dioc/Sub/I, fo. 229v; LRRO, 1D 41.34/2, fo. 43r; LAO, W1690/220; *Cal. Rev.*, 118.
Abraham CLIFFORD	Clendon, Essex, 1662	MD Oxford 1670. Practised medicine in London; *Cal. Rev.*, 122.
Joseph COOPER	Moseley, nr Bromsgrove, Worcs 1662	Adept at natural philosophy, mathematics and medicine; *Cal. Rev.*,134.
Richard COORE	Tong, nr Birstall, Yorks	Presented at assizes with others in 1676 for practising medicine without a licence; antinomian; *Cal. Rev.*, 135; Como, *Blown by the Spirit*, 321–2

John COURTMAN	Thorpe Malsor, Northants, 1662	Practised medicine with great success; particularly renowned for cure of paralytic distempers and distracted people; *Cal. Rev.*, 138–9.
Luke CRANWELL	St Peter's, Derby, 1662	'Cried up for cures among nonconformist party'; *Cal. Rev.*, 142; Baily (ed.), *Account of Revd John Flamsteed*, 11; Porter, *Life of Mr John Hieron*, 33, 53.
Francis CROSS	Charlinch, Somerset, 1662	Leiden MD 1664. Practised medicine at Bristol; *Cal. Rev.*, 148; Innes Smith, 59
Thomas DOUGLAS	St Olave's, London, 1661	Conventicler; swore not to take up weapons against the King, 1666. He described himself as a 'candidate', RCPL, 1674; *Cal. Rev.*, 168; CLRO, SF 169, 28 March 1666; LPL, VX 1A/10/68.
Roger DRAKE	St Peter Cheap, London, 1660	MD Leiden, 1640; candidate, RCPL 1643 (resigned 1646). An early proponent of Harveian circulation, he gave up medicine for a career in church. Took up medicine again after 1660 at Stepney; *Cal. Rev.*, 171; Innes Smith, 72; *ODNB*.
Lewis DU MOULIN	Camden Prof of History, Oxford, 1660	MD Leiden, 1630 (incorp. Cambridge, 1634). Practised medicine in London before the civil war. Returned to medical practice after 1660. Imprisoned in 1673 for publishing 'a treasonable and seditious book'; *Cal. Rev.*, 172; Innes Smith, 74; Munk, i, 227; *ODNB*; *CSPD, 1673*, 380.
John EATON*	Bridport, Dorset, 1661	Canterbury medical licence, 1663, signed by puritan doctors Nathan Paget and Thomas Coxe; LPL, FII/4/50; F1/C, fo. 121v.
Richard EDWARDS*		Reluctant conformist according to friend, Philip Henry. Made extra-lic, RCPL, December 1662, possibly as insurance in event that he declined preferment in restored church.
Nathaniel FAIRFAX	Willisham, Suffolk, 1662	Licensed to practise medicine in the Diocese of Norwich, 1665; MD Leiden, 1670. Corresponded with RS; *Cal. Rev.*, 189; Innes Smith, 82; *ODNB*; Oldenburg, *Correspondence*.

Continued

Name	When and where ejected	Notes
Giles FIRMIN	Shelford, Essex, 1662	Practised medicine in America before returning to Essex. Returned to medical practice after 1662, when prescribing *gratis* to the poor; *Cal. Rev.*, 197; Calamy, *Abridgment*, ii, 296.
William FLOYDE	Woodford, Northants, 1660	MD Cambridge, 1661. Practised medicine at Ipswich, Suffolk. Dedicatee of Leiden theses of the sons of two nonconformist ministers, Thomas Fones and Robert Brinsley.
Daniel FOOT(E)	Swaffham Bulbeck, Cambs, 1662	MD Cambridge, 1654. Helmontian.
John FRENCH	Wenvoe, Glamorgan, 1662	Practised medicine at Cardiff.
Tobias GARBRAND	Principal of Gloucester Hall, Oxford, 1660	MD Oxford, 1648. After 1660, he practised medicine at Abingdon, where he was frequently prosecuted for his nonconformity; *Cal. Rev.*, 217.
Richard GILPIN	Greystoke, Cumberland, 1660	MD Leiden 1676. He combined a role as a leading nonconformist preacher in the north of England with a medical career after 1660; *Cal. Rev.*, 223–4; Innes Smith, 94; *ODNB*.
Henry GODMAN	Godmell, Sussex, 1660	Ex-lic RCPL 1664. Later settled at Deptford, Kent, where licensed to preach, 1672; *Cal. Rev.*, 225.
James GREENWOOD	Old Hutton, Kendal, 1662	Accused of using medicine as pretence in order to proselytize for nonconformist cause in NW England; *Cal. Rev.*, 234.
Richard GRIFFITHS	King's Coll., Cambridge, fellow	Originally destined for church, he was 'not minded to conform'. MD Caen, 1664; Hon Fell RCPL, 1664; fellow 1687.
Thomas GUNNS	Birling, Kent, 1660	Licensed to practise medicine in archdeaconry of Essex (at Great Burstead), 1666; *Cal. Rev.*, 238.
Cuthbert HARRISON	Tullaman, Tipperary	Prosecuted in 1678 for practising medicine without a licence in his native Lancashire; *Cal. Rev.*, 249; Harley,'Licensed Physicians', 406.
Leonard HOAR	Wanstead, Essex, 1660	MD Cambridge by royal letters, 1671; Returned to America, where appointed President of Harvard, 1672; *Cal. Rev.*, 269.

Paul HOBSON	Chaplain of Eton, 1660	Chemical physician and barber surgeon; leading figure among Restoration Baptists and frequently imprisoned for plotting; *Cal. Rev.*, 269.
Richard HOLBROOKE	Trinity Chapel, Salford, Lancs 1662	Licensed to practise medicine in diocese of Chester, 1673; *Cal. Rev.*, 271.
Edward HULSE	Emmanuel Coll., Cambridge, fellow, 1662	Nonconformity in question, but certainly sympathetic to dissent and physician to many nonconformists. Leiden MD, 1668 (incorp. Oxford, 1670); fellow RCPL 1677; *Cal. Rev.*, 283; Innes Smith, 123; Munk, i, 397–8.
John HUTCHINSON	Trinity Coll., Cambridge, 1660	Licensed to practise medicine by puritan president of RCPL, Dr John Micklethwaite; 1662; *Cal. Rev.*, 287.
Richard INGLETT	Exeter Coll, Oxford, 1662 fellow	Extra-lic RCPL 1661. He practised medicine at Plymouth; *Cal. Rev.*, 289; Munk, i, 298.
Timothy JORDAN	Eckington, Worcs, 1661	Practised medicine in London after ejection; *Cal. Rev.*, 303; TNA, PROB 11/330, fo. 86.
John LAUGHTON	place uncertain? Hunts?	*Cal. Rev.*, 316.
Robert LAW	Hennock, Devon, 1662	Addicted to study and practice of medicine, he was licensed to practise medicine in the diocese of Exeter, 1662; *Cal. Rev.*, 317; DRO, 518, *sub* Hennock; Mortimer, 'Index', 119.
John LOMAX	Wooler, Northumberland, 1660	Practised as doctor, surgeon and apothecary at North Shields; harassed for nonconformity; *Cal. Rev.*, 327
George LONG	Newcastle-under-Lyme, Staffs, 1661	MD Leiden 1668; practised medicine at Newcastle and Leicester; *Cal. Rev.*, 327; Innes Smith, 144.
John LYDSTON*	St Mellion, Corn'l, 1662	He may have practised physick after 1662, as he owned a manuscript volume of medical and surgical recipes; *Cal. Rev.*, 331; BL. Sloane MS 500.
John MANSHIP	St Nicholas, Guildford, Surrey, 1660	Extra-lic RCPL 1663. He also received a licence to practise in the province of Canterbury in 1665; *Cal. Rev.*, 337–8; Munk, i, 308; LPL, VG 1/1, fo. 185; Sheldon, fo. 204.

Continued

Name	When and where ejected	Notes
William MARSHALL	Lancaster, 1660	MD Cambridge 1652; candidate RCPL 1669; *Cal. Rev.*, 341; Munk, i, 358.
Edmund MATTHEWS	Wollaston, Northants, 1662	Practised at Wellingborough; *Cal. Rev.*, 344–5.
Henry MAURICE*	Conformed 1662, but subsequently resigned out of conscience, *c.*1671	Occasionally practised physic while simultaneously enjoining spiritual counsel; Palmer, *Nonconformist's Memorial*, ii, 341.
Richard MORTON Snr	Kinver, Staffs, 1662	MD Oxford, 1670 (incorp. Cambridge, 1680); fellow RCPL 1679; physician to Prince of Orange and later physician in ordinary to same as William III; *Cal. Rev.*, 357; Munk, 398–400.
Samuel OGDEN	Mackworth, Derbys, 1662	Well versed in all branches of natural philosophy, including medicine, botany and anatomy, and early adherent of Cartesianism; *Cal. Rev.*, 371–2.
Samuel OLDERSHAW	Coleorton, Leics, 1660	Chaplain and physician; *Cal. Rev.*, 373.
John PANTON	All Souls, Oxford, fellow, 1660	His brother Henry was also a physician and nonconformist; *Cal. Rev.*, 380–1.
John PEACHY	St Paul's Walden, Herts, 1662	MD Caen, *c.*1683. Practised medicine at Gloucester and Oxford; licensed RCPL 1683. Chemical physician; *Cal. Rev.*, 384; Munk, i, 430–1; SAL, MS 202, fo. 173.
William PELL	Gt Staunton, Durham, 1662	Practised physick in north Yorkshire and later served as assistant to Richard Gilpin at Newcastle; Calamy, *Abridgment*, ii, 288–90.
Richard PERROT	York Cathedral, 1660	Extra-lic RCPL 1670; *Cal. Rev.*, 387; Munk, i, 360.
Robert PERROT	Nether Dean, Beds, 1662	B. Med Cambridge, 1642. Combined preaching and medicine after ejection, at Kettering, Nottingham and Maidstone; *Cal. Rev.*, 387.
John PRATT	Trinity Coll., Cambridge, fellow, 1660	MD Cambridge, 1645; candidate RCPL 1649. He practised medicine at Abingdon before the civil war, and served the parliamentary forces in 1640s; *Cal. Rev.*, 398; Munk, i, 252; Berkshire RO, D/A2/c/162, fo. 6; TNA, SP 28/35/III, fo. 380; Adair, 'Court Martial', 210–11.

John PRINGLE	Eglington, Northumberland, 1662	Extra-lic RCPL 1662. Practised with fellow physician and ejected minister, Richard Gilpin at Newcaste. Imprisoned 1665; *Cal. Rev.*, 400; Munk, i, 307.
Richard RESBURY	Oundle, Northants, 1662	Practised physic at Oundle after Ejection; *Cal. Rev.*, 407.
John REYNER	Emmanuel Coll., Cambridge, fellow, 1662	Practised medicine at Nottingham after ejection; *Cal. Rev.*, 408.
John REYNOLDS	Wolverhampton, Staffs, 1660	MD Leiden 1682. Shortly before, he was prosecuted for practising medicine without a licence at Stourbridge in Worcestershire. Executor of the will of Joseph Cooper (above); *Cal. Rev.*, 409; Innes Smith, 193; WRO, 795.02/ BA 2302/33/7390; Birmingham City Archives, MS 3440/Acc 1933-029/412046.
Edward RICHARDSON	Ripon, Yorks, 1660	Extra-lic RCPL 1662; MD Leiden 1664; *Cal. Rev.*, 410–11; Munk, i, 307; Innes Smith, 144; see also above pp. ???–???.
John RICHARDSON	Stamford, Lincs, 1662	Practised at Stamford after ejection; *Cal. Rev.*, 411.
Edward RIGGS*	St John's Thanet, 1660	Radical turncoat, who under cover of acting as a physician spied on former comrades in the Netherlands; Marshall, *Intelligence and Espionage*, 145–6.
Thomas RISLEY*	Pembroke Coll., Oxford, fellow	Practised medicine at Risley, Warks, where he also preached and taught school; *ODNB*.
Samuel ROLLS	Dunton, Bucks, 1661 or 1662	Claimed to have taken up medicine 'by the great Suspition which I had of the Approaching ruine of Schollars in the late times'; MD Cambridge, 1675; *Cal. Rev.*, 415–6; Cooper, *Annals of Cambridge*, iii, 570.
Thomas ROSEWELL*	Sutton Mandeville, Wilts, 1662	Probably did not practise medicine, but clearly possessed wide interest in the Subject. Author of tract on plague, 1665. Also refuted king's ability to heal those afflicted with king's evil for which he was tried, found guilty, but pardoned; *Cal. Rev.*, 418.

Continued

Name	When and where ejected	Notes
Gilbert RULE	Alnwick, Northumberland, 1660	Leiden MD, 1665. Accused of plotting, often prosecuted. In 1678, described as unlicensed physician living at Berwick-upon-Tweed; *Cal. Rev.*, 420; Innes Smith, 200; *CSPD, 1678*, 553.
Henry SAMPSON	Framlingham, Suffolk, 1660	MD Leiden, 1668; Hon Fell RCPL, 1680. Dedicatee of numerous Leiden theses; *Cal. Rev.*, 425; Innes Smith, 30, 58, 66, 102, 204; Munk, i, 410–12.
John SINGLETON	Christ Church, Oxford, 1660	MD Utrecht 1671. Nephew of Congregationalist, John Owen; *Cal. Rev.*, 443–4; Innes Smith, 214.
John SKINNER*	Weston under Penyard with Hope Mansell, Herefordshire 1660	Described as a 'medical practitioner' when prosecuted for preaching at a conventicle in Abingdon, 1670. Baptist; Capp, *Fifth Monarchy Men*, 262; Berkshire RO, A/JQ/z/11, *sub* 15 May 1670.
Richard SMITH*	Whitestaunton, Somerset, 1662	Physician after ejection; Calamy, *Abridgment*, ii, 613.
Samuel SMITH*	St Olave, Southwark, 1662	Surgeon and chemical physician. Licensed to practise medicine in diocese of Winchester, 1667, and province of Canterbury, 1685. Frequently prosecuted for preaching, and refused parish office 1672; Bax, 'Marriage and Other Licences', 240; LPL, VX 1A/10/225/1–2; VG 1/3, fo. 88v; Sancroft, fo. 256; SHC, QR 2/5, Epiph'y, 1683, 55, 101; QS 2/1/3, 69.
Philip STEPHENS	Principal, Hart Hall, Oxford, 1660	MD Oxford 1656; candidate RCPL, 1659; Birken, 'Dissenting Tradition', 216; Munk, i, 296 [medical career not noted in *Cal. Rev.*].
Anthony STEPHENSON	Roos, Yorkshire, 1662	Schoolmaster, clergyman and physician; *Cal. Rev.*, 462–3; Bickford and Bickford, *Medical Profession in Hull*, 123.
James STEPHENSON	Martock, Somerset, 1662	Studied medicine at Leiden 1650 but did not graduate. Combined medical practice with clerical duties both before and after ejection. Licensed to practise in dioceses of Bath and Wells, Exeter and Gloucester, 1662. Son, John (d.1656), a physician; *Cal. Rev.*, 463; LPL, FII/3/252; F1/C, fo. 108.

Samuel STODDON	West Buckland, Somerset	Specialized in cure and treatment of distracted; *Cal. Rev.*, 464–5.
John SWAN	Ickham, Kent, 1662	Licensed to practise medicine in diocese of Canterbury, 1662. Possibly same as JS, appointed physician in extraordinary to Charles II, 1670; CCAL, DCb/L/R/17; TNA, LC 3/26, fo. 143.
Titus THOMAS	Aston, Salop	Practised medicine at Shrewsbury after ejection; *Cal. Rev.*, 481.
William TREVETHECK*	Petrockstow, Cornwall 1662	In all probability the same as the WT, BA, of Horwood, Devon, who was licensed to practise medicine by the Archbishop of Canterbury in 1681 (with the testimonials of two Cornish medics); LPL, VX 1A/10/158/1–3; Sancroft, fo. 237v.
Andrew TRISTRAM	Bridgnorth, Salop, 1662	Extra-lic RCPL 1667. Licensed to preach 1672; *Cal. Rev.*, 493; Munk, i, 355.
Thomas TROIT	Owermoigne, Dorset, 1660	Practised medicine at Coningsby, Lincs, after ejection; *Cal. Rev.*, 494–5.
John TROTTLE*	Spettisbury, Dorset, 1660	Practised medicine at Thorncombe, Dorset, after the Restoration; DRO, PR 362–364/33/9.
Edward WARREN	St Peter's, Colchester, 1662	Extra-lic RCPL 1667. Practised medicine at Colchester after ejection; *Cal. Rev.*, 511; Munk, i, 355; Calamy, *Abridgment*, ii, 293.
Bartholomew WESTLEY	Allington, Bridport, Dorset, 1662	Practised medicine before and after ejection. Licensed to practise in the diocese of Bristol, 1662; *Cal. Rev.*, 521; LPL, FII/3/277; F1/C, fo. 107v.
Edmund WHINCOP*	Leiston, Suffolk	Practised medicine before civil war; practice after Restoration speculative; *Cal. Rev.*, 523.
John WILSON	Hulcott, Bucks, 1660	*Cal. Rev.*, 536.
Robert WOOD	Lincoln Coll, Oxford, fellow, 1660	Licensed to practise medicine by Univ. of Oxford, 1656; Birken, 'Dissenting Tradition', 216; *ODNB*; Foster, iv, 1672.

Note: Birken includes in his sample the name of Thomas Woodcock (*Cal. Rev.*, 543–4). However, I have not found any reference to Woodcock's practice of medicine at any stage in his career. In all probability, Birken has confused Thomas with his son, Samuel, who enrolled as a medical student at Leiden; see Appendix 2 (a).

APPENDIX 2 (B)

Sons of ejected ministers who studied and/or practised medicine after the Restoration (those unnoticed by Birken are marked with an asterisk)

Name	Father	Notes
Bezaliel ANGIER*	Samuel Angier	MD Utrecht, 1703; licentiate RCPL,1710; *Cal. Rev.*, 12–13; Innes Smith, 6; Munk, ii, 33.
John BAGLEY*	William Bagley	MD Utrecht, 1682. Practised medicine at Worcester; physician to godly Harley family of Brampton Bryan; *Cal. Rev.*, 21; Innes Smith, 11; *HMC.14th Report, Appx, Part III: MSS of Duke of Portland, vol.3*, 438, 483.
John BALL*	William Ball	MD Utrecht, 1688. Combined medicine with ministry to nonconformist congregation at Honiton, Devon; *Cal. Rev.*, 25; Innes Smith, 14.
Nicholas BARBON	Praisegod Barbon	MD Utrecht, 1661; Hon Fell RCPL, 1664. Did not practice; Innes Smith, 14; Munk, i, 345.
William BELCHER*	William Belcher	B. Med Cambridge, 1680; MD 1708. Practised medicine at Maidstone, Kent; *Cal. Rev.*, 45–6; Venn, i, 126.
Nathaniel BLINMAN*	Richard Blinman	Practised at Bridgwater, Somerset. Licensed for province of Canterbury, 1680 (supported by two nonconformist medics); *Cal. Rev.*, 61; LPL, VX 1A/10/143/1–4; Sancroft, fo. 231.
William BOSSE*	Thomas Bosse	Practised at Blaby, Leics. Licensed to practise medicine and surgery in the archdeaconry of Leicester, 1677; *Cal. Rev.*, 65; LRRO, 1D 41/34/2, fo. 38r.

Thomas BOWLES*	Edward Bowles	Medical student at Leiden (enrolled same day, and lodged with fellow Yorkshire student Daniel Richardson (below). No evidence of practice; *Cal. Rev.*, 67; Innes Smith, p.28; LUA, ASF 12, 60.
Robert BRINSLEY*	John Brinsley	See Appendix 2 (a).
Thomas BROWNE*	Edward Brown(e)?	Practised at Stamford, Lincs. Extra-lic RCPL, 1662 (father, Edward, ejected at Stamford); *Cal. Rev.*, 80; Munk, i, 306.
Timothy BYFIELD	Richard Byfield	Described himself as MD. Fellow of College of Physicians, Dublin, 1676. Author of various works in which he showed a preference for chemical medicines over Galenic, and cited van Helmont favourably. He practised in London and was later attracted to the French Prophets, entering into a partnership to sell patent medicines with fellow supporter of the Prophets and chemist, Francis Moult; *Cal. Rev.*, 97; Byfield, *Short and Plain Account* (1687), 6–7, 11–12, 12–13; Wales and Hartley (eds), *Visitation of London, 1687*, ii, 623; *The Honest Quaker* (1707), 4–6, 8–9; TNA, PROB 11/594, fos 217v–218r.
Daniel CAPEL*	Daniel Capel	He practised, like his father, at Stroud, Gloucs. Licensed to practise in the diocese of Gloucester, 1680; *Cal. Rev.*, 101; *m. i.*, St Lawrence's, Stroud; GRO, GDR 226A, 61. NB. There is some doubt as to whether his father was ejected or voluntarily quit the church.
John CART(E)*	John Carte	Ex-lic RCPL, 1674. Practised medicine at Manchester; *Cal. Rev.*, 102; Munk, i, 368.
John CHESTER Jnr	John Chester	Practised at Guildford, Surrey (father, above, also a physician); *Cal. Rev.*, 114.
John CHISHULL	John Chishull	*Cal. Rev.*, 115.
Mathew CLARKE	Mathew Clarke	Birken, 'Dissenting Tradition', 217.

Continued

Name	Father	Notes
Robert COURTMAN	John Courtman	B Med Cambridge, 1684. He probably practised at Bedford; *Cal. Rev.*, 138–9; Venn, i, 406.
Samuel CRADOCK*	Samuel Cradock	MD Leiden, 1693; *Cal. Rev.*, 140–1; Innes Smith, p.55.
John CROFTS	John Crofts	Practised at Romsey, Hants; *Cal. Rev.*, 145; Hampshire RO, 1708B/17.
Christopher DOMINICK*	John Dominick?	MD Oxford 1675; practised medicine at Dublin. Elected MP Ardfert 1692, but died the same year. Probably the son of John D, ejected at King's Lynn; Foster, i, 413; *N & Q*, 6 (1912), 477.
John DURANT	William Durant	MD Leiden 1671; *Cal. Rev.*, 174; Innes Smith, 76.
Blackerby FAIRFAX	Nathaniel Fairfax	Medical student Leiden 1696. MD Cambridge, 1728. Author of works on history, politics, botany and medicine; *Cal. Rev.*, 189; Innes Smith, 82.
Nathaniel FAIRFAX	Benjamin Fairfax	see Appendix 2 (a).
Thomas FAIRFAX*	John Fairfax	Practised at Needham Market, Suffolk; Licensed in province of Canterbury (with signatures of two nonconformist physicians of RCPL), 1687; *ODNB*, sub Fairfax, John; LPL, VX 1A/10/239/1–2.
Nathaniel FIRMIN	Giles Firmin	Licentiate RCPL 1676. He or his son, of Castle Hedingham, Essex, licensed to practise medicine in province of Canterbury, 1704; Venn, ii, 140; Munk, i, 389; LPL, VX 1A/10/376; VG 1/6, fo. 199v; Tenison 1, fo. 155.
John and Samuel FISHER*	James Fisher	Both physicians, practising at Sheffield; Oldenburg, *Correspondence*, vii, 387n.
Thomas FONES	Samuel Fones	MD Leiden, 1669. Practised medicine at Ipswich; *Cal. Rev.*, 204; Innes Smith, 86.
Francis FULLER*	Francis Fuller	Author of medical work on the therapeutic virtues of exercise. No evidence of medical practice; *Cal. Rev.*, 215; *ODNB*; Fuller, *Medicina Gymnastica* (1705).
Joseph GAYLARD*	Robert Gaylard	MD Leiden 1688 (incorp. Cambridge, 1693); candidate RCPL, 1694. Fought at Sedgmoor; *Cal. Rev.*, 218–9; Innes Smith, 92; Munk, i, 504.

John GILES or GYLES	John Giles or Gyles	Giles' father was a nonconformist minister, but not ejected. JG Jnr MD Utrecht, 1699. Succeeded Samuel Benion as pastor of Presbyterian academy at Shrewsbury, 1708?; Innes Smith, 104; *ODNB*, sub Reynolds, John.
Thomas GOLDHAM	Thomas Goldham	Physician, of Burwash, Sussex (d.1679). Probably the son of Thomas Goldham, ejected minister of Burwash, 1662; *Cal. Rev.*, 226.
Nehemiah GREW	Obadiah Grew	MD Leiden, 1671; FRS 1671; Hon Fell RCPL 1680; *Cal. Rev.*, 236; Innes Smith, 102; Munk, i, 406–9; *ODNB*.
Thomas GROVE	Edward Grove	Practised medicine at Taunton; *Cal. Rev.*, 237.
Joseph HALLET(T)*	Joseph Hallet(t)	Medical student, Leiden, 1685. No evidence of medical practice; *Cal. Rev.*, 243; Innes Smith, 105.
Joseph HALSEY	Joseph Halsey	MD Utrecht 1691. Thesis dedicated to Hugh Boscawen, Whig exclusionist MP, Presbyterian and father's patron; *Cal. Rev.*, 244; Innes Smith, 105.
Edward HARDING	John Harding	Extra-lic RCPL 1661. Practised at Northampton. Father translated works of Paracelsus in 1650s; *Cal. Rev.*, 247; Munk, i, 302; Webster, *Great Instauration*, 281.
Clopton HAVERS	Henry Havers	MD Utrecht, 1685; FRS 1686; extra-lic, RCPL, 1684; licentiate 1687; *Cal. Rev.*, 252; *ODNB*; Innes Smith, 110; Munk, i, 477.
Samuel HAWORTH	William Haworth	Extra-lic RCPL, 1680 and physician to duke of York. Author of numerous works; *Cal. Rev.*, 254; Munk, i, 416–7; *ODNB*.
William HICKMAN*	Henry Hickman	WH probably a medical student at Leiden in 1680s, when father Henry served as pastor to English church there; *Cal. Rev.*, 260–1; Innes Smith, 117.
William HOLBROOKE	Richard Holbrooke	B. Med Cambridge, 1686. Practised medicine at Salford; *Cal. Rev.*, 271; Venn, ii, 388.
Adam HOLLAND*	Thomas Holland	MD Leiden, 1687. Combined medical with nonconformist ministry at Macclesfield; *Cal. Rev.*, 272–3; Innes Smith, 119.

Continued

Name	Father	Notes
George HOWE	John Howe	MD Leiden 1679; licentiate RCPL, 1679; fellow 1687; *ODNB.*
Sir Edward HULSE	Edward Hulse	MD Cambridge, 1717; fellow RCPL, 1718; Venn, ii, 429.
Samuel JOLLYor JOLLIE*	Thomas Jolly or Jollie	Extra-lic RCPL, 1680; *Cal. Rev.*, 301; Munk, i, 405.
Diodat LAWSON*	Thomas Lawson	physician in ordinary without fee, 1672. Emigrated to New England, where pastor to congregation at Scituate; *Cal. Rev.*, 319; TNA, LC 3/27, fo. 46v.
Gershom LEVERTON*	Nicholas Leverton	Surgeon, at Plymouth, who died there while attending Dutch prisoners of war; *Cal. Rev.*, 324.
Theophilus LOBB	Stephen Lobb	Practised medicine at Shaftesbury, Dorset. Licensed to practise throughout the province of Canterbury, 1707; Birken, 'Dissenting Tradition', 217; LPL, VX 1A/10/415; VG 1/6, fo. 225; Tenison, fo. 268.
John LUFF	John Luff	MD Oxford, 1673; regius prof. of medicine, Oxford, 1681–98; *Cal. Rev.*, 330–1; Foster, iii, 949.
John MARTIN or MARTYN*	Thomas Martyn	Licentiate RCPL, 1683; *Cal. Rev.*, 342 (ejected Plymouth, 1661); Foster, iii, 979; Munk, i, 428.
Samuel MAYNE*	Zachary Mayne	B. Med Oxford, 1708. Physician to pioneering hospital at Northampton; *Cal. Rev.*, 346–7; Foster, iii, 995.
Richard MEAD(E)	Matthew Mead(e)	MD Padua, 1695; FRS 1703; fellow RCPL, 1716; physician in ordinary to George II. Celebrated Whig physician; *Cal. Rev.*, 348; *ODNB.*
Sir John MICKLETHWAITE*	Thomas Micklethwaite	MD Padua 1638. Leading figure in RCPL, acting as its President, 1676–1681. A nonconformist sympathizer who probably used his authority to assist medics from dissenting backgrounds; *Cal. Rev.*, 349; *ODNB.*
Joseph MORLAND	Martin Morland	MD Leiden 1699; FRS 1703. He practised at Epsom in Surrey; *Cal. Rev.*, 355; Innes Smith, 164.
Richard MORTON Jnr	Richard Morton Snr	MD Cambridge, 1695; fellow RCPL 1707; Venn, iii, 218; Munk, ii, 20.

Charles NICHOLS*	Charles Nichols	MD Caen, 1679; licentiate RCPL, 1687. Practised medicine at Faversham, Kent, and Stepney, Middlesex; *Cal. Rev.*, 365–6; Munk, i, 476.
Rupert NYE	Philip Nye	*Cal. Rev.*, 370.
William OLIVER*	William Oliver	MD Rheims 1699, previously medical student at Leiden in 1680s. Licentiate RCPL, 1692; FRS 1704. Served as surgeon to rebel forces of duke of Monmouth, 1685; *Cal. Rev.*, 373–4; *ODNB*; Innes Smith, 173; Munk, i, 493–4.
Daniel OXENBRIDGE	John Oxenbridge	MD Leiden, 1662, dedicated to nonconformist medic Richard Burthogge; *Cal. Rev.*, 377–8; Birken, 'Dissenting Tradition, 377–8; Innes Smith, 175.
Matthew POOLE	Matthew Poole	MD Cambridge by royal mandate 1684. Earlier enrolled as a medical student at Leiden, 1675; *Cal. Rev.*, 394–5; Innes Smith, 185.
Daniel RICHARDSON*	Edward Richardson	Entered Leiden as medical student, 1678 *Cal. Rev.*, 410–11; Innes Smith, 193.
Gilbert RULE Jnr	Gilbert Rule Snr	MD Harderwyck, 1683; *Cal. Rev.*, 420; Innes Smith, 200.
John SHARP*	Thomas Sharp	Medical student at Leiden; *Cal. Rev.*, 434; Innes Smith, 208.
Samuel SHAW*	Samuel Shaw	MD Utrecht, 1692, thesis dedicated to former Whig plotter, Thomas Grey, 2nd Earl of Stamford. Master of Free Grammar Schhol, Tamworth, 1708, a position previously held by his father; *Cal. Rev.*, 435; Innes Smith, 209.
Nicholas SHERWILL*	Nicholas Sherwill	Medical student at Leiden, 1699, 1701; *Cal. Rev.*, 439; Innes Smith, 210.
Nathaniel SMITH*	Samuel Smith, ejected St Bennet Gracechurch, London	Surgeon at St Bartholomew's Hospital; *Cal. Rev.*, 568.
Augustine SWIFT*	Richard Swift	Licensed to practise medicine by the archbishop of Canterbury, 1684. He practised at Hendon, Middlesex; LPL, VX 1A/10/216/1–2; VG 1/3, fo. 110; Sancroft, fo. 251v.

Continued

Name	Father	Notes
Edmund THORPE*	Edmund Thorpe.	Licensed to practise medicine by the archbishop of Canterbury, 1677. He practised at Wokingham, Berks; LPL, VX 1A/10/106; VG 1/3, 320; Venn, iv, 236; ESxRO, DUN 51/74; SAS-RF/3/66; TNA, PROB 11/557, fos 27v–28r. Brother of Thomas, below.
Thomas THORPE	Edmund Thorpe.	Intended for ministry; B. Med Cambridge, 1666. Practised medicine at Ashford, Kent, where he actively supported the local Presbyterian church; *Cal. Rev.*, 485; Venn, iv, 237. Brother of Edmund, above.
Matthew TOOGOOD*	Matthew Toogood.	Practised medicine at Axminster, Somerset, where he was also ruling elder of dissenting congregation. In 1694, he applied for a medical licence from the archbishop of Canterbury (with support of the vicar and churchwardens of the parish); no licence registered. Extra-licentiate RCPL, 1694. His son John, MD Leiden, 1718; *Cal. Rev.*, 489; LPL, VX 1A/10/285; Munk, i, 511–12; Innes Smith, 234.
Elias TRAVERS*	Thomas Travers	Studied medicine and divinity in 1670s. Nonconformist minister in Ireland. No evidence of medical practice; *Cal. Rev.*, 490; Venn, iv, 261.
William TREIS*	William Treis?	Medical student at Leiden, 1687. Son of William Treis, ejected at St Mabyn, Cornwall, 1660?; *Cal. Rev.*, 491–2; Innes Smith, 235.
John WALROND*	Thomas Walrond	Practised physic at Exeter; *Cal. Rev.*, 508; Foster, iv, 1563; TNA, PROB 11/472, fos 124v–125r.
Matthew WESTLEY*	John Westley	Practised medicine and surgery in London (d.1737). Uncle of founder of Methodism; *Cal. Rev.*, 521.
William WESTMACOTT*	William Westmacott	Practised medicine at Newcastle under Lyme, Staffs. Author of two medical Works, 1694; *Cal. Rev.*, 521–22; FSL, MS V.a.441; Krivatsky, William Westmacott's *Memorabilia*', 331–8.

Samuel WOODCOCK	Thomas Woodcock.	Medical student at Leiden, 1685. No evidence of medical practice; *Cal. Rev.*, 543–4; Innes Smith, 252.
John WOODHOUSE*	John Woodhouse	MD Leiden 1700, thesis dedicated to father. Practised at Nottingham and buried alongside father at Rearsby, Leics, 1733; *Cal. Rev.*, 544; Innes Smith, 252; TNA, PROB 11/458, fos 190r–191r.
John WORTH*	John Worth	According to Palmer, Worth took a degree in physic and practised at Marlborough in Wiltshire, where he was also minister to a dissenting congregation; *Cal. Rev.*, p546–7; Palmer, *Nonconformist's Memorial*, ii, 229–30.
John YARDLEY*	John Yardley	MD Padua, *c.*1662; previously studied medicine at Leiden. Hon Fell, RCPL, 1664. Practised medicine at Bishop's Stortford; JP Hertfordshire; *Cal. Rev.*, 550; Venn, iv, 487; Innes Smith, 255; Munk, i, 350–1.

Note: Also included in Birken's list were Nicholas Munckley (son of John), Robert Nesbitt (son of John) and John Oldfield (son of Joshua), all the offspring of men who only became dissenting ministers after 1662. The list of men falling in this category could also be expanded greatly with further research.

APPENDIX 2 (C)

Sons of ejected ministers apprenticed to London apothecaries after the Restoration

Name	Father	Master	Date
William AMES	William Ames	David Clarke	1665
Joseph BATT	Timothy Batt	Jonathan Leigh	1682
Elijah BEANE	Alexander Beane	Richard Worcester	1677

Beane practised as an apothecary in Stepney, Middlesex, where he was a member of the congregation of the ejected minister George Day; TNA, PROB 11/420, fos 7r–8r [will of Elijah Beane, apothecary, of Ratcliffe in Stepney, Middlesex, 25 November 1693, pr. 24 May 1694].

Samuel BOHEME	Maurice Boheme	Isaac Dover	1673
Samuel CLARKE	John Clarke	Edward Baker	1674
Nathaniel COLLINS	George Collins	David Clarke	1670
John COOPER	Joseph Cooper	William Beckwith	1677

Cooper sold his father's posthumous *A Prospect of Heavenly Glory* (London, 1700) from his shop in Whitechapel, Middlesex; *Cal. Rev.*, 134.

William CORNISH	Henry Cornish	Simon Lloyd	1677

Described as a student of medicine at Oxford, he was admitted as an extra licentiate of the London College of Physicians in 1686. 'Doctor' Cornish later settled at Chertsey, Surrey and was buried in the dissenter burial ground there in 1733; Munk, i, 438; SHC, CHY/1/4 [parish registers of Chertsey, Surrey, 1721–1755]; TNA, PROB 11/656, fos 39v–41r [will of William Cornish of Chertsey, 14 July 1732, pr. 15 January 1732/3].

Peter CROUCH	John Crouch	William Booker	1674

Peter Crouch, apothecary, was buried at Bunhill Fields, 21 August 1710; Booker's own son Samuel was apprenticed to William Sell, apothecary, of London who was himself the son of an ejected schoolmaster; *Cal. Rev.*, 433.

Josias FRENCH	John French	Robert Phelpes	1672
Samuel FRENCH	John French	Belliver Davies	1674
Samuel HARDY	Samuel Hardy	Robert Phelpes	1691
John HAWORTH	William Haworth	Mark Stratton	1678
Isaac HUNT	Edward Hunt	Simon Lloyd	1680
John HUTCHINSON	John Hutchinson	Zachary Allen	1695
John KESTIN	Nicholas Kestin	Jeremiah Lawry/Lowry	1671
Jeremiah LAWRY/LOWRY	Thomas Lawry/Lowry	John Rogers	1662
Vincent LAWSON	Vincent Lawson	William Phillipps	1675
Henry LUKIN	Henry Lukin	Robert Porter	1689

Henry Lukin Snr (1628–1719) was an author of devotional guides and a friend of John Locke; *ODNB*, sub Lukin, Henry; *Cal. Rev.*, 331.

Samuel MALTHUS	Robert Malthus	John Thorpe	1663

Samuel's brother Daniel Malthus (1652–1717) was made free as a London apothecary in 1678 (no record of an apprenticeship has been found). He set up shop next to his close friend Dr Thomas Sydenham (he named a son Sydenham after him) in Pall Mall and became exceedingly wealthy, serving as apothecary to Queen Anne; P. James, *Population Malthus: His Life and Times* (London & New York, 2006; 1st ed., 1979), 5–6.

Walter MARSHALL	Walter Marshall	Simon Brinsmead	1672
Joseph NICHOLLS	Charles Nicholls	Edward Baker	1671

Brother of the physician Charles Nicholls, he was probably dead before 1679 as he is not mentioned in his father's will.

John NOTT	John Nott	Belliver Davies	1669
Andrew PARSONS	Andrew Parsons	Mark Stratton	1664
Elias PLEDGER	Elias Pledger	Mark Stratton	1680
Joseph SACHEVERELL	John Sacheverell	George Wright	1675
Nathaniel SCARLETT	William Scarlett	Mark Stratton	1685
Philip SHERWOOD	Joseph Sherwood	Jonathan Wilson	1684

Wilson was the son of Thomas Wilson, the puritan minister of Stratford upon Avon, Warwickshire.

Samuel SILVESTER	Matthew Silvester	Jonathan Dodsworth	1687
John STALHAM	John Stalham	William Sell	1668
John STARR	Comfort Starr	David Clarke	1679

His father Comfort Starr was said to be living with his son John on Tower Hill in 1690; *Cal. Rev.*, 460.

Jonathan TRAY	William Tray	Thomas Rolfe/Rolphe	1676

Rolfe was a nonconformist and was buried at Bunhill Fields; TNA, PROB 11/379, fo. 71r–72r [will of Thomas Rolfe, citizen and apothecary, of London, 13 October 1683, pr. 7 January 1684/5]; PROB 11/397, fos 201v–203r [will of Susanna Rolfe, widow, 5 May 1688, pr. 30 November 1689].

Edward TREDCROFT	John Tredcroft	Thomas Hotchkis	1666
Thomas TREGOSSE	Thomas Tregosse	Robert Phelpes	1678
John TROTT	John Trott	Joseph Pawlett	1688
Matthew WESTLEY	John Westley	Thomas Fox	1679
Thomas WILSON	John Wilson	Daniel Freeman	1682

Freeman was a close friend of the prominent nonconformist minister and physician, Henry Sampson; TNA, PROB 11/440, fos 45v–46r [will of Daniel Freeman, citizen and apothecary, of London, 28 November 1696, pr. 13 September 1697]. Another of his apprentices Edmund Frost married the daughter of the ejected minister John Meadows of Eusden, Suffolk. Frost himself was made an extra licentiate of the College of Physicians in 1704 and practised medicine at Hunston, Suffolk; Munk, ii, 14. Wilson (d.1699) himself was a nonconformist and like his father was a great admirer of Richard Baxter; TNA, PROB 11/452, fos 97r–98r [will of Thomas Wilson, apothecary, of London, 20 March 1698/9, pr. 1 August 1699].

Continued

Name	Father	Master	Date
George WOODMAN	Matthew Woodman	Thomas Hotchkis	1670
Richard WRAGG	Christopher Wragg	Edward Pilkington	1674
Jonathan WRIGHT	Robert Wright	Thomas Hotchkis	1674

In addition:

William Grace, the son of the ejected minister Walter Grace, was apprenticed to Richard Baily, apothecary, of London, in 1652.

Benjamin King (d.1703), apothecary, of Sleaford, Lincolnshire, was the son of the ejected minister of the same name.

Thomas Marshall, the son of the dissenting minister and physician Thomas Marshall (1639–1693) of Ilminster, Somerset, was apprenticed to Robert Jackson, apothecary, of London in 1686.

Edward Prince, the son of Edward Prince, the Whig and nonconformist town clerk of Oxford, was apprenticed to Jonathan Wilson, apothecary, of London in 1667. Prince Jnr set up in medical practice in Barbados.

William Sell, the son of the ejected schoolmaster William Sell, was apprenticed to Ann Glover, apothecary, of London in 1650.

Nathaniel Smart, the son of Ithiell Smart (d.1661), the Presbyterian minister of Ashby de la Zouch, Leicestershire, was apprenticed to his uncle Richard Litler, apothecary, of London in 1661. Smart's death in 1661 almost certainly prevented his ejection. Litler himself was on friendly terms with the nonconformist Thomas Watson (d.1686); TNA, PROB 11/346, fos 332v–334v [will of Richard Lytler, citizen and apothecary, of London, 8 August 1673 & 26 November 1674, pr. 5 December 1674].

APPENDIX 3

Medical Mayors

Thomas Agar	Apothecary	Kingston u Thames	1685–6
George Allat	Apothecary	Coventry, Wks	1684–5
John Allington	Apothecary	Banbury, Oxon	1680–1
John Archer	Physician	Kendal, Westm'd	1706–7
Thomas Archer	Physician	Hertford, Herts	1681–2, 1694–5
Henry Arnold alias Groves	Surgeon	Malmesbury, Wilts	1670–1
James Arthur Snr	Surgeon	Hythe, Kent	1657–8
Francis Banister	Physician	Bedford, Beds	1635–6
Lawrence Banyer	Physician	Wisbech, Cambs	1705–6
Peter Baro	Physician	Boston, Lincs	1610–11
Charles Baron	Chemist/ druggist	Wells, Somerset [p.r., St Cuthbert, Wells]	'8 times mayor'
Francis Bave	Apothecary	Bath, Somerset	1729–30
Robert Bent	Apothecary	Reading, Berks	1634–5, 1640–1
John Bigg	Physician	Wycombe, Bucks	1686–7, 1692–3, 1701–2
George Birch	Apothecary	Norwich, Norfolk	1621–2
Sampson Birch	Apothecary	Stafford, Staffs	1671–2, 1681–2, 1685–6
Robert Blease	Apothecary	Chester, Cheshire	1603–4
Thomas Bliss	Surgeon	Maidstone, Kent	1682–3
Septimus Bott	Apothecary	Coventry, Wks	1686–7
John Boyce	Apothecary	Bath, Somerset	1655–6
Abel Brookesby	Apoth'y/ physician	Coventry, Wks	1671–2
Moses Bruch	Apothecary/ physician	Windsor, Berks	1690–1
William Bubb	Apothecary	Gloucester, Glos	1671–2
Benjamin Bullivant	Apoth'y/ physician	Northampton, Nts	1702–3
John Bullack/Bullock	Surgeon	Dover, Kent	1674–6, 1689–90
Thomas Burford	Apothecary	Bath, Somerset	1642–3
John Burrell	Druggist	Exeter, Devon	1698–9, 1718–19

William Callis	Apothecary	Leicester, Leics	1664–5
Samuel Case	Apothecary	Stratford u Avon, Wks	1693–4
William Chamberlen	Physician	Shaftesbury, Dorset	1664–5, 1674–5 1685–6
Cuthbert Chambers	Apothecary	Ripon, Yorks	1675–6, 1706–7 & 2 other occasions
William Chambers	Apothecary	Ripon, Yorks	1688–9, 1699–1700 1709–10
Robert Chapman	Apothecary	Bath, Somerset	1668–9, 1678–9, 1689–90
Charles Child	Apothecary	Bath, Somerset	1709–10
William Clarke	Apothecary	Grantham, Lincs	1651–2, 1657–8
Tobias Cleare/Cleere	Apoth'y/surgeon	Sandwich, Kent	1649–50, 1654–5, 1660–1, 1670–1
William Clemson	Apothecary	Shrewsbury, Salop	1709–10
Joseph Colfe	Apothecary	Canterbury, Kent	1611–12
William Collibee	Apothecary	Bath, Somerset	1719–20
Edward Collins	Apothecary	Exeter, Devon	1709–10
John Collins	Apothecary	Exeter, Devon	1679–80
Christiopher Concett	Apothecary	York, Yorks	1599–1600, 1609–10
John Conny	Surgeon	Rochester, Kent	1676–7, 1696–7, 1699–1700
Robert Cowne	Druggist	Plymouth, Devon	1711 (died)
John Craycroft	Apoth'y/ physician	Leicester, Leics	1698–9
William Cropp	Apoth'y/ physician	Southampton, Hants	1696–7
John Crosse	Physician	Totnes, Devon	1687–8
Nicholas Curtis	Apothecary	Doncaster, Yorks	1686–7
Robert Dabynett	Apothecary	Exeter, Devon	1685–6, 1694–5
George Davies/Davis	Apothecary	Beverley, Yorks	1701–2, 1721–2
Thomas Day	Surgeon	Dover, Kent	1638–40
George Demountfryart	Physician	Bodmin, Cornwall	1691–2, 1694–5 1700–1, 1712, 1716–17
John Dimsdale	Surgeon	Hertford, Herts	1706–7, 1711–12
William Dobson	Apothecary	York, Yorks	1729–30

Robert Dodge	Barber	Exeter, Devon	1752–3 (died)
Edward Elwick	Apothecary	York, Yorks	1664–5
George Essex	Apothecary	York, Yorks	1509
Robert Fielding	Physician	Gloucester, Glos	1664, Aug-Sept 1669
Thomas Flay/Fley	Apoth'y/ physician	Exeter, Devon	1630–1
Richard Ford	Apothecary	Bath, Somerset	1713–14, 1730–1
Henry Fowler	Physician	Gloucester, Glos	1670–72, 1679–80
Henry France	Apothecary	Doncaster, Yorks	1715–16
William Francis	Apothecary	Derby, Derbys	1697–8, 1699–1701
Thomas Gale	Apothecary	Taunton, Somerset	1712–13 (died)
Francis Gardiner	Physician	Southampton, Hants	1712–13, 1723–4
Jacob Gater	Physician	Winchester, Hants	1738–9, 1748–9
Rosewell Gibbs	Apothecary	Bath, Somerset	1725–6
Thomas Gibbs	Apothecary	Bath, Somerset	1699–1700, 1711–12
John Golder	Physician	Dover, Kent	1644–6, 1661–2
William Goodridge	Surgeon	Salisbury, Wilts	1619–1620
John Goodwin	Surgeon	King's Lynn, Nk	1721–2, 1728–9
William Greaves	Apothecary	Nottingham, Notts	1692–3, 1698–9
Michael Greenstreet	Physician	Faversham, Kent	1666–7, 1673–4, 1684–5
John Grove	Surgeon	Hythe, Kent	before 1618
Anthony Gunson	Apoth'y/grocer	Stamford, Lincs	1588–9
Bridstock Harford	Physician	Hereford, Hfs	1697–8
Francis Harriman	Apothecary	Coventry, Wks	1673–4
David Harris	Apoth'y/grocer	Bristol, Glos	1550–1
Thomas Harwood	Apothecary	Shrewsbury, Salop	1702–3
Robert Haslen	Apoth'y/ physician	Chichester, Sussex.	1687–8, 1699–1700
William Hewett	Apothecary	Tiverton, Devon	1670–1
Thomas Hiern	Surgeon	Okehampton, Devon	1718–19, 1721–2
John Hoar	Apothecary	Northampton, Nts	1699–1700
Henry Holmes	Apothecary	Derby, Derbyshire	1694–5
Robert Jeffery	Apothecary	Barnstaple, Devon	1656–7
Matthew Jenison	Apothecary	Newark, Notts	1654–5
Benjamin Jones	Apothecary	Stratford u Avon, Wks	1669–70
William Jordan	Apothecary	Gloucester, Glos	1685–6

Edward Knighton	Apothecary	Northampton, Nts	1675–6
Thomas Knowler	Physician	Canterbury, Kent	1673–4, 1687–8
Henry Lambe	Apothecary	Colchester, Essex	1662–3, 1674–5
Nicholas Lane	Apothecary	Gloucester, Glos	1703–4
George Langford	Surgeon	Nottingham, Notts	1688–9
Jonah Lavington	Apoth'y/ druggist/ physician	Plymouth, Devon	1705–6
William Leverett	Physician	Newark, Notts	1558–9, 1563–4, 1574–5
William Levins	Apothecary	Oxford, Oxon	1572–3, 1579–80, 1586–7, 1594–5, July-Sept 1601
Martin Llewellyn	Physician	Wycombe, Bucks	1671–2
Henry Lucas	Surgeon	Banbury, Oxon	1710–11
William Maundy	Physician	Sandwich, Kent	1701 (died)
Anthony Maynard	Apothecary	Newport, I of W, Hants	1626–7, 1635–6
John Merrick	Physician	Reading, Berks	1702–3, 1713–14
Robert Morrey	Surgeon	Chester, Cheshire	1669–70
Thomas Moseley/Mosley	Apothecary	York, Yorkshire	1687–8
John Neale	Physician	Doncaster, Yorks	1723–4
Robert Norman	Apoth'y/ physician	Beverley, Yorks	1664–5, 1667
Joseph Palmer	Surgeon	South Molton, Devon	1720–1, 1732–3
Henry Parker	Apothecary	Bath, Somerset	1673–4
Philip Pear	Druggist	Exeter, Devon	1717–18
Roger Perkins	Apothecary	Doncaster, Yorks	1719–20
John Philipps	Apothecary	Exeter, Devon	1721–2
Thomas Pidgeon	Apothecary	Coventry, Wks	1661–2
Edmund Pitt	Apothecary	Worcester, Worcs	1656–7
John Pond	Apoth'y/surgeon	Maldon, Essex	March 1687–Jan'y 1688
Peter Proby	Barber surgeon/ grocer	London	1622–3
Abia Qui	Surgeon/ physician	Malmesbury, Wilts	1672–3
George Rasin/Rasine	Apothecary	Doncaster, Yorks	1665–6, 1674–5, 1683–4
Henry Ravening	Surgeon	Barnstaple, Devon	1687–8

Christopher Richardson	Surgeon	Kingston u Hull, Yorks	1660–1, 1678–9
Silvester Richmond	Surgeon/ physician	Liverpool, Lancs	1672–3
John Robinson	Surgeon	Berwick u Tweed, Nd	1649–50
Caleb Rocket	Apoth'y/ physician	Dartmouth, Devon	1714–15
John Rolfe	Surgeon	Harwich, Essex	1636–7, 1642–3 (died)
Francis Rushworth	Apoth'y	Northampton, Nts	1643–4
Arnold de Salanova	Surgeon	Weymouth, Dorset	1672–3
Anthony Salter	Physician	Exeter, Devon	April-Sept 1665
Robert Seaman	Surgeon	Harwich, Essex.	1672–3, 1681–2, 1690–1
Andrew Slee	Physician	Boston, Lincs	1662–3, 1664–5, 1675–6
Aquila Smith/Smyth	Physician	Malmesbury, Wilts	1686–7
Bernard Smith	Apothecary	Taunton, Somerset	1685–6, 1694–5
William Smith	Apothecary	Shrewsbury, Salop	1707/8
Walter Southwell	Apoth'y/grocer	Canterbury, Kent	1634–5
John Speed	Physician	Southampton, Hants	1681–2, 1694–5
Hugh Starkey	Surgeon	Chester, Cheshire	1687–8, 1700–1
Thomas Tiddeman	Surgeon	Dover, Kent	1684–5
Francis Tomkies	Surgeon	Oswestry, Salop	1700–1
Thomas Tomkies	Surgeon	Oswestry, Salop	1708–9
Thomas Trainter	Apothecary	Hereford, Hfs	1717–18
William Trevett/Trevitt	Apothecary	Exeter, Devon	1573–4
Francis Tuthill	Apothecary	Bridgwater, Somerset	1649 (removed)
Daniel Tyas	Apothecary	Worcester, Worcs	1639–40, 1643–4
Hannibal Vivian	Physician	Lostwithiel, C'wall	1632–3, 1636–8, 1640–1
John Watkinson	Surgeon	Kingston u Hull, Yks	1610–11
John Welchman	Apothecary	Banbury, Oxon	1675–6, 1689–90, 1699
John Welch/Welsh	Surgeon/ physician	Rye, Sussex	1662–4, 1668–9, 1673–4
Robert Weller	Apothecary	Rochester, Kent	1719–1720
Simon Westcott	Apothecary	Taunton, Somerset	1707 (died)
Anthony Westwood	Surgeon/ physician	Arundel, Sussex	1665–6, 1669–70

William Wheatley	Apothecary	Banbury, Oxon	1648–9
John Williams	Apothecary	Oxford, Oxon	1598–9
John Windebank	Physician	Guildford, Surrey	1663–4
Robert Wood	Apothecary	Shrewsbury, Salop	1684–5
Christopher Woodhouse	Physician	Berkhamsted, Herts	1662–3
Edward Woolmer	Apothecary	Bath, Somerset	1706–7, 1720–1
Collins Wolrich/Woolrich	Apothecary	Shrewsbury, Salop	1683–4, 1688–9
John Wright	Surgeon	Rochester, Kent	1704–5
Joseph Wright	Apothecary	Nottingham, Notts	1667–8, 1674–5 (died)
Joseph Wright	Physician	Maidstone, Kent	1687–8
Richard Wye	Surgeon	Rochester, Kent	1652–3, 1656–7
John Yardley	Surgeon	Coventry, Wks	1689–90
Thomas Yate	Apothecary	Gloucester, Glos	1665–6
James Yonge	Surgeon	Plymouth, Devon	1694–5

Bibliography

1. Manuscripts

Angus Library, Regent's Park College, Oxford

Church Book of the Glasshouse Yard Baptist meeting, 1680–1740.
Church book of the White's Alley Baptist meeting, 1680–1700.

Bedfordshire and Luton Archives and Records Service

HSA/1671 W/15 and S22: records of High Sheriff, Bedfordshire, assizes.

Berkshire Record office, Reading

D/A1/201/35: administration of the will of Manasses King, physician, of Newbury, Berkshire, 1696.
W1/AC1/1/1: minutes book of the corporation of Windsor, 1653–1725.

Bodleian Library, Oxford

Add. MS C.303 and 308: correspondence and papers of archbishop Gilbert Sheldon.
Ashmole MS 419.
Ashmole MS 826.
Carte MSS 35, 79, and 219.
Lister MSS 3 and 35: correspondence of Dr Martin Lister.
MS Eng. hist. c. 478: Herrick family papers.
MS Eng. hist. c. 711: diary of Roger Whitley, 1684–97.
Oxford University Archives, NEP/supra/Reg Qa: Register of Congregation, 1647–1659.
Rawlinson Letters 51 and 109: correspondence of Philip, Lord Wharton.
Rawlinson MS A 176 and 188: papers of Samuel Pepys.
Rawlinson MS B 239: accounts of the sale of episcopal estates, 1647–55.
Rawlinson MSS C 948 and D 1137: casebooks of Thomas Sclater, J. P.
Tanner MSS 32, 36, 38, 40, 52, 54, 55, 62A, 148: papers of Thomas Tanner (1674–1735).

British Library, London

Additional MS 4460: Birch papers, including extracts from the day books of Dr Henry Sampson.
Additional MS 5829: proceedings of the committee for scandalous ministers, Essex.
Additional MS 15,642: Journal of John Locke, 1679.
Additional MS 17,677: state papers and correspondence related to the United Provinces, 1576–1764.
Additional MS 28,037: minutes of the corporation of Dover, 1674–8.
Additional MS 35,104: letter book of Edward Conway, 1681–3.
Additional MS 41,803–41,818: Middleton papers.
Additional MS 61,681: papers of the Boteler family.
Additional MS 78,298 and 78,311: correspondence of John Evelyn.
Lansdowne MS 821–823: correspondence of Henry Cromwell, 1654–9.

Sloane MS 123: miscellaneous correspondence, 1660–83.
Sloane MS 203: correspondence and collections of Dr John Downes.
Sloane MSS 1256–1280, 1282–1294, 1297–1299: manuscript notes and papers of Dr Christopher Love Morley.
Sloane MS 1326: correspondence and papers of Dr Henry Power.
Sloane MS 1393: correspondence and papers of Dr Henry Power.
Sloane MS 1968: miscellaneous letters and papers.
Sloane MS 3299: miscellaneous correspondence of James Petiver and others.
Sloane MS 3505, fos 99v–100r: 'Praxis pro maniacis curandis'.
Sloane MS 3515: miscellaneous correspondence.
Sloane MS 4036: correspondence of John Northleigh.

Cambridge University Library

Cambridge University Archives, Grace Book H (1645–1668).
MS LI v 8: collection of medical receipts of Augustine Kueffler.
MS Mm.I.45 [Baker MS 35]: volume of transcripts made by Thomas Baker (1656–1740).
EDR, E12: loose bundles of indictments and recognizances, assize files, 1642–9.

Canterbury Cathedral Archives and Library

DCb/L/B/Box 1, no. 17 [17 April 1662].
DCb/L/R/17–27: register of general licences.
U3/267: parish registers of Eastry, Kent, 1559–1736.

Derbyshire Record Office, Matlock

D 239 M/O 1082, 1121, 1617, 1619, 1637, and 1649: correspondence and papers of George Treby.

Devon Record Office, Exeter

C 772: Consistory Court Act Book, 1675–1683.
Chanter MS 45: act book of the diocese of Exeter, 1668–1679.
ECA, C/1/65 and 66: Exeter City Archives, Quarter Sessions Order Book, 1660–1672; 1682–1688.
ECA 10: Exeter City Archives, Act Book of Exeter Chamber, 1652–1663.
ECA 11: Exeter City Archives, Act Book of Exeter Chamber, 1663–1684.
ECA 11, 38, 56, 60, 62, 63, 64, 66; ECA,
ECA, File 1/6: petitions for relief.
PR 518: surgeons' licences issued in the diocese of Exeter.
PR 362–364/33/1–29.
3167A/PR/1/1: parish registers of Farringdon.

Doctor Williams' Library, London

Harmer MS 76.7: Records of the Congregational Church at Wrentham, Suffolk.

Dorset Record Office, Dorchester

B2/8/1: Dorchester Offenders' Book.

Durham University Library

DPRI/1/1642/B7/1–6 [will of William Broad, doctor of physic, of Berwick upon Tweed, Northumberland, undated, pr.24 December 1642; inventory dated 29 December 1642].

East Sussex Record Office, Brighton

FRE 606: Medical commonplace book of Philip Frith.
FRE 5421–5634: correspondence of John Allin with Philip Frith and others, 1663–1680.
RYE 1/15: assembly book of the corporation of Rye, 1662–1666.
RYE 19/7: appointment of James Welsh as captain of the trained bands and clerk of the passage, 1673.
RYE 47/169/14: correspondence of the corporation of Rye.
RYE 82/82, 52, 55: precept and rate made for paying off the armed forces, Rye, 1660.
SAS-M/1/692 and 774.
SAS-WH/201 [will of John Braman, 1703].

East Suffolk Record Office, Ipswich

HD 36/A/213.

Essex Record Office, Chelmsford

D/ABW 63/61: will of Reuben Robinson, gent, of Maldon, 3 February 1664/5 and 6 April 1665, pr. 5 June 1665.
D/ABW 68/33; will of Peter Mark Sparke, doctor in physic, of Bishop's Stortford, Hertfordshire, 24 February 1675/6, pr. 3 May 1676.
D/DPb T2/21–23: Wiston Hall estate and family records, marriage settlement of William Gurnell, clerk, and Sarah Mott, witnessed by Roger Goodyear, doctor of physic, of Lavenham, Suffolk, 1646.
D/P 201/1/1: parish registers of Maldon.

Folger Shakespeare Library, Washington DC

V.a.284–299: diaries of John Ward, vicar of Stratford-upon-Avon, Warwickshire.
V.a.441: account of William Westmacott.

Friends House Library, London

Martin Mason MSS.
Swarthmore MSS.

Gemeente Archief, Amsterdam

318/2: Notulen van het Consistory or Book of Discipline, 1621–1627].

Gloucestershire Record office, Gloucester

D 3117/151, 153: lease agreements, 16 December 1672 and 1 October 1676.
GBR 3/3: Gloucester corporation minute book, 1656–1686.
GBR 3/4: Gloucester corporation minute book, 1668–1673.
GBR 3/6: Gloucester corporation minute book, 1681–1690.
GBR 3/7: Gloucester corporation minute book, 1690–1700.
GBR 3/8: Gloucester corporation minute book, 1700–1716.
GBR K1/31: case papers, Lent assizes; William Jordan v. corporation.
P154/14 IN 1/1: parish registers of St Michael's, Gloucester, 1553–1663.
Q/SO 1: Gloucestershire quarter sessions order book, 1672–1681.

Guildhall Library, London

MS 5265/1 [Barber Surgeons' Company, Freedom and Admissions, 1522–1664].
MS 10,116: medical testimonials, diocese of London.

Hampshire Record Office, Winchester

18M51/636/22: 'To the Right Honourable Sir John Lawson', 1664.
Q1/5: QS Order Book, Hampshire, 1672–1679.

House of Lords Record Office, London

HL/PO/JO/10/1: main papers.

Kent History and Library Centre, Maidstone

Fa/I/12: grant of incorporation, borough of Faversham, 1685.
PRC 19/3/39; 1/11/41; 2/36/43; 2/37/66.

Kingston Museum and Heritage Service, Kingston upon Thames, Surrey

KE2/7/5; 2/7/12/1; 2/7/15/7: prosecutions under the Conventicle Acts, 1665–1677.

Lambeth Palace Library, London

FI and FII: medical licenses issued by the Faculty Office of the archbishop of Canterbury.
MS 639: returns of diocesan surveys.
MS 941, no. 124 [The Case of St Thomas' Hospital, 17 April 1703].
Registers of the archbishops of Canterbury.
VX IA/10: applications and testimonials for medical licences issued by the office of the Vicar General of the archbishop of Canterbury, 1663–1775.

Lancashire Record Office, Preston

DP 353: unpublished sermons of Christopher Hudson.

Leicestershire and Rutland Record Office, Wigston Magna

archdeaconry court of Leicester wills, will of Richard Farmer, gent, of Kilby, Leicestershire, 10 September 1687, pr. 1688.
1D 41/13/82: archdeaconry of Leicester papers.
1D 41/34/1: subscription book, archdeaconry of Leicester, 1624–1683.

Leiden University Library, Leiden

ASF 12: enrolment register, Leiden University.

Lincolnshire Archives Office, Lincoln

Dioc/Sub/I: subscription Book, diocese of Lincoln, 1563–77; 1613–1679.

London Metropolitan Archives, Clerkenwell, London

archdeaconry court of London, will of Blaze Allen, citizen and doctor of physic, of St Botolph Aldgate, London, 2 March 1702/3; pr. 11 June 1703.
Corporation of London quarter sessions file 163 (1662), 202 (1670).
MS 09540/1: subscription book, diocese of London, 1662–1683/4.
MS 9172/122/103: will of Roger Grant, esquire, of St Dunstan's, Stepney, Middlesex, 2 April 1724, pr. 9 April 1724.
DL/C/314: commissary court of the bishop of London, office act book, 1617–19.
DL/C/343: vicar general's register, consistory court of London, 1627–37.
P69/AND4/A/001/MS04107/002: parish registers of St Andrew Undershaft, London, 1634–1692.

P69/BOT4/A/002/MS04516/001: parish registers of St Botolph Bishopsgate, London, 1677–1701.
P69/GIS/A/002/MS06419/013: parish registers of St Giles Cripplegate, London, 1703–1711].
P69/MGT1/A/001/MS04346/001: parish registers of St Margaret, Lothbury, London, 1558–1736.
P69/TRI2/A/010/MS 09245: parish registers of Holy Trinity, Minories, London, 1694–1713.
P92/GEO/143: parish registers of St George the Martyr, Southwark, Surrey, 1695–1732.
P93/DUN/128, 278, 279: parish registers of St Dunstan's, Stepney, Middlesex, 1702–1709; 1666–1684; 1622–1666.

Malmesbury Borough Archives, Malmesbury

Malmesbury corporation minute book, 1600–1721.

National Archives, Kew, London

ADM 1/5257/5: courts martial papers, Board of Admiralty.
ASSI 24/1: bail book, assizes, western circuit, 1654–7.
ASSI 24/22: order books, assizes, western circuit, 1652–1677.
ASSI 35: home circuit, assizes: indictment files, 1559–1688.
ASSI 44/25: indictment file, northern and north-east circuits, 1677.
C6/305/28: Chancery proceedings, John Russell v. Clement Halsey and others, 1694.
C 10/477/110: Chancery proceedings, William Goddard v. Marchamont Nedham and others, 1666.
C 111/190/31.
LC 3/2: papers of Lord Chamberlain's office.
LC 3/24: enrolment of household officials during the reign of Charles II, 1660–85.
LC 3/25, 26 and 27: registers of the Lord Chamberlain, 1666, 1671.
LC 3/28: appointments to royal household, 1674–85.
LC 3/56: registers and appointments made by Lord Chamberlain, 1685.
LS 13/197: Board of Green Cloth, 1660–1685.
PC 2/57, 58, 59, 62, 63, 66, 67, 68, 69 and 70: Privy Council registers, February-December 1664; 1665-1666; 1666–1667; 1669–1671; 1671–1675; May 1677–1678; January-April 1679; April 1679-May 1680; 1680–1683; 1683–1685.
PROB 11: administrations and wills proved in the Prerogative Court of Canterbury.
RG6/499: register of Quaker burials, London and environs, 1660–1700.
SP 28: Commonwealth Exchequer papers.
SP 29: state papers of the reign of Charles II, 1660–1685.

National Library of Ireland, Dublin

MS 11,959: orders in council, 1651–5.
MS 11,961: answers to petitions, 1655–6.

New College, Oxford

MS 9502: diary of Robert Woodford, 1637–1641.

Northamptonshire Record Office, Northampton

Peterborough Diocesan Records, CB 44: Correction Book, Consistory Court, Western Division, 1614–1616.

Norwich and Norfolk Record Office, Norwich

MC 1/17 386x5: Sir Allen Apsley to Humphrey Henchman, 1660.
PD 499/2: parish registers of St Mary in the Marsh, Norwich, i.e., Cathedral Close, 1667–1724.
Traf 3286x5: Trafford family papers.
Y/S1/4: Great Yarmouth Sessions Book, 1679–1732.

Nottinghamshire Archives, Nottingham

DD/N/201/26: indenture and deed of sale, 26 May 1682.

Oxfordshire Record Office, Oxford

PAR 213/1/R1/1: parish registers of St Peter's in the East, Oxford, 1559–1653.

Representative Church Body Library, Dublin

GS 2/7/3/20: notes relating to ministers of the gospel appointed by the Commonwealth government in Ireland, abstracted by the Rev. St John D. Seymour.

Royal College of Physicians Library, London

MS 2293: Liber Annalium Collegii Medicorum Londinsensium [Annals], 5 vols.
LEGAC/ENV 79: prosecution of John Harborough, 1702.
LEGAC/ENV 81: prosecution of Gabriel Hubbard, 1682.
LEGAC/ENV98: prosecution of George Pope, 1688.
LEGAC/ENV 100: prosecution of William Russell, 1683.

Royal Society, London

Boyle Letters, vol. 5.
Boyle Papers 25.
RB/1/29/8.

Shakespeare Birthplace Trust Record Office, Stratford-upon-Avon

BRU 2/2: council minute book, Stratford-upon-Avon, 1593–1628.
BRU 2/3: council minute book, Stratford-upon-Avon, 1628–1657.
ER1/1/94: Sydrak Davenport to John Hall, July 1632.

Sheffield University Library

Hartlib Papers: papers of Samuel Hartib (*c.*1600–62) [available on CD-ROM].

Society of Antiquaries, London

MS 202, no. 101.

Society of Apothecaries, London

MS 8200/2: court minutes, 1651–1680
MS 8200/3: court minutes 1680–1694

Somerset Heritage Centre, Taunton

DD\Bs/39: subscription book, diocese of Bath and Wells, 1660–69.
D\D/Bs/42: subscription book, diocese of Bath and Wells, 1672–1695.
D\D\Ca 310: comperta, Taunton and Bath archdeaconry, 1636.
DD\S\BT: Butleigh Court papers.
DD\SP/319/6: annuity out of lands at Bishops Hull, 1697.

D\P\BEC/2/1/2: parish registers of Beckington, Somerset, 1653–1741.
D\P\PET/S/2/1/1: parish registers of South Petherton, Somerset, 1574–1674.
Q/SR/99, 104, 106: Somerset Quarter Sessions rolls.

Southampton City Archives, Southampton

SC2/1/8: Southampton Assembly Book, 1642–1679.
SC2/1/9: Southampton Assembly Book, 1679–1734.
SC3/1/1: Southampton Burgess Admissions Book, 1496–1704.

Staffordshire Record Office, Stafford

B/V/1/72: visitation, comperta, and acta, diocese of Coventry and Lichfield, 1665.

Surrey History Centre, Woking

K174/6/2.
QR 2/5: Surrey Quarter Sessions rolls.
QS 2/1/2 and 3: Surrey quarter sessions order books, 1664–1671 and 1672–1676.
SW 23/423: will of Henry Forty, gospel minister, of St Olave, Southwark, Surrey, 14 May 1692, pr. 13 January 1692/3.
SW/25/730: will of Edmund Yalden, clerk and rector, of Compton, Surrey, 25 December 1684, pr. 27 May 1685.

Trinity College, Dublin

MS 889: papers and correspondence of William Molyneux.

Wellcome Library, London

MS 5334–5340: register of episcopal medical licences compiled by A. W. Haggis.
MS 7671/6 [White to Chamberlen the elder, 18 February 1673/4].

West Suffolk Record Office, Bury St Edmunds

EE/501/17/26.
IC500: archdeaconry of Sudbury probate records.

West Sussex Record Office, Chichester

Additional MS 8759: conveyance, 16 December 1690.
Additional MS 8935: award of arbitration, 30 October 1691.
Ep I/3/1: subscription book, diocese of Chichester, 1635–1685.
Ep.II/1/1: subscription book, diocese of Chichester, 1604–1751.
Par/214/1/1/1: parish registers of Woodmancote.

Wiltshire and Swindon Archives

A1/110: Wiltshire quarter sessions rolls.
D1/14/1/1a-e: testimonials for medical licences, 1660–93.
D1/14/2/1: testimonials for surgeons, diocese of Salisbury, *c.*1690–1708.
D1/22/2: subscription book, diocese of Salisbury, 1664–1668.
D1/22/4: subscription book, diocese of Salisbury, 1662–1687.
D1/54/5: churchwardens' presentments from various deaneries, diocese of Salisbury, 1669–71.
D5/9/2: subscription book, peculiar of dean of Salisbury, 1674–1731.
G23/1/4: Salisbury Borough Ledger Book, 1640–1723.

P4/1700/8: will of John Feak or Feake of Salisbury, 29 September 1699, pr. 16 July 1700.
P23/406: will of Timothy Boyce, physician, of Wantage, Berkshire, pr. 1721.
1589/47: parish registers of Westport St Mary, 1678–1795.
1597/2: parish registers of St John the Baptist, Devizes, 1653–1705.
1901/2 and 3: parish registers of St Edmund's, Salisbury, 1653–1699; 1699–1767.

Worcestershire County Record Office, Worcester

795.02/BA2302/11.
795.02/BA2302/11/2491 and 33/7390.

2. Printed Primary Sources (Pre-1800)

Account of a Miraculous Cure of a Young Man in Newington (London, 1709).
Acton, G., *Physical Reflections upon a Letter Written by J. Denis... to Monsieur de Montmor ... Concerning a New Way of Curing Sundry Diseases by Transfusion of Blood* (London, 1668).
A Letter in Answer to Certain Quaeries and Objections Made by a Learned Galenist, Against the Theorie and Practice of Chymical Physick (London, 1670).
Agate, J., *The Plain Truth: Or, An Answer to Mr Withers His Defense, &c. Part 1* (Exeter, 1708).
Ambrose, I., *Media: The Middle Things, in Reference to the First and Last Things* (London, 1650).
Ashmole, E., *The Antiquities of Berkshire*, 3 vols (London, 1719).
Aston, T., *Satan in Samuels Mantle, or the Cruelty of Germany Acted in Jersey* (London, 1659).
Atkins, W., *A Discourse Showing the Nature of Gout* (London, 1694).
Aubrey, J., *The Natural History and Antiquities of Surrey*, 5 vols (London, 1729).
Aut Helmont, Aut Asinus: Or, St. George Untrust Being a Full Answer to His Smart Scourge (London, 1665).
Bacon, W., *A Key to Helmont, or, a Short Introduction to the Better Understanding of the Theory and Method of the Most Profound Chymical Physicians* (London, 1682).
Baker, R., *A Chronicle of the Kings of England* (London, 1684).
Banister, J., *Compendius Chirurgerie* (London, 1585).
Barker, R., *Consilium Anti-Pestilentiale* (London, 1665).
Barnes, J., *The History of the Most Victorious Monarch Edward III* (Cambridge, 1688).
Baston, S., *Baston's Case Vindicated, or a Brief Account of Some Evil Practices of the Present Commissioners for Sick and Wounded* (London, 1695).
[Bastwick, J.], *Flagellum Pontificiis et Episcoporum Latialium* (Amsterdam?, 1635).
The Second Part of the Book Called Independency Not Gods Ordinance (London, 1645).
Baxter, R., *The Certainty of the Worlds of Spirits* (London, 1691).
Reliquiae Baxterianae... Faithfully Publish'd... by Matthew Silvester (London, 1696).
B[eadle], J., *The Journal or Diary of a Thankful Christian, Presented in Some Meditations upon Numb[ers] 33:2* (London, 1656).
Beaton, N., *No Treason to say, Kings Are God's Subjects... In Some Sermons Preached at Lurgarshal in Sussex* (London, 1661).
Bentham, J., *The Societie of the Saints: Or, A Treatise of Goode Fellowes, with Their Good Fellowship: Delivered in the Lecture of Kettering in Northampton-shire, in Foureteene Sermons* (London, 1630).

Besse, J., *A Collection of the Sufferings of the People Called Quakers... from 1650, to... 1689*, 2 vols (London, 1753).
Betts, J., *De Ortu et Natura Sanguinis* (London, 1669).
Biggs, N., *Matæotechnia Medicinae Praxeωs. The Vanity of the Craft of Physick* (London, 1651).
Bishop, J., *The Marrow of Astrology in Two Books* (London, 1687).
Bolnest, E., *Medicina Instaurata, or, a Brief Account of the True Grounds and Principles of the Art of Physick* (London, 1665).
Aurora Chymica. Or a Rational Way of Preparing Animals, Vegetables, and Minerals, for a Physicall Use (London, 1672).
Bolton, J., *A Justification of the Righteous Judgement of God on Nathaniel Smith* (London?, 1669).
Bolton, R., *Two Sermons Preached at Northampton at Two Severall Assises There... 1621... 1629* (London, 1639).
Bond, J., *A Doore of Hope, also Holy and Loyall Activity. Two Treatises Delivered in Severall Sermons in Excester* (London, 1641).
Occasus Occidentalis: Or, Job in the West. As it was Laid Forth in Two Severall Sermons at Two Publike Fasts, for the Five Associated Westerne Counties (London, 1645).
Border, D., *ΠΟΛΥΦΑΡΜΑΚΟΣ κάι ΧΥΜΙΣΤΗΣ, or, The English Unparallel'd Physitian and Chyrurgian* (London, 1651).
B[ostocke], R., *The Difference Betwene the Auncient Phisicke... and the Latter Phisicke* (London, 1585).
Bourne, H., *The History of Newcastle upon Tyne. Or, the Ancient and Present State of the Town* (Newcastle, 1736).
Boys, E., *Sixteen Sermons* (London, 1672).
Bradwell, S., *A Detection of Ed. Glovers Hereticall Confection* (London, 1585).
The Rasing of the Foundations of Brownisme (London, 1588).
Brady, R., *Complete History of England* (London, 1685).
Treatise of Cities and Boroughs (London, 1690).
Brinsley, J., *The First Booke of Tullies Offices Translated Gramatically* (London, 1616).
Brinsley, J., *The Healing of Israels Breaches. Wherein is Set Forth Israels Disease, Cure, Physitian, Danger... As They Were Delivered in Six Sermons at the Weekly Lecture in the Church of Great Yarmouth* [23 February–13 April 1642] (London, 1642).
A Parlie with the Sword About a Cessation [Yarmouth, 28 December 1642] (London, 1643).
Prayer and Praise. A Two-fold Tribute, to be Payed by All Loyal Subjects to their Supream and Subordinate Soveraign [23 April 1661] (London, 1661).
Bromfield, M., *A Brief Discovery of the True Causes, Symptoms, and Effects of that Most Reigning Disease, the Scurvy. Whereunto is added a Short Account of those Incomparable and Most Highly Approved Pills, called Pillulae in Omnes Morbos* (London, 1675 and 1678).
[Brooke, H.], *Cautionary Rules for Preventing the Sickness* (London, 1665).
The Durable Legacy (London, 1681).
Buck, J., *St Paul's Thanksgiving set forth in a Sermon Preached before the Right Honorable House of Peers* [10 May 1660] ... *Being the Day of Solemn Thanksgiving to Almighty God for His Late Blessings upon this Kingdom* (London, 1660).
Burges, A., *The Magistrates Commission from Heaven. Declared in a Sermon Preached in Laurencejury, London* [28 September 1644] (London, 1644).
Burthogge, R., *De Lithiasi et Calculo* (Leiden, 1662).
Of the Soul of the World, and of Particular Souls. In a Letter to Mr Lock Occasion'd by Mr Keil's Reflections upon an Essay Lately Published concerning Reason (London, 1699).

Calamy, E., *An Abridgment of Mr Baxter's History of His Life and Times. With an Account of the Ministers, &c who were Ejected after the Restauration of King Charles II*, 2 vols (2nd ed., London, 1713).
Carter, J., 'A Rare Sight, or the Lyon' [18 June 1650] in *The Tomb-stone, or a Rare Sight* (London, 1653).
Cary, P., *A Disputation between a Doctor and an Apothecary, or, a Reply to the New Argument of Dr R. Burthogge, MD. for Infant's Baptism* (London, 1684).
A Solemn Call unto All That Would Be Owned as Christ's Faithful Witnesses... Or, A Discourse Concerning Baptism (London, 1690).
A Just Reply to Mr John Flavell's Arguments: By Way of Answer to a Discourse Lately Published, Entituled, A Solemn Call (London, 1690).
Capua, L. di, *The Uncertainty of the Art of Physick*, trans. J. Lancaster (London, 1684).
Casaubon, M., *Of Credulity and Incredulity in Things Natural, Civil, and Divine* (London, 1668).
Castle, G., *The Chymical Galenist: A Treatise wherein the Practise of the Ancients is Reconcil'd to the New Discoveries in the Theory of Physick* (London, 1667).
Cawdrey, D., *Church-Reformation Promoted in a Sermon on Matth[ew].18. vers[e].15,16,17: Preached at Northampton... Before the Association of Ministers* (London, 1657).
[Chaderton, L.], *A Fruitfull Sermon, upon the 3, 4, 5, 6, 7, 8 Verses of the 12. Chapiter of the Epistle of S.Paul to the Romanes* (London, 1584).
Charles II, *A Proclamation Against Vicious, Debauch'd, and Prophane Persons* (London, 30 May 1660).
Charleton, W., *The Immortality of the Human Soul, Demonstrated by the Light of Nature. In Two Dialogues* (London, 1657).
Natural History of the Passions (London, 1674).
Chauncey, I., *Innocence Vindicated: by a Brief and Impartial Narrative of the Proceedings of the Court of Sessions in Bristol against Ichabod Chauncey, Physician in that City* (London, 1684).
Chauncy, Sir H., *The Historical Antiquities of Hertfordshire* (London, 1720).
Clagett, W., *Of the Humanity and Charity of Christians, a Sermon Preached at the Suffolk Feast in St Michael Cornhill, London* [30 November 1686] (London, 1687).
Clarke, J., *Ill Newes from New England: Or, A Narrative of New-Englands Persecution* (London, 1652).
Clarke, W., *The Natural History of Nitre: Or, a Philosophical Discourse of... Nitre, with Its Vertues and Uses* (London, 1670).
Clarkson, L., *The Lost Sheep Found* (London, 1660).
Coelson, L., *Speculum Perspicuum Uranicum: Or, an Almanck* [sic]... *1678* (London, 1678).
Speculum Perspicuum Uranicum, or, An Almanack for the Year... 1680 (London, 1680).
Speculum Perspicuum Uranicum... 1685 (London, 1685).
Colbatch, J., *A Physico-Medical Essay, Concerning Alkaly and Acid* (London, 1696).
A Collection of Voyages and Travels... in Six Volumes. Volume V (3rd ed., London, 1746).
Colley, A., *Nature's Champion, Sounding a Challenge to Her Stoutest Assailants: Or, a More Ample Explanation of the Virtue and Use of My Pillulae Aureae Purgantes* (London, 1670).
C[ollop], J., *Medici Catholicon* (London, 1656).
Consett, J., *The Olive Branch, or The Miraculous Restauration of Peace, both to Church and State in Great Britain and Ireland* (London, 1660).
The Rod of Recompence (London, 1660).

Cook, J., *Unum Necessarium: Or, The Poore Mans Case* (London, 1648).
Cooper, E., *The Asse Beaten for Bawling; or, A Replie from the Citie, to the Crie of the Country* (London, 1661).
On the Recovery of Our Most Gracious Queen Katherine from Her Late Grievous and Deplorable Fit of Sicknesse (London, 1664).
Cooper, W., *Collectanea Chymica* (London, 1684).
Corbett, E., *Gods Providence. A Sermon Preached Before the Honourable House of Commons, at their Late Solemne Fast* [28 December 1642] (London, 1642).
Cotta, J., *Cotta Contra Antonium* (London, 1623).
Cox, N., *Vindiciae Veritatis, or a Confutation of the Heresies and Gross Errours Attested by Thomas Collier* (London, 1677).
[Coxe, D.], *A Discourse, Wherein the Interest of the Patient in Reference to Physick and Physicians is Soberly Debated* (London, 1669).
Cranwell, L., *The Holding the Bishop and Presbyter Equall, Vindicated from Heresie* (London, 1661).
Croese, G., *The General History of the Quakers*, 2 vols (London, 1696).
Crosby, T., *The History of the English Baptists*, 4 vols (London, 1738–40).
Curtis, T., *Essays on the Preservation and Recovery of Health* (London, 1704).
Dale, S., *The History and Antiquities of Harwich and Dovercourt* (London, 1730).
D[awes], L., *Two Sermons Preached at the Assises Holden at Carlile, Touching Sundry Corruptions of These Times* (Oxford, 1614).
De Graaf, R., *De Succo Pancreatico; or, A Physical and Anatomical Treatise of the Nature and Office of the Pancreatice Juice*, trans. C. Packe (London, 1676).
[Deantry, E, and Davis, N.], *The Resolution of Those Physitians Presented by the Colledge to the Right Honourable the Lord Mayor and Court of Aldermen . . . for the Prevention and Cure of the Plague* (London, 1665).
Denton, W., *Jus Regiminis: Being a Justification of Defensive Arms in General and Consequently of Our Late Revolutions and Transactions to be the Just Right of the Kingdom* (London 1689).
Diurnall Occurrences in Parliament (London, 1642).
Dixon, R., *Consultum Sanitatis, A Directory to Health* (London, 1663).
D[oughty], J., *A Discourse Concerning the Abstrusenesse of Divine Mysteries . . . Another Touching Church-Schismes* (Oxford, 1628).
Du Laurens, A., *A Discourse of the Preservation of the Sight: of Melancholike Diseases; of Rheumes, and of Old Age . . . Translated . . . by . . . Richard Surphlet* (London, 1599).
Du Moulin, L., *La Tyrannie des Prejugez, ou, Reflexions sur le Fragment d'une Lettre de Mademoiselle Marie du Moulin* (London, 1678).
Dudley, D., *Metallum Martis* (London, 1665).
Dunton, J., *The Life and Errors of John Dunton Late Citizen of London* (London, 1705).
Edwards, T., *Gangraena* (London, 1646).
Ellis, J., *S. Austin Imitated: Or Retractions and Repentings in Reference unto the Late Civil and Ecclesiastical Changes in the Nation . . . in II Books* (London, 1662).
Ellwood, T., *The History of the Life of Thomas Ellwood . . . The Second Edition* (London, 1714).
Erastus, T., *The Nullity of Church Censures* (London, 1659).
Faber, A. O., *De Auro Potabile Medicinali, ad Potentissimum Principem, Carolum II* (London, 1677).
Fido, J., Jeanes, T., and Shaw, W., *The Parliament Justified in Their Late Proceedings Against Charles Stuart* (London, 1649).

Flavell, J., *The Whole Works of the Reverend Mr. John Flavel* (London, 1701).
Fletcher, R., *The Character of a True Physician* (London, 1676).
Starkey Revived, or, Collections out of Nature's Explication, and Helmont's Vindication, Being a Short Examination of the State of Physick as Now Practised (London, 1676).
Ford, S., *Primitiae Regiminis Davidici. Or, the First Fruits of David's Government... Represented in a Sermon at the Assises held at Reading* [28 February 1654] (London, 1654).
Frankland, R., *The Honours of the Lords Spiritual Asserted: and Their Priviledges to Vote in Capital Cases in Parliament* (London, 1679).
The Annals of King James and King Charles the First (London, 1681).
French, J., *The Yorkshire Spaw, or a Treatise of Four Famous Medicinal Wells* (London, 1652).
F[ydge], T., *The Citizens Sacred Entertainment: Being an Essay to Ingratiate the Practice of Vertue, to Consummate the Happiness of Humane Nature, and to Gratifie Ingenuous and Religious Spirits* (London, 1666).
Gayton, E., *The Religion of a Physician, or Divine Meditations upon the Grand and Lesser Festivals, Commanded to be Observed in the Church of England* (London, 1663).
Gee, J., *The Foot out of the Snare* (London, 1624).
Gell, R., *EIPHNIKON: Or, a Treatise of Peace Between the Two Visible Divided Parties* (London, 1660).
Gerard, J., *Herbal* (London, 1597).
Gilpin, R., *De Hysterica Passione* (Leiden, 1676).
The Comforts of Divine Love Preach'd upon the Occasion of the Much Lamented Death of the Reverend Mr Timothy Manlove (London, 1700).
Glanvill, J., *Sadducismus Triumphatus: Or, Full and Plain Evidence Concerning Witches and Apparitions* (London, 1681).
Glauber, J. R., *Works*, ed. C. Packe (London, 1687).
Godfrey, R., *Various Injuries and Abuses in Chymical and Galenical Physick* (London, 1674).
Goodall, C., *The Colledge of Physicians Vindicated, and the True State of Physick in this Nation Faithfully Represented* (London, 1676).
Gouge, W., *The Right Way: Or a Direction for Obtaining Good Successe in a Weighty Enterprise* (London, 1648).
Granger, T., *The Application of Scripture or The Maner How to Use the Word to Most Edifying* (London, 1616).
[Greaves, E.], *Morbus Epidemicus Anni 1643. Or, The New Disease with the Signes, Causes, Remedies, &c* (Oxford, 1643).
Grew, N., *A Treatise of the Nature and Use of the Bitter Purging Salt* (London, 1697).
Griffiths, R., *A-la-mode Phlebotomy No Good Fashion, or, The Copy of a Letter to Dr Hungerford* (London, 1681).
Guidott, T., *A Discourse of the Bathe... With an Account of the Lives, and Character, of the Physicians of Bathe* (London, 1676).
Gulter, G., *The Archbishops Crueltie, Made Knowne in a True Story of One Mr. Edward Rood* (London, 1641).
Hall, J., *Select Observations on English Bodies* (London, 1657).
Hargrave, A., *Reason in Season: Or, a Word on the Behalf of the Non-Collegiate Physicians and of the Right of the People in the Choice of Their Physicians* (London, 1676).
Hart, J., *KAINIKH, or the Diet of the Diseased* (London, 1633).
Hasted, E., *The History and Topographical Survey of the County of Kent*, 12 vols (2nd ed., Canterbury, 1798).

Haworth, S., *A Philosophic Discourse Concerning Man* (London, 1680).
A Description of the Duke's Bagnio (London, 1683).
The True Method of Curing Consumptions (London, 1683).
Hayward, E., *The Answer of Edward Hayward... to a Most Abusive and Scandalous Pamphlet... by George Kendall, MA* (London, 1656).
Headrich, J., *Arcana Philosophia, or Chymical Secrets Containing the Noted and Useful Chymical Medicines of Dr Wil[lliam] and Rich[ard] Russel Chymists* (London, 1697).
Henchman, R., *A Peace-Offering in the Temple; Or, A Seasonable Plea for Unity among Dissenting Brethren* [14 October 1660] (London, 1661).
Herle, C., *A Payre of Compasses for Church and State. Delivered in a Sermon Preached at St. Margarets in Westminster, Before the Honourable House of Commons at their Monethly Fast November the Last, 1642* (London, 1642).
Herring, F., *A Modest Defence of the Caveat Given to Wearers of Impoisoned Amulets* (London, 1604).
Hester, J., *The Pearle of Practise, or, Practisers Pearl for Physick and Chirurgerie* (London, 1594).
[Heywood, O.], *Some Remarks upon the Life of... Mr. Nathanael Heywood, Minister of the Gospel of Christ at Ormeskirk in Lancashire* (London, 1695).
Hickeringill, E., *Works*, 3 vols (London, 1716).
[Hickes, J.], *A True and Faithful Narrative, of the Unjust and Illegal Sufferings, and Oppressions of Many Christians... in the County of Devon* (1671).
Hodges, N., *Vindiciae Medicinae & Medicorum: Or An Apology for the Profession and Professors of Physick in Answer to the Several Pleas of Illegal Practitioners* (London, 1665).
[Holles, D.], *Some Considerations upon the Question, Whether the Parliament is Dissolved by It's Prorogation for 15 Months* (London?, 1676).
Holyday, B., *Against Disloyalty, Fower Sermons Preach'd in the Times of the Late Troubles* (Oxford, 1661).
H[ookes], N., *Amanda, A Sacrifice to an Unknown Goddesse, or, A Free-Will Offering of a Loving Heart to a Sweet-Heart* (London, 1653).
Hotham, C., *A True State of the Case of Mr Hotham* (London, 1651).
[Hubbard, T.], *A Briefe and True Relation of the Great Disorders and Riot Attempted and Committed upon the House and Goods of Thomas Hubbert Esquire... in Moore-fields on the 21 Day of March Last* (London, 1647).
Pilula ad Expurgandam Hypocrisin. A Pill to Purge Formality. Wherein is Discovered the Sad and Useful Condition of All Formal Professors of Religion (London, 1650).
Humble Petition of Divers Inhabitants of the County of Hertford, who have Faithfully Adhered to the Good Old Cause. Presented to Parliament by Dr.Barber... May 13. 1659 (London, 1659).
Huyberts, A., *A Corner-Stone Laid Towards the Building of a New Colledge... in London* (London, 1675).
Izacke, R., *Remarkable Antiquities of the City of Exeter* (London, 1723).
Jackson, J., *Enchiridion Medicum Theoretico-Practicum; sive Tractatus de Morborum Theoria & Praxi* (London, 1695).
Jacombe, S., *Moses His Death: Opened and Applied, in a Sermon at Christ-Church in London at the Funeral of Mr Edward Bright* [23 December 1656] (London, 1657).
Johnson, R., *An Almanack for the Year 1683* (London, 1683).
Enchiridion Medicum; or a Manual of Physick (London, 1684).
Praxis Medicinae Reformata: Or, The Practice of Physick Reformed (London, 1700).

Johnson, W., 'Short Animadversions upon the Book Lately Published by one who stiles himselfe NOAH BIGGS, Helmontii Psittacum', appended to Johnson's edition of John Hester's *Three Exact Pieces of Leonard Phioravant* (London, 1652).

Α'γυρτο-Μάςτιξ: Or, Some Brief Animadversions upon Two Late Treatises (London, 1665).

Johnston, N., *The Excellency of Monarchical Government* (London, 1686).

Jones, G., *Hell's Cabal, or the Devilish Plots of Envy and Malice, against Dr Jones, and His Friendly Pills Discovered* (London, 1674?).

George Jones of London, Student in the Art of Physick and Chyrurgery (London?, 1675?).

George Jones of Hatton Garden, Holborn... His Book of Mighty Cures (London?, 1675?).

Kendall, G., *The Clerk of the Surveigh Surveighed and His Rigging Cast* (1656).

An Appendix to the Unlearned Alchimist (London, 1663?).

Kennedy, P., *An Essay on External Remedies* (London, 1715).

Knollys, H., *The Life and Death of... Mr Hanserd Knollys* (London, 1692).

L., J., *The New Disease or a Rational Account of the Great Colds and Coughs now Raging Amongst Us* (London, 1676).

Lamport, J., *A Direct Method of Ordering and Curing... the Smallpox* (London, 1685).

Langley, J., *Gemitus Colombae: The Mournfull Note of the Dove. A Sermon... Before the Honourable House of Commons, at Their Solemn Fast* [25 December 1644] (London, 1645).

L'Estrange, R., *The Accompt Clear'd: In Answer to a Libel Intituled A True Account from Chichester Concerning the Death of Habin the Informer* (London, 1682).

Love, C., *Englands Distemper, Having Division and Error, as Its Cause. Wanting Peace and Truth for Its Cure. Set Forth in a Sermon Preacht at Uxbridge on January 30th being the First Day of the Treaty* (London, 1645).

The Loyall Scout (London, 1659).

Mackerell, B., *The History and Antiquities of... King's Lynn in the County of Norfolk* (London, 1738).

Marshall, C., *A Plain and Candid Relation of the Nature, Use, and Dose of Several Approved Medicines* (London, 1670; 2nd ed., 1681).

Marshall, S., *A Sermon Preached Before the Honourable House of Commons... at their Publike Fast* [17 November 1640] (London, 1641).

The Right Understanding of the Times: Opened in a Sermon Preached to the... House of Commons [30 December 1646] (London, 1647).

Marston, J., *A Sermon Preached at St. Margaretts in Westminster... before Many of the Worthy Members of the Honourable House of Commons* [6 February 1642/3] (London, 1643).

Matthews, R., *The Unlearned Alchymist* (1st ed., London, 1660).

The Unlearned Alchymist (3rd ed., London, 1663).

Maynwaring, E., *Tutela Sanitatis. Sive Vita Protracta. The Protection of Long Life, and Detection of Its Brevity* (London, 1664).

Morbus Polyrhizos et Polymorphaeus (London, 1665).

Solamen Ægrorum, sive Ternarius Medicamentorum Chymicorum (London, 1665).

Mercurius Elencticus (London, 1649).

Mercurius Pragmaticus (London, 1649).

Merret, M., *Self-Conviction; or an Enumeration of the Absurdities, Railings, against the College, and Physicians in General* (London, 1670).

Moore, J., *A Leaf Pull'd from the Tree of Life: Medicinall for the Healing of Englands Divisions. Or a Glimpse of the Excellency of a Kingly Government* (London, 1660).

Morant, P., *The History and Antiquities of the County of Essex*, 2 vols (London, 1768).

Morley, C. L., *De Morbo Epidemico* (London, 1680).

Mossom, R., *Englands Gratulation for the King and His Subjects Happy Union. First Preach't on the Day of Publique Thanksgiving* [10 May 1660] (London, 1660).
A Most Learned, Conscientious, and Devout-Exercise; held forth the last Lords-Day, at Sir Peter Temples, in Lincolnes-Inne-Fields; by Lieut-Generall Crumwell. As it was Faithfully Taken Down in Characters by Aaron Guerdon (London, 1649).
Mountagu, Z., *The Jus Divinum of Government; or Magistracy Proved to be God's Ordinance, and Justice the Magistrates Duty. In a Plain Sermon Preached Before the Judges of Assize at East-Grinsted in the County of Sussex* (London, 1652).
Nye, P., *A Sermon Preached to the Honourable Citizens of London* [29 September 1659] (London, 1661).
[Mowlin, J.], *The Divell in Kent, or His Strange Delusion at Sandwitch* (London, 1647).
The Mystery of the Good Old Cause Briefly Unfolded (London, 1660).
The Names of the Iustices of Peace, of England and Wales... 1650 (London, 1650).
N[edham], M., *Medela Medicinae: A Plea for the Free Profession, and a Renovation of the Art of Physick* (London, 1665).
Needham, W., *Disquisitio Anatomica de Formato Foetu* (London, 1667).
Neville, R., *The Poor Scholar. A Comedy* (London, 1662).
An English Inquisition for a Heretick Or, The Punishment due to Hereticks [visitation sermon, Ware, 19 April 1672] (London, 1673).
The Necessity of Receiving the Holy Sacrament... Declared in a Sermon [Ware, 28 August 1678] (London, 1679).
The Nature and Causes of Hardness of Heart, Together with the Remedies Against It. Discovered in a Sermon [St Mary's, Cambridge, n.d.] (London, 1683).
TÀ ANΩ. The Things Above Proved to be the Most Proper Objects of the Mind and Affections, in a Sermon Preached before the University in Great St Maries Church in Cambridge (London, 1683).
Northleigh, J., *The Parallel: Or, The New Specious Association, an Old Rebellious Covenant* (London, 1682).
The Triumph of Our Monarchy, over the Plotts and Principles of Our Rebels and Republicans (London, 1685).
Oberndorffer, J., *Anatomyes of the True Physition and Counterfeit Mounte-Banke... Translated into English by F[rancis] H[erring]... Hereunto is Annexed: A Short Discourse or Discovery of Certaine Stratagems* (London, 1602); the latter republished as *Beware of Pick-purses* (London, 1605).
O'Dowde, T., *The Poor Man's Physician... The Third Edition* (London, 1665).
Two Letters Concerning the Cure of the Plague. The One to Thomas Eliot Esq.... The Other the Mayor of the Town of Southampton (London, 1665).
Ogilby, J., *The Fables of Aesop Paraphras'd in Verse, and Adorn'd with Sculpture* (London, 1651).
Okey, T. T., *Disputatio Medica Inauguralis de Febre Quartana* (Harderwyck, 1704).
Oldmixon, J., *The History of England, During the Reigns of the Royal House of Stuart* (London, 1730).
Owen, J., *A Complete Collection of the Sermons of the Reverend and Learned John Owen, D. D.* (London, 1721).
P., C., *A Dissertation Concerning the Pre-Existency of Souls* (London, 1684).
Packe, C., *Mineralogia, or, An Account of the Preparation, Manifold Vertues, and Uses of a Mineral Salt, Both in Physick and Chyrurgery* (London, 1693).
Medela Chymica or, an Account of the Vertues and Uses of a Select Number of Chymical Medicines (London, 1708).

Parker, G., *An Account of a Portable Barometer, with Reasons and Rules for the Use of It* (London, 1699).

Partridge, J., *Merlinus Liberatus. An Almanack... 1697* (London, 1697).

Paxton, P., *An Essay Concerning the Body of Man, Wherein Its Changes or Diseases are Consider'd, and the Operations of Medicines Observ'd* (London, 1701).

A Directory Physico-Medical, Composed for the Benefit of all Such as Deign to Study and Practise the Art of Physick (London, 1707).

Peachey, J., *Some Observations Made Upon the Root Cassummuniar Called otherwise Rysagone, Imported from the East Indies. Shewing Its Nature and Virtues, and Its Usefulness... in Apoplexies, Convulsions, Fits of the Mother, the Griping of the Gutts* (London, 1679).

Some Observations Made Upon the Barbado Seeds, Shewing their Admirable Virtue in Curing Dropsies (London, 1694).

Some Observations Upon the Herb Called Perigua, Imported from the Indies: Shewing Its Admirable Virtue in Curing the Diabetes (London, 1694).

Some Observations upon the Serpent Stones, Imported from the Indies: Shewing Their Admirable Virtues in Curing Malignant Spotted Feavers (London, 1694).

Some Observations Made Upon the Russia Seed. Shewing Its Admirable Virtues in Curing the Rickets in Children. Written by a Doctor of Physick in the Countrey to Esq. Boyle at London, 1674 (London, 1694).

Some Observations Made Upon the Cyclonian Plant. Shewing Its Admirable Virtues against Deafness. Written by a Physitian to the Honourable Esq. Boyle (London, 1695).

Some Observations Upon the Herb Cassiny Imported from Carolina. Shewing Its Admirable Virtue in Curing the Small-pox. Written by a Doctor of Physick in the Countrey to Esq. Boyle at London (London, 1695).

Penot, B., *Penotus Παλίμξθ: or The Alchymists Enchiridion. In Two Parts... Faithfully Englished... by B. P. Philalethes* (London, 1692).

A Perfect Diurnall of Some Passages in Parliament (London, 1649).

P[eters], H., *Good Work for a Good Magistrate* (London, 1651).

Phillips, D., *A Dissertation of the Small Pox... Translated by T. E.* (London, 1702).

Phillips, E., *The New World of English Words: Or, A General Dictionary* (London, 1658).

Pickering, B., *A Firebrand Pluckt Out of the Burning. A Sermon Preached... Before the Honourable House of Commons, at their Late Solemne Fast* [27 November 1644] (London, 1645).

[Pitman, H.], *A Relation of the Great Sufferings and Strange Adventures of Henry Pitman, Chyrurgion to the Late Duke of Monmouth* (London, 1689).

Plukenet, L., *Almagestum Botanicum sive Phytographiae* (London, 1696).

Pope, W., *The Life of the Right Reverend Father in God Seth, Lord Bishop of Salisbury* (London, 1697).

Pordage, J., *Innocencie Appearing, Through the Dark Mists of Pretended Guilt. Or, A Full and True Narration of the Unjust and Illegal Proceedings of the Commissioners of Berks... against John Pordage of Bradfield* (London, 1655).

Porter, R., *The Life of Mr John Hieron* (London, 1691).

The Principles of the Chymists of London Stated, with the Reasons of Their Dissent from the Colledge of Physicians; As They were Unanimously Agreed on by Them, at a Meeting in London... In Two Parts (London?, 1676).

Prynne, W., *A Fresh Discovery of Some Prodigious New Wandring-Blasing-Stars, & Firebrands Stiling Themselves New-Lights* (London, 1645).

R., J., *The Innocent Assemblies, and Good Order of the People of God (called Quakers) Vindicated* (London?, 1669).

The Ranters' Creed: Being a True Copie of the Examination of a Blasphemous Sort of People, Commonly Called Ranters... Taken Before Thomas Hubbert Esquire (London, 1651).

Raunce, J., *Astrologia Accusata Pariter & Condemnata. Or the Diabolical Art of Judicial Astrologie, Receiving the Definitive Sentence of Final Condemnation* (London, 1650).

Rawlinson, J., *Vivat Rex. A Sermon Preached at Pauls Crosse on the Day of His Majesties Happie Inauguration* [24 March 1614] (Oxford, 1619).

Reading, J., *A Faire Warning. Declaring the Comfortable Use Both of Sicknesse and Health. Delivered in Several Sermons at Saint Maries in Dover* (London, 1621).

A Relation of the Miraculous Cure of Susannah Arch, of a Leprosy and Ptysick (London, 1695).

Reyner, E., *Rules for the Government of the Tongue* (London, 1656).

Reynolds, J., *A Discourse upon Prodigious Abstinence* (London, 1669).

Rhodocanaces, C., *Carmina Graeca Rythmica Gratulatoria de reditu Serenissimi Sacratissimi & Theophylactou Principis Caroli II* (Oxford, 1660).

Alexicacus, or Spirit of the True Salt (London, 1664).

Riolan, J., *A Sure Guide; or, the Best and Nearest Way to Physick and Chyrurgery... in Six Books... Englished by Nich. Culpeper, Gent., and W. R. Doctor of the Liberal Arts, and of Physick* (London, 1657).

Rogers, J., *ΔΙΑΠΟΛΙΤΕΙΆ. A Christian Concertation with Mr. Prin, Mr. Baxter, Mr. Harrington, for the True Cause of the Commonwealth* (London, 1659).

Rusden, M., *A Further Discovery of Bees, Treating of the Nature, Government, Generation and Preservation of the Bee* (London, 1679; 2nd ed., 1685).

Russell, W., *A Physical Treatise, Grounded Not Upon Tradition, nor Phancy, but Experience* (London, 1684).

Ryves, B., *Mercurius Rusticus* (Oxford?, 1646).

St John, O., *An Argument of Law Concerning the Bill of Attainder of Thomas, Earl of Strafford* (London, 1641).

Salmon, W., *An Apology for the Innocency and Justice of the Quakers Cause* (London, 1674).

Doron Medicum (London, 1683).

Saunders, R., *Plenary Possession Makes a Lawfull Power: or Subjection to Powers that are in Being Proved to be Lawfull and Necessary, in a Sermon Preached Before the Judges in Exeter* [23 March 1650/1] (London, 1651).

Schroeder, J., *The Compleat Chymical Dispensatory in Five Books* (London, 1669).

Sclater, W., *Civil Magistracy by Divine Authority, Asserted, and Laid Forth in a Sermon, Preached at the Assizes Holden at Winchester* [4 March 1652/3] (London, 1653).

A Divine Cordiall for a Devout Soule... In a Sermon Preached at Taunton in the Assize Week [4 April 1653] (London, 1653).

Scot, T., *Vox Dei: Iniustice Cast and Condemned. In a Sermon Preached... at the Assises Holden in St. Edmunds Bury in Suffolke* [20 March 1622/3] (London, 1623).

God and the King in a Sermon Preached at the Assises Holden at Bury S.Edmonds [13 June 1631] (Cambridge, 1633).

Seaman, L., *Solomons Choice, or, a President for Kings and Princes, and All that are in Authority Presented in a Sermon before the Honourable House of Commons... at their Publique Fast* [25 September 1644] (London, 1644).

Sedgwick, O., *England's Preservation or, a Sermon Discovering the Onely Way to Prevent Destroying Judgements: Preached to the Honourable House of Commons at their Late Solemne Fast* [25 May 1642] (London, 1642).

Sherley, T., *A Philosophical Essay: Declaring the Probable Causes, whence Stones are Produced in the Greater World* (London, 1673).

Simpson, W., *Philosophical Dialogues Concerning the Principle of Natural Bodies* (London, 1677).

Skinner, T., *Elenchi Motuum Nuperorum in Anglia, Pars III. Sive, Motus Compositi* (London, 1676).

Skippon, P., 'An Account of a Journey Made Thru' Part of the Low Countries, Germany, Italy, and France [1663–1665]', in *A Collection of Voyages and Travels... in Six Volumes* (London, 1732).

Slater, S., *The Protector's Protection: Or, The Pious Prince Guarded by a Praying People. A Sermon Preached at St. Edmundsbury in Suffolk...Being a Day Set Apart for Solemn Fasting and Humiliation and Seeking a Blessing upon His Highness the Lord Protector* [13 October 1658] (London, 1659).

Smith, N., *The Quakers Spiritual Court Proclaim'd* (London, 1668).

Speciall Newes from the Army at Warwicke since the Fight: Sent from a Minister of Good Note, to an Alderman Here in London (London, 1642).

Spencer, J., *A Discourse of Divers Petitions of High Government, and Great Consequence, delivered by the Authour into the Hands of King James... and King Charles... A Treatise of Melancholie* (London, 1641).

Sprackling, R., *Medela Ignorantiae: Or a Just and Plain Vindication of Hippocrates and Galen from the Groundless Imputations of M[archamont] N[edham]* (London, 1665).

Sprigge, J., *Anglia Rediviva Englands Recovery being the History of the Motions, Actions, and Successes of the Army* (London, 1647).

Stanley, E., *Three Sermons Preached in the Cathedral Church of Winchester* [19 August 1660] (London, 1662).

Starkey, G., *The Admirable Efficacy, and Almost Incredible Virtue of True Oyl, which is made of Sulphur-Vive*, in W. Cooper (ed.), Collectanea Chymica: A Collection of Ten Several Treatises in Chymistry (London, 1684).

Starsmare, J., *ΠΑΙΔΩΝ ΝΟΣΗΜΑΤΑ or Children's Diseases Both Outward and Inward* (London, 1664).

Stennett, J., *Works*, 4 vols (London, 1731–2).

Streater, A., *An Ague, which Hitherto Amongst All Sorts Hath Beene Accounted the Physitians Shame* (London, 1641).

A Letter Sent to My Lord Mayor (London, 1642).

Stubbe, H., *Malice Rebuked, or A Character of Mr. Richard Baxters Abilities* (London, 1659).

Sutton, T., *Jethroes Counsell to Moses: Or, a Direction for Magistrates. A Sermon Preached at St Saviours in Southwarke... Before the Honourable Iudges* [5 March 1621/2] (London, 1631).

Swinnock, G., *Men are Gods, or the Dignity of Magistracy, and the Duty of the Magistrate: As it was Presented in a Sermon at the Assize Holden at Hertford* [2 August 1653] (London, 1660).

Sydenham, T., *Epistolae Responsoriae* (London, 1680).

Tractatus de Podagra et Hydrope (London, 1683).

Sylvius, F. de la Boë, *A New Idea of the Practice of Physic... Whereunto is Prefixed a Preface... by Dr. Mar[chamont] Nedham. Translated... by Richard Gower* (London, 1675).

Terry, E., *ΨΕΥΔΕΛΕΥΘΕΡΙΑ. Or, Lawlesse Liberty Set Forth in a Sermon Preached Before the Right Honourable the Lord Mayor of London* [16 August 1646] (London, 1646).

Thomas, M., *Two Assize Sermons Preached at Bridgnorth... Salop... 1657* (London, 1659).

Thomas, W., *The Regulating of Law-Suits, Evidences, and Pleadings. An Assize Sermon Preacht at Carmarthen* [16 March 1656/7] (London, 1657).

Thompson, T., *A Diet for a Drunkard: Delivered in Two Sermons at Saint Nicholas Church in Bristol… 1608* (London, 1612).
Thomson, G., *Loimologia. A Consolatory Advice, and Some Brief Observations Concerning the Present Pest* (London, 1665).
ΠΛΑ'ΝΟ-ΠΝΙΓΜΟ'Σ. Or, A Gag for Johnson (London, 1665).
ΆΟΙΜΟΤΟΜΙΑ or The Pest Anatomized (London, 1666).
Μισοχυμίας 'ΕλεΓχθ: or, A Check Given to the Insolent Garrulity of Henry Stubbe (London, 1671).
A Letter Sent to Mr Henry Stubbe (London, 1672).
Ορθο-μιθοδος ίατω-χυμυεή: Or The Direct Method of Curing Chymically (London, 1675).
Thoresby, R., *Ducatus Leodiensis: or, the Topography of the Ancient and Populous Town and Parish of Leedes* (London, 1715).
Thoroton, R., *The Antiquities of Nottinghamshire* (London, 1677).
Tonge, S., *The Narrative and Case of Simson Tonge, Gent* (London, 1681).
Tonstall, G., *A New-Years-Gift for Doctor Witty* (London, 1672).
Torbuck, J., *Ημέως παρ Ημέως. Extraordinary Dayes, Or, Sermons on the Most Solemn Feasts* (Oxford, 1671).
Treasons Anatomie or the Duty of the Loyall Subject (1647).
A True and Exact Diurnall of the Proceedings in Parliament (London, 1642).
Tuckney, A., *The Balme of Gilead, for the Wounds of England: Applied in a Sermon Preached at Westminster, Before the Honourable House of Commons at the Late Solemne Fast* [30 August 1643] (London, 1643).
Turner, P., *The Opinion of Peter Turner… Concerning Amulets or Plague Cakes* (London, 1603).
Turner, R., *ΒΟΤΑΝΟΛΟ'ΤΙΑ, or, The Brittish Physician* (London, 1664).
V., J., *Golgotha, or a Looking-Glass for London, and the Suburbs Thereof* (London, 1665).
Van Helmont, F. M., *The Paradoxal Discourses of F. M. van Helmont Concerning the Macrocosm and Microcosm, or the Greater and Lesser World and Their Union* (London, 1685).
Van Helmont, J. B., *A Ternary of Paradoxes… Translated, Illustrated, and Ampliated by Walter Charleton, Doctor in Physick, and Physician to the Late King* (London, 1650).
Deliramenta Catarrhi: Or, The Incongruities, Impossibilities, and Absurdities Couched Under the Vulgar Opinion of Defluxions. The Author that Great Philosopher, by Fire, Joh. Bapt. Van Helmont… The Translator and Paraphrast Dr. Charleton (London, 1650).
Vines, R., *The Impostures of Seducing Teachers Discovered; in a Sermon Before the Right Honorable the Lord Mayor and Aldermen of the City of London* [23 April 1644] (London, 1644).
ΠΕΡΙΑΜΜΑ 'ΕΠΙΔΗ'ΜΙΟΝ: Or, Vulgar Errours in Practice Censured (London, 1659).
W., J., *The Royall Entertainment of the King, by the Royalists of Huntingdon* (London, 1645).
W., S., *Medela Medicorum, or, an Enquiry into the Reasons & Grounds of the Contempt of Physicians* (London, 1678).
Walker, A., *God Save the King: or Pious and Loyal Joy, the Subjects Duty, for their Soveraign's Safety. Opened in a Sermon at Aldermanbury* [30 May 1660] (London, 1660).
Walsall, F., *The Bowing the Hearts of Subjects to Their Sovereign* [24 May 1660] (London, 1660).
W[alwyn], W., *Health's New Store-House Opened* (London, 1661).
Warly, J., *The Natural Fanatick, or, Reason Consider'd in its Extravagancy in Religion* (London, 1676).

The Reasoning Apostate: or Modern Latitude-Man Considered, as He Opposeth the Authority of the King and Church (London, 1677).

Warren, J., *The Unprofitable Servant: a Sermon Preached at the Assize Holden at Chelmesford* [26 March 1655] (London, 1655).

Warton, T., *The Life and Literary Remains of Ralph Bathurst, MD, Dean of Wells, and President of Trinity College in Oxford* (London, 1761).

Weale, J., *A Preparative for the Fast; or, a Sovereigne Balsome for the Cure of the Distemper of the Times* (London, 1642).

Westmacott, W., *Θεολοβοτανολογια: sive, Historia Vegetabilium Sacra: or, A Scripture Herbal* (London, 1694).

The Weekly Post (London, 1659).

Wharton, T., *Adenographia: sive, Glandularum Totius Corporis Descriptio* (London, 1656).

Whincop, J., *Gods Call to Weeping and Mourning. Set out in a Sermon before the House of Commons... Being the Day Before the Treaty (at Uxbridge) Began* [29 January 1644/5] (London, 1645).

Whitaker, J., *The Christians Great Design on Earth is to Attain Assurance for Heaven... Set forth in a Sermon Preached Before the Right Honourable the Lord Mayor... of London* [8 April 1645] (London, 1645).

The Danger of Greatnesse: or Uzziah his Exultation and Destruction Set forth in a Sermon Before the Right Honourable the Lords and Commons Assembled in Parliament [14 January 1645/6] (London, 1646).

Whitaker, T., *An Elenchus of Opinions Concerning the Cure of the Small Pox* (London, 1661).

White, J., *A Sermon Preached at Dorchester... at the Generall Assizes* [7 March 1633] (London, 1648).

Whitmore, H., *Febris Anomala or, The New Disease that Now Rageth Throughout England* (London, 1659).

Wilkinson, H., *Miranda, Stupenda. Or, The Wonderfull and Astonishing Mercies which the Lord Hath Wrought for England... Presented in a Sermon Preached Before the Honorable House of Commons* [21 July 1646] (London, 1646).

Willan, E., *Beatitas Britanniae: Or, King Charles the Second, Englands Beatitude, as Preached to the Incorporation of Eye, in the County of Suffolk, March 31 1661* (London, 1661).

Willis, B., *The History and Antiquities of the Town, Hundred, and Deanery of Buckingham* (London, 1755).

Windet, J., *Ad Majestatem Caroli Secundi Sylvae Duae* (London, 1660).

Winter, S., *Directions for the Use of My Elixir, My Philosophical Petza or Plaister, and My Balsam* (London, 1664?).

Wiseman, R., *Severall Chirurgicall Treatises* (London, 1676).

Wolferstan, S., *An Enquiry into the Causes of Diseases in General, and the Disturbances of the Humors in Mans Body* (London, 1692).

Wolveridge, J., *Speculum Matricis Hybernicum* (London, 1670).

Wynell, J., *Lues Venerea* (London, 1660).

Yarwood, J., *Physick Refin'd: Or, A Little Stream of Medicinal Marrow, Flowing from the Bones of Nature* (London, 1683).

Yonge, J., *Currus Triumphalis, è Terebinthô... Or an Account of the Many Admirable Vertues of Oleum Terebinthinae* (London, 1679).

Wounds of the Brain proved Curable (London, 1682).

Medicaster Medicatus, or a Remedy for the Itch of Scribling. The First Part (London, 1685).

3. Printed Primary Sources (Post-1800)

Acts of the Privy Council of England 1625–1626 (London, 1934).
Album Studiosorum Academiae Lugduno Bataviae MDLXXV–MDCCCLXXV (The Hague, 1875).
Aubrey, J., *Brief Lives*, ed. A. Clark, 2 vols (Oxford, 1898).
Baily, F. (ed.), *An Account of the Revd John Flamsteed, the First Astronomer Royal* (London, 1835).
Barlow, J. (ed.), *A Calendar of the Registers of Apprentices of the City of Gloucester 1595–1700* (Gloucestershire Rec. Soc., vol. 14, 2001).
Bate, F., *The Declaration of Indulgence 1672: A Study in the Rise of Organised Dissent* (London, 1908).
Bax, A. R., 'Marriage and Other Licences in the Commissary Court of Surrey', *Surrey Archaeological Collections*, 11 (1893), 204–43.
Bickford, J. A. R., and Bickford, M. E. (eds), *The Medical Profession in Hull 1400– 1900: A Biographical Dictionary* (Kingston upon Hull, 1983).
Blencowe, R. W., 'Extracts from the Parish Registers and Other Parochial Documents of East Sussex', *Sussex Archaeological Collections*, 4 (1851), 280–3.
Blomefield, F., *An Essay Towards a Topographical History of the County of Norfolk*, 11 vols (London, 1805–1811).
Bloom, J.H., and James, R. R., *Medical Practitioners in the Diocese of London... 1529–1725* (Cambridge, 1935).
Bowler, H. (ed.), *London Sessions Records, 1605–1685* (London, Catholic Rec. Soc., 1934).
Boyse, J., *The Works of the Reverend and Learned Mr. Joseph Boyse, of Dublin*, 2 vols (London, 1728).
Bruce, J. (ed.), *Diary of John Manningham, of the Middle Temple, and of Bradbourne, Kent, Barrister-at-Law, 1602–1603* (London, Camden Soc., vol. 99, 1868).
Calamy Revised. Being a Revision of Edmund Calamy's Account of the Ministers and Others Ejected and Silenced, 1660–2, ed. A. G. Matthews (Oxford, 1934; reissued 1988).
Calendar of Treasury Books, vol. 1 [1660–1667] (London, 1904).
Calendar of Treasury Books, vol. 3 [1669–1672] (London, 1908).
Calendar of Treasury Books, vol. 7 [1685–1689] (London, 1923).
Calendar of Treasury Books, vol. 8 [1689–1692] (London, 1931).
Chalk, T. (ed.), *The Journal, Together with Sundry Epistles and Other Writings of Charles Marshall* (London, 1844).
Chester, J. L. (ed), *The Parish Registers of St Thomas the Apostle, London, 1558 to 1754* (London, Harleian Soc., 1881).
Clark, A. (ed.), *The Life and Times of Anthony Wood, Antiquary, at Oxford, 1632– 1695*, 5 vols (Oxford, Oxford Hist. Soc., 1891–1900).
Cockburn, J. S. (ed.), *Calendar of Assize Records, Kent Indictments, Charles II 1676–1688* (London, 1997).
Commons' Journal, vols 2, 6 and 7 [1640–1643; 1648–1651; 1651–1660] (London, 1802).
Conway Letters: The Correspondence of Anne, Viscountess Conway, Henry More, and Their Friends, 1642–1684, ed. M. H. Nicholson (New Haven, 1930; rev. ed., S. Hutton, Oxford, 1992).
Cooper, C. H., *Annals of Cambridge*, 5 vols (Cambridge, 1842–53).
Crittall, E. (ed.), *Victoria County History of Wiltshire. Vol. 8* (London, 1965).
De Beer, E. S. (ed.), *The Diary of John Evelyn*, 6 vols (Oxford, 1955).
De Beer, E. S. (ed), *The Correspondence of John Locke*, 7 vols (Oxford, OUP, 1976–82).

Dennett, J. (ed.), *Beverley Borough Records 1575–1821* (Wakefield, Yorkshire Archaeological Soc., vol. 84, 1932).

Dooley, B. M. (ed.), *Italy in the Baroque: Selected Readings* (New York & London, 1995).

Douglas, D. C. (ed.), *English Historical Documents*, 10 vols (London, 1995), vi [1660–1714].

Fenwick, T. F., and Metcalfe, W. C. (eds), *The Visitation of the County of Gloucester, 1682–1683* (Exeter, 1884).

Ferguson, J., *Bibliotheca Chemica*, 2 vols (Glasgow, 1906).

Firth, C. H., and Rait, R. S. (eds), *Acts and Ordinances of the Interregnum, 1642–1660*, 3 vols (London, 1911).

Fockema Andraea, S. J., and Meijer, T. J. (eds), *Album Studiosorum Academiae Franekerensis (1585–1811, 1816–1844)* (Franeker, 1968).

Goldie, M., *et al.* (eds), *The Entring Book of Roger Morrice 1677–1691*, 6 vols (Woodbridge & New York, 2007).

Greaves, R. W. (ed.), *The First Ledger Book of High Wycombe* (London, Buckinghamshire Rec. Soc., vol. 11, 1947).

Green, M. A. E. (ed.), *The Diary of John Rous, Incumbent of Santon Downham, Suffolk, from 1625 to 1642* (London, Camden Soc., vol. 66, 1856).

Calendar of the Proceedings of The Committee for Compounding, &c, 1643–1660, 5 vols (London, 1889–92).

Hardy, W. J., (ed.), *Hertford County Records. Notes and Extracts from the Sessions Rolls 1581 to 1698* (Hertford, 1905).

Middlesex County Records. Calendar of Sessions Books, 1689–1709 (1905).

Henning, B. (ed.), *The History of Parliament: The House of Commons, 1660–1690*, 3 vols (London, 1983).

Herbert, N. M. (ed.), *Victoria County History of Gloucestershire, vol. 4* (London, 1988).

Historical Manuscripts Commission. Sixth Report, Part 1, Report & Appendix (London, 1877).

Historical Manuscripts Commission. Eleventh Report, Appendix, Part II. The Manuscripts of the House of Lords, 1678–1688 (London, 1887).

Historical Manuscripts Commission. Eleventh Report, Appendix, Part VII (London, 1888).

Historical Manuscripts Commission. Thirteenth Report, Appendix, Part 1. The Manuscripts of... the Duke of Portland. Vol. 1 (London, 1891).

Historical Manuscripts Commission, Thirteenth Report, Appendix, Part IV (London, 1892).

Historical Manuscripts Commission. Fourteenth Report, Appendix, Part III. Manuscripts of the Duke of Portland, vol. 3 (London, 1894).

Historical Manuscripts Commission. Fourteenth Report, Appendix, Part II. Manuscripts of the Duke of Portland, vol. 4 (London, 1894).

Historical Manuscripts Commission. Reports on the Manuscripts of the Marquess of Downshire... Vol. 1... Part 1 (London, 1924).

Holmes, C. (ed.), *The Suffolk Committees for Scandalous Ministers, 1644–1646* (Ipswich, Suffolk Rec. Soc., vol. 12, 1970).

Howard, J. J. (ed.), *A Visitation of the County of Essex. Begun 1664, Finished 1668* (London, 1888).

Hunter, Rev. J., *The Rise of the Old Dissent, Exemplified in the Life of Oliver Heywood... 1630–1702* (London, 1842).

Hughes Clarke, A. W., and Campling, A. (eds), *The Visitation of Norfolk... 1664* (London, Harleian Soc., vol. 86, 1934).

Hunter, M., and Gregory, A. (eds), *An Astrological Diary of the Seventeenth Century: Samuel Jeake of Rye 1652–1699* (Oxford, 1988).

Hunter, M., Mandelbrote, G., Ovenden, R., and Smith, N. (eds), *A Radical's Books: The Library Catalogue of Samuel Jeake of Rye, 1623–90* (Woodbridge, 1999).
Hunter, M., Clericuzio, A., and Principe, L. (eds), *The Correspondence of Robert Boyle*, 6 vols (London, 2001).
Innes Smith, R. W., *English-Speaking Students of Medicine at the University of Leyden* (Edinburgh, 1932).
Irvine, W. F. (ed.), *Marriage Licences Granted Within the Archdeaconry of Chester in the Diocese of Chester*, 4 vols (Lancashire and Cheshire Rec. Soc., vols 65, 69, 73, 77, 1912–24).
Jeaffreson, J. C. (ed.), *Middlesex County Records*, 4 vols (London, Middlesex County Rec. Soc., 1888–92).
Jenkinson, H., and Powell, D. L. (eds), *Surrey Quarter Sessions Records... 1659–1661* (Frome & London, Surrey Rec. Soc., vol. 13, 1934).
Josten, C. H. (ed.), *Elias Ashmole (1617–1672): His Autobiographical and Historical Notes, His Correspondence, and Other Contemporary Sources Relating to His Life and Work*, 5 vols (Oxford, 1966).
Juřica, J. (ed.), *A Calendar of the Freemen of the City of Gloucester 1641–1838* (Bristol, Gloucestershire Record Series, vol. 4, 1991).
Le Hardy, W. (ed.), *Hertfordshire County Records. Calendar to the Sessions Books and Sessions Minute Books... 1658 to 1700*, 6 vols (Hertford, 1930).
Buckinghamshire Sessions Records. Vol. 1 1678 to 1694 (Aylesbury, 1933).
Lloyd Thomas, J. M. (ed.), *The Autobiography of Richard Baxter, Being the Reliquiae Baxterianae Abridged from the Folio (1696)* (London, 1925).
Longden, H. I. (ed.), *Northamptonshire and Rutland Clergy*, 16 vols (Northampton, 1938–52).
Lords' Journal, vols 11 and 13 [1660–1666; 1675–1681].
McGrath, P. (ed.), *Merchants and Merchandise in Seventeenth-Century Bristol* (Bristol, Bristol Record Soc., vol. 19, 1955).
McKinley, R. A. (ed.), *Victoria County History of Leicestershire. Vol. 4* (London, 1858).
Mayo, C. H. (ed.), *The Municipal Records of the Borough of Dorchester, Dorset* (Exeter, 1908).
Mayor, J. E. B. (ed.), *The Life of Matthew Robinson* (Cambridge, 1856).
Meekings, C. A. F. (ed.), *Dorset Hearth Tax Assessments 1662–1664* (Dorchester, 1951).
Metcalfe, W. C. (ed.), *Visitations of Hertfordshire... 1572... 1634* (London, Harleian Soc., vol. 22, 1886).
Morland, C. (ed.), *The Somersetshire Quarterly Meeting of the Society of Friends, 1668–1699* (Woking, Somerset Rec. Soc., vol. 75, 1978).
Mortimer, R. (ed.), *Minute Book of the Men's Meeting of the Society of Friends in Bristol 1686–1704* (Bristol, Bristol Rec. Soc., vol. 30, 1977).
Munk, W., *The Roll of the Royal College of Physicians of London, 1518–1800*, 3 vols (London, 1878).
Napier, A. (ed.), *The Theological Works of Isaac Barrow, D. D.*, 9 vols (Cambridge, 1859).
Nichols, J., *The History and Antiquities of the County of Leicester*, 4 vols (London, 1795–1815).
The Correspondence of Henry Oldenburg, eds A. R. and M. B. Hall, 13 vols (Madison, Milwaukee, London & Philadelphia, 1965–86).
Ormerod, G. (ed.), *Epistolary Relics of Lancashire and Cheshire Antiquaries, 1653–1673* (Manchester, Chetham Soc., vol. 24, 1850).
Parsloe, G. (ed.), *The Minute Book of Bedford Corporation 1647–1664* (Luton, Bedfordshire Rec. Soc., vol. 26, 1949).

Raine, J. (ed.), *Depositions from the Castle of York Relating to Offences Committed in the Northern Counties in the Seventeenth Century* (Durham, Surtees Soc., vol. 40, 1861).
Robinson, H. W., and Adams, W. (eds), *The Diary of Robert Hooke, 1672–1680* (London, 1935).
Rutt, J. T. (ed.), *Diary of Thomas Burton, Esq., Member in the Parliaments of Oliver and Richard Cromwell from 1656 to 1659*, 4 vols (London, 1828).
Rylands, W. H. (ed.), *The Visitation of the County of Warwick, 1682–1683* (London, Harleian Soc., vol. 62, 1911).
Salzman, L. F., *Victoria County History of Sussex*, vols 3 and 4 (London, 1935 and 1953).
Scott, M. (ed.), *Apprenticeship Disputes in the Lord Mayor's Court of London 1573–1723* (London, British Rec. Soc., Apprenticeship Series, vol. 1, Part 2, 2016).
Shaw, W. A., *A History of the English Church During the Civil Wars and Under the Commonwealth, 1640–1660*, 2 vols (London, 1900).
Letters of Denization and Acts of Naturalization for Aliens in England and Ireland, 1603–1700 (Lymington, Huguenot Society, vol. 18, 1911).
Snell, B. S. (ed.), *The Minute Book of the Monthly Meeting of the Society of Friends for the Upperside of Buckinghamshire, 1669–1690* (High Wycombe, Buckinghamshire Rec. Soc., vol. 1, 1937).
Snow, V. F., and Young, A. S. (eds), *Private Journals of the Long Parliament*, 3 vols (New Haven and London, 1982–92).
Spalding, R. (ed.), *The Diary of Bulstrode Whitelocke 1605–1675* (Oxford, 1990).
Squibb, G. D. (ed.), *The Visitation of Somerset and the City of Bristol 1672* (London, Harleian Soc., vol. 11, 1992).
Sykes-McLean, H. (ed.), *The Registers of Woodmancote, 1582–1812* (Brighton, 1932).
A Collection of the State Papers of John Thurloe, Esq., ed. T. Birch, 7 vols (London, 1742).
Tonge, I., 'Journal of the Plot, 1678', in *Diaries of the Popish Plot*, ed. D. G. Greene (New York, 1977).
Toon, P. (ed.), *The Correspondence of John Owen (1616–1683)* (Cambridge & London, 1970).
Wales, T. C., and Hartley, C. P. (eds), *The Visitation of London Begun in 1687*, 2 vols (London, Harleian Society, vols 16 and 17, 2004).
Walker Revised Being a Revision of John Walker's Sufferings of the Clergy During the Grand Rebellion 1642–60, ed. A. G. Matthews (Oxford, 1948).
Webster, T., and Shipps, K. (ed.), *The Diary of Samuel Rogers, 1634–1638* (Woodbridge and Rochester, NY, 2004).
Wigfield, W. M., *The Monmouth Rebels 1685* (Gloucester, 1985).
Wilkin, S. (ed.), *Sir Thomas Browne's Works. Including his Life and Correspondence*, 4 vols (London & Norwich, 1836).
Wilkinson, C. H. (ed.), *The Poems of Richard Lovelace* (Oxford, 1930).
Woodhead, J. R., *The Rulers of London 1660–1689: A Biographical Record of the Aldermen and Common Councilmen of the City of London* (London, 1965).
Worth, R. N., 'The Siege Accounts of Plymouth, *Transactions of the Devonshire Association*, 17 (1885), 215–39.
The Diary and Correspondence of Dr John Worthington, ed. J. Crossley, 3 vols (Manchester, Chetham Soc., vols 13, 36, 114, 1847–1886).

4. Printed Secondary Works

Adair, J., 'The Court Martial Papers of Sir William Waller's Army', *Journal of the Society for Army Historical Research*, 44 (1966), 205–26.

Agnew, L. R. C., 'De Sanguine Episcopoque: A Discussion of Bishop Robert Grove [1634–1696] and his *Carmen de Sanguinis Circuitu, &c* (1685)', *Bulletin of the History of Medicine*, 34 (1960), 318–30.
Akkerman, N., *Invisible Agents: Women and Espionage in Seventeenth-Century Britain* (Oxford, 2018).
Andrews, J., 'The Politics of Committal to Early Modern Bethlem', in R. Porter (ed.), *Medicine in the Enlightenment* (Amsterdam, 1995), 6–63.
Ashcraft, R., *Revolutionary Politics and Locke's* Two Treatises of Government (Princeton, NJ, 1986).
Ashley Montagu, M. F., *Edward Tyson, MD, FRS, 1650–1708 and the Rise of Human and Comparative Anatomy in England* (Philadelphia, Memoirs of the American Philosophical Society, vol. 20, 1943).
Austin, R., 'The City of Gloucester and the Regulation of Corporations, 1662–63', *Transactions of the Bristol and Gloucestershire Archaeological Society*, 58 (1936), 257–74.
Aylmer, G., *The State's Servants: The Civil Service of the English Republic 1649–1660* (London and Boston, 1973).
Baines, A. H. J., 'The Signatories of the Orthodox Confession of 1679', *Baptist Quarterly*, 18 (1957–8), 80–1.
Barnard, T., *Cromwellian Ireland: English Government and Reform in Ireland 1649–1660* (Oxford, 1975).
Beddard, R. A., 'Tory Oxford', in N. Tyacke (ed.), *The History of the University of Oxford: Seventeenth-Century Oxford* (Oxford, 1997), 863–905.
Bell, W. G., *The Great Plague of London in 1665* (London, 1951).
Bellany, A., and Cogswell, T., *The Murder of King James I* (New Haven & London, 2015).
Betteridge, A., 'Early Baptists in Leicestershire and Rutland', *Baptist Quarterly*, 26 (1976), 209–23.
Bettey, J. H., 'Contrasts among the Dorset Clergy during the Seventeenth Century', *Notes and Queries for Somerset and Dorset*, 32 (1986–1990), 846.
Biagioli, M., *Galileo, Courtier: The Practice of Science in the Age of Absolutism* (Chicago, 1993).
'Etiquette, Interdependence, and Sociability in Seventeenth-Century Science', *Critical Inquiry*, 22 (1996), 193–238.
Birken, W. J., 'The Royal College of Physicians of London and Its Support of the Parliamentary Cause in the English Civil War', *Journal of British Studies*, 23 (1983), 47–62.
'The Dissenting Tradition in English Medicine of the Seventeenth and Eighteenth Centuries', *Medical History*, 39 (1995), 197–218.
'Merton Revisited: English Independency and Medical Conservatism in the Seventeenth Century', in E. L. Furdell (ed.), *Textual Healing: Essays on Medieval and Early Modern Medicine* (Leiden & Boston, MA, 2005), 259–83.
Blatchly, J., *The Town Library of Ipswich* (Woodbridge, 1989).
Brent, C., *Pre-Georgian Lewes c.690–1714; The Emergence of a County Town* (2004).
Brown, C., *History of Newark-upon-Trent*, 2 vols (Newark, 1907).
Bussby, F., 'George Morley, Bishop of Worcester, 1660–62', *Transactions of the Worcestershire Archaeological Society*, 37 (1960), 11–23.
Calder, I. M., 'A Seventeenth-Century Attempt to Purify the Anglican Church', *American Historical Review*, 53 (1948), 760–75.
Capp, B. S., *The Fifth Monarchy Men: A Study in Seventeenth-Century Millenarianism* (London, 1972).

Astrology and the Popular Press: English Almanacs 1500–1800 (London & Boston, 1979).
Caron, L., 'Thomas Willis, the Restoration and the First Works of Neurology', *Medical History*, 59 (2015), 525–53.
Carpenter, E., *Thomas Tenison, Archbishop of Canterbury: His Life and Times* (London, 1948).
Carter, A. C., *The English Reformed Church in Amsterdam in the Seventeenth Century* (Amsterdam, 1964).
Champion, J. T. I., *The Pillars of Priestcraft Shaken: The Church of England and Its Enemies, 1660–1730* (Cambridge, 1992).
Champion, J. T. I., and McNulty, L., 'Making Orthodoxy in Late Restoration England: The Trials of Edmund Hickeringill, 1662–1710', in M. J. Braddick and J. Walter (eds), *Negotiating Power in Early Modern Society: Order, Hierarchy and Subordination in Britain and Ireland* (Cambridge, 2001), 227–48.
Christy, J. M., 'Dr Benjamin Allen (1663–1738) of Braintree: A Forgotten Essex Naturalist', *The Essex Naturalist*, 16 (1911), 145–75.
'More about Dr Benjamin Allen (1663–1738) of Braintree, Naturalist', *The Essex Naturalist*, 17 (1912), 1–14.
Clapp, S. L. C., 'Subscription Publishers Prior to Jacob Tonson', *The Library*, 19 (1932), 158–83.
Clarke, A., *Prelude to Restoration in Ireland: The End of the Commonwealth, 1659–1660* (Cambridge, 1999).
Clericuzio, A., 'From Van Helmont to Boyle. A Study of the Transmission of Helmontian Chemical and Medical Theories in Seventeenth-Century England', *British Journal for the History of Science*, 16 (1993), 303–34.
Coffey, J., and Lim, P. C. H. (eds), *The Cambridge Companion to Puritanism* (Cambridge, 2008).
Cohen. I. B., (ed.), *Puritanism and the Rise of Modern Science: The Merton Thesis* (New Brunswick, NJ, 1990).
Collins, J. R., *The Allegiance of Thomas Hobbes* (Oxford, 2005).
Collins, S. L., *From Divine Cosmos to Sovereign State: An Intellectual History of Consciousness and the Idea of Order in Renaissance England* (Oxford, 1989).
Como, D. R., *Blown by the Spirit: Puritanism and the Emergence of an Antinomian Underground in Pre-Civil-War England* (Stanford, 2004).
Considine, J., 'In Praise of Edward Phillips', *Studia Linguistica Universitatis Iagellonicae Cracoviensis*, 132 (2015), 211–28.
Cook, H., *The Decline of the Old Medical Regime in Stuart London* (Ithaca, NY, and London, 1986).
'The Society of Chemical Physicians, the New Philosophy, and the Restoration Court', *Bulletin of the History of Medicine*, 61 (1987), 61–77.
'Policing the Health of London: The College of Physicians and the Early Stuart Monarchy', *Social History of Medicine*, 2 (1989), 1–33.
'Medical Innovation or Medical Malpractice? Or, a Dutch Physician in London: Joannes Groenvelt, 1694–1700', *Tractrix*, 2 (1990), 63–91.
'Practical Medicine and the British Armed Forces after the "Glorious Revolution"', *Medical History*, 34 (1990), 1–26.
Trials of an Ordinary Doctor: Joannes Groenevelt in Seventeenth-Century London (Baltimore, MD, 1994).
'Sir John Colbatch and Augustan Medicine: Experimentalism, Character and Entrepreneuralism', *Annals of Science*, 47 (2006), 475–505.

Cooke, M. A. L., 'Richard Surflet, Translator and Practitioner in Physic', *Medical History*, 25 (1981), 41–56.
Cooper, T., 'Richard Baxter and His Physicians', *Social History of Medicine*, 20 (2007), 1–19.
Cooper, W. D., 'Notices of the Last Great Plague, 1665–6', *Archaeologia*, 37 (1857), 1–22.
Cregan, D. F., 'The Confederate Catholics of Ireland: The Personnel of the Confederation, 1642–9', *Irish Historical Studies*, 29 (1995), 490–512.
Cressy, D., *England on Edge: Crisis and Revolution 1640–1642* (Oxford, 2006).
Cunningham, A., 'The Transformation of Hippocrates in Seventeenth-Century Britain', in D. Cantor (ed.), *Reinventing Hippocrates* (Aldershot, 2002), 91–115.
Dalton, R. J., 'Gerrard Winstanley: The Experience of Fraud 1641', *The Historical Journal*, 34 (1991), 973–84.
Daly, J., 'Cosmic Harmony and Political Thinking in Early Stuart England', *Transactions of the American Philosophical Society*, 69 (1979), 1–40.
Davies, C. S. L., 'Conspiracy, Kinship, and Preferment in the Interregnum and Restoration: the Brunsells and Holders of Nottinghamshire', *Midland History*, 31 (2006), 1–17.
Dawbarn, F., 'Patronage and Power: The College of Physicians and the Jacobean Court', *British Journal for the History of Science*, 31 (1998), 1–19.
'New Light on Dr Thomas Moffet: The Triple Roles of an Early Modern Physician, Client and Patronage Broker', *Medical History*, 47 (2003), 3–22.
De Krey, G. S., *London and the Restoration 1659–1683* (Cambridge, 2005).
Debus, A. G., *The French Paracelsians: The Chemical Challenge to Medical and Scientific Tradition in Early Modern France* (Cambridge, 1991).
Decamp, E., *Civic and Medical Worlds in Early Modern England: Performing Barbery and Surgery* (London, 2016).
Diamond, W. C., 'Natural Philosophy in Harrington's Political Thought', *Journal of the History of Philosophy*, 16 (1978), 387–98.
Dickson, D. R., 'Thomas Henshaw and Sir Robert Paston's Pursuit of the Red Elixir: An Early Collaboration Between Fellows of the Royal Society', *Notes and Records of the Royal Society of London*, 51 (1997), 57–76.
Eccleshall, R., *Order and Reason in Politics: Theories of Absolute and Limited Monarchy in Early Modern England* (Oxford, 1978).
Ellis, F. H., 'The Author of Wing C6727: Daniel Coxe, F. R. S., or Thomas Coxe, F. R. S.', *Notes and Records of the Royal Society of London*, 18 (1963), 36–8.
Elmer, P., 'Medicine, Science and the Quakers: the "Puritanism-Science" Debate Reconsidered', *Journal of the Friends Historical Society*, 54 (1981), 265–86.
'Medicine, Religion and the Puritan Revolution', in R. French and A. Wear (eds), *The Medical Revolution of the Seventeenth Century* (Cambridge, 1989), 10–45.
The Miraculous Conformist: Valentine Greatrakes, the Body Politic, and the Politics of Healing in Restoration Britain (Oxford, 2013).
Witchcraft, Witch-Hunting, and Politics in Early Modern England (Oxford, 2016).
'Promoting Medical Change in Restoration Ireland: The Chemical Revolution and the Patronage of James Butler, duke of Ormond (1610–88)' in J. Cunningham (ed.), *Early Modern Ireland and the World of Medicine: Practitioners, Collectors and Contexts* (Manchester, 2019), 84–101.
'"Under the Operation of a Higher and Exalted Mind": Medicine, Mysticism and Social Reform in Restoration England', in H. C. Powell and C. J. Saunders (eds), *Visions and Voice-Hearing in Medieval and Early Modern Contexts* (Cham, Switzerland, 2021), 281–304.
Elwyn-Hughes, R., 'The Rise and Fall of the "Antiscorbutics": Some Notes on the Traditional Cures for "Land Scurvy"', *Medical History*, 34 (1990), 52–64.

Farr, D., 'John Blackwell and Daniel Cox: Further Notes on Their Activities in Restoration England and British North America', *Pennsylvania Magazine of History and Biography*, 123 (1999), 227–33.
John Lambert, Parliamentary Soldier and Cromwellian Major General, 1619–1684 (Woodbridge, 2003).
Fissell, M., *Patients, Power, and the Poor in Eighteenth-Century Bristol* (Cambridge, 1991).
Frank Jnr, R. G., 'The Physician as Virtuoso in Seventeenth-Century England', in B. Shapiro and R. G. Frank (eds), *English Scientific Virtuosi in the Sixteenth and Seventeenth Centuries* (Los Angeles, 1979), 57–114.
'Medicine', in N. Tyacke (ed.), *The History of the University of Oxford. Volume IV. Seventeenth Century Oxford* (Oxford, 1997), 505–58.
French, H. R., '"Ingenious and Learned Gentlemen': Social Perceptions and Self-Fashioning among Parish Elites in Essex, 1680–1740', *Social History*, 25 (2000), 44–66.
Furdell, E. L., *James Welwood: Physician to the Glorious Revolution* (Conshohocken, PA, 1998).
The Royal Doctors, 1485–1714: Medical Personnel at the Tudor and Stuart Courts (Rochester, NY, 2001).
Publishing and Medicine in Early Modern England (Rochester, NY, 2002).
Gascoigne, J., *Cambridge in the Age of the Enlightenment: Science, Religion and Politics from the Restoration to the French Revolution* (Cambridge, 1989).
Gaskill, M., *Witchfinders: A Seventeenth-Century English Tragedy* (London, 2005).
Goldie, M., 'John Locke's Circle and James II', *The Historical Journal*, 35 (1992), 579–84.
'James II and the Dissenters' Revenge: The Commission of Enquiry of 1688', *Bulletin of the Institute of Historical Research*, 66 (1993), 53–88.
Goldie, M., and Spurr, J., 'Politics and the Restoration Parish: Edward Fowler and the Struggle for St Giles Cripplegate', *English Historical Review*, 109 (1994), 572–96.
Greaves, R. L., *Deliver Us from Evil: The Radical Underground in Britain, 1660–1663* (Oxford and New York, 1986).
Enemies Under His Feet: Radicals and Nonconformists in Britain, 1664–1677 (Stanford, CA, 1990).
Secrets of the Kingdom: British Radicals from the Popish Plot to the Revolution of 1688–1689 (Stanford, 1992).
Gruber von Arni, E., *Justice to the Maimed Soldier: Nursing, Medical Care and Welfare for Sick and Wounded Soldiers and Their Families during the English Civil Wars and Interregnum, 1642–1660* (Aldershot, 2001).
Gunn, J. A. W., 'The *Civil Polity* of Peter Paxton', *Past and Present*, 40 (1968), 42–57.
Gunther, R. T., *Early Science in Cambridge* (Oxford, 1937).
Hale, D. G., *The Body Politic: A Political Metaphor in Renaissance English Literature* (The Hague & Paris, 1971).
'Analogy of the Body Politic' in P. P. Wiener (ed.), *Dictionary of the History of Ideas*, 5 vols (New York, 1973–4), i, 69.
Haley, K. H. D., *The First Earl of Shaftesbury* (Oxford, 1968).
Halliday, P. D., *Dismembering the Body Politic: Partisan Politics in England's Towns 1650–1730* (Cambridge, 1998).
Harkness, D. E., *The Jewel House: Elizabethan London and the Scientific Revolution* (New Haven & London, 2007).
Harley, D., '"Bred Up in the Study of That Faculty": Licensed Physicians in North- West England, 1660–1760', *Medical History*, 38 (1994), 398–420.

'Rychard Bostok of Tandridge, Surrey (*c.*1530–1605), M.P., Paracelsian Propagandist and Friend of John Dee', *Ambix*, 47 (2000), 29–34.

Harris, J. G., *Foreign Bodies and the Body Politic: Discourses of Social Pathology in Early Modern England* (Cambridge, 1998).

Harris, T., *London Crowds in the Reign of Charles II: Propaganda and Politics from the Restoration to the Exclusion Crisis* (Cambridge, 1987).

Hawkins, M., 'Piss Profits: Thomas Willis, His *Diatribae Duae* and the Formation of His Professional Identity', *History of Science*, 49 (2011), 1–24.

Hay, A., *The History of Chichester* (Chichester & London, 1804).

Hessayon, A., 'Lead's Life and Times (Part Two): The Woman in the Wilderness', in A. Hessayon (ed.), *Jane Lead and Her Transnational Legacy* (London, 2016).

Hilberry, C., 'Medical Poems from John Collop's *Poesis Rediviva* (1656)', *Journal of the History of Medicine and Allied Sciences*, 11 (1956), 384–411.

Hill, J. E. C., 'The Medical Profession and Its Critics', in *idem*, *Change and Continuity in Seventeenth-Century England* (London, 1974), 157–78.

Hughes, A., 'Religion and Society in Stratford-upon-Avon, 1619–1638', *Midland History*, 19 (1994), 58–84.

Hull, W. I., *Benjamin Furly and Quakerism in Rotterdam* (Swarthmore, PA, 1941).

Hunter, M., *Science and Society in Restoration England* (London & New York, 1981).

'Introduction. Fifteen Essays and a New Theory of Intellectual Change', in *idem*, Science *and the Shape of Orthodoxy: Intellectual Change in Late Seventeenth-Century Britain* (Woodbridge, 1995), 11–18.

Hurwich, J. J., '"A Fanatick Town": The Political Influence of Dissenters in Coventry, 1660–1720', *Midland History*, 4 (1977–8), 15–47.

Ivimey, J., *A History of the English Baptists*, 4 vols (London, 1811–20).

James, A., *Poets, Players and Preachers: Remembering the Gunpowder Plot in Seventeenth-Century England* (Toronto, 2016).

Jenner, M. S. R., 'The Roasting of the Rump: Scatology and the Body Politic in Restoration England', *Past and Present*, 177 (2002), 84–120.

Jenner, M. S. R., and Wallis, P. (eds), *Medicine and the Market in England and Its Colonies, c.1450–c.1850* (Houndmills, Basingstoke, 2007).

Jodziewicz, W., 'A Stranger in the Land: Gershom Bulkeley of Connecticut', *Transactions of the American Philosophical Society*, 78 (1988).

Kingston, A., *East Anglia and the Great Civil War: The Rising of Cromwell's Ironsides in the Associated Counties of Cambridge, Huntingdon, Lincoln, Norfolk, Suffolk, Essex, and Hertford* (London, 1897).

Knights, M., 'Petitioning and the Political Theorists: John Locke, Algernon Sidney and London's "Monster Petition" of 1680', *Past and Present*, 138 (1993), 94–111.

Representation and Misrepresentation in Later Stuart Britain: Partisanship and Political Culture (Oxford & New York, 2005).

The Devil in Disguise: Deception, Delusion, and Fanaticism in the Early English Enlightenment (Oxford, 2011).

Knott, O., 'The Baptists of Liverpool in the Seventeenth Century', *Baptist Quarterly*, 4 (1928–9), 219–22.

Lake, P., *Moderate Puritans and the Elizabethan Church* (Cambridge, 1982).

'The Laudian Style: Order, Uniformity and the Pursuit of the Beauty of Holiness in the 1630s', in K. Fincham (ed.), *The Early Stuart Church, 1603–1642* (Basingstoke, 1993), 161–85.

Lane, J., *John Hall and His Patients: The Medical Practice of Shakespeare's Son-in-law* (Stroud, 1996).

Leng, T., *Benjamin Worsley (1618–1677): Trade, Interest and the Spirit in Revolutionary England* (Woodbridge, 2008).
Levitin, D., '"Made Up from Many Experimentall Notions": The Society of Apothecaries, Medical Humanism, and the Rhetoric of Experience in 1630s London', *Journal of Medical History and Allied Sciences*, 70 (2015), 549–87.
Lindley, K., 'Whitechapel Independents and the English Revolution', *The Historical Journal*, 41 (1998), 283–91.
MacDonald, M., *Mystical Bedlam: Madness, Anxiety, and Healing in Seventeenth- Century England* (Cambridge, 1981).
McLachlan, H. J., *Socinianism in Seventeenth-Century England* (Oxford, 1951).
Mahony, M., 'Presbyterianism in the City of London, 1645–1647', *The Historical Journal*, 22 (1979), 93–114.
Malcolm, J. L., 'Charles II and the Reconstruction of Royal Power', *The Historical Journal*, 35 (1992), 307–30.
Mann, S., 'Physic and Divinity; the Case of Dr John Downes, M.D. (1627–1694)', *The Seventeenth Century*, 31 (2016), 451–70.
Marshall, A., 'Colonel Thomas Blood and the Restoration Political Scene', *The Historical Journal*, 32 (1989), 561–82.
Intelligence and Espionage in the Reign of Charles II, 1660–1685 (Cambridge, 1994).
Martensen, R. L., *The Brain Takes Shape: An Early History* (Oxford & New York, 2004).
'Hippocrates and the Politics of Medical Knowledge in Early Modern England', in D. Cantor (ed.), *Reinventing Hippocrates* (Aldershot, 2002), 116–35.
Martin, L., 'John Crane (1571–1652): The Cambridge Apothecary and Philanthropist', *Medical History*, 24 (1980), 432–46.
Mears, N., 'The Culture of Fasting in Early Stuart Parliaments', *Parliamentary History*, 39 (2020), 423–41.
Mendelsohn, A., 'Alchemy and Politics in England 1649–1665', *Past and Present*, 135 (1992), 30–78.
Merritt, J. F., *Westminster 1640–60: A Royal City in a Time of Revolution* (Manchester & New York, 2013).
Miller, J., *Politics and Religion in English Provincial Towns 1660–1722* (Oxford, 2007).
Money, W., *The History of the Ancient Town and Borough of Newbury in the County of Berks* (Oxford, 1887).
Monod, P. K., *The Murder of Mr. Grebell: Madness and Civility in an English Town* (New Haven & London, 2003).
Moran, B. T., *The Alchemical World of the German Court: Occult Philosophy and Chemical Medicine in the Circle of Moritz of Hessen (1572–1632)* (Stuttgart, 1991).
Morgan, V., *A History of the University of Cambridge*, 4 vols (Cambridge, 1989–2004), ii [1546–1750].
Morrill, J., *The Nature of the English Revolution. Essays by John Morrill* (London & New York, 1993).
Morris, G. C. R., 'On the Identity of Jaques du Moulin, F.R.S., 1667', *Notes and Records of the Royal Society*, 45 (1991), 1–10.
Mortimer, I., 'Index of Medical Licentiates, Applicants, Referees and Examiners in the Diocese of Exeter, 1586–1783', *Transactions of the Devonshire Association*, 136 (2004), 99–134.
'A Directory of Medical Personnel Qualified and Practising in the Diocese of Canterbury, *c.*1560–1730', *Archaeologia Cantiana*, 126 (2006), 135–70.
The Dying and the Doctors: The Medical Revolution in Seventeenth-Century England (London, 2009).

Morton, A. L., *The World of the Ranters* (London, 1970).
Mowrer, L. T., *The Indomitable John Scott* (New York, 1960).
Mullett, M., '"To Dwell Together in Unity": The Search for Agreement in Preston Politics, 1660–1690', *Transactions of the Historic Society of Lancashire and Cheshire*, 125 (1974), 64–5.
'Conflict, Politics and Elections in Lancaster, 1660–1688', *Northern History*, 19 (1983), 61–83.
Newman, W. R., *Gehennical Fire: The Lives of George Starkey, an American Alchemist in the Scientific Revolution* (Cambridge, MA, 1994).
Newman, W. R., and Principe, L. M., *Alchemy Tried in the Fire: Starkey, Boyle, and the Fate of Helmontian Chemistry* (Chicago & London, 2002).
Nutton, V. (ed.), *Medicine at the Courts of Europe, 1500–1837* (London and New York, 1990).
Palmer, W. M., 'The Reformation of the Corporation of Cambridge, July 1662', *Proceedings of the Cambridgeshire Antiquarian Society*, 17 (1912–13), 75–136.
Parsons, F. G., *The History of St Thomas's Hospital*, 2 vols (London, 1934).
Peachey, G. C., 'Thomas Trapham—Cromwell's Surgeon—and Others', *Proceedings of the Royal Society of Medicine*, 24 (1931), 1441–9.
Pelling, M., 'Politics, Medicine, and Masculinity: Physicians and Office-bearing in Early Modern England', in M. Pelling and S. Mandelbrote (eds), *The Practice of Reform in Health, Medicine and Science, 1500–2000* (Aldershot, 2005), 81–105.
Pells, I., 'Reassessing Frontline Medical Practitioners of the British Civil Wars in the Context of the Seventeenth-Century Medical World', *Historical Journal*, 62 (2019), 399–425.
Peters, E., 'Trauma Narratives of the English Civil War', *Journal for Early Modern Cultural Studies*, 16 (2016), 78–94.
Pocock, J. G. A., 'Robert Brady, 1627–1700: A Cambridge Historian of the Restoration', *Cambridge Historical Journal*, 10 (1950–52), 186–204.
Porter, R., *Quacks: Fakers & Charlatans in English Medicine* (Stroud, 2000).
Poynter, F. N. L., 'An Unnoticed Contemporary English Poem in Praise of Harvey and Its Author', *Journal of the History of Medicine and Allied Sciences*, 11 (1956), 374–83.
Poynter, F. N. L., and Bishop, W. J., *A Seventeenth-Century Doctor and His Patients: John Symcotts, 1592?–1662* (Bedfordshire Historical Records Society, vol. 31, 1951).
Prendergast, J. P., *The Cromwellian Settlement of Ireland* (Dublin, 1922).
Principe, L. M., *The Aspiring Adept: Robert Boyle and His Alchemical Quest* (Princeton, NJ, 1998).
Principe, L., and Newman, W., 'Alchemy vs Chemistry: The Etymological Origins of a Historiographic Mistake', *Early Science and Medicine*, 3 (1998), 32–65.
Ransome, D. R., 'Wives for Virginia, 1621', *William and Mary Quarterly*, 48 (1991), 3–18.
Rattansi, P., 'The Helmontian-Galenist Controversy in Restoration England', *Ambix*, 12 (1964), 1–23.
Redwood, J., *Reason, Ridicule and Religion: The Age of Enlightenment in England, 1660–1750* (London, 1976).
Romanell, P., *John Locke and Medicine: A New Key to Locke* (Buffalo, NY, 1984).
Roos, A. M., 'Lodestones and Gallstones: The Magnetic Iatrochemistry of Martin Lister (1639–1712)', *History of Science*, 46 (2008), 343–64.
Web of Nature: Martin Lister (1639–1712) (Leiden, 2011).
'The Chymistry of Francis Willughby (1635–72): The Trinity College, Cambridge Community', in T. Birkhead (ed.), *Virtuoso by Nature: The Scientific Worlds of Francis Willughby FRS (1635–1672)* (Leiden, 2016), 99–121.

Rose, C., 'Politics and the London Royal Hospitals, 1683–1692', in L. Granshaw and R. Porter (eds), *The Hospital in History* (London & New York, 1989), 123–48.

Rosenberg, A., 'The Sarah Stout Murder Case: An Early Example of the Doctor as an Expert Witness', *Journal of the History of Medicine and Allied Sciences*, 12 (1957), 61–70.

Sakula, A., 'Dr John Radcliffe, Court Physician, and the Death of Queen Anne', *Journal of the Royal College of Physicians of London*, 19 (1985), 255–60.

Sampson, H., 'Dr Faber and His Celebrated Cordial', *Isis*, 34 (1942–3), 472–96.

Sawday, J., *The Body Emblazoned: Dissection and the Human Body in Renaissance Culture* (London & New York, 1995).

Schoenfeldt, M., 'Reading Bodies', in K. Sharpe and S. N. Zwicker (eds), *Reading, Society and Politics in Early Modern England* (Cambridge, 2003), 215–43.

Serjeantson, R., 'The Education of Francis Willughby', in T. Birkhead (ed.), *Virtuoso by Nature: The Scientific Worlds of Francis Willughby FRS (1635–1672)* (Leiden, 2016), 44–98.

Shannon, W. D., *Seventeenth-Century Lancashire Restored: The Life and Work of Dr Richard Kuerdon, Antiquary and Topographer, 1623–1702* (Manchester, Chetham Soc., vol. 54, 2020).

Sharpe, K., *Politics and Ideas in Early Stuart England* (London & New York, 1989).

'An Image Doting Rabble: The Failure of Republican Culture in Seventeenth-Century England', in K. Sharpe and S. N. Zwicker (eds), *Refiguring Revolutions: Aesthetics and Politics from the English Revolution to the Romantic Revolution* (Berkeley and Los Angeles, 1998), 25–56.

Shaw, J., *Miracles in Enlightenment England* (New Haven & London, 2006).

Shawcross, J. T., *The Arms of the Family: The Significance of John Milton's Relatives and Associates* (Lexington, KY, 2004).

Siraisi, N., *History, Medicine, and the Traditions of Renaissance Learning* (Ann Arbor, MICH, 2007).

Smith, N., *Literature and Revolution in England, 1640–1660* (New Haven & London, 1994).

'Popular Republicanism in the 1650s: John Streater's *Heroic Mechanicks*', in Q. Skinner and D. Armitage (eds), *Milton and Republicanism* (Cambridge, 1995), 137–55.

Soll, J., 'Healing the Body Politic: French Royal Doctors, History, and the Birth of a Nation 1560–1634', *Renaissance Quarterly*, 55 (2002), 1259–1286.

Spurr, J., *English Puritanism, 1603–1689* (Houndmills, 1998).

Tanes, R. G. S., 'The "New Disease" and the Parliamentary Army at Ottery St Mary November/December 1645', *Devon and Cornwall Notes and Queries*, 34 (1978–81), 110–20.

Thomas, Sir H., 'The Society of Chymical Physitians. An Echo of the Great Plague at London, 1665', in E. A. Underwood (ed.), *Science, Medicine and History*, 2 vols (London, 1953), ii, 56–71.

Thomas, K. V., *Religion and the Decline of Magic: Studies in Popular Beliefs in Sixteenth and Seventeenth-Century England* (London, 1971).

Thorley, D., 'Daniel Foote, M. D., of Cambridge: The Evidence in Print and from the Sloane Collection', *eBritish Library Journal* (2013), article 15.

Trail, R. R., 'Richard Morton (1637–1698)', *Medical History*, 14 (1970), 166–74.

Turner, G. L., 'Bunyan's Licence under the Indulgence', *Transactions of the Baptist Historical Society*, 6 (1919), 129–37.

Twigg, J., *The University of Cambridge and the English Revolution 1625–1688* (Woodbridge, 1990).

Underdown, D., *Somerset in the Civil War and Interregnum* (Newton Abbot, 1973). *Revel, Riot, and Rebellion: Popular Politics and Culture in England, 1603–1660* (Oxford, 1985).

Fire from Heaven: Life in an English Town in the Seventeenth Century (London, 1992).

Urwick, W., *Nonconformity in Hertfordshire* (London, 1884).

Veenhoff, A., and Smolenaars, M., 'Hugh Goodyear and His Papers', *Transactions of the Lancashire and Cheshire Antiquarian Society*, 95 (1999), 1–22.

Wallis, P., 'Competition and Cooperation in the Early Modern Medical Economy', in M. S. R. Jenner and P. Wallis (eds), *Medicine and the Market in England and Its Colonies*, 47–68.

Walsham, A., *Providence in Early Modern England* (Oxford, 1999).

Walter, J., *Understanding Popular Violence in the English Revolution: The Colchester Plunderers* (Cambridge, 1999).

Walzer, M., *The Revolution of the Saints: A Study in the Origins of Radical Politics* (London, 1966).

Warmington, A., '"Madd, Bedlam Madd": An Incident in Gloucester's Seventeenth-Century Municipal History Reconsidered', *Transactions of the Bristol and Gloucestershire Archaeological Society*, 111 (1993), 165–73.

Wear, A., *Knowledge and Practice in English Medicine, 1550–1680* (Cambridge, 2000).

Webster, C., 'The College of Physicians: "Solomon's House" in Commonwealth England', *Bulletin of the History of Medicine*, 41 (1967), 393–412.

'English Medical Reformers of the Puritan Revolution: A Background to the "Society of Chemical Physitians"', *Ambix*, 14 (1967), 16–41.

'Henry Power's Experimental Philosophy', *Ambix*, 14 (1967), 150–78.

The Great Instauration: Science, Medicine and Reform 1626–1660 (London, 1975).

'Alchemical and Paracelsian Medicine', in *Health, Medicine and Mortality in the Sixteenth Century*, ed. C. Webster (Cambridge, 1979), 328–32.

'Puritanism, Separatism and Science', in R. L. Numbers and D. C. Lindberg (eds), *God and Nature: Historical Essays on the Encounter between Christianity and Science* (Berkeley, CA, 1986), 192–217.

Webster, T., *Godly Clergy in Early Stuart England: The Caroline Puritan Movement, c.1620–1643* (Cambridge, 1997).

Werrett, S., 'Healing the Nation's Wounds: Royal Ritual and Experimental Philosophy in Restoration England', *History of Science*, 38 (2000), 377–99.

Whittet T. D., 'Sir Thomas Clarges, Apothecary and Envoy', *Journal of the Royal Society of Medicine*, 81 (1988), 464–7.

Winsser, J., 'Mary Dyer and the "Monster" Story', *Quaker History*, 79 (1990), 20–34.

Withey, A., 'Medicine and Mortality in Early Modern Monmouthshire: The Commonplace Book of John Gwin', *Welsh History Review*, 23 (2006), 48–73.

'Unhealthy Neglect? The Medicine and Medical Historiography of Early Modern Wales', *Social History of Medicine*, 21 (2008), 163–74.

Woodward, W., *Prospero's America: John Winthrop Jr, Alchemy, and the Creation of New England Culture, 1606–1676* (Chapel Hill, NC, 2010).

Woolley, B., *The Herbalist: Nicholas Culpeper and the Fight for Medical Freedom* (London, 2004).

Wright, S., *The Early English Baptists 1603–1649* (Woodbridge, 2006).

Wykes, D. L., 'The Autobiographical Account of a Leicestershire Apothecary: Samuel Statham, *c*.1673–1732', *The Leicestershire Historian*, 3 (1990), 6–16.

Wyman, A. L., 'Samuel Barrow, MD, Physician to Charles II and Admirer of John Milton', *Medical History*, 18 (1974), 335–48.

Zaller, R., 'Breaking the Vessels: The Desacralization of Monarchy in Early Modern England', *Sixteenth Century Journal*, 29 (1998), 757–78.

5. Unpublished Papers, Theses and Electronic Resources

Andrews, J., 'Bedlam Revisited: A History of Bethlem Hospital, *c.*1634–*c.*1770', Ph. D. (Queen Mary & Westfield College, London, 1991).

Brod, M., 'Dissent and Dissenters in Early Modern Berkshire', D. Phil (Oxford, 2002).

Bucholz, R., www.luc.edu/history/fac_resources/bucholz/DCO/DCO.html [electronic database of court officers, 1660–1837].

Condick, F. M., 'The Life and Works of Dr John Bastwick (1595–1654)', Ph. D. (London, 1983).

Corley, J. M., 'Some Elizabethan Controversies about the Church and the Ministry', D. Phil (Durham, 1959).

Exeter University, Centre for Medical History, 'The Medical World of Early Modern England, Wales and Ireland, *c.*1500–1715', available at practitioners.exeter.ac.uk.

Gentles, I., 'The Debentures Market and Military Purchases of Crown Land, 1649–1660', Ph. D. (London, 1969).

Innes Smith MSS: www.rcpe.ac.uk/library/history/english-students/index

Whiteman, E. A. O., 'The Episcopate of Dr Seth Ward, Bishop of Exeter (1662 to 1667) and Salisbury (1667 to 1688/9)', Ph. D. (Oxford, 1951).

Woodcraft, D. R., 'A "Politick Engine": Astrology and Politics 1678–1715', Ph. D. (Warwick, 1997).

Index

For the benefit of digital users, indexed terms that span two pages (e.g., 52–53) may, on occasion, appear on only one of those pages.